Handbook of Meningococcal Disease

Edited by
Matthias Frosch and
Martin C. J. Maiden

Related Titles

Gillespie, S.H., Hawkey, P. (Eds.)

Principles and Practice of Clinical Bacteriology, 2nd Edition

2006
ISBN 0-470-84976-2

Grandi, G. (Ed.)

Genomics, Proteomics and Vaccines

2004
ISBN 0-470-85616-5

Kaufmann, S.H.E. (Ed.)

Novel Vaccination Strategies

2004
ISBN 3-527-30523-8

Dale, J.W., Park, S.F.

Molecular Genetics of Bacteria, 4th Edition

2004
ISBN 0-470-85084-1

Handbook of Meningococcal Disease

Infection Biology, Vaccination, Clinical Management

Edited by
Matthias Frosch and Martin C. J. Maiden

WILEY-VCH

WILEY-VCH Verlag GmbH & Co. KGaA

The Editors

Prof. Dr. Matthias Frosch
Institute of Hygiene and Microbiology
University of Würzburg
Josef-Schneider-Straße 2
97080 Würzburg
Germany

Prof. Dr. Martin C. J. Maiden
Peter Medawar Building for Pathogen Research
Department of Zoology
University of Oxford
South Parks Road
Oxford OX1 3SY
Great Britain

Cover
Neisseria meningitidis adherent to human brain derived endothelial cell (SEM 10.000 × magnification). Kindly provided by Alexandra Schubert-Unkmeir, Institute for Hygiene and Microbiology, Würzburg.

Library of Congress Card No.: applied for

British Library Cataloguing-in-Publication Data
A catalogue record for this book is available from the British Library.

Bibliographic information published by Die Deutsche Bibliothek
Die Deutsche Bibliothek lists this publication in the Deutsche Nationalbibliografie; detailed bibliographic data is available in the Internet at <http://dnb.ddb.de>

Printed in the Federal Republic of Germany
Printed on acid-free paper

Typesetting K+V Fotosatz GmbH, Beerfelden
Printing Betz-Druck GmbH, Darmstadt
Bookbinding J. Schäffer GmbH, Grünstadt

ISBN-13: 978-3-527-31260-3
ISBN-10: 3-527-31260-9

Contents

Handbook of Meningococcal Disease. Infection Biology, Vaccination, Clinical Management.
Edited by M. Frosch and M.C.J. Maiden

ISBN: 3-527-31260-9

Preface

Meningococcal disease has apparently emerged relatively recently, with definitive descriptions dating only from 1805 in Europe and North America and 1905 in Africa. During the 20th century it attained a global distribution both as an endemic and epidemic disease, with a number of pandemics. At the beginning of the 21st century, the disease remains a major challenge globally with around 500,000 cases a year, 300,000 of which occur in sub-Saharan Africa: these numbers increase substantially in those years when major epidemics occur in Africa.

The basis for this *Handbook of Meningococcal Disease* was the classic book edited by Keith Cartwright entitled *Meningococcal Disease* and published by John Wiley & Sons in 1995. This book brought together up-to-date information on all aspects of meningococcal disease with value for paediatricians microbiologists, infectious disease specialists and professionals in public health medicine. However, since 1995 substantial progress has been made and we look back to a decade with changes in the epidemiology of meningococcal disease, improved understanding of the meningococcal population biology, new options to combat the disease by vaccination and exciting new insights into the basic biology of the meningococcus, which was stimulated by the availability of whole genome sequence data and the novel insights into cell biology. The *Handbook of Meningococcal Disease* covers all these aspects on the recent research on meningococci and meningococcal disease.

This book would not have been possible without the outstanding contributions of a group of internationally respected authors. We would like to thank our colleagues for giving their valuable time and effort toward compilation of this book, but we are also grateful to all those who are engaged in the intensive, and increasingly successful, efforts to eliminate this disease. We are also indebted to Andreas Sendtko at Wiley-VCH for the initial suggestion to put this book together and for the committed and stimulating support and promotion of the project.

Würzburg and Oxford, February 2006 Matthias Frosch and Martin Maiden

Handbook of Meningococcal Disease. Infection Biology, Vaccination, Clinical Management.
Edited by M. Frosch and M.C.J. Maiden

ISBN: 3-527-31260-9

Foreword

This book is welcome, summarizing as it does our current understanding of the microbiology, pathology and epidemiology of meningococcal disease, as well as updating readers on clinical developments. For me, it has been a pleasure and a privilege to work closely with one of the editors over a period of many years, and equally so to be invited to write this Foreword. I hope that readers will both enjoy and learn from the experience of the many contributors to this timely addition to the meningococcal literature.

Meningococcal disease remains perhaps the most fascinating of human bacterial infections. The microbe colonizes only Man, is ubiquitously and commonly distributed and lives harmlessly in the main at the back of the human throat. Yet when it invades, it can cause disease of almost unparalleled ferocity, manifesting mainly as meningitis, but in a substantial minority of patients as septicemia (blood poisoning) without involvement of the meninges.

The meningococcus can cause sporadic, endemic or epidemic disease. In developed countries, there are two quite distinct age peaks (infancy, early adulthood), each with entirely different underlying pathological mechanisms. Different serogroups affect different continents and countries at different times, yet despite burgeoning international travel and the inevitability of incessant introductions of new meningococcal strains into all countries across the globe, the African epidemiology remains persistently dominated by serogroup A disease, whereas in Europe, the Americas and Australasia, serogroups B and C are most common and have been so for years.

Unlike the great majority of other bacterial species that cause human disease, meningococci have remained (with one or two anecdotal exceptions), persistently and thankfully sensitive to antibiotics, in the face of gross exposure, indeed, over-exposure, over the past 60 years. This is despite their highly developed ability to acquire useful genes from other nasopharyngeal bacteria.

Clearly, the disease and its causative microbe present us with problems, conundrums and questions to which we cannot as yet find answers. What is equally clear is that the pace of investigation is quickening. Meningococcal disease is now accorded a high public health priority in most developed countries, perhaps in part because of the fear it evokes in both parents of young children and also in health care professionals, who dread missing a case of this largely treatable condition, thus causing death or avoidable morbidity.

Handbook of Meningococcal Disease. Infection Biology, Vaccination, Clinical Management.
Edited by M. Frosch and M.C.J. Maiden

ISBN: 3-527-31260-9

At governmental level, the disease is important not only for economic reasons but also because the prospects for reduction in morbidity and mortality are excellent, and because there are also good prospects for global disease control through the deployment of effective vaccines for all serotypes within the next few years. The problems in realizing this exciting vision are not just technological, but financial, political and organizational.

Bill Gates, the founder of the Microsoft Corporation, made a striking contribution to the battle against meningococcal disease by promising generous funding for a program to control a range of (mainly vaccine-preventable) infections in the world's poorer countries. Many developed country governments have now followed his example. The support of the Bill and Melinda Gates Foundation includes funding earmarked specifically for the manufacture and deployment of conjugated meningococcal vaccines in the African "meningitis belt".

The manufacture of conjugated vaccines for serogroup A and C meningococci is technically straightforward; and the constraints in controlling meningococcal disease in Africa are now largely financial and organizational. Given goodwill, the Gates' initiative should overcome these problems, thereby addressing by far the most important global public health issue in meningococcal disease control.

The developed world, where thankfully meningococcal disease attack rates are only a fraction of those seen in African epidemics, needs a serogroup B vaccine. Here, the hurdles are still technological. It is immensely frustrating to observe the plain epidemiological fact that meningococcal disease is rare after the age of 25–30 years, indicating that a natural protective process operates, yet to date we have been unable to characterize it and mimic it with a vaccine.

Though the past few years have seen less progress in the development of serogroup B vaccines than one might have hoped for, it seems likely that, with the diverse range of innovative technological approaches now being explored, we may at last be on the brink of identifying and developing a successful men B vaccine candidate. I look forward with some optimism to the global control of meningococcal disease within the next decade, an achievable public health goal.

Brobury, February 2006 Keith Cartwright

List of Contributors

Ole Herman Ambur
Centre for Molecular Biology
and Neuroscience and Institute
of Microbiology
University of Oslo
Rikshospitalet Radiumhospitalet Trust
0027 Oslo
Norway

Colin Block
Clinical Microbiology Unit
Infectious Diseases
Hadassah–Hebrew University Medical
Centres
IL 91120 Jerusalem
Israel

Ray Borrow
Vaccine Evaluation Department
Manchester Medical Microbiology
Partnership
PO Box 209
Clinical Sciences Building
Manchester Royal Infirmary
Manchester, M13 9WZ
Great Britain

Sandrine Bourdoulous
Institut Cochin
Département de Biologie Cellulaire
Université René Descartes Paris V
22 rue Méchain
75014 Paris
France

Petter Brandtzaeg
Department of Pediatrics
Ullevål University Hospital
University of Oslo
0407 Oslo
Norway

Helen Campbell
Immunisation Division
PHLS Communicable Disease
Surveillance Centre
61 Colindale Avenue
London, NW9 5EQ
Great Britain

Keith Cartwright
Brobury House
Brobury
Herefordshire, HR3 6BS
Great Britain

Handbook of Meningococcal Disease. Infection Biology, Vaccination, Clinical Management.
Edited by M. Frosch and M.C.J. Maiden

ISBN: 3-527-31260-9

Dominique A. Caugant
WHO Collaborating
Centre for Reference and Research
on Meningococci
Division of Infectious Disease Control
Norwegian Institute of Public Health
PO Box 4404 Nydalen
0403 Oslo
Norway

Heike Claus
Institute of Hygiene
and Microbiology
University of Würzburg
Josef-Schneider-Straße 2
97080 Würzburg
Germany

Tonje Davidsen
Centre for Molecular Biology
and Neuroscience
and Institute of Microbiology
University of Oslo
Rikshospitalet Radiumhospitalet Trust
0027 Oslo
Norway

Philippe Denoël
GlaxoSmithKline Biologicals
Rue de l'Institut 89
1330 Rixensart
Belgium

Jeremy Derrick
Department of Biomolecular Sciences
Faculty of Life Sciences
UMIST
PO Box 88
Manchester, M60 1QD
Great Britain

Andrew Ekins
Department of Microbiology
and Infectious Diseases
University of Calgary
Calgary
Alberta, T2N 4N1
Canada

Ian M. Feavers
Division of Bacteriology
NIBSC
Blanche Lane
South Mimms
Potters Bar
Hertfordshire, EN6 3QG
Great Britain

Christiane Feron
GlaxoSmithKline Biologicals
Rue de l'Institut 89
1330 Rixensart
Belgium

Matthias Frosch
Institute of Hygiene
and Microbiology
University of Würzburg
Josef-Schneider-Straße 2
97080 Würzburg
Germany

Karine Goraj
GlaxoSmithKline Biologicals
Rue de l'Institut 89
1330 Rixensart
Belgium

Steve J. Gray
Meningococcal Reference Unit
Health Protection Agency
Clinical Science Building
Manchester Royal Infirmary
PO Box 209 Oxford Road
Manchester, M13 9WL
Great Britain

John E. Heckels
Molecular Microbiology Group
Division of Infection, Inflammation and Repair
University of Southampton Medical School
Southampton General Hospital
Southampton, SO16 6YD
Great Britain

Keith A. Jolley
Peter Medawar Building for Pathogen Research
Department of Zoology
University of Oxford
South Parks Road
Oxford, OX1 3SY
Great Britain

Oliver Kurzai
Institute of Hygiene and Microbiology
University of Würzburg
Josef-Schneider-Straße 2
97080 Würzburg
Germany

Rosanna Leuzzi
Chiron Vaccines
Via Fiorentina 1
53100 Siena
Italy

Martin C. J. Maiden
Peter Medawar Building for Pathogen Research
Department of Zoology
University of Oxford
South Parks Road
Oxford, OX1 3SY
Great Britain

Elizabeth Miller
Immunisation Division
PHLS Communicable Disease Surveillance Centre
61 Colindale Avenue
London, NW9 5EQ
Great Britain

Philippe C. Morand
Department of Molecular Biology
Max Planck Institute for Infection Biology
Schumannstr. 21/22
10117 Berlin
Germany

E. Richard Moxon
Weatherall Institute of Molecular Medicine
Department of Paediatrics
Room 4252 ~ Level 4
John Radcliffe Hospital
University of Oxford
Headley Way
Headington
Oxford, OX3 1DU
Great Britain

Simon Nadel
Paediatric Intensive Care Unit
St. Mary's Hospital
Praed Street
London, W2 1NY
Great Britain

Xavier Nassif
Laboratoire de Microbiologie
Faculté de Médecine
Necker-Enfants Malades
156 Rue de Vaugirard
75015 Paris
France

Mariagrazia Pizza
Chiron Vaccines
Via Fiorentina 1
53100 Siena
Italy

Joyce S. Plested
Weatherall Institute of
Molecular Medicine
Department of Paediatrics
Room 4252 ~ Level 4
John Radcliffe Hospital
University of Oxford
Headley Way
Headington
Oxford, OX3 1DU
Great Britain

Andrew J. Pollard
Weatherall Institute of
Molecular Medicine
Department of Paediatrics
Room 4252 ~ Level 4
John Radcliffe Hospital
University of Oxford
Headley Way
Headington
Oxford, OX3 1DU
Great Britain

Jan T. Poolman
GlaxoSmithKline Biologicals
Rue de l'Institut 89
1330 Rixensart
Belgium

Peter M. Power
Weatherall Institute of
Molecular Medicine
Department of Paediatrics
Room 4252 ~ Level 4
John Radcliffe Hospital
University of Oxford
Headley Way
Headington
Oxford, OX3 1DU
Great Britain

Sanjay Ram
Section of Infectious Diseases
Evans Biomedical Research Center
Boston University Medical Center
650 Albany St.
Boston
Massachussetts, 02118
USA

Mary Ramsay
Immunisation Division
PHLS Communicable Disease
Surveillance Centre
61 Colindale Avenue
London, NW9 5EQ
Great Britain

Rino Rappuoli
Chiron Vaccines
Via Fiorentina 1
53100 Siena
Italy

Neil Ravenscoft
Department of Chemistry
University of Cape Town
Rondebosch 7701
Cape Town
South Africa

Thomas Rudel
Department of Molecular Biology
Max-Planck-Institute
for Infection Biology
Schumannstraße 21/22
10117 Berlin
Germany

Silvana Savino
Chiron Vaccines
Via Fiorentina 1
53100 Siena
Italy

Christoph Schoen
Institute of Hygiene
and Microbiology
University of Würzburg
Josef-Schneider-Straße 2
97877 Würzburg
Germany

Anthony B. Schryvers
Department of Microbiology
and Infectious Diseases
University of Calgary
3330 Hospital Drive N.W.
Calgary
Alberta, T2N 4N1
Canada

James Stuart
Health Protection Agency South West
The Wheelhouse
Bond's Mill
Stonehouse
Gloucestershire, GL10 3RF
Great Britain

Janet Suker
NIBSC
Blanche Lane
South Mimms
Potters Bar
Hertfordshire, EN6 3QG
Great Britain

Tone Tønjum
Centre for Molecular Biology
and Neuroscience
and Institute of Microbiology
University of Oslo
Rikshospitalet Radiumhospitalet Trust
0027 Oslo
Norway

Rachel Urwin
Department of Biology
The Pennsylvania State University
Mueller Laboratory
University Park
PA 16802
USA

Julio A. Vázquez
Reference Laboratory for Meningococci
Instituto de Salud Carlos III
National Centre for Microbiology
Ctra Majadahonda–Pozuelo Km 2
28220 Majadahonda – Madrid
Spain

Mumtaz Virji
Department of Pathology
and Microbiology
School of Medical Sciences
University of Bristol
University Walk
Bristol, BS8 1TD
Great Britain

Ulrich Vogel
Institute of Hygiene
and Microbiology
University of Würzburg
Josef-Schneider-Straße 2
97080 Würzburg
Germany

Vincent Weynants
GlaxoSmithKline Biologicals
Rue de l'Institut 89
1330 Rixensart
Belgium

J. Claire Wright
Weatherall Institute of
Molecular Medicine
Department of Paediatrics
Room 4252 ~ Level 4
John Radcliffe Hospital
University of Oxford
Headley Way
Headington
Oxford, OX3 1DU
Great Britain

Color Plates

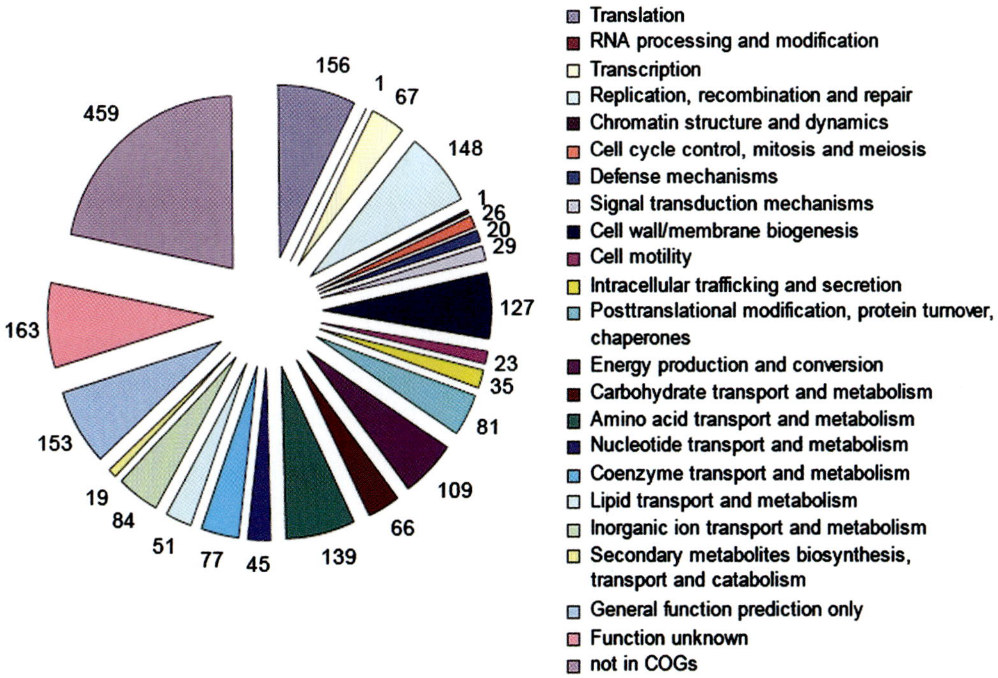

Fig. 5.3 Pie chart showing the percentage of *N. meningitidis* MC58 genes that are represented in each of the role families as indicated. The role category data shown was generated on the COG annotation of encoded proteome.

Handbook of Meningococcal Disease. Infection Biology, Vaccination, Clinical Management.
Edited by M. Frosch and M. C. J. Maiden

ISBN: 3-527-31260-9

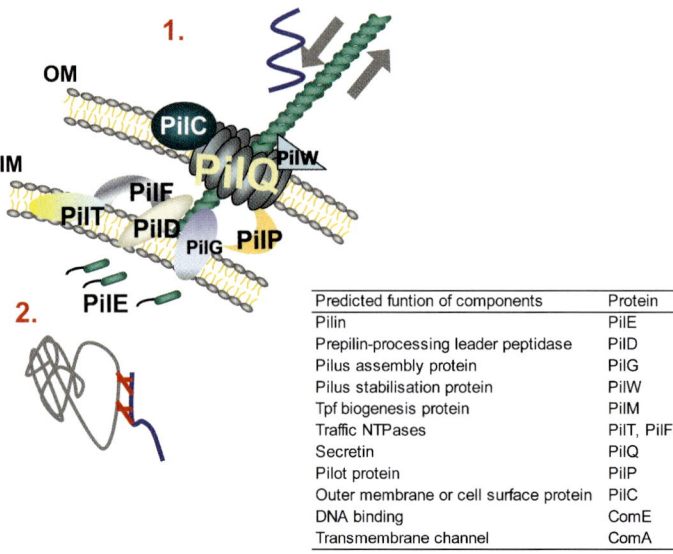

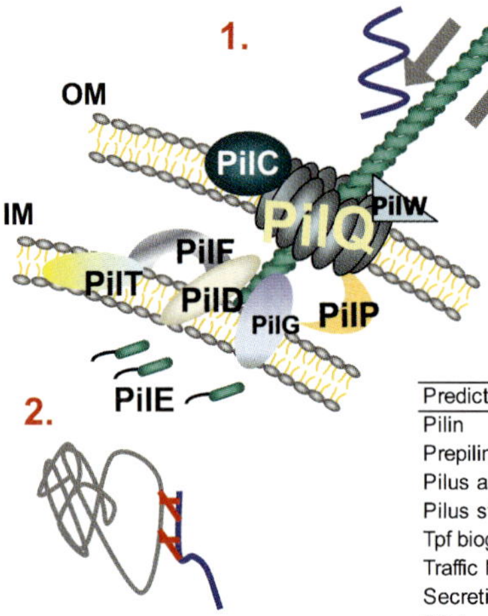

Predicted funtion of components	Protein
Pilin	PilE
Prepilin-processing leader peptidase	PilD
Pilus assembly protein	PilG
Pilus stabilisation protein	PilW
Tpf biogenesis protein	PilM
Traffic NTPases	PilT, PilF
Secretin	PilQ
Pilot protein	PilP
Outer membrane or cell surface protein	PilC
DNA binding	ComE
Transmembrane channel	ComA

Fig. 7.1 Horizontal gene transfer through transformation of exogenous DNA. 1. A schematic model for type IV pilus formation and competence, based on the *Neisseria meningitidis* pilus. The major pilin (PilE) and minor pilins are processed by the prepilin peptidase (PilD) and assembled into the pilus fibre. The polytopic membrane protein (PilG) and the traffic NTPase (PilF) participate in this process. The outer membrane/tip-located protein (PilC) stabilizes the assembled filament. The pilus crosses the outer membrane through a channel that is formed by the secretin (PilQ), with the assistance of its pilot protein (PilP). DNA present in the environment is entangled by retracting pili and introduced into the meningococcal cell through the outer membrane (OM) and inner membrane (IM). The incoming DNA is transported across the outer membrane through a channel that is formed by the secretin (PilQ), with the assistance of its pilot protein (PilP). 2. One strand of the DNA enters the cytosol; the other is degraded and the degradation products are released into the periplasmic space. In the cytoplasm the incoming DNA (blue) is integrated into the genome (gray) by homologous recombination [145].

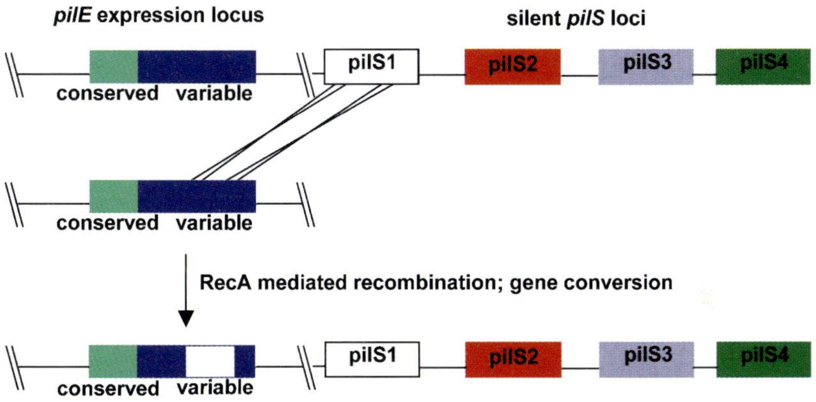

Fig. 7.3 Meningococcal antigenic variation by gene conversion. Meningococcal pilin antigenic variation is mediated by RecA-dependent gene conversion. Pili consist of thousands of pilin (PilE) subunits polymerized into long fibers. The PilE protein contains a highly conserved N-terminal domain and a variable C-terminal domain, the latter determining the antigenicity of the pili. The variable region is the result of a nonreciprocal transfer of DNA from one of a number of silent partial *pilS* loci to the single *pilE* expression locus. The silent loci, sometimes present several hundred basepairs away from the *pilE* expression locus, may donate a stretch of nucleotides, on the basis of short sequence homology. The genetic mechanism proceeds through a form of gene conversion requiring RecA and multiple crossover events during recombination that results in a unidirectional transfer of a *pilS* segment to the *pilE* variable region.

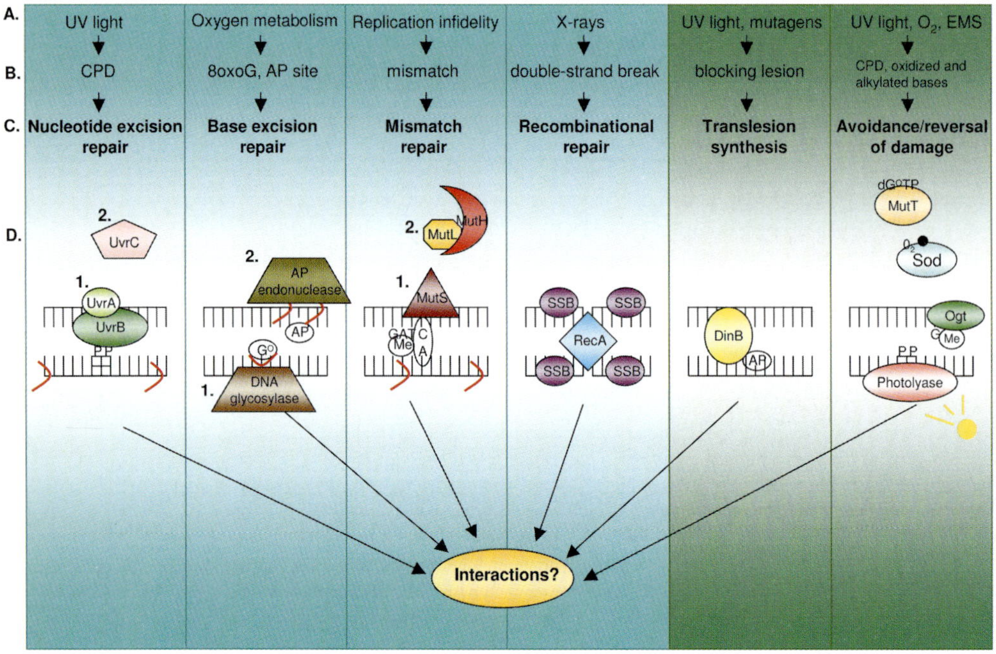

Fig. 7.4 Major DNA repair pathways. A number of repair pathways exist in organisms to manage the cytotoxic and mutagenic effect of DNA damage that can arise through endogenous and exogenous stress. A. Some examples of DNA-damaging agents. EMS – ethanemethyl sulfonate. B. DNA damage typically induced by the agent. CPD – cyclobutane pyrimidine photodimer, 8oxoG (G^{O}) – 7,8-dihydro-8oxo-2′-deoxyguanosine, AP site – abasic site. C. The DNA repair pathway often involved in removing the DNA lesion. Blue-colored pathways represent true repair, green pathways represent avoidance or reversal of a damage or a manner of bypassing a lesion. D. Important components participating in the repair pathway in *E. coli*. Red arrows indicate cleaved DNA strand. Please note that this figure does not show the detailed steps or every component involved in each repair pathway. P – pyrimidine, Me – methyl group, SSB – single-stranded binding protein, $O_2^{\bullet}$ – oxygen radical, SOD – superoxide dismutase.

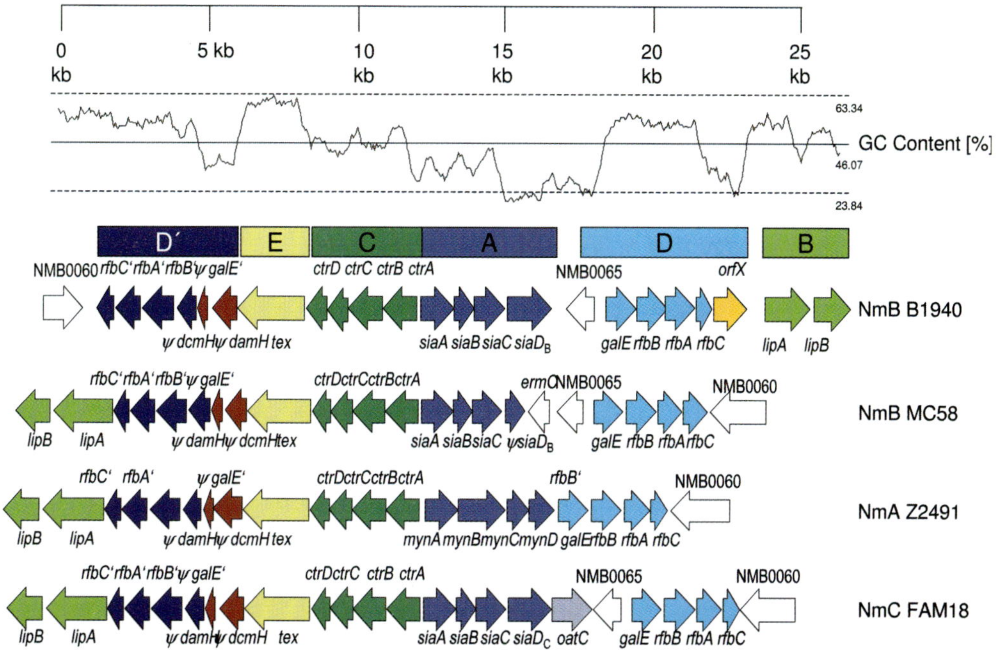

Fig. 8.1 The genetic organization of *cps* locus in serogroup B strains B1940 and MC58, serogroup A strain Z2491 and serogroup C strain FAM18. The plot demonstrates the GC content and the boxes indicate the functional regions A–E refer to strain B1940. Homologous genes in the *cps* locus are indicated by the same colors. The genome sequences of MC58, Z2491 and FAM18 were obtained, respectively, from TIGR (http://www.tigr.org/tigr-scripts/CMR2/GenomePage3.spl?database=gnm) and the Sanger Centre (http://www.sanger.ac.uk/Projects/N_meningitidis/; for references see text). The MC58 derivative subjected to genome sequencing by TIGR carried an inactivated version of the *siaD* gene.

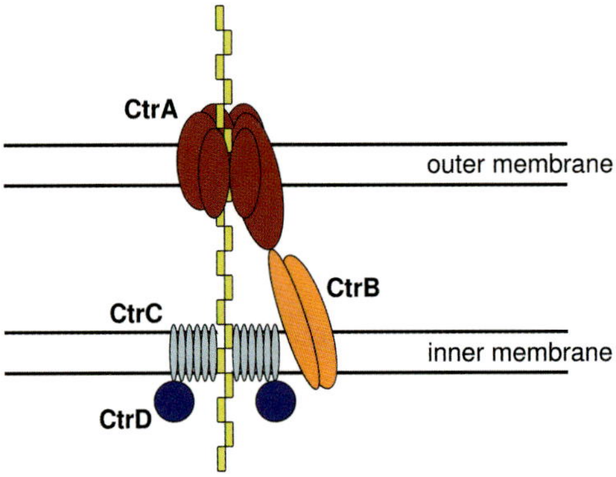

Fig. 8.3 Hypothetical model of the capsular polysaccharide transport system. The ABC transporter proteins CtrC and CtrD direct the translocation of the polysaccharide (yellow chain) through the inner membrane. Transport of the polysaccharide through the inner and outer membranes is tightly coupled. Translocation through the outer membrane is enabled by the auxiliary protein CtrA, which forms a β-barrel structure. The translocation zones of the inner and outer membrane are stabilized through CtrB, which links CtrA to the inner membrane.

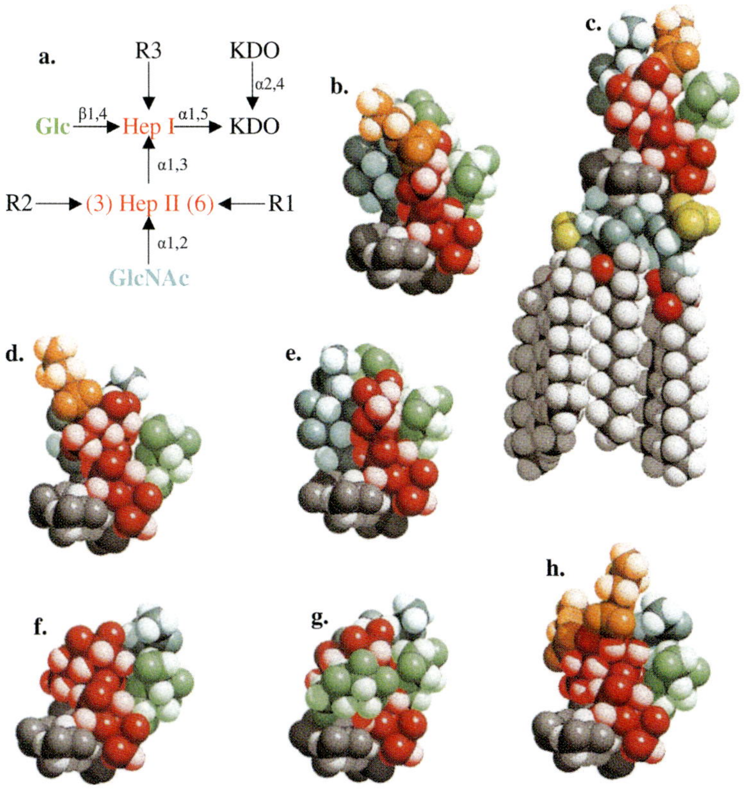

Fig. 9.5 Conserved structures within the inner core LPS region (adapted from Gidney et al. [4]). Seven structural variants are found within the inner core region of *N. meningitidis* LPS. (a) Structural representation of the inner core LPS. Substitutions to the second heptose (Hep II) can occur at the 3- and/or 6-position. (b–h) Three-dimensional space-filling molecular models of the seven LPS inner core structural variants are color-coded as follows: phosphoethanolamine (PEtn, orange), glucose (Glc, green), N-acetyl glucosamine (GlcNAc, pale blue), heptose (Hep, red), 3-deoxy-D-*manno*-2-octulosonic acid (KDO, dark gray), lipid A (pale gray). Molecular models were constructed using a Metropolis Monte-Carlo approach and are drawn with the same orientation for the KDO residue. The lipid A moiety is shown in panel (c) only, (b) immunotype L2 (R1 PEtn, R2 Glc-α1,3), (c) immunotype L3 (R2 PEtn), (d) immunotype L4 (R1 PEtn), (e) immunotype L5 (R2 Glc-α1,3), (f) an *lpt3* mutant of an L3 immunotype (no substitutions), (g) strain 1000 (R3 Glc-α1,2), (h) strain 2220Y (R1 PEtn, R2 PEtn).

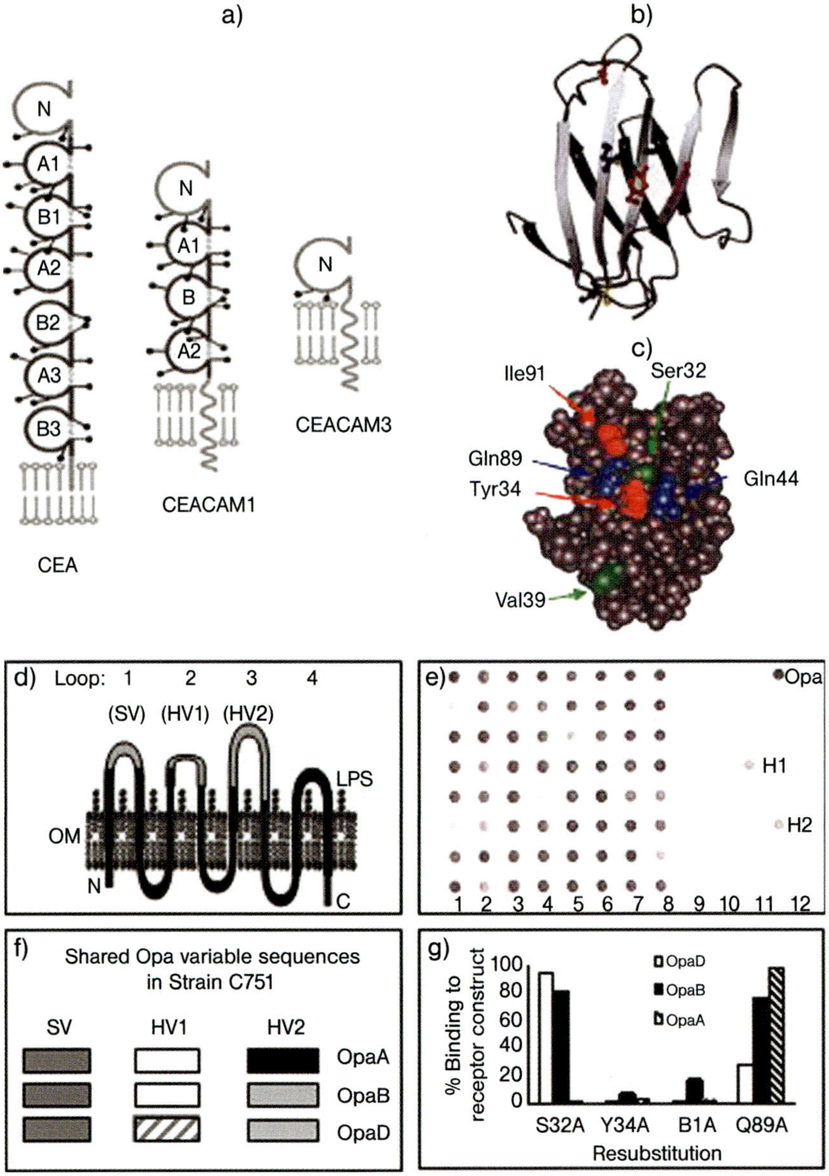

a)
N
A1
B1
A2
B2
A3
B3
CEA
N
A1
B
A2
CEACAM1
N
CEACAM3
b)
c)
Ile91
Ser32
Gln89
Tyr34
Gln44
Val39
d) Loop: 1 2 3 4
(SV) (HV1) (HV2)
LPS
OM
N
C
e)
Opa
H1
H2
1 2 3 4 5 6 7 8 9 10 11 12
f)
Shared Opa variable sequences in Strain C751
SV
HV1
HV2
OpaA
OpaB
OpaD
g)
% Binding to receptor construct
100
80
60
40
20
0
OpaD
OpaB
OpaA
S32A
Y34A
B1A
Q89A
Resubstitution

Fig. 10.2 Structures of CEACAMs, the principal receptors for Opa adhesins and their binding site on the receptor. (A) CEA and CEACAM1, the epithelial receptors and CEACAM3, the granulocyte-specific receptor, each contains a highly homologous N-terminal domain targeted by Opa proteins. Glycosylation sites are depicted by ball and stick representations. CEACAM1 and CEACAM3 contain immunoreceptor tyrosine-based inhibitory (ITIM) and activation (ITAM) motifs respectively in their cytoplasmic regions whilst CEA, the largest member of the family is a GPI-anchored molecule (adapted from CEA website; http://cea.klinikum.uni-muenchen.de). (B) Ribbon diagram showing the arrangement of eight beta strands that make up the N-terminal domain. Residues of importance for Opa targeting on the CFG face of the N-domain are shown. (C) Van der Waals surface representation of the N-domain model showing these residues in color, the key amino acids being shown in red (based on [92]). (D) Two-dimensional arrangement of the semivariable and hypervariable loops of Opa proteins [71]. (E) Whole cell lysates of pathogenic neisseria isolates (columns 1–8) and other mucosal isolates including *P. aeruginosa, E. coli, H. influenzae* were overlaid with a soluble receptor construct containing the N-terminal domain of CEACAM1 linked to human Fc. Receptor binding was detected using anti-Fc alkaline phosphatase conju gate. Binding of the majority of pathogenic Opa-expressing bacteria to the receptor can be seen in addition to two *H. influenzae* strains (H1, H2) as well as purified Opa protein [65]. (F) *N. meningitidis* Strain C751 Opa derivatives contain three different combinations of HV1 and HV2 (OpaA and B share HV1, OpaB and D share HV2, whereas HV1 of Opa D and HV2 of OpaA are unique). (G) Receptor-binding properties of the C751 Opa proteins using single amino acid substituted N-domain constructs show the primary importance of Y34 and I91 and the influence of HV1 and HV2 in adhesion to the receptor with S32A and Q89A substitutions (adapted from [92]).

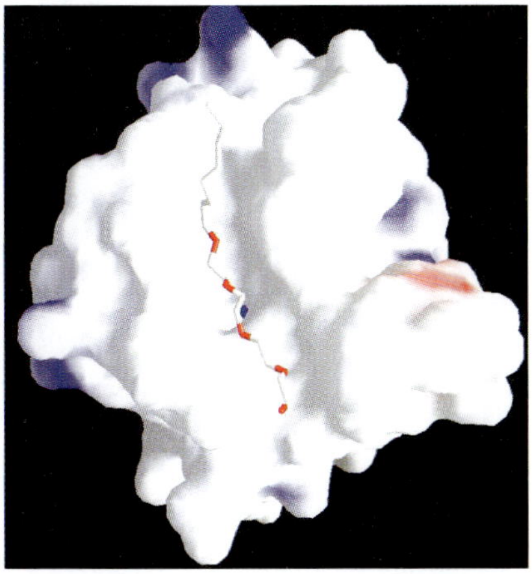

Fig. 10.5 b Surface representation of NspA viewed from the top, prepared using GRASP [175], with basic and acidic residues in blue and red respectively. A $C_{10}E_5$ polyoxyethylene detergent molecule, bound within a hydrophobic groove, is shown superimposed on the structure.

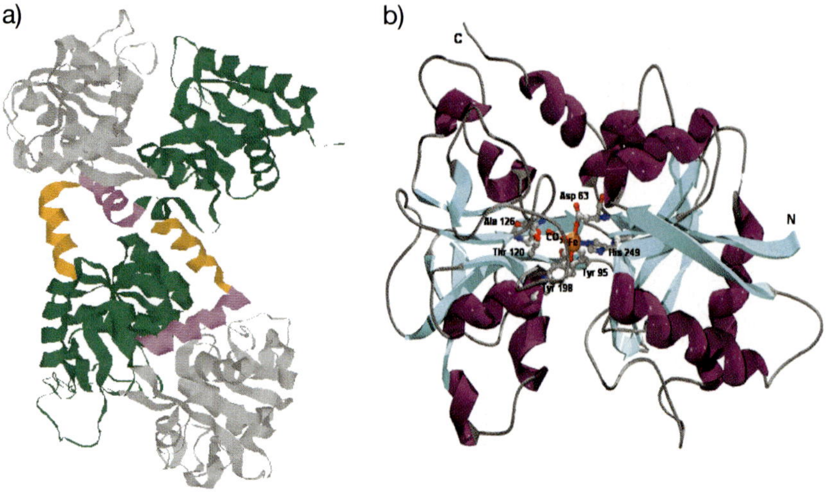

Fig. 11.1 Structure of transferrin and lactoferrin. (A) Ribbon model of human lactoferrin, illustrating the domain structure of both the N-lobe (top) and C-lobe (bottom). Domain 1 (green) is connected to domain 2 (white) by antiparallel beta-strands forming the base of an interdomain cleft. The two lobes are connected by an inter-domain bridge consisting of two alpha-helices (pink and yellow) equivalent to the C-terminal tail of the C-lobe. (B) Ribbon model of the human lactoferrin N-lobe, illustrating the amino acids from both domains and the anion that form the iron coordination complex.

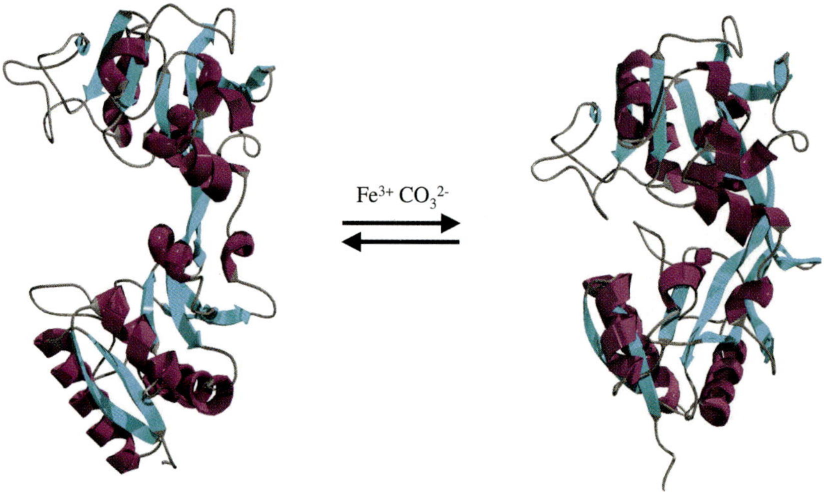

Fig. 11.2 Domain closure associated with iron binding. Ribbon model of the apo-form (left) and iron-loaded form (right) of the human lactoferrin N-lobe.

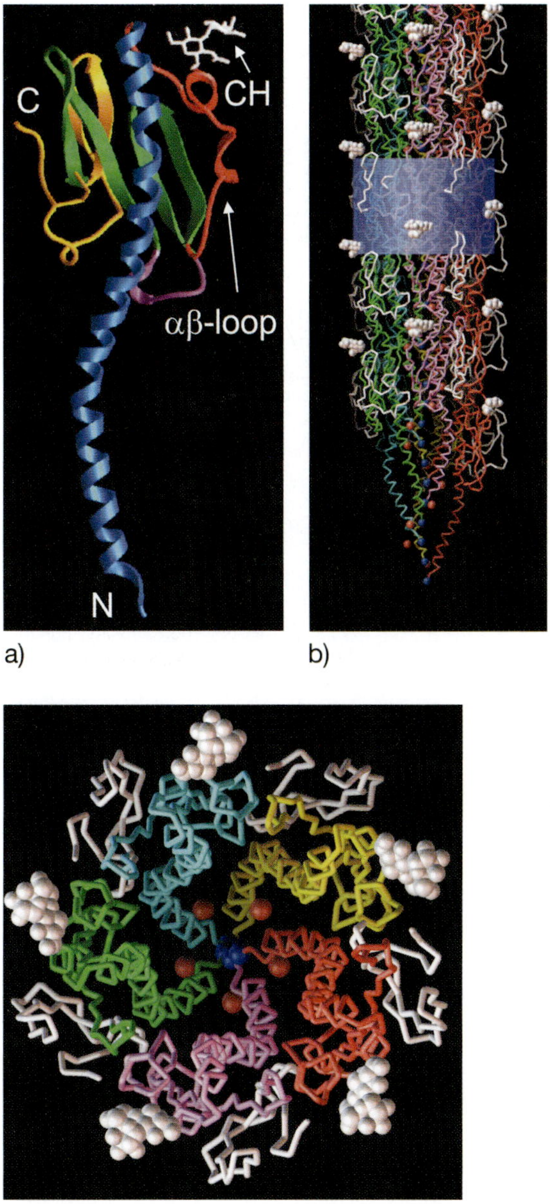

c)

Fig. 12.3 Structural model for pilin (adapted from [11]). (a) Structure of the pilin monomer. Colors indicate different functional parts of pilin. The carbohydrate (CH), N-terminus (N) and C-terminus (C) and the $\alpha\beta$-loop is indicated. (b) The helical assembly of the monomer forms the pilus fiber. (c) Projection of a cross section of the pilus fiber. Different colors indicate individual pilin subunits (by courtesy of J. A. Tainer).

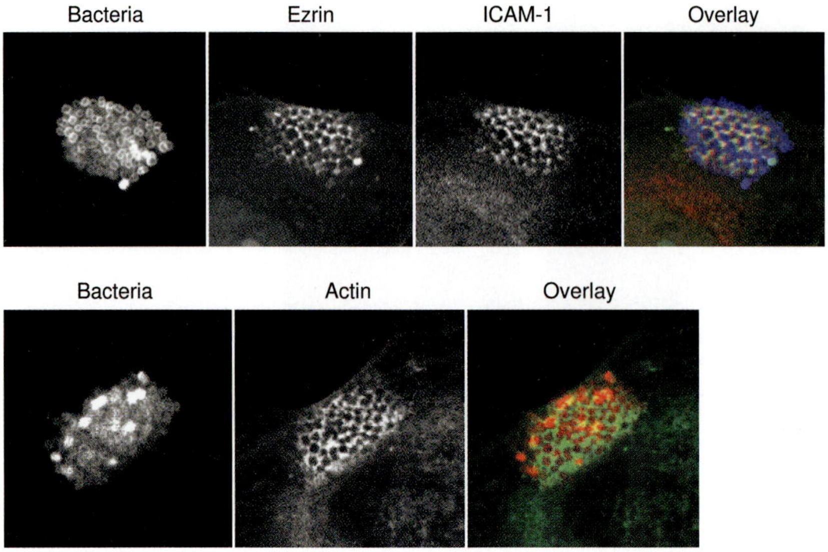

Fig. 13.1 Infection of human endothelial cells by *Neisseria meningitidis* induces the formation of cortical plaques beneath bacterial colonies. Human endothelial cells infected for 3 h with the 2C43 strain of *N. meningitidis* were stained for bacteria (blue), ezrin (green), and ICAM-1 (red), or double-stained for bacteria (red) and actin (green), and were analysed by confocal microscopy.

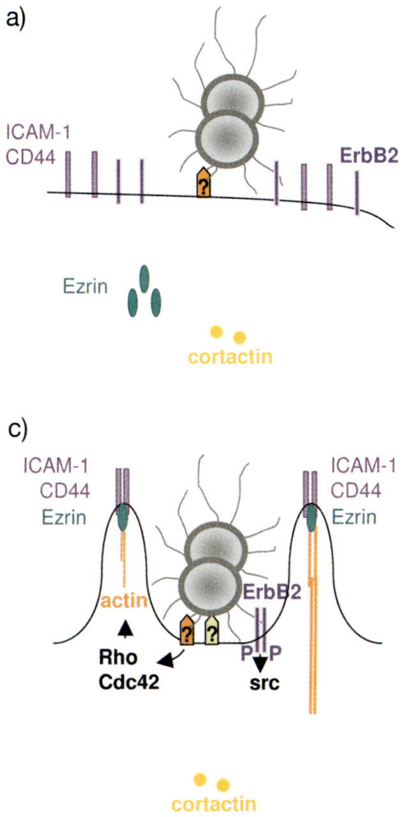

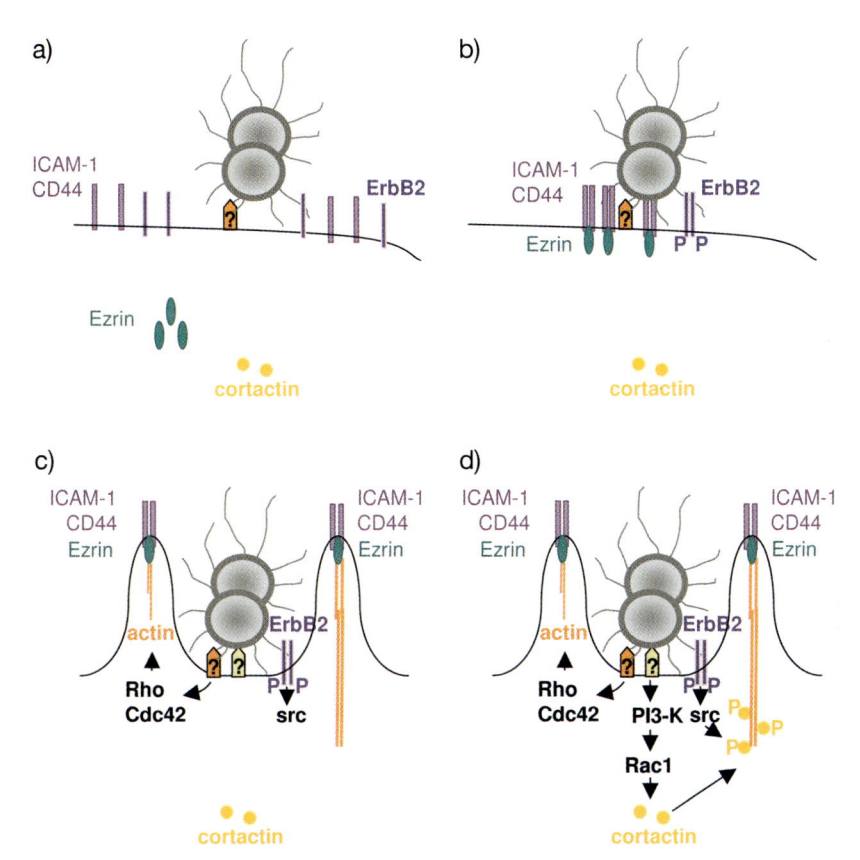

Fig. 13.2 Schematic representation of the signaling pathways activated by *N. meningitidis*, leading to their internalization into human endothelial cells. (A) Type IV pili initiate the interaction of virulent, encapsulated *N. meningitidis* with human endothelial cells by interacting with a cellular receptor, possibly CD46 [17]. (B) This pili-dependent adhesion induces the recruitment of ezrin and the clustering of several transmembrane proteins: the ErbB2 tyrosine kinase receptor and the ezrin-binding proteins CD44 and ICAM-1. (C) The activation of both Rho and Cdc42 GTPases induces a local polymerization of cortical actin. ErbB2 clustering leads to the activation of src tyrosine kinase. (D) In parallel, LOS of *N. meningitidis*, by a mechanism which remains to be identified, provides a costimulatory signal leading to PI3-K and Rac1 activation and the subsequent translocation of cortactin to the site of cortical actin rearrangements. When localized at the cell plasma membrane, cortactin is tyrosine-phosphorylated by src kinase and contributes to the formation of dynamic actin structures, leading to the formation of membrane projections which surround bacteria and induce their internalization within endothelial intracellular vacuoles.

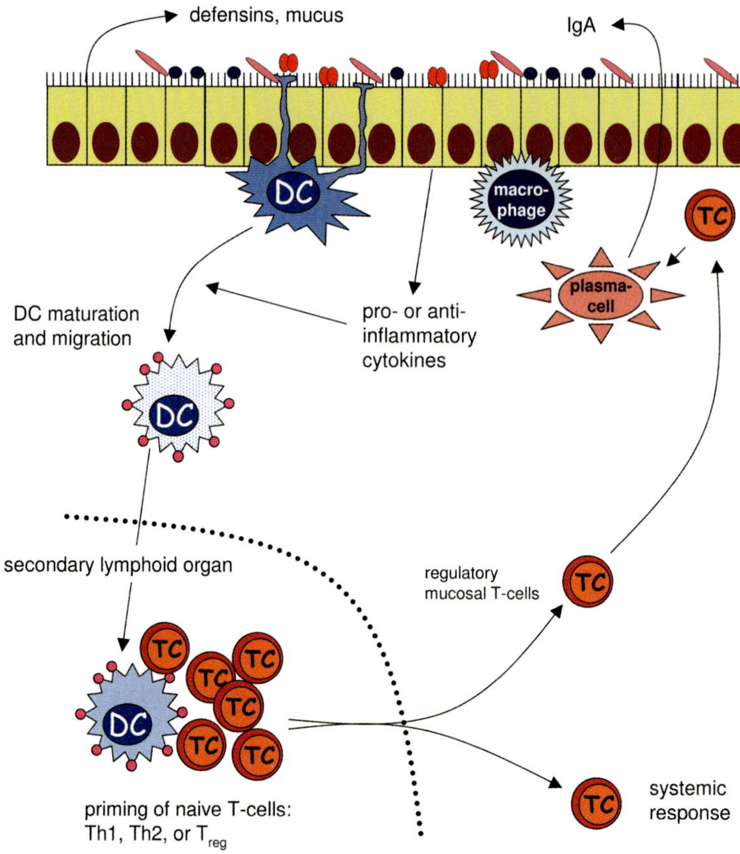

Fig. 15.1 Cells contributing to mucosal immunity. The nasopharyngeal mucosa is the port of entry for invasive *N. meningitidis*. Several mechanisms control immunity at this barrier. Resident macrophages and dendritic cells (DC) can sample antigen from apical and invading bacteria. DC can shuttle ingested antigen to regional secondary lymphoid organs during phenotypic maturation and induce an appropriate T-cell response. T-cells can disseminate further in the case of a systemic response or home to the epithelium (mostly regulatory T-cells contributing to immune homeostasis). The majority of human plasma cells is associated with epithelial barriers and secretes IgA, which is shuttled aross the epithelium and represents a major humoral constituent of mucosal immunity. Epithelial cells also contribute to immune homeostasis. They produce mucus and several antimicrobial peptides or proteins (defensins, lysozyme) regulating the composition of the apical flora. In addition, they can secrete anti-inflammatory as well as proinflammatory mediators in response to environmental stimuli that regulate DC and macrophage activity.

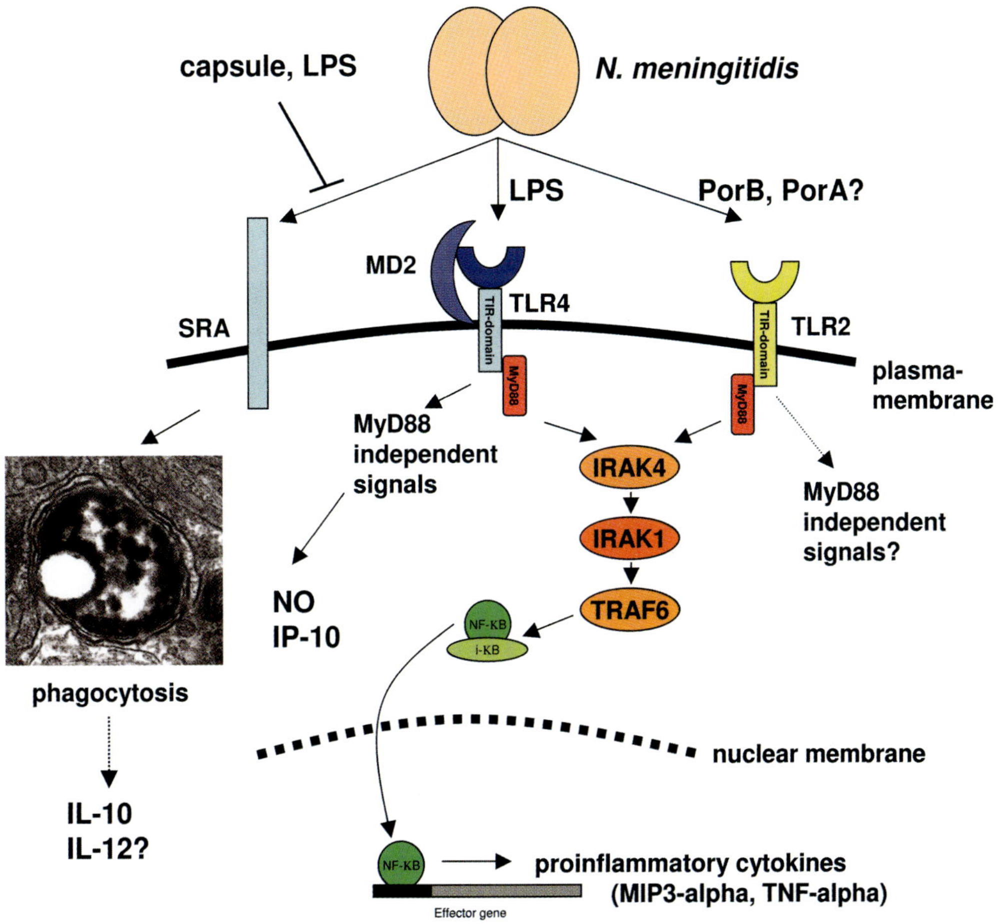

Fig. 15.2 Receptors and signaling events induces by *N. meningitidis* in dendritic cells. Several receptors on the DC surface are involved in recognition of meningococci. LPS interaction with TLR4 requires the TLR4 associated LPS recognition proteins MD2 and CD14 as well as some structural components of the meningococcal LPS (see text). This interaction is probably responsible for rapid activation of the immature DC and the induction of cytokine secretion. Beside LPS, other outer membrane components might also stimulate DC activation. This has been shown for PorB which interacts with TLR2, thereby inducing DC maturation and cytokine secretion. The graphic depicts only the common MyD88 dependent signaling pathway. This cascade can potentially branch to activate MAPK-pathways. In addition, MyD88 independent signaling pathways have been described for TLRs. For phagocytosis of *N. meningitidis*, the Scavenger Receptor A seems to be the predominant receptor on macrophages and dendritic cells. Although the internalization of *N. meningitidis* by DC can potentially lead to signaling, as contact to several TLRs might occur after phagosomal fusion, a direct role of SRA in signaling has yet to be determined.

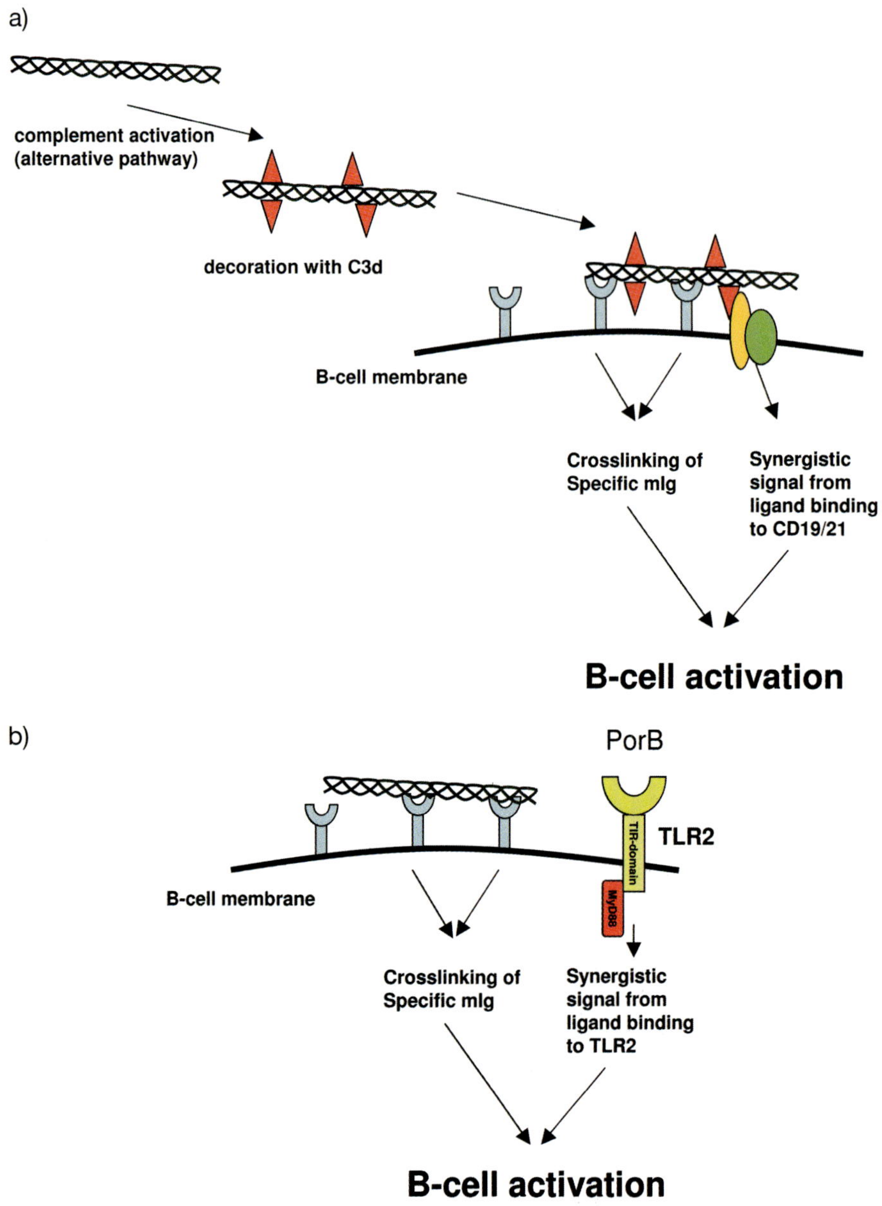

Fig. 15.4 Mechanisms leading to B-cell activation by meningococcal capsular polysaccharide. Crosslinking of B-cell membrane bound immunoglobulin receptors provides the first signal for B-cell activation. Second signals might be provided by the activation of the CD19/CD21 complement receptor complex by proteolytically released C3d, which is attached to capsule polysaccharide after activation of the complement cascade (a). Alternatively, Toll-like receptors might provide a second signal, due to the unique situation, that B-cells simultaneously express antigen-specific and pattern recognition receptors. Meningococcal PorB has been shown to activate B-cells via TLR2 (b).

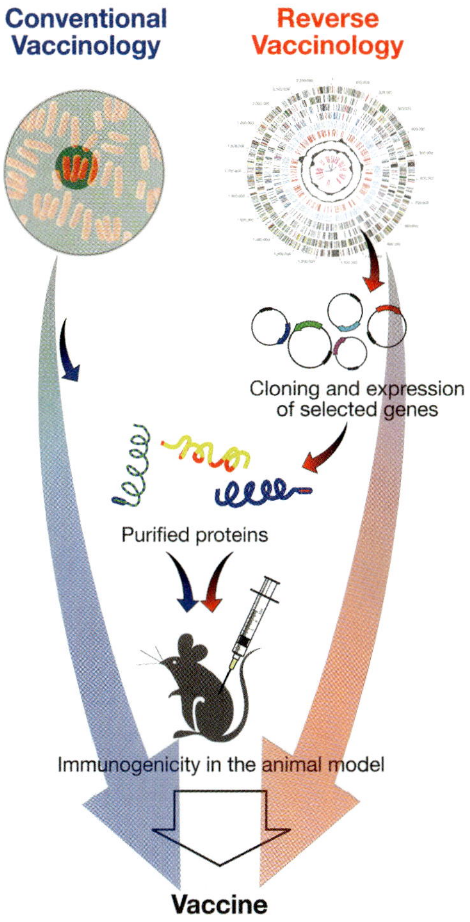

Fig. 19.1 Schematic representation of the conventional and "reverse" genome-based approaches to vaccine development.

1
Historical Aspects

Keith Cartwright

1.1
The Origins of Meningococcal Disease

The story of meningococcal disease has mirrored the scientific and technological developments of the time. Each advance, from early microscopy through bacterial culture and classification techniques to mathematical modelling, genetics, molecular microbiology and proteomics, has been reflected in advances in our understanding of, and latterly, control of meningococcal disease.

For most of the 19th century, communications between scientists were limited and the disciplines of microbiology and epidemiology did not exist. Medicine was primarily observational, much more art than science, and there were few rational, science-based treatments. Without diagnostic tools, it was impossible to differentiate one "spotted fever" from another. In this pre-technological time, it would have been very difficult to differentiate sporadic cases (or even outbreaks) of meningococcal disease from conditions such as typhus, typhoid and smallpox. Thus it is very hard to say whether Vieusseux really was the first to describe an outbreak of meningococcal disease when he documented 33 deaths from a "spotted fever" accompanied in most cases by meningitis in Eaux-Vives, a small suburb of Geneva, Switzerland.

Nevertheless, some early clinicians were capable diagnosticians and the signs and symptoms of meningococcal disease – at least in the form in which we see it today – are in many ways strikingly characteristic, especially in its epidemic form. Could it truly have been a new disease in 1805? This must remain a possibility. We know now that the meningococcus, as well as being highly adapted to the human nasopharynx (suggesting a long and intimate commensal relationship with Man), is also a highly transformable bacterium, capable of acquiring and integrating DNA from a range of microbes with which it comes into contact. It remains a possibility (that cannot be proved or disproved) that, in a small Swiss community in 1805, a nasopharyngeal commensal neisseria acquired by chance the genetic material that allowed it to become the meningococcus we know today.

Handbook of Meningococcal Disease. Infection Biology, Vaccination, Clinical Management.
Edited by M. Frosch and M.C.J. Maiden

ISBN: 3-527-31260-9

1.2
The 19th Century

Epidemiology: Outbreaks and Epidemic Periods with High Case Fatality Rate

For most of the 19th century, meningococcal disease was recognized and described principally when clusters of cases occurred. Many were associated with the military. In this pre-antibiotic era, the disease was associated with very high mortality (70% or more), though not all died swiftly. There are numerous accounts of patients whose rash and fever settled over a week or so, leaving the afflicted individual comatose, lingering for days or even weeks before finally perishing. Presumably in such cases, patients survived long enough to mount a partial or even complete immune response, but by the time the infection was controlled, brain damage was severe and the chance of survival slight. August Hirsch, a medical historian, published by far the most comprehensive account of the disease during this period in 1886.

First Isolation of the Meningococcus

It was only towards the end of the century in 1887 that Anton Weichselbaum, working in Vienna, isolated the putative bacterium causing the disease from six of eight fatal cases. A pneumococcus was isolated from the remaining two. Jaeger, a German microbiologist disputed these findings, attributing the cause of the disease to an intracellular chaining coccus (therefore presumably a streptococcus) from fatal cases in a military outbreak in Stuttgart [1]. This confusion may have arisen either because, as we know now, meningitis can be caused by a range of different microorganisms (Jaeger may have isolated a pneumococcus), or (more likely) Jaeger's cultures were contaminated. Keeping cultures pure was a major problem for early microbiologists. Before long, Weichselbaum's findings were replicated and vindicated and his "*Diplococcus intracellularis meningitidis*" was recognized as the true cause of meningococcal meningitis.

Lumbar Puncture in Living Patients

The demonstration of the practicality of lumbar puncture as an investigative procedure by Quincke in 1893 not only provided a means by which a diagnosis could be established in a significant proportion of patients, but perhaps more importantly paved the way for intrathecal serotherapy.

Isolation of Meningococci from Throat Swabs

An important advance in developing an understanding of the mechanism of spread of the disease was the first isolation of meningococci from throat swabs and its differentiation from gonococci by Kiefer in 1896. The end of the 19th century was a fertile period for traditional medical microbiology, with the isolation and characterization of a host of medically important bacteria, reflecting advances in bacterial culture techniques and in classification methods.

1.3 From 1900 to 1920

Immunotherapy

The first major advance of the new century was the development of meningococcal antisera by German and US researchers. In Germany, Jochmann and his team raised antisera in rabbits and then horses, demonstrated protection in a guinea pig model and then proceeded to human trials, beginning with subcutaneous administration and then utilizing the intrathecal route. By 1908, Flexner and Jobling in the USA were able to report 25% mortality in a large series – a dramatic improvement in outcome when compared with the death rate in untreated patients. Serum sickness and the occasional case of secondary meningitis were among the problems with this new treatment.

Epidemiology: World War I – Investigations in Recruit Training Camps

In the UK, notification of a range of infectious conditions such as cerebrospinal meningitis and typhoid was made a legal requirement for doctors in 1912, having been introduced on a piecemeal basis, city by city, since 1905.

Most combatant countries began to experience upsurges in meningococcal disease incidence with the mobilization of millions of young men into the military establishment. It was quickly recognized that the problem was largely restricted to new recruits. Attack rates were low in seasoned troops. Captain JA Glover of the British Royal Army Medical Corps (RAMC) led a major program of investigation that lasted the duration of the war at the Guards Training Depot at Caterham in south London. Key findings were an association of disease with the winter months, with periods of severe overcrowding and with large rises in the prevalence of meningococcal nasopharyngeal carriage prior to the onset of cases of disease.

Efforts were made to control the disease through interventions that included increasing the space between beds, improving the ventilation in accommodation huts, deferral of typhoid vaccination and the use of zinc sulfate spray as a nasopharyngeal disinfectant for recruit troops where there had already been a case. In retrospect, perhaps the first two of these measures were the most important. For whatever reason, by the time of the 1918–1919 influenza epidemic, the disease had been controlled and there were only two cases of cerebrospinal fever that winter in a still-overcrowded camp. Subsequent work showed that high carriage rates were not always associated with disease and that acquisition rates and the intrinsic virulence of the circulating meningococci were more important.

First Vaccine Trials

The first generation of meningococcal vaccines were crude by today's standards, comprising no more than standardized suspensions of killed meningococci. In 1912, Sophian and Black in the USA used a heat-killed vaccine to immunize first a group of medical students and then larger groups of family case contacts and nurses. Side-effects were similar to those of the newly developed typhoid vaccines. (In view of the likely endotoxin content, a red, swollen and sore arm at the injection site must have been almost universal!)

Greenwood used a similar, but polyvalent vaccine during a large outbreak of disease in and around Salisbury, England, in 1915. Two doses of the vaccine were given to more than 4000 individuals of whom approximately 25% were schoolchildren. Over the next year, there were seven cases among just over 5000 unvaccinated children and no cases in the vaccinated children. The difference in disease attack rates was not significant.

In a US military camp outbreak in 1917, a whole-cell vaccine was given to 4700 soldiers of a total population of 25 000 [2]. After a 5-month follow-up period, there were 43 cases amongst unimmunized troops, compared with a single case in a fully vaccinated recruit and two cases in partially immunized soldiers, giving a short-term efficacy of 87%.

Meningococcal Typing

Gordon and Murray, RAMC microbiologists, raised antisera to meningococci in rabbits and used these to develop a typing system (types I–IV). A French typing system developed a few years later at the Pasteur Institute, Paris, utilized letters rather than numerals (A–D). It took until 1950 for an international committee to unify the two schemes to create the serogroup classification that remains in use today (Table 1.1). All major outbreaks that occurred between 1914 and 1945 were caused by strains that would now be designated as serogroup A.

Table 1.1 Relationships between historical and present-day classifications of meningococcal serogroups.

Reference	Year	Classification
Gordon, Murray [3]	1915	I II III IV
Nicolle, Debains, Jouan [4]	1918	A B A B C D
Recommended (Int. Assoc. Microbiol.)	1950	A B A D C

1.4
From 1921 to 1939

Epidemiology

There were a number of notable outbreaks of meningococcal infection on both sides of the Atlantic during the late 1920s, caused by serogroup A strains. Major serogroup A epidemics occurred in the sub-Saharan region of Africa, the Meningitis Belt, but were poorly documented.

The Meningococcal Capsule

In the US, Geoffrey Rake and his colleagues carried out detailed carriage studies and characterized the nature of the meningococcal capsule. His group showed that "smooth" meningococci were well capsulated and could be agglutinated by specific anticapsular antisera, in contrast to "rough" strains. Freshly isolated meningococci were more likely to be "smooth", i.e. to express abundant capsular material. He and his colleagues went on to demonstrate that the meningococcal capsule was composed of polysaccharide. This work was published in 1935 and it seems inevitable that it would have led to the development of purified capsular polysaccharide vaccines but for the waning of interest (and probably funding) with the discovery of the dramatic therapeutic potential of sulfonamides.

Sulfonamides – The First Specific Therapeutic Agents

Following tests in animals, sulfanilamide (Prontosil), the first sulfa drug used therapeutically, was reported in 1937 to be highly effective in human meningococcal infections. It was followed almost immediately by reports of the use of sulfapyridine – better known as M&B 693 (May & Baker). Not surprisingly, sulfonamide treatment immediately gained widespread acceptance, not only for meningococcal meningitis but also for pneumonia and a whole range of other infections. Sulfonamides formed the mainstay of meningococcal disease treatment throughout World War II.

1.5
From World War II to 1960 – Epidemiology

At the outbreak of World War II, there were again major outbreaks of meningococcal disease in combatant countries. In the UK there were more than 12 000 cases in 1940 and the USA also experienced a major upsurge in disease a little later with a peak of over 18 000 cases. In both countries, though there was a strong association with the military, there were also high rates of disease in civilian populations. Fortunately, sulfonamides and then later penicillin were widely available to treat affected patients. In the UK, case fatality rates dropped to below 20% (and were probably lower than this "headline" figure due to relative under-ascertainment of surviving cases).

With the availability of an increasing range of potent antibiotics in the years after World War II, it must have seemed that meningococcal disease had been defeated. Across the developed world rates of disease were generally low, although major epidemics continued to occur in the Meningitis Belt countries.

In 1950, the International Association of Microbiologists rationalized the classification system for meningococci, opting for the French nomenclature that had been in use since 1918.

During the 1950s, there was a gradual change in the disease epidemiology in many developed countries, with the decline of serogroup A strains and their replacement by a more diverse range of meningococci within which serogroup B strains generally predominated, with serogroup C also present.

Though numbers of cases in most European countries and in the USA remained at levels that were relatively low by historical comparison, case fatality rates remained stubbornly in the region of 15% or so and there was a better understanding of the appreciable morbidity amongst survivors. Meningococcal septicemia was recognized to be associated with very high case fatality rates.

1.6
From 1961 to 2005

Epidemiology

There was a timely reminder in 1963 that meningococcal disease continued to pose a major public health problem when Lapeysonnie documented the major epidemics of the disease that had been occurring (and continued to occur) in the Meningitis Belt. Lapeysonnie characterized the area in geographical terms, extending from northern Nigeria and Upper Volta in the west to Somalia in the east, i.e. stretching right across the continent. Epidemics continued to occur throughout the period with attack rates sometimes briefly in excess of 500 per 10^{5} population.

In the 1980s and 1990s, the incidence of meningococcal disease began to rise again in many countries. Outbreaks of serogroup B disease were documented in Cuba, Brazil, Chile, Norway, the United Kingdom and New Zealand, among other countries. In the 1990s, many European countries, including Spain, the Czech Republic and the United Kingdom, saw increases in the incidence of serogroup C disease caused by a strain of very high virulence. The start of the new millennium was marked by the occurrence of outbreaks of W-135 disease amongst Hajji pilgrims visiting Mecca. The responsible strain belonged to the same clone as that causing the recent serogroup C disease in Europe, suggesting that the clone had acquired a new capsule gene [51].

Meningococcal Typing

Typing of meningococci rose to a fine art with phenotypic characterization reflecting variations in capsular polysaccharide, class I and II/III (porA and porB) outer membrane proteins, lipooligosaccharide moieties and resistance to sulfonamides. Multilocus enzyme electrophoresis (MLEE), a surrogate for a genetic typing system, was used widely for investigation of outbreaks and for characterization of strain collections. In 1998, the development of multilocus sequence typing (MLST) provided a reproducible and unambiguous means of genetically characterizing meningococci. With rapid development of the world wide web, data on meningococcal sequence types are now held on an open-ended, open-access database, available to researchers throughout the world.

Vaccines

Despite many different approaches, the year 2005 was reached without the availability of a universal serogroup B vaccine suitable for most developed countries. Though outer membrane vesicle serogroup B vaccines tailored to specific strains had been made in Cuba and Norway, they proved unsuitable for widespread application. The publication of the sequence of the men B genome by a group led by Rino Rappuoli of the Chiron Corporation lifted hopes that a number of potential vaccine candidate antigens would be identified, but this hope has yet to be translated into reality. Many other approaches to the development of serogroup B vaccines are currently being explored.

There has been more better progress in the control of disease caused by strains of serogroups A and C. Conjugated polysaccharide vaccines have been developed for both of these serogroups, and in the case of the latter, deployed with tremendous success, first in the United Kingdom and then more widely in many European countries. Early in the new millennium, and in a politico-economic development of enormous importance, the Microsoft Corporation founder, Bill Gates, donated many tens of millions of dollars to a program aimed at developing and rolling out conjugated vaccines in the countries of the Meningitis Belt. Serogroup A conjugates are now being manufactured in India at low cost; and the groundwork is being laid for their use in Africa in the next few years.

Clinical Management

With an increasing appreciation of the importance of the host response to meningococcal infection as a factor in tissue damage and poor outcome, there have been a number of new therapeutic modalities developed that aim to block some of the damaging host immune responses that characterize severe meningococcal sepsis. As yet, none has been shown to impact significantly on outcome.

On a more practical note, there has been a dramatic reduction in the meningococcal disease case fatality rate during the past 10–15 years as a consequence

Table 1.2 Milestones in the history of meningococcal disease.

Year	Author(s)	Milestone
Classical	Hippocrates, etc.	Description of headache with fever. Uniformly fatal. Could have been any one of a number of diseases.
1684	Willis	*"A description of an epidemical feaver in 1661"*. English physician described an outbreak of a spotted fever [6]. Could have been typhus or typhoid.
1806	Vieusseux	First well documented description of an outbreak of meningococcal disease in Eaux Vives, near Geneva, Switzerland [7]. Most cases had meningitis.
1806	Danielson, Mann	First description (independent of Vieusseux) of an outbreak of meningococcal disease in the New World (Medfield, Mass., USA) [8].
19th century	Hirsch	Medical historian documented outbreaks in Europe and USA throughout the 19th century (1805–1882) [9]. Described three principal epidemic periods with very high case fatality rates.
1884	Marchiafava, Celli	Italian physicians describe oval micrococci (small round Celli bacteria) within leucocytes in spinal fluid of patients dying with meningitis. Negative cultures [10].
1887	Weichselbaum	Viennese physician isolated "*Diplococus intracellularis meningitidis*" from spinal fluid of six of eight cases of primary, sporadic meningitis. First isolation of a meningococcus [11].
1893	Quincke	German physician carries out first lumbar puncture in a living patient [12].
1894	Voelcker	First report of supra-renal apoplexy (later known as Waterhouse-Friderichsen syndrome) [13].
1896	Heubner	German microbiologist isolated meningococci from spinal fluid of living patient [14].
1896	Kiefer	German microbiologist isolates meningococci from the throat (nasopharyngeal carriage) [15]. Differentiated meningococci from gonococci.
1906	Jochmann	German physician raises animal antisera, tests in animals and attempts intrathecal serotherapy [16]. First rational treatment.
1908	Flexner, Jobling	Extensive use of horse antimeningococcal sera for intrathecal treatment in both USA and Germany [17]. Case fatality rate halved in treated patients (still only a small minority).
1911	Netter, Debré	Updated Hirsch's account of outbreaks [18].
1911	Waterhouse	English physician also described supra-renal apoplexy (but could have been hemorrhagic smallpox) [19].

Table 1.2 (continued)

Year	Author(s)	Milestone
1912		Introduction of a national system of infectious disease notification (including cerebrospinal fever) in the UK.
1912	Sophian, Black	First whole-cell vaccine tested in USA [20].
1914–1918		Major rise in incidence of meningococcal disease in WWI combatant countries.
1915–1916	Greenwood	First whole-cell vaccine deployed during outbreak in Southern England. Attempt at evaluation of efficacy unsuccessful [21].
1915	Gordon, Murray	English army microbiologists developed first serological classification system [3].
1914–1918	Glover	Detailed epidemiological studies in army recruit depots in England linking overcrowding and high rates of carriage with disease [22].
1918	Friderichsen	Also described supra-renal apoplexy (now Waterhouse-Friderichsen syndrome) [23]. The most mis-spelt eponym in the history of meningococcal disease!
1918	Nicolle	Pasteur Institute microbiologists published a new serological classification [4].
1919	Rolleston	Detailed review of meningococcal disease during WWI. Association with respiratory viral infections and influenza recognized [24].
1920s–1930s		Outbreaks of disease in urban communities in Europe and USA. Recognition of major outbreaks in sub-Saharan Africa.
1929	Fleming	Discovered penicillin. Subsequently developed by Florey, Chain, et al. [25].
1933	Rake, Scherp	US microbiologist described rough and smooth (i.e. encapsulated) strains. Subsequently showed that capsule was composed of polysaccharide [26]. Paved the way for development of capsular polysaccharide vaccines.
1937	Schwentker	"*Treatment of meningococcic meningitis with sulfanilamide*" [27]. A major landmark. The first specific and highly effective treatment.
1939	Banks et al.	Use of sulfonamides for treatment becomes widespread and remains so until end of war [28, 29].
1940	Fairbrother	Sulfonamides found to clear nasopharyngeal carriage making chemopropylaxis possible [30].
1940s		Major epidemics of meningococcal disease in combatant countries in WWII.
1950	Intl Assoc. Microbiol.	New meningococcal serogroup nomenclature (A, B, C, etc.), still in use today.
1956	Branham	Canadian microbiologist wrote detailed review of the history of meningococcal infection [31].

Table 1.2 (continued)

Year	Author(s)	Milestone
1963	Lapeysonnie	Documented massive epidemics of meningococcal disease in sub-Saharan Africa from 1940s [32].
1963	Millar	Emergence of sulfonamide resistance [33]. Hampered chemoprophylaxis and sparked vaccine development program in US military.
1969	Hollis	Identification and characterization of *Neisseria lactamica*. Permitted distinction between meningococcus and lactamica in carriage studies [34].
1969	Gotschlich et al.	Major US military research program results in the publication of seminal papers on meningococcal capsular polysaccharides, mechanisms of immunity to infection and the development and testing of the first polysaccharide vaccines [35–39].
1982	DeVoe	Detailed review of understanding of meningococcal disease pathogenesis [40].
1987	Achtman	Electrophoretic typing (MLEE); first genetically based classification system allowing a better understanding of meningococcal evolution [41].
1988	Botha	First report of a penicillinase-producing meningococcus [42].
1991	Sierra	Cuban microbiologists developed strain-specific outer membrane vesicle vaccine for local outbreak of serogroup B disease [43]. Outbreak declined.
1990s	Various	Limitations of plain polysaccharide vaccines appreciated. Technological development of conjugated vaccines.
1991	Kristiansen	First report of PCR test for diagnosis [44].
1995	Cartwright	Updated history of the disease [5].
1997	Levin et al.	Human gene polymorphisms linked to risk of disease [45, 46].
1998	Maiden	Multi-locus sequence typing (MLST) of bacteria [47]. Open-access electronic sequence type database created.
1990s	Levine	Improved clinical management reduced case fatality rate [48].
1999	Miller et al.	Introduction of conjugated serogroup C vaccine in the UK. Men C disease rapidly controlled [49].
1999	Chippaux et al.	Men A+C conjugates enter clinical trials in Africa [50].
2000–2001	Taha	Outbreaks of W-135 disease in Hajji pilgrims [51].
2000	Rappuoli et al.	Men B genome sequenced [52]. Candidates for serogroup B vaccines identified [53].

Table 1.2 (continued)

Year	Author(s)	Milestone
2001	Gates	Computer billionaire funds Meningitis Vaccine Project – a major program of meningococcal vaccination in sub-Saharan Africa. Politics and economics meet microbiology and epidemiology!
2005		Efforts to develop safe and effective men B vaccines continue.

of: (a) familiarity with the symptoms of the disease amongst parents, teenagers and health care professionals leading to earlier recognition and treatment, (b) a better appreciation that time is precious in early management if the disease process is to be arrested – the concept of the "Golden Hour" and (c) the development and widespread implementation of good protocols for case management, leading to a more consistent standard of treatment with fewer mistakes in fewer hospitals. These simple measures have led to a reduction of more than 50% in the case fatality rate in the United Kingdom.

In 2005, meningococcal resistance to penicillin remains no more than a very occasional curiosity. One hopes that it may remain so, at least until we are able to control meningococcal disease through vaccination.

1.7 Conclusion

This is a necessarily brief account of only some of the milestones in the history of meningococcal disease. These are set out in Table 1.2 for ease of reference. Readers wishing for a little more detail are referred to the first chapter in "Meningococcal Disease", a book that I edited in 1995 [5]. Since this book is now out of print, copies of the chapter and a more extended historical bibliography can be obtained directly from the author (Prof. Keith Cartwright, Brobury House, Brobury, Herefordshire, HR3 6BS, United Kingdom).

References

1 Jaeger H **1895**, Zur aetiologie der meningitis cerebrospinalis epidemica, *Zeitschr. Hyg. Infect.* 19, 351–370.

2 Gates FL **1918**, A report on antimeningitis vaccination and observations on agglutinins in the blood of chronic meningococcus carriers, *J. Exp. Med.* 28, 449–474.

3 Gordon MH, Murray EG **1915**, Identification of the meningococcus, *J. R. Army Med. Corps* 25, 411–423.

4 Nicolle M, Debains E, Jouan C **1918**, Etudes sur les méningococciques et les serums anti-méningococciques, *Ann. Inst. Pasteur* 32, 150–169.

5 Cartwright K **1995**, Introduction and historical aspects, in *Meningococcal Disease*, ed. Cartwright K, John Wiley & Sons, Chichester, p. 1–19.
6 Willis T **1684**, A description of an epidemical feaver ... 1661, in *Practice of Physics*, Treatise VIII, T Dring, London, p. 46–54.
7 Vieusseux M **1806**, Memoire sur la maladie qui a régné à Genève au printemps de 1805, *J. Med. Chir. Pharmacol.* 11, 163–182.
8 Danielson L, Mann E **1806**, The history of a singular and very mortal disease, which lately made its appearance in Medfield, *Med. Agric. Reg.* 1, 65.
9 Hirsch A **1886**, Epidemic cerebro-spinal meningitis, in *Handbook of Geographical and Historical Pathology, vol III – Diseases of Organs and Parts* (translated from the German by Creighton C), New Sydenham Society, London, p. 547–594.
10 Marchiafava E, Celli A **1884**, Spra i micrococchi della meningite cerebrospinale epidemica, *Gazz. Osped.* 5, 59.
11 Weichselbaum A **1887**, Ueber die aetiologie der akuten meningitis cerebro-spinalis epidemica, *Fortschr. Med.* 5, 573–583, 620–626.
12 Quincke HI **1893**, Ueber meningitis serosa, *Samml. Klin. Vort.* 67, 655–694.
13 Voelcker AF **1894**, Abstract of post mortem report, *Middx Hosp. Rep. Med. Surg. Pathol. Reg.* 1894, 278.
14 Heubner JOL **1896**, Beobachtungen und versuche über den meningokokkus intracellularis (Weichselbaum-Jaeger), *Jb. Kinderheilk.* 43, 1–22.
15 Kiefer F **1896**, Zur differentialdiagnose des erregers der epidemischen cerebrospinal-meningitis und der gonorrhoe, *Berl. Klin. Woch.* 33, 628–630.
16 Jochmann G **1906**, Versuche zur serodiagnostik und serotherapie der epidemischen genickstarre, *Dtsch Med. Wschr.* 32, 788–793.
17 Flexner S, Jobling JW **1908**, An analysis of four hundred cases of epidemic meningitis treated with the anti-meningitis serum, *J. Exp. Med.* 10, 690–733.
18 Netter A, Debré R **1911**, *La Méningite Cérébrospinale*, Masson, Paris.
19 Waterhouse R **1911**, A case of supra-renal apoplexy, *Lancet* 1911i, 577–578.
20 Sophian A, Black J **1912**, Prophylactic vaccination against epidemic meningitis, *J. Am. Med. Assoc.* 59, 527–532.
21 Greenwood M **1917**, The outbreak of cerebrospinal fever at Salisbury in 1914–15, *Proc. R. Soc. Med.* 10, 44–60.
22 Glover JA **1920**, Observations of the meningococcus carrier rate and their application to the prevention of cerebro-spinal fever, *Spec. Rep. Ser. Med. Res. Council* 50, 133–165.
23 Friderichsen C **1918**, Nebennierenapoplexie bei kleinen kindern, *Jb. Kinderheilk.* 87, 109–125.
24 Rolleston H **1919**, Lumleian lectures on cerebro-spinal fever, Lecture 1, *Lancet* 1919i, 541–549.
25 Fleming A **1929**, On the antibacterial action of cultures of a penicillium with special reference to their use in the isolation of *B. influenzae*, *Br. J. Exp. Pathol.* 10, 226–236.
26 Scherp H, Rake G **1935**, Studies on meningococcus infection, VIII, The type I specific substance, *J. Exp. Med.* 61, 753–769.
27 Schwentker FF **1937**, Treatment of meningococcic meningitis with sulfanilamide, *J. Pediatr.* 11, 874–880.
28 Banks HS **1939**, Chemotherapy of meningococcal meningitis, A review of 147 consecutive cases, *Lancet* 1939i, 921–927.
29 Beeson PB, Westerman E **1943**, Cerebrospinal fever, Analysis of 3,575 case reports, with special reference to sulphonamide therapy, *Br. Med. J.* 1, 497–500.
30 Fairbrother RW **1940**, Cerebrospinal meningitis, The use of sulphonamide derivatives in prophylaxis, *Br. Med. J.* 2, 859–862.
31 Branham SE **1956**, Milestones in the history of the meningococcus, *Can. J. Microbiol.* 2, 175–188.
32 Lapeysonnie L **1963**, La méningite cérébro-spinale en Afrique, *Bull. WHO* 28[suppl], 3–114.
33 Millar JW, Siess EE, Feldman HA, et al. **1963**, In vivo and in vitro resistance to sulfadiazine in strains of *Neisseria meningitidis*, *J. Am. Med. Assoc.* 186, 139–141.

34 Hollis DG, Wiggins GL, Weaver RE **1969**, *Neisseria lactamicus* sp. n., a lactose-fermenting species resembling *Neisseria meningitidis*, *Appl. Microbiol.* 17, 71–77.

35 Goldschneider I, Gotschlich EC, Artenstein MS **1969**, Human immunity to the meningococcus, I, The role of humoral antibodies, *J. Exp. Med.* 129, 1307–1326.

36 Goldschneider I, Gotschlich EC, Artenstein MS **1969**, Human immunity to the meningococcus, II, Development of natural immunity, *J. Exp. Med.* 129, 1327–1348.

37 Gotschlich EC, Teh Yung Liu, Artenstein MS **1969**, Human immunity to the meningococcus, III, Preparation and immunochemical properties of the group A, group B and group C meningococcal polysaccharides, *J. Exp. Med.* 129, 1349–1365.

38 Gotschlich EC, Goldschneider I, Artenstein MS **1969**, Human immunity to the meningococcus, IV, Immunogenicity of group A and group C meningococcal polysaccharides in human volunteers, *J. Exp. Med.* 129, 1367–1384.

39 Goldschneider I, Gotschlich EC, Artenstein MS **1969**, Human immunity to the meningococcus, V, the effect of immunization with meningococcal group C polysaccharide on the carrier state, *J. Exp. Med.* 129, 1385–1395.

40 DeVoe IW **1982**, The meningococcus and mechanisms of pathogenicity, *Microb. Rev.* 46, 162–190.

41 Olyhoek T, Crowe BA, Achtman M **1987**, Clonal population structure of *Neisseria meningitidis* serogroup A isolated from epidemics and pandemics between 1915 and 1983, *Rev. Infect. Dis.* 9, 665–692.

42 Botha P **1988**, Penicillin-resistant *Neisseria meningitidis* in Southern Africa, *Lancet* 1988i, 54.

43 Sierra GVG, Campa HC, Varcacel NM, et al. **1991**, Vaccine against serogroup B *Neisseria meningitidis*, Protection trial and mass vaccination results in Cuba, *Natl Inst. Public Health Ann.* 14, 195–210.

44 Kristiansen B-E, Ask E, Jenkins A, et al. **1991**, Rapid diagnosis of meningococcal meningitis by polymerase chain reaction, Lancet 337, 1568–1569.

45 Nadel S, Newport MJ, Booy R, Levin M **1996**, Variation in the tumor necrosis factor-α gene promoter region may be associated with death from meningococcal disease, *J. Infect. Dis.* 174, 878–880.

46 Westendorp RGJ, Langermans JAM, Huizinga TWJ, et al. **1997**, Genetic influence on cytokine production and fatal meningococcal disease, *Lancet* 349, 170–173.

47 Maiden MCJ, et al. **1998**, Multilocus sequence typing: a portable approach to the identification of clones within populations of pathogenic microorganisms, *Proc. Natl Acad. Sci. USA* 1998, 3140–3145.

48 Booy R, Habibi P, Nadel S, et al. **2001**, Reduction in case fatality rate from meningococcal disease associated with improved healthcare delivery, *Arch. Dis. Child* 85, 386–390.

49 Miller E, Salisbury D, Ramsay M **2001**, Planning, registration, and implementation of an immunisation campaign against meningococcal serogroup C disease in the UK: a success story, *Vaccine* 20[suppl], S58–S67.

50 Campagne G, Garba A, Fabre P, et al. **2000**, Safety and immunogenicity of three doses of a *Neisseria meningitidis* A+C diphtheria conjugate vaccine in infants from Niger, *Pediatr. Infect. Dis. J.* 19, 144–150.

51 Taha MK, Achtman M, Alonso JM, et al. **2000**, Serogroup W135 meningococcal disease in Hajj pilgrims, *Lancet* 356, 2159.

52 Tettelin H, Saunders NJ, Heidelberg J, et al. **2000**, Complete genome sequence of *Neisseria meningitidis* serogroup B strain MC58, *Science* 287, 1809–1815.

53 Pizza M, Scarlato V, Masignani V, et al. **2000**, Identification of vaccine candidates against serogroup B meningococcus by whole-genome sequencing, *Science* 287, 1816–1820.

Part I
Epidemiology of Meningococcal Disease

Handbook of Meningococcal Disease. Infection Biology, Vaccination, Clinical Management.
Edited by M. Frosch and M.C.J. Maiden

ISBN: 3-527-31260-9

2
The Population Biology of *Neisseria meningitidis*: Implications for Meningococcal Disease, Epidemiology and Control

Martin C.J. Maiden and Dominique A. Caugant

2.1
Introduction: The Meningococcus, an Enigmatic Pathogen

2.1.1
The Global Burden of Meningococcal Disease

Meningococcal disease, in both endemic and epidemic forms, is an important cause of morbidity and mortality in developing countries as well as in the industrialized world. In the absence of epidemics, approximately 500 000 cases of invasive meningococcal disease are reported annually worldwide, resulting in more than 50 000 deaths (Tikhomirov et al. 1997). Half of these cases occur in a zone south of the Sahara in Africa, the so-called "Meningitis Belt" (Lapeyssonnie 1963), which comprises 18 countries spreading from Ethiopia in the east to Senegal in the west and includes a population of about 300 million people. While in industrialized countries, the incidence rate of endemic disease is usually around 1–2 cases per 100 000 individuals, explosive epidemics periodically occur in the Meningitis Belt, with incidence rates that may exceed 500 per 100 000 (Schwartz et al. 1989).

Epidemics of meningococcal disease are extremely disruptive to healthcare systems, especially in countries with limited resources; but even in parts of the world where therapy is readily available and affordable, meningococcal disease remains associated with a mortality rate of over 10% (Peltola 1983). Death of a previously healthy individual may occur within a few hours of the first appearance of symptoms and those who survive frequently suffer from permanent tissue damage, persistent neurological sequelae and digit or limb loss (Brandtzaeg 1995). The severity of meningococcal meningitis and septicemia, the two most common disease syndromes, combined with the unpredictability and rapidity of disease onset (Rosenstein et al. 2001), raise much public concern regarding this disease and present a challenge for management at both the clinical and public health levels (Stuart et al. 1997). Disease control is further hampered by the lack of safe and comprehensive vaccines that are efficacious in all age groups (Jodar

Handbook of Meningococcal Disease. Infection Biology, Vaccination, Clinical Management.
Edited by M. Frosch and M.C.J. Maiden

ISBN: 3-527-31260-9

et al. 2002). Many of the features of meningococcal disease that complicate its management are a consequence of the complexities of the population biology of the organism. Thus, investigations of the biology of *Neisseria meningitidis* have been and remain of central importance in unravelling the epidemiology of this fearsome disease and its causative agent.

N. meningitidis is solely associated with humans and has not been isolated elsewhere in nature. It is an encapsulated bacterium, with many isolates enveloped by a polysaccharide capsule, a major antigenic structure that is used to classify meningococcal isolates by immunological means into serogroups. Each serogroup corresponds to a chemically and antigenically distinct capsular polysaccharide and, although 13 distinct serogroups have been described (Vedros 1987), virtually all isolates from invasive disease belong to one of five serogroups, namely: A, B, C, W-135 and Y (Peltola 1983). As shown in Fig. 2.1, the serogroups of the strains causing disease are not uniformly distributed throughout the world (Tikhomirov et al. 1997). Serogroup A meningococci are the major cause of the large, cyclic epidemics in Africa and in Asia, while in industrialized nations 30–70% of the disease is caused by serogroup B organisms. Serogroup C meningococci are particularly associated with, usually, smaller-scale outbreaks worldwide. The importance of serogroup Y disease has been rising in recent years, currently accounting for

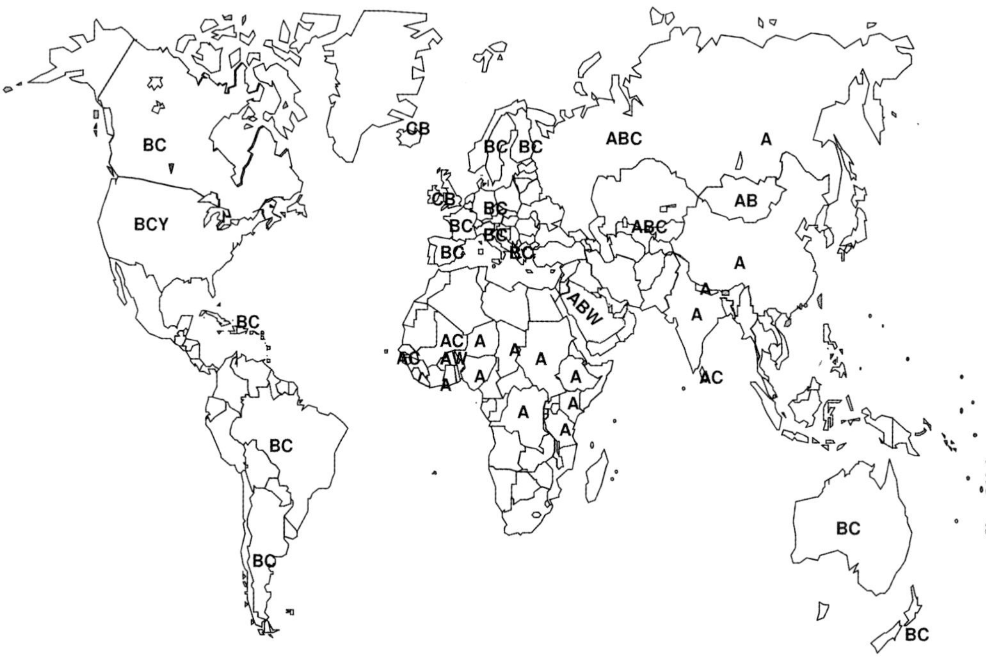

Fig. 2.1 Global distribution of meningococcal disease. The distribution of the various serogroups of meningococci is indicated by the appropriate letters (after Tikhomirov et al. 1997)

over 30% of cases in the USA (McEllistrem et al. 2004; Rosenstein et al. 1999). Serogroup W135 meningococci (Popovic et al. 2000), which until recently mainly caused sporadic cases of disease, was associated with large outbreaks among pilgrims to the Hajj in Saudi Arabia in 2000 and 2001 and was responsible for a severe epidemic in Burkina Faso in 2002 (Decosas and Koama 2002). The remaining capsular serogroups are rarely associated with disease, although outbreaks caused by meningococci of serogroup X have also been described recently in Africa (Djibo et al. 2003; Gagneux et al. 2002).

2.1.2
Paradoxes Arising from Meningococcal Natural History

From the perspective of the natural history of *N. meningitidis*, meningococcal disease presents a number of paradoxes. Whilst disease occurrence is sporadic, unpredictable and, even during large epidemics, affects only a small proportion of the population, the causative agent appears to be common in human populations. The majority of people will, at one time or another and almost certainly on multiple occasions throughout life, harbor the bacterium asymptomatically in the throat. Cross-sectional population studies have shown that, in nonepidemic settings, around 10% of healthy humans carried meningococci in the upper airway (Cartwright et al. 1987; Caugant et al. 1994; Claus et al. 2005; Stephens 1999). In closed and semi-closed populations, such as military recruits and university students, carriage rates increase and may be near 100% (Andersen et al. 1998; Claus et al. 2005). Further, although both carriage rates and disease incidence are dependent on the age of the host, the highest rates of carriage do not correspond to the age-specific disease incidence. In the United Kingdom, for example, a country that can be considered as typical of the industrialized world in this respect, disease incidence peaks in very young children, while carriage rates are highest in young adults (Fig. 2.2; Cartwright et al. 1987; Jones and Mallard 1993).

Part of the explanation of these observations is that *N. meningitidis*, notwithstanding its notoriety as an aggressive pathogen, has evolved as a harmless commensal inhabitant of the nasopharynx of humans. If the very artificial – and extremely rare (Boutet et al. 2001) – situation of laboratory-acquired infection is discounted, neither meningitis nor septicemia presents the meningococcus with an opportunity for person-to-person spread (Maiden 2004). Therefore, while disease is devastating to the individual host, it is of no significance in terms of the spread of meningococci from person to person and is an incidental – or even accidental – occurrence (Fig. 2.3; Maiden 2004). This presents a further paradox: as the disease does not promote spread and indeed is likely to inhibit it by removing hosts from the transmission system, how and why has this ability to cause disease, even infrequently, arisen and persisted in meningococal populations (Stollenwerk et al. 2004)?

Another puzzle is the paucity of historical records that can be unambiguously identified as describing meningococcal disease. The first recognized description

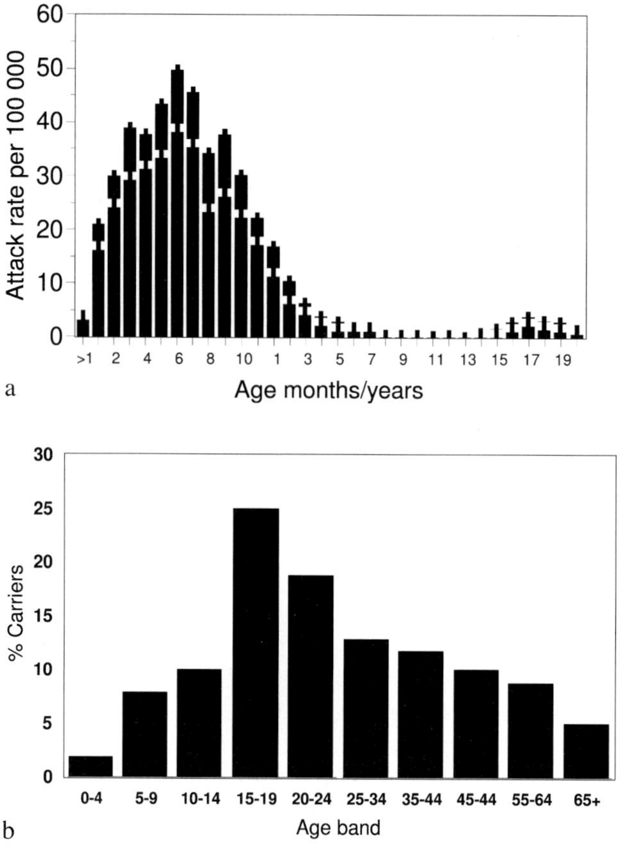

Fig. 2.2 Age-specific rates of (a) carriage and (b) meningococcal disease in the UK in the 1980s. Data from Jones and Mallard (1993; disease) and Cartwright et al. (1987; carriage).

of the disease was at the start of the 19th century in Europe (Vieusseux 1805) and there is little evidence of the disease in Africa before the 20th century (Greenwood 1999), despite the fact that meningococcal disease syndromes are both dramatic and characteristic. In this respect, it is worth noting that descriptions identifiable as gonococcal disease, caused by the closely related but acapsulate gonococcus, are as old as civilization itself, dating to around 4000 years ago (Rothenberg 1993). This raises the prospect that the meningococcus is a relatively recently emerged pathogen, which perhaps derived from an acapsulate ancestor, following the acquisition of the capsule locus (Claus et al. 2002; Dolan-Livengood et al. 2003).

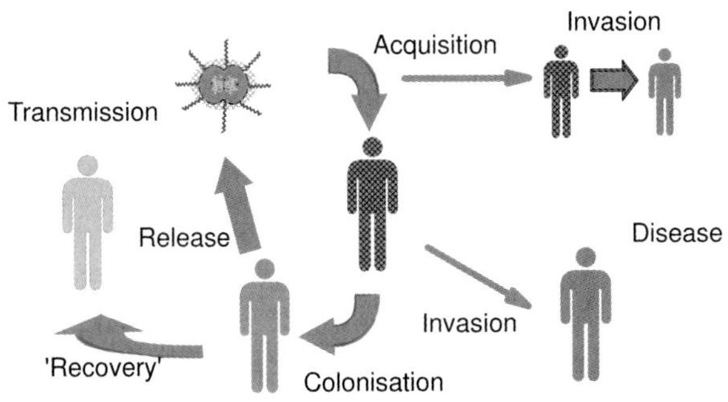

Fig. 2.3 Transmission cycle of meningococci. This illustrates that disease is not part of the normal transmission cycle of meningococci. In adults (represented by the larger figure) acquisition is common but disease is rare, while in the case of children (represented by the smaller figure) acquisition is rare, but disease is relatively more common.

2.2 Meningococcal Diversity and its Consequences

2.2.1 Genetic and Antigenic Diversity

The high diversity of meningococcal populations is a characteristic that complicates both vaccine design and public health monitoring of the disease (Maiden and Frosch 2001). This diversity is evident in both the surface structures of the meningococcus, as indicated by antigenic diversity, and in the genetic variation of genes encoding metabolic functions. While diversifying selection imposed by the host immune system can be invoked to explain the diversity of surface antigens and the genes that encode them, the diversity of genes encoding cellular components that do not interact directly with the host immune system cannot be explained in this way.

There are marked differences in the propensity of particular meningococcal antigenic and genetic variants to cause disease and also, perhaps, in the severity and type of disease that they cause (Caugant 1998). The polysaccharide capsule protects the meningococcus from complement attack and phagocytosis and is essential for systemic invasion into the bloodstream and passage through the blood–brain barrier. Unencapsulated meningococci are only exceptionally isolated from cases of invasive disease, usually only in immunocompromised individuals. In contrast, approximately 50% of the strains isolated from healthy carriers lack capsule and are therefore nonserogroupable by serological means. The loss of capsule enhances the capability of the bacterium to adhere to the mucosal epithelium; and meningococci have developed a number of mechanisms to control capsule production (Dolan-Livengood et al. 2003). A proportion of carried meningococci, those that have the capsule null locus (*cnl*) in place of the capsule region of the chromosome, are genetically incapable of expressing capsule (Claus et al. 2002).

The sub-capsular antigens, the membrane proteins and lipopolysaccharides (LPSs) that make up the outer membrane of the meningococcus, also display a wide variety of antigenic types and are the basis of the serotyping (variation in the PorB porin), serosubtyping (PorA porin) and immunotyping (LPS) schemes (Frasch et al. 1985; Hitchcock 1989). All strains of *N. meningitidis* express PorB and most strains express PorA. Variation in these structures has been evidenced both by the use of extent panels of monoclonal antibodies (Abdillahi and Poolman 1987, 1988) and by sequencing of the genes coding for these antigens (Barlow et al. 1989; Maiden et al. 1991; Russell et al. 2004; Suker et al. 1994; van der Ley et al. 1991). While there is some evidence that particular variants of these sub-capsular components are associated with invasive disease, this is much less clear-cut than the evidence for the involvement of capsular polysaccharides. It is possible, for example, that sialylated LPS can substitute for the anti-phagocytic properties of the capsule during disseminated infection, but this is much less common than disease caused by capsulated meningococci.

A number of studies have shown that numerous meningococcal surface structures are phase-variable and the bacterium is able to change the level of expression of these antigens in response to changing environmental conditions. Thus, these highly variable structures are under diversifying selection and are consequently less attractive for epidemiological studies. However, these and other variable components encoded by so-called "contingency genes", play an important role in pathogenesis (Moxon et al. 1994).

During the past two decades, a variety of techniques have been used to explore the genetic diversity of meningococci. Indeed, studies of meningococcal diversity have been in the forefront of studies of bacterial population biology (Cooper and Feil 2004; Feil 2004; Maiden et al. 1998; Urwin and Maiden 2003). By far the most influential of these techniques have been the related approaches of multilocus enzyme electrophoresis (MLEE; Selander et al. 1986) and multilocus sequence typing (MLST; Maiden et al. 1998). Both of these techniques, which have been used to examine the population structure of a variety of pathogenic and nonpathogenic bacteria (Musser 1996; Urwin and Maiden 2003), assess the diversity of randomly chosen, multiple genes encoding essential metabolic functions. These so-called housekeeping genes are expected to be subject to stabilizing selection for conservation of the metabolic functions of the proteins that they encode. By indexing variation that is not a consequence of positive selection, these approaches aim to obtain data pertinent to establishing the reliable evolutionary relationships among isolates. In the case of MLEE, genetic variation is assessed by examination of the gene products (normally metabolic enzymes) encoded by various loci after starch gel electrophoresis and specific histochemical staining (Selander et al. 1986). This valuable method became obsolete after the development of MLST, which exploits advances in high-throughput DNA sequencing technology to measure the variation of genes directly and definitively (Maiden et al. 1998).

In both MLEE and MLST, genetic variants at multiple loci are determined and assigned an arbitrary allele number. The allele numbers for all loci examined by the scheme are combined into an allelic profile, known as an electrophoretic type (ET) in MLEE or as a sequence type (ST) in the case of MLST. MLST uses fewer loci (seven) than MLEE (15–20 loci), but the degree of resolution of MLST is much higher at each locus, in that all polymorphisms are detected; and, thus, MLST identifies many more alleles per locus. While both of techniques produce equivalent data, MLST data are more easily compared across studies and laboratories. A centralized repository of curated MLST data is available via the Internet (www.pubmlst.org/neisseria; www.neisseria.org/mlst), a fundamental advantage for the analysis of a pathogen that may achieve intercontinental spread (Caugant et al. 1986; Moore et al. 1989). This chapter will use the MLST nomenclature, as used on the MLST website, which defines STs and clonal complexes named after particular STs (e.g. ST-11 complex), with cross-references to the MLEE nomenclature (e.g. ET-37 and ET-37 complex) where necessary.

2.2.2
Structure Within Meningococcal Populations – The Clonal Complex

The application of population genetic approaches, first MLEE and later MLST, identified the extent of genetic diversity in the species. This can be best illustrated by referring to the *Neisseria* MLST website. Although the information accessible at the website is not comprehensive, it is continually updated, providing an indication of meningococcal diversity described to date. At the time of writing this review, the publicly available isolate database contained a total of 4802 meningococcal sequence types, with the number of unique alleles identified at the seven MLST loci ranging from 174 for the least diverse locus, *adk*– to 319 for the most diverse locus, *aroE*.

Despite this bewildering diversity in genes demonstrably subject to stabilizing selection, analysis of the data and especially those obtained by rational sampling of particular populations reveals that the species diversity is highly structured. First, all multilocus genotypes are not equally represented. Indeed, most of them are identified only once, or a few times, while a relatively small proportion of ETs/STs are repeatedly identified in many data sets. Second, a number of the frequent genotypes have a wide temporal and geographic distribution, often being observed on multiple continents and over periods of decades. Finally, when the data are examined by a variety of clustering techniques, these persistent ETs/STs appear to form the centre of clusters of related genotypes. Such groups of related genotypes are referred to as clonal complexes and are pragmatically defined as those genotypes that share identical nucleotide sequences for at least four MLST loci with the central genotype (Fig. 2.4). Grouping of meningococci into clonal complexes has been of major importance in investigating the epidemiology of the disease and has been essential in understanding and meeting the challenges of vaccine development.

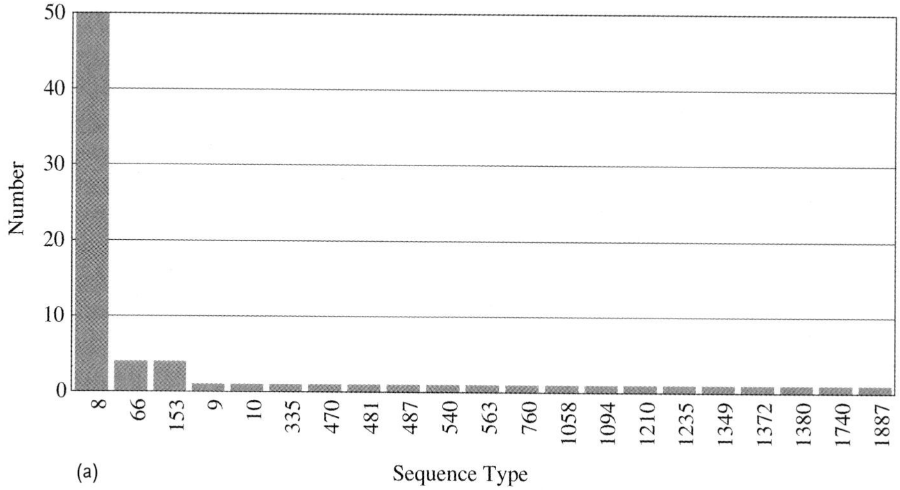

(a)

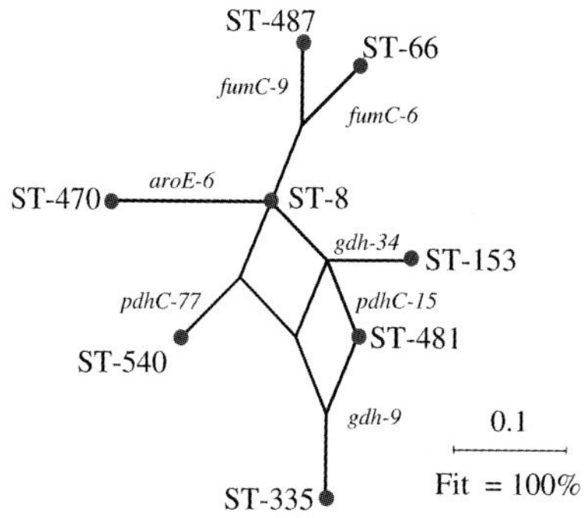

(b)

Fig. 2.4 A meningococcal clonal complex. The figure shows (a) the frequency of variant genotypes in the PubMLST *Neisseria* database and (b) the relationship of the genotypes with Split decomposition analysis of allelic profiles. The Split graph has been annotated with the molecular changes associated with each branch. Most of these changes have been generated by recombination rather than mutation.

2.3 Mechanisms of Diversification and Structuring in Meningococcal Populations

2.3.1 Mutation and Recombination in Bacterial Evolution

Genetic variation can arise in bacterial populations by two mechanisms: (a) mutation, by which we mean principally the accumulation of *de novo* genetic changes by processes such as substitution, insertion and deletion and (b) recombination, the combining of genes with distinct evolutionary histories. Recombination may be intergenomic, where the recombining genes are acquired from a distinct organism, or intragenomic, where multiple copies of the gene exist in the genome.

The *a priori* expectation is that in the haploid, asexual organisms, such as the bacteria, diversity is principally generated by mutation as there is no sexual stage in the life cycle and most genes are only present in one copy in the genome. In the absence of sexual exchange, any novel genetic polymorphism is limited to the descendants of the cell in which the mutation first occurred. Different bacteria therefore accumulate distinct patterns of polymorphisms scattered throughout the genome, depending on their ancestry. This leads to a highly structured population that can be accurately modelled by a tree-like phylogeny in which the branches have been generated by single mutations. During population growth and spread, many of the variant forms are lost as a consequence of selective events ("periodic selection"; Selander and Levin 1980) or stochastic events ("bottlenecking"; Achtman 1997). Under this scenario, a bacterial population becomes structured into a "clonal population", which comprised a number of distinct "lineages", each of which is characterized by a unique pattern of polymorphisms (Orskov and Orskov 1983). Clonal populations have a number of recognisable and indeed testable features: linkage disequilibrium (the nonrandom assortment of genetic polymorphisms), tree-like phylogenetic structure and congruence of phylogenetic trees at each locus.

The clonal model was the predominant paradigm for bacterial population structures for a number of years. In spite of some degree of linkage disequilibrium in the meningococcus, the presence of clusters of closely related genotypes in isolate collections examined by MLEE provided early indication of a high level of recombinational events in this naturally transformable bacterial species. In asexual organisms, horizontal genetic exchange (the transfer of genetic material among bacterial cells that do not necessarily share a mother cell) involves the exchange of relatively small parts of the chromosome of the order of a few kilobase pairs (i.e. less than 1% of the "average" bacterial genome) at any one time. This process has been colorfully referred to as "localized sex" (Maynard Smith et al. 1991). Over a number of generations, this relatively limited "sexual" activity erases the clonal structure, by reassorting genetic variation. *N. meningitidis*, as the majority of bacteria studied to date, are neither fully clonal nor nonclonal, but rather show evidence for both clonal spread and genetic exchange (Spratt and Maiden 1999).

2.3.2
Evidence for Recombination in Meningococcal Populations

Evidence for recombination was first observed in genes encoding antibiotic resistance and surface antigens, in the form of "mosaic genes" (Feavers et al. 1992; Spratt et al. 1992). These are allelic variants that have patterns of polymorphisms most parsimoniously explained by the recombination of two genes with distinct evolutionary histories. Such mosaic genes can easily be explained by positive selection of very rare events that conferred a particular advantage, such as antibiotic resistance. In *N. meningitidis*, however, mosaic structures also occur in housekeeping genes (Zhou and Spratt 1992), where positive section is unlikely to occur (Maiden 1993).

Analyses of MLST data demonstrated that there was little congruence in the phylogenic signals observed at different loci and at the whole genome level (Feil et al. 1999; Holmes et al. 1999). Further, the clonality of meningococcal populations might have been amplified in some collections by sampling bias (Maynard Smith et al. 1993). As some genotypes are more likely to be associated with invasive disease than others, these are over-represented in collections of disease isolates, as opposed to collections obtained from healthy carriers. The degree of linkage disequilibrium in the species as a whole is much reduced in comparison to that in disease-associated isolates.

A modification of the clonal structure model was proposed to explain the over-representation of certain genotypes in meningococcal populations, the epidemic population structure (Maynard Smith et al. 1993). This model envisages the occasional emergence of particularly fit variants that come to transitorily dominate a population. However, as virulence does not equate to fitness, which must be measured in terms of transmission success in the case of the meningococcus, this model does not provide a wholly satisfactory explanation of meningococcal population structure and its relation to epidemiology (Gupta and Maiden 2001; Stollenwerk et al. 2004).

A number of studies have undertaken quantitative or semi-quantitative estimation of the relative impacts of mutation and recombination on meningococcal evolution. Usually, the ratio of changes caused by recombination versus mutation has been estimated at 8–16 to one (Feil et al. 1999; Jolley et al. 2005). For one population of carried meningococci, this rate was shown to be inconsistent with the degree of structuring observed in the population under simple neutral models (Jolley et al. 2005). The same study demonstrated that the structuring was unlikely to be generated by "demographic" factors, such as geographic distribution, or by purely neutral processes, indicating that fitness differences for transmission associated with different STs might be a structuring force (Jolley et al. 2005).

Further levels of structuring are evident in the combinations of antigenic variants observed in association with particular genetic lineages (Gupta et al. 1996). Models of immunological selection can generate such structuring into discrete and "nonoverlapping" structures (those in which antigenic variants are not shared among distinct strains; Urwin et al. 2004), but in the absence of hitchhiking, apparently precluded by high recombination rates, this structuring is again difficult to explain without evoking some form of selection operating on the population (Gupta and Maiden 2001).

In conclusion, meningococcal populations are highly diverse, but extensively structured in spite of rates of horizontal gene transfer that are sufficiently high to disrupt clonal population structures. While the underlying mechanisms have yet to be fully resolved, it is probably that a combination of immune selection imposed by herd immunity and fitness differences among meningococcal strains is responsible for this structuring. This particular population structure of *N. meningitidis* has important implications for both epidemiological monitoring and vaccine design.

2.4
Meningococcal Genotypes in Carriage and Disease

All meningococci must live in a successful commensal association with humans to persist, but some genotypes appear to have a higher propensity to cause disease (Caugant 2001; Maiden et al. 1998; Yazdankhah et al. 2004). This realization has made the analysis of carrier populations an essential step in the study of meningococci. Unfortunately, but for wholly understandable reasons, emphasis has historically been placed on the collection and analysis of isolates from patients with invasive disease and there is a relative paucity of good, well characterized collections of carried meningococci.

Early studies (carried out before the introduction of genetic characterization techniques) established the age distribution of meningococcal carriage in a number of populations and that, while virtually all isolates from disease are capsulate, a large proportion of carried meningococci are acapsulate. It is now known that this can be for essentially two reasons, either (a) these meningococci do not possess the capsule locus (the capsule null or *cnl* meningococci), or (b) the expression of the capsule has been down-regulated by one of a number of genetic mechanisms; and such down-regulation can be temporary or permanent (Claus et al. 2002; Dolan-Livengood et al. 2003; Sadler et al. 2003). As capsulation is highly unlikely to have evolved as a virulence determinant in a normally commensal organism, the down-regulation during carriage suggests that the capsule has a role in transmission rather than long-term carriage. In addition, the prevalence of certain disease-associated capsules, especially serogroups C, is very low in the majority of carriage studies (Caugant et al. 1988; Claus et al. 2005; Maiden and Stuart 2002).

2.4.1
The Hyperinvasive Lineages

When compared to collections of meningococci collected from the nasopharynx of healthy individuals, meningococci from diseased individuals are typically much less diverse (Caugant 2001; Jolley et al. 2005; Yazdankhah et al. 2004). Indeed, a limited number of genotypes, and especially clonal complexes, dominate world-wide collections of meningococci (Caugant 1998; Caugant et al. 1987b; Maiden et al. 1998). These meningococci, belonging to the "hyperinvasive lineages", appear to have an increased propensity to cause invasive disease. Although the definition of such lineages has been informal, comparisons of equivalent collections of disease associated and carried meningococci character-

Table 2.1 Some principal clonal complexes of *Neisseria meningitidis* and their association with disease (odds ratio of disease to carriage prevalence with 95% confidence interval) and serogroup among disease isolates; from Yazdankhah et al. (2004).

Clonal complex	Disease association odds ratio	Serogroup B	Serogroup C	Serogroup W-135	Serogroup Y	Others and not-groupable
ST-11	52 (20–135)	11%	80%	6%		3%
ST-23	0.2 (0.1–0.7)	10%		3%	56%	31%
ST-32	0.9 (0.4–2.2)	82%	5%		3%	10%
ST-35	0.3 (0.1–1.1)	50%				
ST-162	0.8 (0.4–1.18)	82%		6%		12%
ST-269	6.1 (0.5–12.8)	86%			5%	9%
ST41/44	1.1 (0.5–2.3)	79%	2%		2%	17%

ized by MLST have enabled this property to be quantified in terms of the prevalence of particular clonal complexes in point-prevalence carriage studies and among cases of invasive disease (Table 2.1; Yazdankhah et al. 2004); and such calculations show the very large differences in this respect among meningococci, allowing a more formal definition of hyperinvasive meningococci. The global epidemiology of meningococci is best described in terms of these lineages.

2.5 Global Epidemiology of Meningococcal Disease

2.5.1 The Group A Pandemics

Previously described as the "subgroups" of serogroups A (Crowe et al. 1988; Olyhoek et al. 1987), three clonal complexes (the ST-1, ST-4, ST-5 complexes) that are strictly associated with the serogroups A capsular polysaccharide have caused the majority of meningococcal disease in Africa and Asia in the past 40 years (Wang et al. 1992). Two of these, the ST-1 complex (previously known as subgroup I) and the ST-5 complex (subgroup III) have achieved pandemic spread. Organisms of the ST-1 complex were responsible for outbreaks of meningococcal disease in the United States and in Europe during the Second World War. At the beginning of the 1960s, strains of the ST-1 complex were identified in China as well as in the African continent (first in North Africa and in the African meningitis belt, later also in South Africa). During the following decade, these strains were associated with disease in both North and South America; and in the 1980s they were found in Australia and New Zealand (Achtman 1990). Strains of the ST-1 complex were already causing disease in

Russia in the 1970s and have remained present, since several clones of the complex have been associated with a recent increase in serogroups A disease in the Moscow region (Achtman et al. 2001). Meningococci of the ST-5 complex have been responsible for three pandemics since the 1960s. The first one started in China, spread to Eastern Europe, Russia, Scandinavia and then Brazil. The second pandemic started again in China, but spread to Nepal and India and then was imported to Saudi Arabia by pilgrims from South Asia attending the annual Hajj pilgrimage to Mecca. From there, the clone ST-5 was introduced to Europe, the United States and Africa. In the following years, all countries of the meningitis belt experienced severe epidemics, culminating in 1996 with over 150000 reported cases. Since the mid-1990s, ST-5 has gradually been replaced in Africa by a new clone of the ST-5 complex, ST-7, which has resulted in a new wave of disease (Nicolas et al. 2001). A few ST-7 strains had previously been identified in the early 1990s in China, Mongolia and Russia. The large epidemics in Africa caused by members of the ST-5 complex have stimulated the "Meningitis Vaccine Project" (Soriano-Gabarro et al. 2004) which aims to develop affordable conjugate polysaccharide vaccines that could be used effectively in infant immunization campaigns.

2.5.2 The ST-11 (ET-37) Complex Epidemics

This clonal complex has caused a number of epidemics and pandemics, but unlike the ST-1 and ST-5 complexes, it has been associated with various serogroups (although principally those containing sialic acid), corresponding to serogroups B, C, Y and W-135 (Wang et al. 1993). Sulfonamide-resistant serogroup B ST-11 complex meningococci caused an epidemic of meningococcal disease among US service personnel in US recruitment camps during the Vietnam war period (Brundage and Zollinger 1987), triggering the development of the first effective meningococcal vaccines. Interestingly, this was facilitated by a capsule replacement event in 1967 in which the predominant strain switched from serogroup B, against which a "plain" polysaccharide vaccine is ineffective, to a serogroup C epidemic which could be interrupted with polysaccharide vaccines. During the 1990s, a new variant member of the ST-11 complex (first identified in Canada and designated using the MLEE terminology as the ET-15 variant of the ET-37 complex; Ashton et al. 1991) spread throughout Europe, resulting in an increased incidence of disease and outbreaks among teenagers (Caugant 2001). This event prompted the development and licensure of serogroup C conjugate vaccines, then leading a number of countries, including the UK (Miller et al. 2001), Spain (Larrauri et al. 2005) and the Netherlands (Welte et al. 2005), to introduce these vaccines into national immunization programs. In 2000 and 2001, another variant of this ST-11 clonal complex was responsible for outbreaks of serogroup W135 disease in Saudi Arabia, again associated with the Hajj pilgrimage. Then, this variant spread to Europe and the USA, causing cases among returning pilgrims and their close contacts (Taha et al. 2000). In 2002, the first large epidemic caused by W135 occurred in Burkina Faso, resulting in more than 12 000 cases (Decosas and Koama 2002). Reactive mass vaccination campaigns with the meningococcal A+C polysaccharide vaccine, the epidemic control measure recommended by the WHO, were stopped when serogroup W135 was confirmed to be the main capsular type involved in the epidemic. Because of global shortage in supply of the meningococcal ACYW polysaccharide vaccine, mass vaccination of the population could not be undertaken. This alarming situation appears to have been only transient, as most outbreaks in the meningitis belt since 2002 have been again caused by serogroup A strains of the ST-5 complex.

2.5.3 The ST-32 (ET-5) Pandemic

Starting in the mid-1970s, a clone of a novel genotype, frequently expressing serogroup B capsules, the ST-32 (originally identified as ET-5) complex, spread throughout Europe and the Americas (Caugant et al. 1987 a). Numerous variants have since been reported (Bygraves et al. 1999), but ST-32 complex strains associated with three distinct serosubtypes have been responsible for epidemics in Norway, Cuba and Chile, respectively. Norway (Bjune et al. 1991) and Cuba (Sierra et al. 1991) developed and implemented outer membrane vesicle (OMV) vaccines against the variant prevalent in these countries: the "Norwegian" strain (typically B:15:P1.7,16) and the "Spanish" strain (B:4:P19,15), respectively. Both of these vaccines had some success against the respective outbreak strain, but offered limited cross-protection against other members of the same clonal complex harboring different serosubtypes in infants and young children (Perkins et al. 1998). These strain-specific vaccines did, however, provide a model for the development of other "strain-specific" OMV vaccines (Frasch et al. 2001).

2.5.4 The ST-41/44 Complex (Lineage 3)

During the 1990s, members of the ST-41/44 complex displaced the ST-32 complex meningococci as the major cause of serogroup B meningococcal disease in many European countries. This is a highly diverse clonal complex, the only one for which it has been necessary to define two "central" genotypes. A particular variant of this clonal complex was responsible for a protracted hyperendemic wave of disease in New Zealand, which especially affected the Maoris and Pacific Islanders (Dyet et al. 2005; Martin et al. 1998). This epidemic stimulated the development of another OMV vaccine, directed against this particular strain; and mass vaccination of the New Zealand population is ongoing (Oster et al. 2005).

2.5.5 Other Complexes

A variety of other clonal complex/serogroup combinations have caused epidemics and hyperendemics of various scales. The ST-8 complex meningococci (cluster A4), which are apparently related to the ST-11 complex meningococci, were predominant in Europe and in the Americas in the 1970s and 1980s in association with both the serogroups B and the serogroups C polysaccharides. A recent rise in serogroup Y meningococcal disease in the United States has been caused by members of the ST-23 complex (cluster A3), a group of clone specifically associated with carriage in Europe. Several newly defined clone complexes, such as the ST-269, ST-213 and ST-162 complexes, have been associated with increases in disease incidence in one or several countries and may warrant careful surveillance.

In summary, a picture has emerged of meningococcal disease caused by the spread by asymptomatic carriage of various combinations of serogroup and clonal complex, with subcapsular antigens often associated with particular clonal complexes (Urwin et al. 2004). It is likely that these successive waves of different meningococcal types are driven by factors that include the immunity of particular human populations to particular meningococcal types. The different clonal complexes are often associated with different epidemiological behavior and geographic distribution.

2.6 Conclusions: Implications of Meningococcal Population Biology for Disease Control

Immunological differences in meningococci attributable to the serogroup (i.e. the capsular polysaccharide type) have been known for many years, but more sophisticated characterization has been required to further refine meningococcal epidemiology. The concept of the clonal complex has proved especially valuable and it is now well established that several clonal complexes may express different serogroups at different times, resulting in different patterns of disease. Meningococci belonging to the ST-1 and ST-5 complexes, which have been responsible for major pandemics, appear to be an exception, as they are invariably associated with expression of serogroup A and particular subcapsular antigens (Suker et al. 1994). Most other meningococci are apparently more flexible and can express alternative capsular and subcapsular antigens, so that continued surveillance is necessary, even if vaccines are available.

Population studies have major contributions to make at all stages of the development and implementation of vaccines. In the case of the development of the "tailor-made" OMV vaccines for the Norwegian, Cuban and New Zealand outbreaks, it was necessary to choose an appropriate isolate to form the basis of the vaccine. The ability of certain meningococcal clones to "capsule-switch" – i.e. to change their capsules by means of genetic transformation – means that, in the absence of comprehensive meningococcal vaccines, it is necessary to monitor the genotypes and serogroups of meningococcal isolates after the introduction of vaccines (Maiden and Spratt 1999).

The question of why some meningococci are more virulent than others remains to be satisfactorily resolved. However, the existence of comparable well characterized meningococcal isolate collections from both asymptomatic carriers and disease, allied to recent advances in whole genome analyses, provides powerful novel approaches to this question. It is now possible to compare disease and carrier isolate collections for the presence or absence of genetic elements that are thought to be associated with disease. An example of such an analysis identified a "meningococcal disease-associated island" (MDA), probably a bacteriophage that is over-represented in disease compared to carrier isolates (Bille et al. 2005). It is likely that such approaches will add a number of further genetic elements to the list of virulence determinants known for the meningococcus over the next few years.

Much has been achieved in the past 20 years by analyzing meningococci and meningococcal populations from the perspective of their natural history and evolution. Important insights, crucial to improved public health monitoring and disease eradication, have been obtained. However, a number of important issues remain to be resolved. With the exception of the capsule, the factors that lead some meningococcal lineages to be far more virulent (in terms of their ability to cause invasive disease) than others remain to be determined. Once identified, these may be attractive vaccine components. Models explaining the extensive structuring of meningococcal populations need to be further refined and these too may provide valuable insights that can be exploited in public health interventions. The increasing availability of genomic technology, allied to ever-improving collections of isolates that accurately sample defined meningococcal populations, provides the prospect that these advances can be made in the foreseeable future. The immediate prospect for population and evolutionary studies of the meningococcus remains an exciting one.

References

Abdillahi, H., Poolman, J. T. **1987**, *FEMS Microbiol. Lett.* 48, 367–371.

Abdillahi, H., Poolman, J. T. **1988**, *FEMS Microbiol. Immunol.* 47, 139–144.

Achtman, M. **1990**, *Rev. Med. Microbiol.* 1, 29–38.

Achtman, M. **1997**, *Gene* 192, 135–140.

Achtman, M., van der Ende, A., Zhu, P., Koroleva, I. S., Kusecek, B., Morelli, G., Schuurman, I. G., Brieske, N., Zurth, K., Kostyukova, N. N., Platonov, A. E. **2001**, *Emerg. Infect. Dis.* 7, 420–427.

Andersen, J., Berthelsen, L., Bech Jensen, B., Lind, I. **1998**, *Epidemiol. Infect.* 121, 85–94.

Ashton, F. E., Ryan, J. A., Borczyk, A., Caugant, D. A., Mancino, L., Huang, D. **1991**, *J. Clin. Microbiol.* 29, 2489–2493.

Barlow, A. K., Heckels, J. E., Clarke, I. N. **1989**, *Mol. Microbiol.* 3, 131–139.

Bille, E., Zahar, J. R., Perrin, A., Morelle, S., Kriz, P., Jolley, K. A., Maiden, M. C., Dervin, C., Nassif, X., Tinsley, C. R. **2005**, *J. Exp. Med.* 201, 1905–1913.

Bjune, G., Høiby, E. A., Grønnesby, J. K., Arnesen, O., Fredriksen, J. H., Halstensen, A., Holten, E., Lindbak, A. K., Nøkleby, H., Rosenqvist, E., Solberg, L. K., Closs, O., Eng, J., Frøholm, L. O., Lystad, A., Bakketeig, L. S., Hareide, B. **1991**, *Lancet* 338, 1093–1096.

Boutet, R., Stuart, J. M., Kaczmarski, E. B., Gray, S. J., Jones, D. M., Andrews, N. **2001**, *J. Hosp. Infect.* 49, 282–284.

Brandtzaeg, P. **1995**, in *Meningococcal Disease*, ed. Cartwright, K. A. V., John Wiley and Sons, Chichester, p. 71–114.

Brundage, J. F., Zollinger, W. D. **1987**, in *Evolution of Meningococcal Disease*, vol. I, ed. Vedros, N. A., CRC Press, Boca Raton, p. 5–25.

Bygraves, J. A., Urwin, R., Fox, A. J., Gray, S. J., Russell, J. E., Feavers, I. M., Maiden, M. C. J. **1999**, *J. Bacteriol.* 181, 5551–5556.

Cartwright, K. A. V., Stuart, J. M., Jones, D. M., Noah, N. D. **1987**, *Epidemiol. Infect.* 99, 591–601.

Caugant, D. A. **1998**, *APMIS* 106, 505–525.

Caugant, D. A. **2001**, in *Meningococcal Disease: Methods and Protocols*, eds. Pollard, A. J., Maiden, M. C. J., Humana Press, Totowa, N.J., p. 273–294.

Caugant, D. A., Frøholm, L. O., Bovre, K., Holten, E., Frasch, C. E., Mocca, L. F., Zollinger, W. D., Selander, R. K. **1986**, *Proc. Natl Acad. Sci. USA* 83, 4927–4931.

Caugant, D. A., Frøholm, L. O., Bovre, K., Holten, E., Frasch, C. E., Mocca, L. F., Zollinger, W. D., Selander, R. K. **1987a**, *Antonie van Leeuwenhoek J. Microbiol.* 53, 389–394.

Caugant, D. A., Høiby, E. A., Magnus, P., Scheel, O., Hoel, T., Bjune, G., Wedege, E., Eng, J., Frøholm, L. O. **1994**, *J. Clin. Microbiol.* 32, 323–330.

Caugant, D. A., Kristiansen, B. E., Frøholm, L. O., Bovre, K., Selander, R. K. **1988**, *Infect. Immun.* 56, 2060–2068.

Caugant, D. A., Mocca, L. F., Frasch, C. E., Frøholm, L. O., Zollinger, W. D., Selander, R. K. **1987b**, *J. Bacteriol.* 169, 2781–2792.

Claus, H., Maiden, M. C., Maag, R., Frosch, M., Vogel, U. **2002**, *Microbiology* 148, 1813–1819.

Claus, H., Maiden, M. C., Wilson, D. J., McCarthy, N. D., Jolley, K. A., Urwin, R., Hessler, F., Frosch, M., Vogel, U. **2005**, *J. Infect. Dis.* 191, 1263–1271.

Cooper, J. E., Feil, E. J. **2004**, *Trends Microbiol.* 12, 373–377.

Crowe, B. A., Abdillahi, H., Poolman, J. T., Achtman, M. **1988**, *J. Med. Microbiol.* 26, 183–187.

Decosas, J., Koama, J. B. **2002**, *Lancet Infect. Dis.* 2, 763–765.

Djibo, S., Nicolas, P., Alonso, J. M., Djibo, A., Couret, D., Riou, J. Y., Chippaux, J. P. **2003**, *Trop. Med. Int. Health* 8, 1118–1123.

Dolan-Livengood, J. M., Miller, Y. K., Martin, L. E., Urwin, R., Stephens, D. S. **2003**, *J. Infect. Dis.* 187, 1616–1628.

Dyet, K., Devoy, A., McDowell, R., Martin, D. **2005**, *Vaccine* 23, 2228–2230.

Feavers, I. M., Heath, A. B., Bygraves, J. A., Maiden, M. C. **1992**, *Mol. Microbiol.* 6, 489–495.

Feil, E. J. **2004**, *Nat. Rev. Microbiol.* 2, 483–495.

Feil, E. J., Maiden, M. C. J., Achtman, M., Spratt, B. G. **1999**, *Mol. Biol. Evol.* 16, 1496–1502.

Frasch, C. E., van Alphen, L., Poolman, J. T., Rosenqvist, E. **2001**, in *Meningococcal vaccines*, eds. Pollard, A. J., Maiden, M. C. J., Humana Press, Totowa, N.J., p. 81–108.

Frasch, C. E., Zollinger, W. D., Poolman, J. T. **1985**, *Rev. Infect. Dis.* 7, 504–510.

Gagneux, S. P., Hodgson, A., Smith, T. A., Wirth, T., Ehrhard, I., Morelli, G., Genton, B., Binka, F. N., Achtman, M., Pluschke, G. **2002**, *J. Infect. Dis.* 185, 618–626.

Greenwood, B. (1999) *Trans. R. Soc. Trop. Med. Hyg.* 93, 341–353.

Gupta, S., Maiden, M. C. J. **2001**, *Trends Microbiol.* 9, 147–192.

Gupta, S., Maiden, M. C. J., Feavers, I. M., Nee, S., May, R. M., Anderson, R. M. **1996**, *Nat. Med.* 2, 437–442.

Hitchcock, P. J. **1989**, *Clin. Microbiol. Rev.* 2, S64–S65.

Holmes, E. C., Urwin, R., Maiden, M. C. J. **1999**, *Mol. Biol. Evol.* 16, 741–749.

Jodar, L., Feavers, I. M., Salisbury, D., Granoff, D. M. **2002**, *Lancet* 359, 1499–1508.

Jolley, K. A., Wilson, D. J., Kriz, P., McVean, G., Maiden, M. C. **2005**, *Mol. Biol. Evol.* 22, 562–569.

Jones, D. M., Mallard, R. H. **1993**, *J. Infect.* 27, 83–88.

Lapeyssonnie, L. **1963**, *Bull. WHO* 28[Suppl], 53–114.

Larrauri, A., Cano, R., Garcia, M., Mateo, S. **2005**, *Vaccine* 23, 4097–4100.

Maiden, M.C. **2004**, *Adv. Exp. Med. Biol.* 549, 23–29.

Maiden, M.C., Frosch, M. **2001**, *Mol. Biotechnol.* 18, 119–134.

Maiden, M.C., Stuart, J.M. **2002**, *Lancet* 359, 1829–1831.

Maiden, M.C.J. **1993**, *FEMS Microbiol. Lett.* 112, 243–250.

Maiden, M.C.J., Bygraves, J.A., Feil, E., Morelli, G., Russell, J.E., Urwin, R., Zhang, Q., Zhou, J., Zurth, K., Caugant, D.A., Feavers, I.M., Achtman, M., Spratt, B.G. **1998**, *Proc. Natl Acad. Sci. USA* 95, 3140–3145.

Maiden, M.C.J., Spratt, B.G. **1999**, *Lancet* 354, 615–616.

Maiden, M.C.J., Suker, J., McKenna, A.J., Bygraves, J.A., Feavers, I.M. **1991**, *Mol. Microbiol.* 5, 727–736.

Martin, D.R., Walker, S.J., Baker, M.G., Lennon, D.R. **1998**, *J. Infect. Dis.* 177, 497–500.

Maynard Smith, J., Dowson, C.G., Spratt, B.G. **1991**, *Nature* 349, 29–31.

Maynard Smith, J., Smith, N.H., O'Rourke, M., Spratt, B.G. **1993**, *Proc. Natl Acad. Sci. USA* 90, 4384–4388.

McEllistrem, M.C., Kolano, J.A., Pass, M.A., Caugant, D.A., Mendelsohn, A.B., Fonseca Pacheco, A.G., Shutt, K.A., Razeq, J., Harrison, L.H. **2004**, *Emerg. Infect. Dis.* 10, 451–456.

Miller, E., Salisbury, D., Ramsay, M. **2001**, *Vaccine* 20[Suppl. 1], S58–S67.

Moore, P.S., Reeves, M.W., Schwartz, B., Gellin, B.G., Broome, C.V. **1989**, *Lancet* 1989ii, 260–262.

Moxon, E.R., Rainey, P.B., Nowak, M.A., Lenski, R.E. **1994**, *Curr. Biol.* 4, 24–32.

Musser, J.M. **1996**, *Emerg. Infect. Dis.* 2, 1–17.

Nicolas, P., Decousset, L., Riglet, V., Castelli, P., Stor, R., Blanchet, G. **2001**, *Emerg. Infect. Dis.* 7, 849–854.

Olyhoek, T., Crowe, B.A., Achtman, M. **1987**, *Rev. Infect. Dis.* 9, 665–682.

Orskov, F., Orskov, I. **1983**, *J. Infect. Dis.* 148, 346–357.

Oster, P., Lennon, D., O'Hallahan, J., Mulholland, K., Reid, S., Martin, D. **2005**, *Vaccine* 23, 2191–2196.

Peltola, H. **1983**, *Rev. Infect. Dis.* 5, 71–91.

Perkins, B.A., Jonsdottir, K., Briem, H., Griffiths, E., Plikaytis, B.D., Høiby, E.A., Rosenqvist, E., Holst, J., Nokleby, H., Sotolongo, F., Sierra, G., Campa, H.C., Carlone, G.M., Williams, D., Dykes, J., Kapczynski, D., Tikhomirov, E., Wenger, J.D., Broome, C.V. **1998**, *J. Infect. Dis.* 177, 683–691.

Popovic, T., Sacchi, C.T., Reeves, M.W., Whitney, A.M., Mayer, L.W., Noble, C.A., Ajello, G.W., Mostashari, F., Bendana, N., Lingappa, J., Hajjeh, R., Rosenstein, N.E. **2000**, *Emerg. Infect. Dis.* 6, 428–429.

Rosenstein, N.E., Perkins, B.A., Stephens, D.S., Lefkowitz, L., Cartter, M.L., Danila, R., Cieslak, P., Shutt, K.A., Popovic, T., Schuchat, A., Harrison, L.H., Reingold, A.L., et al. **1999**, *J. Infect. Dis.* 180, 1894–1901.

Rosenstein, N.E., Perkins, B.A., Stephens, D.S., Popovic, T., Hughes, J.M. **2001**, *N. Engl. J. Med.* 344, 1378–1388.

Rothenberg, R.B. **1993**, in *The Cambridge World History of Human Disease*, ed. Kipple, K.F., Cambridge University Press, Cambridge, p. 756–763.

Russell, J.E., Jolley, K.A., Feavers, I.M., Maiden, M.C., Suker, J.S. **2004**, *Emerg. Infect. Dis.* 10, 674–678.

Sadler, F., Fox, A., Neal, K., Dawson, M., Cartwright, K., Borrow, R. **2003**, *Epidemiol. Infect.* 130, 59–70.

Schwartz, B., Moore, P.S., Broome, C.V. **1989**, *Clin. Microbiol. Rev.* 2, S118–S124.

Selander, R.K., Levin, B.R. **1980**, *Science* 210, 545–547.

Selander, R.K., Caugant, D.A., Ochman, H., Musser, J.M., Gilmour, M.N., Whittam, T.S. **1986**, *Appl. Environ. Microbiol.* 51, 837–884.

Sierra, G.V.G., Campa, H.C., Varcacel, N.M., Garcia, I.L., Izquierdo, P.L., Sotolongo, P.F., Casanueva, G.V., Rico, C.O., Rodriguez, C.R., Terry, M.H. **1991**, *Natl Inst. Public Health Ann.* 14, 195–207.

Soriano-Gabarro, M., Rosenstein, N., LaForce, F.M. **2004**, *J. Health Pop. Nutr.* 22, 275–285.

Spratt, B.G., Maiden, M.C.J., **1999**, *Proc. R. Soc. Lond. B* 354, 701–710.

Spratt, B.G., Bowler, L.D., Zhang, Q.Y., Zhou, J., Smith, J.M. **1992**, *J. Mol. Evol.* 34, 115–125.

Stephens, D.S. **1999**, *Lancet* 353, 941–942.

Stollenwerk, N., Maiden, M.C., Jansen, V.A. **2004**, *Proc. Natl Acad. Sci. USA* 101, 10229–10234.

Stuart, J.M., Monk, P.N., Lewis, D.A., Constantine, C., Kaczmarski, E.B., Cartwright, K.A. **1997**, *Commun. Dis. Rep. CDR Rev.* 7, R3–R5.

Suker, J., Feavers, I.M., Achtman, M., Morelli, G., Wang, J.-F., Maiden, M.C.J. **1994**, *Mol. Microbiol.* 12, 253–265.

Taha, M.K., Achtman, M., Alonso, J.M., Greenwood, B., Ramsay, M., Fox, A., Gray, S., Kaczmarski, E. **2000**, *Lancet* 356, 2159.

Tikhomirov, E., Santamaria, M., Esteves, K. **1997**, *World Health Stat. Q.* 50, 170–177.

Urwin, R., Maiden, M.C. **2003**, *Trends Microbiol.* 11, 479–487.

Urwin, R., Russell, J.E., Thompson, E.A., Holmes, E.C., Feavers, I.M., Maiden, M.C. **2004**, *Infect. Immun.* 72, 5955–5962.

van der Ley, P., Heckels, J.E., Virji, M., Hoogerhout, P., Poolman, J.T. **1991**, *Infect. Immun.* 59, 2963–2971.

Vedros, N.A. **1987**, in *Evolution of Meningococcal Disease*, vol. II, ed. Vedros, N.A., CRC Press, Boca Raton, p. 33–37.

Vieusseux, G. **1805**, *J. Med. Chir. Pharm.* 2, 163–165.

Wang, J.-F., Caugant, D.A., Li, X., Hu, X., Poolman, J.T., Crowe, B.A., Achtman, M. **1992**, *Infect. Immun.* 60, 5267–5282.

Wang, J.-F., Caugant, D.A., Morelli, G., Koumaré, B., Achtman, M. **1993**, *J. Infect. Dis.* 167, 1320–1329.

Welte, R., Trotter, C.L., Edmunds, W.J., Postma, M.J., Beutels, P. **2005**, *Pharmacoeconomics* 23, 855–874.

Yazdankhah, S.P., Kriz, P., Tzanakaki, G., Kremastinou, J., Kalmusova, J., Musilek, M., Alvestad, T., Jolley, K.A., Wilson, D.J., McCarthy, N.D., Caugant, D.A., Maiden, M.C. **2004**, *J. Clin. Microbiol.* 42, 5146–5153.

Zhou, J., Spratt, B.G. **1992**, *Mol. Microbiol.* 6, 2135–2146.

3
Methods for Typing of Meningococci

Keith A. Jolley, Steve J. Gray, Janet Suker and Rachel Urwin

3.1
Introduction

The characterization, or typing, of microorganisms has been defined as "any of a variety of methods used to distinguish between closely related strains of a given microorganism which exhibit minimal biochemical and biological differences" [1]. This "variety of methods" may include bacteriocin typing, phage typing, serological typing, antibiotic sensitivity testing and an increasing number of molecular-based typing schemes. Such methods are an essential component of infectious disease surveillance and epidemiology, with the accurate and timely characterization of pathogenic organisms representing an essential step in the identification and potential management of disease outbreaks.

Since *Neisseria meningitidis* was recognized as a global pathogen, responsible for localized outbreaks of infection as well as pandemic disease, microbiologists have attempted to differentiate meningococcal isolates, generally using serological methods. The development of serological typing schemes for meningococci has been extensively reviewed [2, 3] and historically has been the most commonly used method for classifying meningococcal isolates. Serology is still used widely in many local hospital and reference laboratories but recent advances in biotechnology have led to the introduction and application of genotypic characterization of meningococcal isolates in an increasing number of them. These methods have not only enhanced the epidemiological surveillance of meningococcal disease but have challenged many of the paradigms of *N. meningitidis* evolution and population biology.

This chapter will focus on the principle methods available for typing meningococci and their most appropriate use. Not every typing method is appropriate in every case, for example a different method may be required for the effective local management of disease cases or clusters compared to large-scale epidemiological or population studies where the goal is the elucidation of global patterns of disease or carriage over time. For the individual patient or case, the characterization of the infecting meningococcus is not pertinent to their treatment but is

Handbook of Meningococcal Disease. Infection Biology, Vaccination, Clinical Management.
Edited by M. Frosch and M. C. J. Maiden

ISBN: 3-527-31260-9

essential for contact management and long-term development of population-based interventions such as vaccine programs.

3.2 Phenotypic Typing Methods

The correct speciation of *N. meningitidis* and isolate characterization are necessary for optimal disease management when cases of meningococcal disease occur. All *N. meningitidis* case isolates are gamma glutamyl aminopeptidase positive (a feature exploited in most commercial identification kits) but may show variable carbohydrate utilization. The majority of meningococci are glucose- and maltose-positive but lactose- and sucrose-negative in the pre-formed enzyme tests found in the commercial kits or in the semi-solid oxidative cysteine trypticase agar (CTA) tests. The glucose- or maltose-negative variants allow for initial phenotypic characterization of isolates. This is not a particularly useful difference as only 2–3% are glucose-negative and about 10% maltose-negative, although rarely is a glucose- and maltose-negative variant observed. The significance or relevance of the biochemical variants is uncertain, as they do not appear associated with any other differentiating characteristic or disease presentation.

Susceptibilities to therapeutic antibiotics (such as penicillin, cefotaxime or ceftriaxone) and prophylactic antibiotics (such as rifampicin or ciprofloxacin) are easily determined for all isolates where the minimum inhibitory concentrations (MICs) may be used to characterize the organism. Resistance to sulfonamides (for example sulfadiazine) is a useful epidemiological phenotypic marker that may be readily determined by local and reference laboratories, although these are not used frequently for therapy or contact management due to the variable MICs within the meningococcal population. Antibiotic susceptibilities and MIC testing are described more fully in the following chapter. The determination of the extremely rare meningococci harboring a β-lactamase-producing plasmid is important and their surveillance essential.

Once the identification of *N. meningitidis* is confirmed, it is necessary to obtain as much information as possible about the surface antigens expressed by the isolate for epidemiological analysis. This is traditionally achieved through the use of specific polyclonal or monoclonal sera. Serological typing of meningococci has followed the International Code of Nomenclature of Bacteria [4], whereby the primary division of classification is referred to as "group" and subdivisions are designated as "type". Chemical and genetic methods have been used to define the antigens that are responsible for specific serological determinants so that the characterization scheme for meningococci comprises: (a) serogroup, based on variants in the capsular polysaccharide, (b) serotype, based on variants of the PorB outer membrane protein (OMP); serosubtype, based on variants of the PorA OMP, (c) immunotype, based on variants in the lipooligosaccharide (Fig. 3.1).

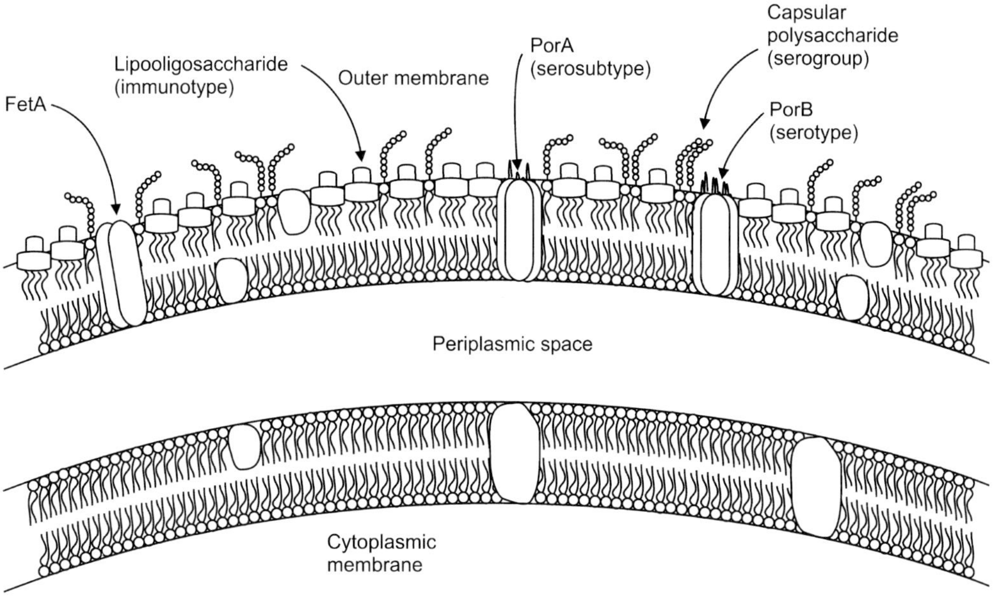

Fig. 3.1 Representation of the meningococcal structures involved in serological typing.

3.3 Serological Typing Methods

3.3.1 Serogrouping of Meningococci

In 1909, serological differences between meningococci were observed and the presence of antigenically distinct polysaccharide capsules first reported in 1933. These were later described as the meningococcal serogroup determinants that were identified by co-agglutination with polyclonal anti-sera [5].

Up to 14 variants of the meningococcal serogroup have been described [2] and the chemical structures of some of the component polysaccharides have been elucidated [6, 7]. Most cases of meningococcal disease are attributable to serogroups A, B, C, Y, or W-135, although cases caused by serogroup X and 29E continue to be identified rarely. Few case isolates from normally sterile sites (CSF, blood, joint fluids) are nonserogroupable using current reagents, although meningococci isolated from nonsterile sites associated with carriage (e.g. nose, throat) often do not express capsule and are therefore nonserogroupable. Indeed it is thought that downregulation of capsule production may be preferred for carriage.

Determining the serogroup of a meningococcal disease isolate is crucial for case contact management, as it establishes whether a serogroup-specific vaccine is available for prophylaxis of contacts to prevent further cases. Furthermore, serogrouping data are an essential part of the population-based epidemiological surveillance of endemic and epidemic meningococcal disease that informs vaccine design and immunization strategies. The identification of serogroups that are rarely associated with disease (such as serogroup Z) may be an indicator of possible immune deficiency in the patient.

A number of commercial agglutination kits for the detection and identification of meningococcal serogroup are available for direct use on cerebrospinal fluid (CSF) or serum. The kits vary from those able to discriminate individual serogroups (A, B, C) to those able to distinguish the current vaccine-preventable serogroups (A, C, Y, W-135) in a single reagent. Other kits may allow the discrimination of serogroups Y and W-135. The kits utilize either rabbit polyclonal antisera (slide agglutination) or mouse monoclonal antibodies (Mabs) in latex agglutination assays. The availability of a serogroup D slide agglutination reagent may account for the continued notation of this serogroup. It is important to note that serogroup B elicits a poor IgG response in humans and other species such that reagents for its detection are mostly based on IgM antibodies (specifically monoclonal antibodies). Only one monoclonal antibody of the IgG2a isotype has been described so far [7a]. Furthermore, a number of kits utilize the cross-reactivity of the *Escherichia coli* KI capsule and the Mabs used for serogroup B detection are actually derived against the *E. coli* organism. The suitability of the serological methods for the confirmation of serogroup is that they are rapid and may be used on killed material (either by heat or by formalin solution). The reagents offer suitable specificity when applied to the testing of meningococcal material, and specifically cultures, but there can be a lack of sensitivity when applied directly to clinical samples.

The mouse monoclonal antibodies that have been isolated against groups A, B, C, W-135, Y and Z may be utilized in the agglutination or enzyme linked immunosorbent assay (ELISA) [8, 9], which is seen to be the preferred method for screening large numbers of samples (or retrospective surveillance). Details of these Mabs can be found at http://neisseria.org/nm/typing/mabs/panel.shtml.

3.3.2 Serotyping and Serosubtyping

Early bactericidal assays first showed evidence for several distinct antigenic types within a single meningococcal serogroup [10]. A serotyping scheme, introduced to identify the heterogeneity of group C meningococci and then extended to include group B organisms, was developed without characterization of the antigens involved [11, 12] but was subsequently shown to be based on both the outer membrane protein (OMP) and the lipopolysaccharide (LPS) antigens [13, 14]. SDS-PAGE outer membrane profiles of the group A meningococcus were found to be homogeneous relative to other meningococcal groups, although some novel LPS and OMP antigens were identified [15]. Antisera to these group A LPS and protein serotypes were incorporated into the solid-phase radioimmunoassay inhibition assay (SPIRA) which had been developed to classify group B and C strains [16]. In 1985, previous schemes were integrated into a single serotyping scheme [17] so that, on the basis of the reactivity of the PorA and PorB porin proteins with immunological reagents, each meningococcal strain was designated a serosubtype and serotype, respectively (Fig. 3.1). This scheme, which uses heat-killed suspensions of meningococci as the antigen with serotype- and serosubtype-specific monoclonal antibodies (MAbs) in a whole-cell or dot-blot ELISA format has been widely adopted [9, 18] (Fig. 3.2).

Molecular characterization of the genes encoding the PorA and PorB proteins has elucidated the basis of serological typing. Structural models of the meningococcal porin proteins propose eight surface-exposed loops interspersed with highly conserved outer membrane-spanning sequences that form a β-barrel tertiary structure similar to that seen in the *E. coli* outer membrane proteins [19]. The antigenically important variable epitopes reside in the exposed loops and are targeted in the host immune response and by serological typing reagents [20]. The meningococcal serosubtype determining epitopes are restricted to two discreet variable regions (VRs) corresponding to loops I (VR1) and IV (VR2) of the PorA protein. All meningococci express either a class 2 (PorB2) or a class 3 (PorB3) serotype-determining PorB protein, which are mutually exclusive and are encoded by alternate alleles at the *porB* locus. Serotyping epitopes can reside in one of at least four of the eight PorB variable loops [21]. Furthermore, some PorB epitopes are difficult to mimic with linear peptides, suggesting that they

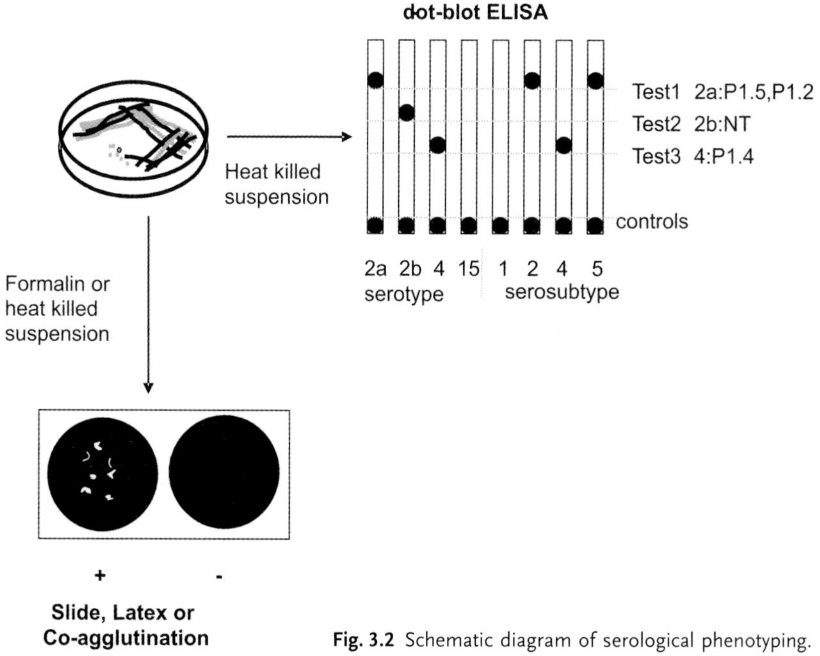

Fig. 3.2 Schematic diagram of serological phenotyping.

are conformational in nature, with one or more surface loops forming the epitopes recognized by serotyping MAbs.

Although many isolates are serotyped and serosubtyped by ELISA, antigenic variants with similar binding affinities are often impossible to distinguish and antigenically divergent novel epitopes fail to react with the current panel of MAbs, leading to an increase in the number of meningococcal isolates defined as not-typable (NT). As it is unlikely that the panel of serotyping MAbs will be expanded to cover all potential PorA and PorB variants, alternative DNA-based typing schemes have been developed for characterization of the serotype and serosubtype determining gene sequences (see below).

3.4
Immunotyping

Thirteen major lipooligosaccharide types have been determined using whole cell ELISA [22, 23] and can be used to characterize meningococci. Most meningococcal isolates express one or more of the L1–L12 immunotypes, with L3, 7, 9 most commonly associated with disease, although they are not routinely used as epidemiological markers. They may, however, be used to define meningococci used in vaccine manufacture or during host-response investigations.

3.5
Multilocus Enzyme Electrophoresis

Multilocus enzyme electrophoresis (MLEE or MEE) is a technique used to identify the phenotypic relationships within a bacterial species irrespective of the antigenic variability targeted by serological typing methods [24, 25]. Allelic variation within slowly evolving metabolic enzymes is determined by measuring variation in the electrophoretic mobility of as many as 25 of these housekeeping loci. This method requires enzyme (protein) extractions from each bacterial isolate that are separated by starch gel electrophoresis and the differences in the mobility of bands are then visualized following treatment with enzyme-specific substrates [26]. Each novel combination of allelic variants (known as electromorphs or allozymes) is referred to as an electrophoretic type, or ET, and cluster analyses can be performed to identify the relationships among bacterial strains with different ETs.

MLEE was first used to investigate global meningococcal epidemiology and population structure in the mid-1980s but has been utilized in only a few specialist laboratories as a result of the level of technical expertise required. Meningococcal strains possessing similar ETs can be assigned to genetically related groups or "clonal complexes" of strains [27]. Although largely superseded by the introduction of multilocus sequence typing (MLST), MLEE studies were the first to describe the major serogroup A (pandemic) clones circulating worldwide and also identified the major clonal complexes associated with serogroups B and C meningococcal disease in Europe and the Americas: ET-37, Lineage III, ET-5 and cluster A4.

3.6 Genetic Characterization

Before the relatively recent advances and increased availability of the technology used for nucleotide sequence determination, a number of derivative and sometimes arbitrary approaches were employed to examine the genetic relatedness of meningococcal isolates, with varying degrees of success. These included DNA-based methodologies that often used gel-based fragment sizing, with inherent problems of reproducibility and standardization, such as ribotyping, restriction fragment length polymorphism (RFLP) and pulsed field gel electrophoresis (PFGE). The increased number of reports describing novel and unrelated genetic typing methods that were difficult to reproduce outside of the original laboratory led to the assertion that, while often useful for the rapid analysis of a potential outbreak, such methods were unlikely to enhance long-term epidemiological studies [28]. Some of these methods, however, have helped in elucidating the molecular basis for serological typing schemes and have greatly advanced the understanding of meningococcal epidemiology.

The use of nucleotide sequencing for genetic characterization offers considerable advantages over the phenotypic methods used traditionally in typing laboratories. The data produced are unambiguous and highly portable by electronic means. Furthermore, the whole sequencing procedure, now performed widely using PCR-based methodology, is amenable to automation and scales readily for high throughput. Sample preparation and reactions can be performed in multi-well plates and use robotics if available. Downstream processing of data, including the assembling of contiguous double-stranded sequences from electropherograms and sequence variant identification, can also largely be automated.

At the same time as PCR technology was developing, parenteral administration of antibiotics in cases of suspected meningococcal infection was leading to a decrease in the number of cases that were confirmed by positive culture. Genetic characterization, unlike phenotypic methods, can be employed without the necessity to culture the organism first. In many cases, nucleotide sequencing can be performed on PCR products obtained directly from clinical specimens [29, 30], an advantage of increasing importance as the proportion of culture-confirmed cases reduces due to early administration of antibiotic therapy. Thus, by targeting a genetic locus of epidemiological importance, confirmation of meningococcal infection and strain characterization can be performed in a single assay.

3.6.1
Antigen Gene PCR and Sequencing for Meningococcal Typing

The further molecular characterization of culture-negative but DNA-positive cases may be achieved by antigen sequencing (described below) to determine the potential type or subtype. This is important in the UK, as approximately 50% of cases in England and Wales are confirmed by PCR alone and, as a result, any cluster or incident of two or more cases is likely to include at least one nonculture case for characterization. Since the UK has successfully introduced the serogroup C conjugate vaccine, typing beyond group for the predominant group B cases is now essential to define and manage related cases. The diversity of several meningococcal antigen genes, in particular those encoding the polysaccharide capsule and the major outer membrane proteins (OMPs), have been exploited for strain characterization.

3.6.2
Genogrouping (PCR-based Designation of Group)

Nonculture (PCR-based) grouping of meningococci has been introduced to some local and most reference laboratories in recent years. Genogrouping was designed to counter the increasing discrepancy between clinically notified cases of meningococcal disease and those microbiologically confirmed by positive meningococcal cultures.

The genetic basis for the chemical and immunological differences in the meningococcal polysaccharide has been elucidated [31, 32] and the variation identified in the capsule biosynthesis operon exploited for PCR and nucleotide sequence-based group identification. The PCR assays are based on genes required for specific capsule production and transport to the cell surface, but there are no internationally agreed PCR targets or primers for the detection and group characterization of meningococci by DNA-based methods. For meningococci that have sialylated polysaccharide capsules (groups B, C, Y, W-135), the *siaD* target may be used [33–35], while group A is chemically distinct where the *mynA* target may be used [36]. A major advantage of the genetic methods of grouping is that they can determine the group of isolates where capsule expression has been switched off, for example during long-term carriage of the meningococcus in the nasopharynx, or when no isolate culture can be obtained from clinical specimens [33]. PCR and sequencing primers have also been designed to amplify the truncated capsule null locus (*cnl*) that many avirulent meningococci possess in place of the capsule biosynthesis operon [37].

3.6.3
Genotyping and Genosubtyping – *porB* and *porA* Sequencing

A meningococcal *porA* gene sequence was first determined in 1989 [38]. Using PCR-based methodology, additional *porA* and *porB* genes were characterized among collections of meningococcal isolates to help elicit structural models and to identify the genetic basis for the failure of serological typing reagents [39, 40]. Nonserosubtypable PorA variants possessed novel gene sequences in one or both of two variable regions (VRs), which encode the linear epitopes VR1 and VR2 and correspond to surface-exposed loops 1 and 4 of the mature protein. Consequently, sequence-based typing of *porA* usually targets only these two regions, as variation in the remainder of the gene is limited and usually does not affect the serosubtype of the isolate. Nucleotide sequences encoding the PorA epitopes VR1 and VR2 can be translated and identified by querying the PorA VR sequence database, located at http://neisseria.org/nm/typing/pora/ [41]. A short semi-variable PorA epitope, VR3, has also been used to help characterize strains [42], although the level of peptide variation seen is considerably less than that for the other variable regions and is not widely used.

The serotype-determining epitopes of PorB have been less easy to identify as these proteins often have discontinuous epitopes, where several of the eight surface-exposed variable loops are involved in epitope formation. As only loops II and III are essentially invariant in PorB, it is necessary to identify amino acid sequence variation in loop I and also loops IV–VIII when determining PorB epitope diversity. A number of nomenclature schemes have been proposed but, as they consist of a string of 5–8 variables (representing some or all eight of the surface-exposed loops), they are unwieldy and not easy to digest. A *porB* sequence database containing whole *porB* gene sequences and corresponding translated PorB amino acid sequences can be queried to determine whether newly characterized sequences are identical or divergent from known alleles (http://neisseria.org/nm/typing/porb).

3.6.4
FetA

Several additional meningococcal antigen genes that may be candidates as genetic, rather than serological, markers have been extensively characterized. For example, the *fetA* gene encodes a major outer membrane protein, FetA (previously known as FrpB), a protein that is expressed by the meningococcus in the iron-limited conditions prevalent in vivo [43]. Several surveys of FetA diversity have indicated that the protein is quite well conserved within hyper-invasive lineages and therefore has potential as an epidemiological marker [44, 45]. The immunodominant FetA epitope resides in a single variable region (VR) located in loop 7 out of 13 surface-exposed loops. Genetic characterization of the short VR-encoding region of *fetA* can therefore be performed using one pair of sequencing primers and the translated VR amino acid sequence identified by database interrogation at: http://neisseria.org/nm/typing/feta.

3.6.5
Multilocus Sequence Typing

Many typing schemes that use genetic characterization rely on cataloguing the variation seen at a single locus. The problem with such schemes in determining phylogeny is that they are inaccurate where horizontal genetic exchange is frequent, since the locus, or parts of it, can be randomly exchanged within the population. Furthermore, antigen genes should be examined with particular care, as they are often subject to strong positive selection for amino acid change, leading to additional sequence variability that can obscure the evolutionary relationships among strains. Multilocus sequence typing (MLST) indexes the neutral variation of housekeeping genes distributed around the genome [46, 47]. As such, it provides a robust method of typing organisms such as the meningococcus that exhibit high levels of horizontal genetic exchange. Housekeeping genes are chosen that are distant enough on the genome that they are unlikely to be co-inherited through a single recombination event and generally not positioned close to genes that are under strong selective pressures, such as the surface antigens exposed to host immune responses.

MLST is a DNA sequence-based version of multilocus enzyme electrophoresis (MLEE) [24]. MLEE suffers from a lack of portability of primary data, the requirement to calibrate with standard strains and a high investment in training. More importantly, any technique that uses a phenotypic marker as the basis for classification will be less sensitive than a sequence-based method for any given number of loci analyzed, as in the case of MLEE a small change in sequence will not necessarily affect the migration rate of a protein. In contrast, nucleotide sequence data provide a fundamental measure of genetic diversity and its interpretation should be unambiguous, while the technique itself is entirely generic. The higher resolution of MLST means that fewer loci are required than in MLEE to achieve similar levels of discrimination.

The MLST scheme for *Neisseria* species is defined by the sequences of fragments, ranging over 433–501 base pairs in length, from seven housekeeping genes: *abcZ* (putative ABC transporter), *adk* (adenylate kinase), *aroE* (shikimate dehydrogenase), *fumC* (fumarate hydratase), *gdh* (glucose-6-phosphate dehydrogenase), *pdhC* (pyruvate dehydrogenase subunit) and *pgm* (phosphoglucomutase) [46]. The lengths of the fragments were chosen as they contained sufficient variable sites to provide the required discrimination while being readily sequenced using a single run on an automated sequencer. The gene fragments are first amplified by PCR, purified and then sequenced on both strands using nested primers [48] (Fig. 3.3). The use of nested primers for sequencing has the advantage that the stringency of the initial PCR reaction can be lowered while maintaining specific sequencing of the gene. This results in higher yields of amplified gene product and clean sequence traces. Use of a lower stringency in the initial PCR also enables the use of MLST with noncultured samples from clinical specimens [29]. Each unique sequence at each locus is assigned an allele number in the order of discovery, and every unique combination of alleles, or

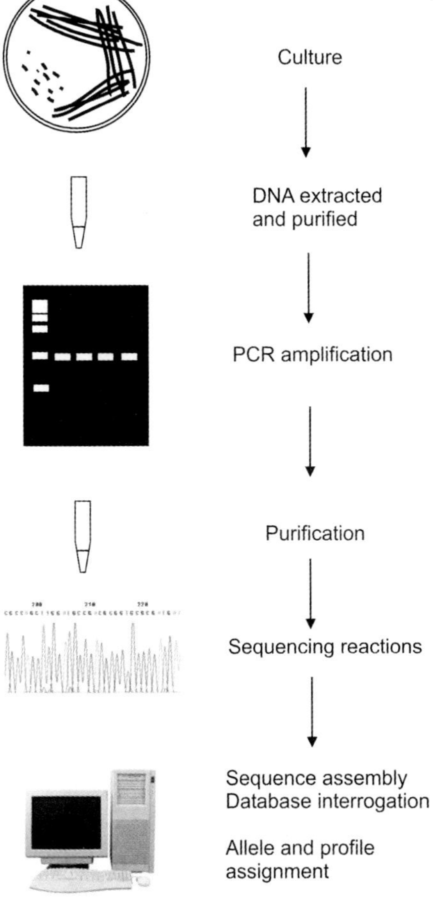

Fig. 3.3 The MLST procedure.

allelic profile, is assigned a sequence type (ST) number. These designations are made by the curator of the MLST database (http://pubmlst.org/neisseria/) [49] and are made immediately available on the web. It is important to note that the numbering of alleles and STs is arbitrary and therefore makes no assumption as to the relatedness of individual sequences or profiles.

As of February 2006, over 5300 STs had been identified, with most loci having over 300 unique allele sequences defined. Individual STs, however, are not equally prevalent. Some STs have been isolated repeatedly over long time spans and wide geographical locations while others are found only infrequently, perhaps only once. Using heuristic methods such as split decomposition [50] or based upon related sequence types (BURST) [51], it can be shown that the highly prevalent STs are usually found to have the highest number of related STs that differ at only one or two loci. They can consequently be thought of as "central genotypes". These genetically related STs, surrounding a central genotype, can be grouped into clonal complexes, as first introduced using MLEE [27]. The clonal complex provides a means of grouping the otherwise enormous diversity seen when looking at individual STs into manageable units of related genotypes. Official definition of clonal complexes is not arbitrary and involves an international management committee of experts in the field, who agree on the central genotypes. The definition of a clonal complex, as used on the Neisseria MLST website (http://pubmlst.org/neisseria/), is those STs that match a central genotype at four or more loci. This is a pragmatic definition that results in groupings that have proved useful for epidemiological analysis and which are also largely in concordance with the genetic lineages initially defined using MLEE. A recent study has also shown that cluster analyses of multiple antigen genes were congruent with the clonal complex groupings identified by MLST [45]. These data suggested that, although deeper phylogenetic relationships among distantly related strains could not be resolved as a result of recombination, both MLST and multiple antigen gene sequences were useful markers for the identification of meningococcal clonal complexes that have emerged relatively recently in evolutionary time.

3.6.6
Variable-number Tandem Repeats

The identification of repetitive sequence motifs with variable-number tandem repeats (VNTR) within the meningococcal genome has enabled a finer level typing method to be developed that can complement the broader typing provided by MLST [52]. It has been shown that isolates from epidemiologically linked cases of a particular sequence type or clonal complex are more likely to have similar VNTR patterns than similar isolates from nonlinked cases.

VNTR loci can be identified by an automated analysis of the genome and primers designed to amplify these regions. The number of tandem repeats at each locus can be determined by running amplification products on agarose gels. Alternatively, DNA sequencer technology can be harnessed to accurately and quickly size DNA fragments.

3.6.7
Pulsed Field Gel Electrophoresis

Pulsed field gel electrophoresis (PFGE) utilizes "rare site" restriction enzymes to produce DNA fingerprints by cutting chromosomal DNA into relatively large pieces. These pieces of DNA can be resolved on a gel by applying an electric field that regularly changes direction allowing the DNA fragments to reptate (snake) through the gel. Fingerprints produced by test strains may be compared by eye but the availability of digital imaging and software packages allow fragment sizes of samples within gels to be compared and allow gel to gel comparisons.

PFGE has been shown to be useful for meningococcal cluster associated isolates. Direct comparisons to the index case may be made or the sample screened for a predominant pattern. PFGE appears to be highly discriminatory but, unless fragments are probed or assigned, it is often unclear what the differences relate to. Problems can arise due to the chromosomal DNA quality, sample loading and gel conditions. It is essential to run fragment size standards in multiple lanes on each gel and a direct comparison to the index case pattern is preferred over inter-gel comparisons. To minimize artefacts, software normalization of the gels is required to accommodate gel "smiling". Differences between isolate fingerprints are often observed and rules have been suggested to assist in the interpretation of genetic relatedness, such as the "4-band differences" rule to allow for single genetic events.

Good quality, intact chromosomal DNA from isolates is required for PFGE, so the method is not applicable to nonculture (PCR) proven cases. Like VNTR, the technique may be suitable to discriminate isolates that have been shown to be closely associated by other techniques, such as MLST.

3.6.8 Databases

The use of nucleotide sequencing in the genetic characterization of bacteria provides a significant benefit in the storage, comparison and dissemination of typing data. Nucleotide sequence data, at its most fundamental level, can be represented as simple text and the relatively small file sizes of trace electropherograms, the primary data, allow them to be attached to e-mail messages for instant comparison or to be archived. The sequences can be compared easily with other sequence data electronically, over the Internet, and without the need for calibration with reference strains. MLST database software has been developed [49] that makes it possible to set up distributed, interconnected isolate databases that query a central profiles database to make ST and clonal complex assignments. The distributed structure enables individual isolate databases to be constructed, each with their own particular structure (fields, allowed values, links to other data sources) and access restrictions, while maintaining the benefit of having a centrally curated, definitive database containing the "dictionary" of allele sequences and profiles. The PubMLST database and website (http://pubmlst.org/neisseria) also provides a range of tools to allow an investigator to further analyze their data.

Similarly, the databases for PorA variable regions, FetA variable regions and PorB (http://neisseria.org/nm/typing) are all compatible with each other and allow, for instance, an MLST isolate database to retrieve sequence information automatically from them. The antigen databases incorporate searching by BLAST to quickly identify known sequences or related variants if the sequence is new. These databases allow information from serological and genetic typing methods to be linked and the integration of such data will become increasingly prevalent.

3.7
Conclusion

The application of meningococcal typing methods and designations depends on the questions being asked. For outbreaks or cluster management, the direct comparison of isolates (and nonculture, DNA material) may necessitate a range of techniques for discrimination (such as PFGE and VNTR) rather than accurate strain designation. This is because the primary question is: "are these two cases different"?

Current nomenclature largely focuses on the serological (or antigenic) characterization of meningococci. This is likely to remain important for a number of reasons, not least the use of effective polysaccharide (serogroup) vaccines and the continuing assessment of OMP or outer membrane vesicle (serotype, serosubtype) based vaccines. Undoubtedly, DNA sequencing improves the typability and confirms the failings of the Mab-based typing schemes but may require further development to improve the timeliness of results. This may in part be achieved by developing rapid, sensitive and cost effective hybridization assays to screen out some of the antigen sequencing.

Current experience suggests that MLST lacks sensitivity for cluster management but is essential for long-term population studies. However, in some instances, MLST may differentiate disease-causing meningococci that have the same antigenic profile due to the naturally transformable nature of the organism. MLST is rapidly becoming the method of choice for clonal and population studies and a sequence type designation is increasingly seen as a requirement for publishable studies, although it may lack the sensitivity provided by methods such as PFGE that may be used to detect differences between genetically related isolates. Combining a MLST profile with sequence data from one or more surface antigens can, however, significantly enhance the discrimination of strains.

There is still a prevailing view in many quarters that nucleotide sequencing is considerably more expensive than many of the techniques it is replacing. While in the past this may have been true and start-up costs may be relatively high, consumable costs are lowering continually, especially with the increased sensitivity of the latest generation of sequencers requiring less reagent. Nucleotide sequencing is also a generic technique, so the same procedure is used whatever the gene target or organism being looked at. This has implications for reducing the costs of training and also the centralization of sequencing facilities that can service the differing needs of a wide range of researchers and public health personnel. It is tempting to think that genetic characterization will become predominant, as sequencing technology becomes cheaper. One advantage of phenotypic characterization, however, is that when positive results are obtained, it confirms the expression of polysaccharide and/or proteins that are available to interact with the host immune system. This feature should not be overlooked with regard to vaccine studies where 100% typability is not the only consideration.

The recent explosion in the use of DNA sequencing of antigen genes and MLST has benefited development of microarrays where PCR amplification of specific genes can be detected by hybridization using sensitive fluorescent photochemistry. Anecdotal evidence suggests that not all gene targets make suitable detection probes for complete characterization although some success with *porA* and *porB* has been found. Conversely, generating a MLST profile by such techniques has proven more difficult due to the enormous range of diversity seen within the housekeeping genes of this organism.

In an ideal world, strains could be characterized using a wide selection of the available typing techniques to build up as full a picture as possible of the organism. In practice, this is rarely necessary and time and financial restraints limit the choices available and so consideration needs to be made to which procedure is the most suitable for a specific situation.

References

1 P. Singleton, D. Sainsbury **2001**, *Dictionary of Microbiology and Molecular Biology* 3rd edn., Wiley, Chichester.

2 N.A. Vedros **1987**, Development of meningococcal serogroups, in *Evolution of meningococcal disease*, ed. N.A. Vedros, CRC Press, Boca Raton, p. 33–37.

3 M.C.J. Maiden, I.M. Feavers **1994**, *J. Med. Microbiol.* 40, 157–158.

4 S.P. Lapage, P.H.A. Sneath, International Union of Microbiological Societies. International Committee on Systematic Bacteriology, International Union of Microbiological Societies. Bacteriology and Applied Microbiology Section **1992**, *International Code of Nomenclature of Bacteria, and Statutes of the International Committee on Systematic Bacteriology, and Statutes of the Bacteriology and Applied Microbiology Section of the International Union of Microbiological Societies: Bacteriological Code*, International Union of Microbiological Societies/ American Society for Microbiology, Washington, D.C.

5 J. Eldridge, E.M. Sutcliffe, J.D. Abbott, D.M. Jones **1978**, *Med. Lab. Sci.* 35, 63–66.

6 S.K. Gudlavalleti, A.K. Datta, Y.L. Tzeng, C. Noble, R.W. Carlson, D.S. Stephens **2004**, *J. Biol. Chem.* 279, 42765–42773.

7 C. Jones, X. Lemercinier **2002**, *J. Pharm. Biomed. Anal.* 30, 1233–1247.

7a M. Frosch, I. Görgen, G.J. Boulnois, K.N. Timmis, D. Bitter-Suermann **1985**, *Proc. Natl Acad. Sci. USA* 82, 1194–1198.

8 E. Rosenqvist, E. Wedege, E.A. Høiby, L.O. Froholm **1990**, *Apmis* 98, 501–506.

9 B. Kuipers, G. van den Dobbelsteen, E. Wedege, L. van Alphen **2001**, Serological characterization, in *Meningococcal Disease: Methods and Protocols*, eds. A.J. Pollard, M.C. Maiden, Humana Press, Totowa, N.J., p. 131–145.

10 I. Goldschneider, E.C. Gotschlich, M.S. Artenstein **1969**, *J. Exp. Med.* 129, 1307–1326.

11 R. Gold, F.A. Wyle **1970**, *Infect. Immun.* 1, 479–484.

12 C.E. Frasch, S. Chapman **1972**, *Infect. Immun.* 5, 98–102.

13 R.E. Mandrell, W.D. Zollinger **1977**, *Infect. Immun.* 16, 471–475.

14 J.T. Poolman, S. De Marie, H.C. Zanen **1980**, *Infect. Immun.* 30, 642–648.

15 W.D. Zollinger, R.E. Mandrell **1980**, *Infect. Immun.* 28, 451–458.

16 W.D. Zollinger, R.E. Mandrell **1977**, *Infect. Immun.* 18, 424–433.

17 C.E. Frasch, W.D. Zollinger, J.T. Poolman **1985**, *Rev. Infect. Dis* 7, 504–510.

18 E. Wedege, E.A. Høiby, E. Rosenqvist, L.O. Frøholm **1990**, *J. Med. Microbiol.* 31, 195–201.

19 D. Jeanteur, J.H. Lakey, F. Pattus **1991**, *Mol. Microbiol.* 5, 2153–2164.

20 K. Saukkonen, M. Leinonen, H. Abdillahi, J.T. Poolman **1989**, *Vaccine* 7, 325–328.

21 C.T. Sacchi, A.P.S. Lemos, A.M. Whitney, C.A. Solari, M.E. Brandt, C.E.A.

Melles, C. E. Frasch, L. W. Mayer **1998**, *Clin. Diagn. Lab. Immunol.* 5, 348–354.
22 H. Abdillahi, J. T. Poolman **1988**, *J. Med. Microbiol.* 26, 177–180.
23 R. J. Scholten, B. Kuipers, H. A. Valkenburg, J. Dankert, W. D. Zollinger, J. T. Poolman **1994**, *J. Med. Microbiol.* 41, 236–243.
24 R. K. Selander, D. A. Caugant, H. Ochman, J. M. Musser, M. N. Gilmour, T. S. Whittam **1986**, *Appl. Environ. Microbiol.* 51, 837–884.
25 P. Boerlin, J. C. Piffaretti **1995**, *Methods Mol. Biol.* 46, 63–78.
26 D. A. Caugant **2001**, Global trends in meningococcal disease, in *Meningococcal Disease: Methods and Protocols*, eds. A. J. Pollard, M. C. J. Maiden, Humana Press, Totowa, N.J., p. 273–294.
27 D. A. Caugant, L. F. Mocca, C. E. Frasch, L. O. Frøholm, W. D. Zollinger, R. K. Selander **1987**, *J. Bacteriol.* 169, 2781–2792.
28 M. Achtman **1996**, *J. Clin. Microbiol.* 34, 1870.
29 P. Kriz, J. Kalmusova, J. Felsberg **2002**, *Epidemiol. Infect.* 128, 157–160.
30 M. A. Diggle, C. M. Bell, S. C. Clarke **2003**, *J. Med. Microbiol.* 52, 505–508.
31 J. S. Swartley, D. S. Stephens **1994**, *J. Bacteriol.* 176, 1530–1534.
32 J. S. Swartley, L. J. Liu, Y. K. Miller, L. E. Martin, S. Edupuganti, D. S. Stephens **1998**, *J. Bacteriol.* 180, 1533–1539.
33 R. Borrow, H. Claus, M. Guiver, L. Smart, D. M. Jones, E. B. Kaczmarski, M. Frosch, A. J. Fox **1997**, *Epidemiol. Infect.* 118, 111–117.
34 R. Borrow, H. Claus, U. Chaudhry, M. Guiver, E. B. Kaczmarski, M. Frosch, A. J. Fox **1998**, *FEMS Microbiol. Lett.* 159, 209–214.
35 M. Guiver, R. Borrow **2001**, PCR diagnosis, in *Meningococcal Disease*, eds. A. J. Pollard, M. C. J. Maiden, Humana Press, Totowa, N.J., p. 23–39.
36 M. A. Diggle, K. Smith, E. K. Girvan, S. C. Clarke **2003**, *J. Clin. Microbiol.* 41, 1766–1768.
37 H. Claus, M. C. Maiden, R. Maag, M. Frosch, U. Vogel **2002**, *Microbiology* 148, 1813–1819.
38 A. K. Barlow, J. E. Heckels, I. N. Clarke **1989**, *Mol. Microbiol.* 3, 131–139.
39 B. McGuinness, A. K. Barlow, I. N. Clarke, J. E. Farley, A. Anilionis, J. T. Poolman, J. E. Heckels **1990**, *J. Exp. Med.* 171, 1871–1882.
40 J. Suker, I. M. Feavers, M. C. J. Maiden, *Microbiology* **1996**, 142, 63–69.
41 J. E. Russell, K. A. Jolley, I. M. Feavers, M. C. Maiden, J. S. Suker **2004**, *Emerg. Infect. Dis.* 10, 674–678.
42 S. C. Clarke, M. A. Diggle, P. Molling, M. Unemo, P. Olcen **2003**, *Vaccine* 21, 2468–2473.
43 M. Beucher, P. F. Sparling **1995**, *J. Bacteriol.* 177, 2041–2049.
44 E. A. Thompson, I. M. Feavers, M. C. Maiden **2003**, *Microbiology* 149, 1849–1858.
45 R. Urwin, J. E. Russell, E. A. Thompson, E. C. Holmes, I. M. Feavers, M. C. Maiden **2004**, *Infect. Immun.* 72, 5955–5962.
46 M. C. J. Maiden, J. A. Bygraves, E. Feil, G. Morelli, J. E. Russell, R. Urwin, Q. Zhang, J. Zhou, K. Zurth, D. A. Caugant, I. M. Feavers, M. Achtman, B. G. Spratt **1998**, *Proc. Natl Acad. Sci. USA* 95, 3140–3145.
47 R. Urwin, M. C. Maiden **2003**, *Trends Microbiol.* 11, 479–487.
48 K. A. Jolley **2001**, Multi-locus sequence typing, in *Meningococcal Disease: Methods and Protocols*, eds. A. J. Pollard, M. C. Maiden, Humana Press, Totowa, N. J., p. 173–186.
49 K. A. Jolley, M. S. Chan, M. C. Maiden **2004**, *Bioinformatics* 5, 86.
50 D. H. Huson **1998**, *Bioinformatics* 14, 68–73.
51 E. J. Feil, B. C. Li, D. M. Aanensen, W. P. Hanage, B. G. Spratt **2004**, *J. Bacteriol.* 186, 1518–1530.
52 S. P. Yazdankhah, B. A. Lindstedt, D. A. Caugant **2005**, *J. Clin. Microbiol.* 43, 1699–1705.

4
Antibiotic Resistance

Colin Block and Julio A. Vázquez

4.1
Introduction

The evolution of antibiotic resistance in pathogenic bacterial species has been and still is a major concern for professionals involved in health, including clinicians, microbiologists and epidemiologists. The widespread use of antibiotics in both hospital and community acquired infections, linked with inter- and intra-species interchange of genetic material, has resulted in a significant reduction in the utility of most antimicrobial agents. Some pathogenic species seem to have a tremendous capacity to acquire as well as to develop different mechanisms of antimicrobial resistance. A good example is *Neisseria gonorrhoeae*, for which treatment guidelines are continuously changing. Gonococci acquire extrachromosomal DNA from other species, exchange chromosomal DNA among themselves and develop their own resistance mechanisms. These phenomena are most important for the survival of the species, and enable the widespread resistance we observe in the gonococcal population. However, the closely related species *N. meningitidis* has in general remained susceptible to antibiotics. Thus, among the clinically important bacteria, the meningococci do not appear to be particularly efficient in developing resistance to antimicrobial agents. The reasons for this are poorly understood; and there are indications that the situation might be changing. In spite of this general susceptibility to currently used agents and considering the seriousness of the disease, changes in the degree of antibiotic susceptibility among clinical isolates of meningococci are raising difficult issues regarding the detection of resistance or reduced susceptibility and interpretation of laboratory results. The determination of breakpoint concentrations that can accurately predict failure of treatment for a particular drug depends on the availability of adequate clinical, pharmacokinetic and microbiological data. Such information is unlikely to be forthcoming for agents such as penicillin in the treatment of meningococcal disease, while the incidence of isolates with reduced susceptibility continues to rise world-wide. Advances in molecular techniques have added a new dimension to our ability to detect organisms that respond poorly to therapy.

Handbook of Meningococcal Disease. Infection Biology, Vaccination, Clinical Management.
Edited by M. Frosch and M.C.J. Maiden

ISBN: 3-527-31260-9

4.2
Testing Antibiotics Against *N. meningitidis*

4.2.1
Methodological Issues in *N. meningitidis* Susceptibility Testing

Meningococcal susceptibility testing has long been plagued by a lack of standardization and a plethora of different methods [1]. In recent years, attempts have been made to address this issue, both by formal studies [2] and by authoritative bodies such as the Clinical and Laboratory Standards Institute (CLSI, formerly the NCCLS) [3], the British Society for Antimicrobial Chemotherapy (BSAC), the Comite de l'Antibiogramme de la Societe Francaise de Microbiologie (SFM), the Swedish Reference Group for Antibiotics (SRGA) and the European Committee on Antimicrobial Susceptibility Testing (EUCAST) of the European Society for Clinical Microbiology and Infectious Diseases. A process of harmonization of methods is in progress in Europe which might contribute substantially to improving the situation in years to come.

In the meanwhile, differences remain in methods and interpretative criteria. The range of culture media in use for testing meningococcal susceptibilities has narrowed in recent years; and there has been a general acceptance of the need for supplementation of the chosen medium with blood. Differences persist, however, some of which are briefly summarized in Table 4.1.

Internet links for access to recommendations
(all accessed successfully in August 2005)
BSAC guide to antimicrobial susceptibility testing:
http://www.bsac.org.uk/susceptibility_testing/guide_to_antimicrobial_susceptibility_testing.cfm
BSAC standardized disc diffusion susceptibility testing:
http://bsac.test.tmg.co.uk/_db/_documents/version_4_january_2005_final_NH_april_2.pdf
EUCAST: http://www.escmid.org/sites/index_f.asp?par=2.4
"Clinical" breakpoints at: http://www.srga.org/eucastwt/MICTAB/index.html
SFM: Communique 2005 at http://www.sfm.asso.fr/nouv/general.php?pa=2
SRGA: http://www.srga.org/

In an interlaboratory study undertaken by the European Monitoring Group on Meningococci (EMGM), Vázquez et al., using a defined set of 17 well characterized clinical isolates of *N. meningitidis*, demonstrated that Mueller-Hinton agar supplemented with sheep blood provided the best results when compared with unsupplemented agar and Mueller-Hinton with heated sheep blood [2]. This study yielded the important observation that one of 11 isolates with *penA* gene sequences typical of strains with reduced susceptibility to penicillin was found in nine of 14 laboratories to have an MIC in the susceptible range. This finding

Table 4.1 Major culture conditions for antimicrobial susceptibility testing of *N. meningitidis* – recommendations of selected authoritative bodies (as of May 2005). a)

		BSAC	CLSI	EUCAST	SFM	SRGA
Media b)	Agar	ISA	MH	MH	MH	ISA
	Broth	ISB	CA-MHB			
Supplements b)		Agar: 5% DF-HB Broth: 5% LHB	Agar: 5% DF-SB Broth: 2–5% LHB	5% DF	5% DF-SB	5% DF-SB+NAD
Incubation	CO_2 (%)	4–6	5 c)	5	5	5
	Temp. (°C)	35–37	35±2	35–37	35–37	35–37
	Duration (h)	18–20	20–24	18	18–20	16–20

a) BSAC = British Society for Antimicrobial Chemotherapy, CLSI = Clinical & Laboratory Standards Institute (USA), EUCAST = European Committee on Antimicrobial Susceptibility Testing, SFM = Societe Francaise de Microbiologie, SRGA = Swedish Reference Group for Antibiotics. Internet links or references are noted in the box above

b) ISA = Iso-Sensitest agar (Oxoid), ISB = Iso-Sensitest broth, MH = Mueller-Hinton agar, CA-MHB = cation-adjusted Mueller-Hinton broth, DF = defibrinated, HB = horse blood, SB = sheep blood, LHB = lysed horse blood, NAD = β-nicotinamide adenine dinucleotide

c) For azithromycin, incubate in air.

emphasises both the need to supplement conventional testing with molecular diagnosis of reduced susceptibility and the inherent limitations of information provided by such conventional testing.

4.2.1.1 The "Invasion" of the Etest

The Etest appeared in the late 1980s [4] and proved to be a valuable tool in the clinical microbiology laboratory. In diagnostic practice, it has replaced recommended standardized methods in many laboratories since, among other things, it provides a convenient and flexible technique that has all but eliminated the substantial preparatory work required for conventional methods. The Etest is not recommended as a standard reference method but, despite this, the publications in which it has served to measure MICs for a wide range of bacteria and fungi are legion. Studies of its application specifically to meningococcal susceptibility testing began in the early 1990s [5–10].

For all the enthusiasm with which the Etest has been received, users would do well to bear in mind its limitations, especially its vulnerability to operator technique and experience. There may also be some antimicrobial agents that give somewhat less accurate and reproducible results, such as penicillin [11], ciprofloxacin [9], ofloxacin and rifampicin [2] or rifampicin [12], although variations generally tend to be minor when compared with agar dilution. As if to remind us of the fallibilities of our primitive methods, these apparent drug-related difficulties are not consistent between studies.

4.2.1.2 The Breakpoint Issue

The publication of recommended susceptibility and resistance breakpoints for *N. meningitidis* does not necessarily reflect a robust evidence base, but quite likely the perceived need to provide diagnostic and reference laboratories with unambiguous interpretative criteria. While there clearly are data which can unerringly indicate susceptibility or resistance for some antibiotics, in many cases it is extremely difficult to distinguish organisms likely to respond to treatment with a certain agent from those likely not to respond. For example, isolates with very high MICs to rifampicin, chloramphenicol and sulfonamides may easily be predicted to be resistant; and there still exist drugs that are uniformly active against meningococci, such as ceftriaxone or cefotaxime. β-Lactamase-producing meningococci with their very high MICs have remained a curiosity (four reports of five isolates published between 1983 and 1996 [13–16]). However, the continuing rise in MICs to penicillin among meningococci in many countries, to values that spell certain clinical resistance for *Streptococcus pneumoniae* meningitis, has not resulted in a clear rise of treatment failures.

These difficulties notwithstanding, most organizations have provided recommended susceptibility breakpoints for *N. meningitidis*. Even the CLSI (NCCLS), which for many years did not specifically include *N. meningitidis* in its recommendations, has finally added breakpoints in its January 2005 tables [3]. Their recommended MIC values are proving controversial however, particularly for the definition of resistance ($MIC \geq 0.5$ mg l^{-1}). Groups investigating penicillin resistance have generally used $MIC > 1.0$ mg l^{-1} to denote resistance, so a significant conceptual readjustment will be required if the CLSI breakpoints are widely adopted. The evidence base for the criteria chosen by the CLSI is not presented, raising important questions of their appropriateness.

Despite such breakpoint preferences among researchers, there remain many material differences between breakpoints recommended by the authoritative bodies mentioned previously (Table 4.2). Noteworthy disagreements are evident concerning breakpoint values, the use of disk-diffusion tests and the drugs for which recommendations are given.

It is quite likely that no satisfactory uniform set of criteria will be achieved, due to the complexity of the issues involved: the vulnerability of *in vitro* testing to multiple technical influences, the variability of organism-related factors, pharmacological considerations, host-related factors and, not least, differing approaches of clinical microbiologists and clinicians.

Table 4.2 MIC and zone breakpoints for *N. meningitidis* – recommendations of selected authoritative bodies (as of May 2005).[a]

Antibiotic	Country/ organization	MIC breakpoints (mg l^{-1})		Disc content (µg unless stated)	Zone diameter breakpoints (mm)		
		R >	S ≤		R ≤	I	S ≥
Penicillin (G)	BSAC	0.06	0.06	1 unit	24	–	25
	CLSI (NCCLS)	0.25	0.06		nr[b]	nr	nr
	EUCAST						
	SFM	1	0.06	Oxacillin 5[c]			18
				Oxacillin 1			11
	SRGA	1	0.25		nr	nr	nr
Penicillin (V)	BSAC						
	CLSI (NCCLS)						
	EUCAST						
	SFM						
	SRGA	1	1		nr	nr	nr
Ampicillin	BSAC						
	CLSI (NCCLS)	1	0.12		nr	nr	nr
	EUCAST						
	SFM	2	0.25				
	SRGA						
Cefuroxime	BSAC						
	CLSI (NCCLS)						
	EUCAST						
	SFM						
	SRGA	1	0.25		nr	nr	nr
Ceftriaxone	BSAC						
	CLSI (NCCLS)		0.12		nr	nr	nr
	EUCAST						
	SFM		0.25				
	SRGA	1	0.06		nr	nr	nr
Cefotaxime	BSAC	1	1	5	29	–	30
	CLSI (NCCLS)		0.12		nr	nr	nr
	EUCAST						
	SFM		0.25				
	SRGA	1	0.06		nr	nr	nr

Table 4.2 (continued)

Antibiotic	Country/ organization	MIC breakpoints (mg l^{-1})		Disc content (μg unless stated)	Zone diameter breakpoints (mm)		
		R >	S ≤		R ≤	I	S ≥
Meropenem	BSAC						
	CLSI (NCCLS)		0.25		nr	nr	nr
	EUCAST						
	SFM						
	SRGA	0.5	0.06		nr	nr	nr
Chloramphenicol	BSAC	2	2	10	19	–	20
	CLSI (NCCLS)	4	2		nr	nr	nr
	EUCAST						
	SFM	4	2	30			30
	SRGA	8	2		nr	nr	nr
Ciprofloxacin [e)]	BSAC [d)]	0.06	0.03	1	31	–	32
	CLSI (NCCLS) [f)]	0.06	0.03		nr	nr	nr
	EUCAST	0.06	0.03				
	SFM						
	SRGA	0.06	0.03		nr	nr	nr
Levofloxacin	BSAC						
	CLSI (NCCLS) [f)]	0.06	0.03		nr	nr	nr
	EUCAST						
	SFM						
	SRGA						
Erythromycin	BSAC	0.5	0.5	5.0	26.0	–	27.0
	CLSI (NCCLS)						
	EUCAST						
	SFM						
	SRGA						
Azithromycin	BSAC						
	CLSI (NCCLS) [g)]	2	0.25		nr	nr	nr
	EUCAST						
	SFM						
	SRGA						
Rifampicin	BSAC	1	1	2	29	–	30
	CLSI (NCCLS)	1.0	0.5		nr	nr	nr
	EUCAST						
	SFM		0.25	30			30
	SRGA	1	1		nr	nr	nr

Table 4.2 (continued)

Antibiotic	Country/ organization	MIC breakpoints (mg l^{-1})		Disc content (µg unless stated)	Zone diameter break-points (mm)		
		R >	S ≤		R ≤	I	S ≥
Tetracycline	BSAC	1	1	10	21	–	22
	CLSI (NCCLS)						
	EUCAST						
	SFM						
	SRGA						
Minocycline	BSAC						
	CLSI (NCCLS)		2		nr	nr	nr
	EUCAST						
	SFM						
	SRGA						
Sulfisoxazole	BSAC						
	CLSI (NCCLS)	4	2		nr	nr	nr
	EUCAST						
	SFM						
	SRGA						
Trimethoprim – sulfameth-oxazole	BSAC						
	CLSI (NCCLS)	0.25/4.8	0.12/2.3		nr	nr	nr
	EUCAST						
	SFM						
	SRGA						

a) Please note that the manner of showing the values by each organization have been adapted to fit a uniform presentation format. The list comprises all antimicrobial agents included by any of the recommending organizations for *N. meningitidis*. BSAC = British Society for Antimicrobial Chemotherapy, CLSI = Clinical & Laboratory Standards Institute (USA), EUCAST = European Committee on Antimicrobial Susceptibility Testing, SFM = Societe Francaise de Microbiologie, SRGA = Swedish Reference Group for Antibiotics. Internet links or references are noted in the text.

b) nr = not recommended.

c) Oxacillin discs may be used to detect reduced susceptibility to penicillin: < 11 mm with 1-µg disk, < 18 mm with 5-µg disk.

d) Quinolone resistance is most reliably detected with nalidixic acid. Isolates with reduced susceptibility to fluoroquinolones have no zone of inhibition with nalidixic acid.

e) At the time of writing, ciprofloxacin was the only agent for which European harmonization had been agreed.

f) For surveillance purposes, a nalidixic acid MIC ≥ 8 mg l^{-1} may correlate with diminished fluoroquinolone susceptibility.

g) CLSI recommendations for azithromycin determined by incubation in ambient air.

4.3
Clinical Impact and Spread of Antibiotic Resistance in Meningococcal Disease

Up to now, only one group of antimicrobial agents has substantially lost its usefulness against *N. meningitidis* – the sulfonamides. This is quite remarkable considering the widespread use of alternative agents for prophylaxis and therapy, especially penicillin and rifampicin, over the two or three decades since the eclipse of the sulfonamides. Furthermore, the massive and prolonged exposure of meningococci to antimicrobial agents administered in the community for other indications has not so far produced reduced susceptibility to third generation cephalosporins, as it has for pneumococci [17, 18]. The position of the fluoroquinolones has become less certain as will be indicated below. The extreme rarity of β-lactamase production has been a welcome surprise, but the slow incremental rise in many countries of penicillin MICs has given us the dilemma of the correct initial choice of treatment when initial diagnostic tricks indicate a meningococcal etiology. High-order resistance to rifampicin has remained a somewhat enigmatic phenomenon and has not become widespread among clinical isolates of *N. meningitidis*. However, "reduced susceptibility" or lower-order resistance to this agent has contributed to its replacement in some countries as the drug of choice for chemoprophylaxis by fluoroquinolones, with ceftriaxone for pregnant women and young children. This significant move has not until now found a solid evidence base.

4.3.1
Antibiotic Resistance in the Chemoprophylaxis of Meningococcal Disease

Rifampicin

Rifampicin resistance in *N. meningitidis* is a much-studied topic. In a recent systematic review and meta-analysis [19, 20], it was concluded that the only drug used for prophylaxis against which resistance developed was rifampicin. Resistance to rifampicin among meningococci is determined largely by mutations in the *rpoB* gene which encodes DNA-dependent RNA polymerase [21–23], although other mechanisms might also play a role [24].

The tendency of rifampicin resistant meningococci to appear following prophylaxis has been recognized since the earliest studies [25–36], although this phenomenon has not been universal [37–41]. Deal and Sanders' publication [37] is frequently misquoted as showing emergence of resistance after prophylaxis. The MIC values of post-prophylaxis resistant isolates have ranged from low-order (up to 10 mg l^{-1}) to high-order resistance (from 100 mg l^{-1} to $\geq$500 mg l^{-1}). Low-order resistance showed up post-prophylaxis in several studies: e.g. in the USA, one study yielded 37/57 isolates having elevated MICs of 2–6 mg l^{-1} but the 20 remaining isolates had MICs of 100–200 mg l^{-1} [27]. In a Nigerian investigation [31], three strains had MICs of 3.2 mg l^{-1} and one had 6.4 mg l^{-1}, whereas pre-prophylaxis MICs in carrier isolates were all <0.1 mg l^{-1}. High-order resistance was the dominant finding in most studies. Claims of non-emergence of resistance have to be evaluated with caution: a New Zealand study the authors concluded that seven meningococci recovered after prophylaxis were susceptible with MICs in the range 0.004 mg l^{-1} to 2.0 mg l^{-1} [41]. This statement highlights the breakpoint issue again: all the official recommendations in Table 4.2 define 2 mg l^{-1} as resistant.

The clinical importance of resistance to this drug has been made clear by the occurrence of invasive disease due to highly resistant organisms, usually occurring after administration of rifampicin for secondary prevention [33, 42–47]. Of course, prophylaxis failures unassociated with rifampicin resistance have also been documented [48, 49].

In spite of wide interest in and frequent reporting of rifampicin resistance in meningococci, the actual frequency of such isolates is usually very low [50]. This suggests that the propagation of resistance in meningococcal populations might be too hard a task for the bacteria. It might be speculated that changes in the *rpoB* gene might generate strains which are resistant but badly adapted for survival for reasons poorly understood. Another crucial factor might be the absence of antibiotic selective pressure: rifampicin is not commonly used in the community, being generally reserved for treatment of tuberculosis.

This drug is still among the preferred agents for chemoprophylaxis of meningococcal disease: it heads the list in the most recent guideline issued by the US Centers for Disease Control and Prevention (CDC) in May 2005 [51].

Quinolones

There are signs that the up-to-now exquisite susceptibility of meningococci to the fluoroquinolone group of antibiotics, chiefly ciprofloxacin, has begun to decline. In 1992, a Greek isolate with an MIC of ≥1 mg l^{-1} was reported in a study of antibiotic susceptibilities [52]. The next data to appear in this less-than-desirable scenario appeared in reports from the UK of *N. meningitidis* isolates with MICs of 0.12 mg l^{-1} [53], a serogroup B isolate from France with an MIC of 0.125 mg l^{-1} [54], a clinical isolate from Australia of a serogroup C meningococcus [55], a case from Spain of a group B organism from CSF with an MIC of 0.12 mg l^{-1} [56] and most recently two strains from Argentina with MICs of 0.06 mg l^{-1} (group B) and 0.12 mg l^{-1} (group Y) [57]. In a portentous glimpse of what may be in store, Shultz and colleagues have produced ciprofloxacin MICs of 8–16 mg l^{-1} by exposure of two strains to the drug *in vitro*, demonstrating the accumulation of mutations in the quinolone resistance determining regions (QRDRs) of the *gyrA* and *parC* genes [58]. Despite the limitations of the study (one isolate had a starting MIC of 0.12 mg l^{-1}; and the other had a tendency to produce colonies in the ciprofloxacin inhibition zone around a disk), the findings give cause for concern. The authors also discuss the possibility of other mechanisms such as efflux pumps which are well described in *N. gonorrhoeae*, as are the QRDRs.

So far, in comparison with its gonococcal cousin, resistance or reduced susceptibility to these agents among meningococci seem to have advanced very slowly; this in spite of the extensive use of these agents in some parts of the world in the treatment of common community acquired infections, particularly of the urinary and respiratory tracts.

Third Generation Cephalosporins

There have been no reports as yet of reduced susceptibility to this group of agents.

Sulfonamides and Trimethoprim-Sulfamethoxazole

This group of agents has essentially been abandoned in the treatment and prophylaxis of meningococcal disease. Resistance became widespread over a period of about 20 years after their massive application; its frequency has been shown to vary widely in different countries, ranging from 6.35% to 100% [50, 59]. In some areas, the frequency of sulfonamide resistance has fallen in recent years, for example in South Australia [12], though whether resistance rates will become sufficiently reduced in the future to allow renewed prudent and selective deployment of these drugs remains an open question.

Minocycline and Other Tetracyclines

Few authorities include this group of drugs in their testing menus (see Table 4.2). Although minocycline appeared to be effective in eradicating pharyngeal carriage, its use was accompanied by frequent side-effects and it never came into general use for chemoprophylaxis [60]. It should be noted, however, that such side-effects were not a consistent accompaniment of minocycline administration, for example in the Finnish military [30]. Furthermore, many studies with post-prophylaxis follow-up have not shown the emergence of resistance. The data are well summarized in a systematic review and meta-analysis [19, 20]. Hansman et al. [12] suggested that 3% of meningococci in South Australia were not susceptible to minocycline. These investigators used a somewhat esoteric breakpoint of 1 mg l^{-1} ($\geq MIC_{50} \times 4$), and all their 133 isolates would have been considered susceptible (≤ 2 mg l^{-1}) by the CLSI (Table 4.2). So it is possible that, if necessary sometime in the future, this agent could be reconsidered for prophylaxis.

Spiramycin

Despite data which cast doubt on its efficacy [61] and other unconvincing studies [62], spiramycin is still recommended for chemoprophylaxis by the World Health Organization [63, 64]. It is therefore necessary to consider this agent in some detail.

While data regarding resistance to spiramycin are truly scarce, pharmacokinetic data really raise the question of whether meningococci should be regarded as realistically susceptible to this agent [61, 65]. Furthermore, meningococci have been

Table 4.3 Susceptibility of *N. meningitidis* to spiramycin.

Reference	n	MIC_{50} (mg l^{-1})	MIC_{90} (mg l^{-1})	CO_2 [a)]
Kamme et al. [65]	>80 [b)]	2.4 [c)]	9.6 [c)]	8%
Nicolas et al. [66]	137	8	16	5%
Dabernat et al. [67]	92	8	16	5–10%
	45	1	1	None
Rohner et al. [97]	174	1	2	None

a) CO_2 supplementation of incubation atmosphere.
b) Not specified. Several species were tested, 80–100 of each.
c) Values estimated from Fig. 5 in [65].

shown to be less susceptible than gonococci and various upper respiratory tract pathogens [65]. Kamme et al. [61] showed that the success of spiramycin in eradicating *N. meningitidis* from the pharynx is dependent on salivary concentrations in excess of the MIC for an extended period. Although reported MIC values vary, probably due to technical variations (Table 4.3), those reported by Nicolas et al. [66], Dabernat et al. [67] and Kamme et al. [65] (MIC_{50}=8.0, 8.0, 2.4 mg l^{-1}, respectively; MIC_{90}=16.0, 16.0, 9.6 mg l^{-1}, respectively) are consistent with the incomplete success of meningococcal eradication from the pharynx [61]. Furthermore, in an extensive study from the Pasteur Institute only 77% of 2153 isolates were regarded as fully susceptible using a disk diffusion test [68]. This paper gives disc breakpoints of 22 mm and <17 mm. A more recent review from the Pasteur Institute [69] presented less optimistic data: only 60.4% of 675 meningococcal isolates were fully susceptible to spiramycin (technical details were not given). Part of the explanation may lie in the different breakpoints currently recommended by the Antibiogramme Committee of the French Society for Microbiology in their 2005 Communique: zone diameters of ≥24 mm (*S*) and <19 mm (*R*), corresponding with MICs of ≤1 mg l^{-1} (*S*) and >4 mg l^{-1} (*R*; accessed at http://www.sfm.asso.fr/nouv/general.php?pa=2 in May 2005).

It is not appropriate to review here all the data available regarding spiramycin as a desirable anti-meningococcal agent. The intention is to raise doubt as to the correctness of the continuing recommendation for its use in chemoprophylaxis.

4.3.2 Antibiotic Resistance in the Treatment of Meningococcal Disease

4.3.2.1 Penicillin

True resistance with high MICs (from 4 mg l^{-1} to ≥256 mg l^{-1}) due to the production of *β*-lactamase has remained rare, having been described only four times [13–15]. *β*-Lactamase-positive strains only retain the plasmid carrying the *β*-lactamase gene under penicillin pressure, growing in media with low concentrations of the antibiotic. This finding might suggest both a low number of copies of the extrachromosomal DNA and/or the poor ability of meningococci to carry plasmids. This view is supported by studies that showed that the percentage of strains of *N. meningitidis* harboring extrachromosomal elements is very low [70, 71].

Meningococcal strains with reduced penicillin susceptibility began to appear only in the 1980s, after a long period of a widespread use. Now, more than 20 years later, the frequency of such strains with "intermediate" resistance to penicillin has dramatically increased but the degree of resistance seem to be quite similar, with MICs of ≥ 1 mg l^{-1} or higher being reported in a few isolated instances. It seems that the biological cost for altering the penicillin-binding proteins (PBPs) is too high for the bacteria, a hypothesis that has been proposed after *in vitro* experiments. In a 1947 study, using a technique of selecting less susceptible mutants on media containing increasing concentrations of penicillin, Miller and Bohnhoff [72] succeeded in increasing the concentration of penicillin required to inhibit the growth of a clinical isolate of *N. meningitidis* by four orders of magnitude. The price this isolate paid for this change was revealed by its gradual reversion to penicillin susceptibility by passage on penicillin-free medium. Nevertheless, an observation with seminal relevance to this discussion of antibiotic resistance was their demonstration that, in a mouse model with a meningococcal inoculum of 100 000 MLD, higher doses of penicillin were required to protect mice challenged with less susceptible organisms (Table 4.4).

The acquisition and persistence of the intermediate degrees of resistance to penicillin has probably allowed the species to survive better in environments

Table 4.4 Protection of mice from challenge of 10^5 MLD meningococci: increased "resistance" required higher doses of penicillin (adapted from Miller and Bohnhoff [72]).

Penicillin resistance (µg ml^{-1})[a]	Penicillin dose (µg)[a]	Outcome (died/total)
0.18	6	8/10
	12	5/10
	24	0/28
6.0	60	24/24
	120	21/36
	180	1/19
12.6	180	1/4
	240	3/16
	300	0/4
300.0	600	3/4
	1200	3/4
	3000	0/3

[a] Converted from units (10 units = 6 µg).

suffused with low concentrations of penicillin and perhaps other β-lactam agents. In this way, costs and benefits to the organism might be reasonably balanced, allowing the spread of intermediate resistance in the meningococcal population in a relative short period of time. However, alterations in the same or other PBPs that might result in higher levels of resistance might affect the cellular membrane in a negative way, producing organisms less able to survive and propagate as new lineages. A very slow advance in the degree of resistance can only be explained with an hypothesis of this sort.

Understanding what actually represents resistance in *N. meningitidis* is problematic. It is well established that meningococci with reduced susceptibility to penicillin (Table 4.2) can cause disease, but the scarcity of reports of failure of treatment with penicillin is noteworthy. In 1974, eight cases were reported in a letter from Greece in which CSF cultures were still positive on the third day of penicillin therapy at 15×10^6 units day^{-1} [73]. Although stated that the isolates were resistant to penicillin, no data were given. Some additional information may be gleaned from the literature, though such publications are largely anecdotal or retrospective collections of data. Turner et al. [74] described a clear treatment failure in a patient who received penicillin in a low dose. A further case in which CSF culture in a 16-year-old youth was positive on the third day of penicillin at a dose of 300 000 units kg^{-1} day^{-1} was encountered in Argentina [75]. An especially interesting case was the development of meningitis in a patient already on high dose treatment for meningococcemia [76]. Selected information from these and other publications that include clinical data are given in Table 4.5.

What remains from such "soft" data nicely demonstrates the difficulty in determining breakpoints when MICs are in a range that clearly put other organisms out of therapeutic reach in meningitis (e.g. 0.12–1.0 mg l^{-1} for pneumococci), but that yield conflicting information for meningococcal infections. The very widespread use of third generation cephalosporins for initial treatment of meningitis in the developed world will doubtless preclude the design and execution of adequate controlled trials that address this issue.

Some Spanish data hinted at a worse outcome due to reduced penicillin susceptibility [77]. A study from the UK addressed this issue and found that a fatal outcome was not associated with penicillin susceptibility but rather with organism characteristics [78]. The chief relevant difficulty of this study was that no data were available as to which patients were treated with penicillin alone, whereas the Spanish data were insufficient for clear-cut conclusions to be drawn.

Given the degree of uncertainty, the nasty nature of the disease and the need for starting antibiotic therapy before an etiological diagnosis is available, initial therapy will most likely continue to be based on advanced cephalosporins. Clinicians should demand of their laboratories the quickest possible determination of MICs to allow a timely consideration of a change to penicillin for fully susceptible strains, thus reducing the use of advanced cephalosporins with their wider ecological impact. Slow laboratory responses will eliminate the usefulness of MICs for the clinician, especially if current urges to shorten the duration of treatment of meningitis take hold [79, 80].

Table 4.5 Patients on record who received penicillin treatment of meningococcal infection due to organisms with reduced susceptibility to penicillin.

Reference	Patients	MICs (mg l^{-1})	Treatment	Outcome	Comments
Turner et al. [74]	1	0.64	penicillin G 500 000 units every 6 h, replaced by chloramphenicol	Survived	Relapse of meningitis on day 5 with positive CSF culture
Bardi et al. [75]	1	0.12–1.0	penicillin G 300 000 units kg^{-1} day^{-1}, replaced by ceftriaxone	Survived	Positive CSF culture after 72 h treatment. Only the abstract was available
Perez-Trallero et al. [98]	12	0.25–1.0	penicillin G 250 000 units kg^{-1} day^{-1} or ampicillin 240–300 mg kg^{-1} day^{-1}	One patient died with fulminant disease	Retrospective case-control comparison of children with susceptible organisms. Fatal case had MIC of 1 mg l^{-1}
Casado-Flores et al. [76]	1	0.25	penicillin G 300 000 units kg^{-1} day^{-1}, replaced by cefotaxime	Survived	Meningitis on day 4 of treatment for meningococcemia. Initial CSF clear. Repeat CSF: 2100 wbc µL^{-1}, Gram-negative diplococci, culture negative
Uriz et al. [99]	10	0.1–0.4	Four children: penicillin G 120–300 mg kg^{-1} day^{-1} 6 children: cefotaxime or other	All survived	Retrospective matched case-control comparison of children with susceptible organisms
Ellis-Pegler et al. [80] Briggs et al. [79]	4	0.125–0.25	Two patients: penicillin G 12×10^6 units day^{-1} Two patients: ceftriaxone ×1 then penicillin G 12×10^6 units day^{-1}	One patient only on penicillin died with fulminant disease	Study of 3-day treatment schedule. (Treatment details of the four patients by personal communication: R. B. Ellis-Pegler and S. Briggs, New Zealand)

4.3.2.2 Chloramphenicol

Chloramphenicol is no longer frequently used for the treatment of meningococcal disease in developed countries [81, 82]. Resistance to this agent is more likely to be of significance in less developed areas, where it is still recommended, and single intramuscular injections of chloramphenicol in oil may constitute the entire course of treatment [63]. High-order resistance to this drug, which is determined in meningococci by a chloramphenicol acetyl transferase encoded by the *catP* gene, has been described in 11 Vietnamese, one French [83] and two Australian isolates [82]. The complete gene was not found in 33 serogroup A isolates from Africa [81], though the authors caution that resistance to chloramphenicol has not been systematically sought in that continent. A recent study of 118 Nigerian isolates using an agar disk diffusion method indicated that 8% were resistant [84].

4.3.2.3 Quinolones

Fluoroquinolones have not yet come to the fore in the therapy of meningococcal disease. In view of the spectre of fluoroquinolone resistance, as outlined above, their use for this purpose should be approached with circumspection. One trial has shown that trovafloxacin was effective in childhood meningitis in comparison with ceftriaxone with or without vancomycin [85]. Trovafloxacin has since been removed from the market in the USA.

4.4
Are There New Drugs or New Strategies on the Horizon?

Consideration of the information above suggests that drug resistance among disease causing meningococci has not reached threatening proportions. Realistic options are available for both antibiotic prophylaxis and treatment of invasive disease. Nevertheless, the future should feature in our forward planning and further research is necessary if further options are to be devised.

In the area of prophylaxis, azithromycin has shown promising results [86], although confirmatory studies are needed, and older agents such as minocycline have retained their activity. Several new agents or variants of older drug groups have been studied, such as peptide deformylase (PDF) inhibitors [87], furylethylene derivatives [88], and glycylcyclines [89].

4.5
Molecular Tools for Definition of Antimicrobial Susceptibility in *N. meningitidis*

Two reasons underpin the need to develop molecular tools to help define the level of antibiotic susceptibility in *N. meningitidis*. The first is the difficulty of determining accurately the category of susceptibility by conventional methods, so a technology offering an objective measure will be very useful. In fact, it has been shown that the ability of different laboratories to detect meningococcal strains with intermediate resistance to penicillin (Pen^I) ranged from 18.2% to 100% in a standardization study [2]. The second and perhaps the most important reason is that with the increasing application of pre-hospital treatment, negative cultures are occurring with greater frequency in clinically diagnosed meningococcal infections. In this setting, molecular techniques enable identification of the pathogen and now can be applied to predict its susceptibility. The implications for both the patient and the public health and epidemiology sectors are clear.

Reduced susceptibility of meningococcal strains to penicillin is due, at least in part, to a decrease in the affinity of penicillin-binding protein 2 (PBP2) [90]. Altered forms of PBP2 are the result of the expression of different sequences of the *penA* gene encoding that protein: susceptible strains have *penA* genes with highly uniform sequences, while *penA* sequences from Pen^I isolates are quite diverse [91]. In order to develop a PCR based strategy to define this intermediate level of resistance, it is essential to define those mutations responsible for it. Significant advances have been made to this end, though some controversy exists as to whether eight [92] or five [93] positions in C-terminal part of PBP2 (amino acids 427–581) are correlated with this level of resistance. Despite this disagreement, we now have molecular markers of reduced penicillin susceptibility. Based on this information three different strategies have been developed. With the first, a 500-bp fragment of the 3′ part of the *penA* gene is amplified with specific primers and submitted to restriction fragment length polymorphism analysis to reveal alterations of *penA* and predict decreased susceptibility to penicillin G by generating specific pattern profiles [94]. The second method uses a real-time PCR assay to detect one of the five marker alterations in the *penA* gene [93]; and discrimination between Pen^I and Pen^S isolates is based on different melting temperatures of probe hybridization. The third strategy deploys a conventional PCR which uses primers designed to obtain a positive amplification only for susceptible strains; meningococci with intermediate level susceptibility give no reaction [95].

All of these strategies have been applied on defined reference strains and studies attempting to validate them are ongoing, certainly offering the hope of clinical application in the near future. Further studies will be necessary to make the connection between susceptibility *in vitro*, response *in vivo* and pharmacokinetic parameters, and to determine clinical test performance in terms of sensitivity, specificity and predictive values.

However, as progress is made, new challenges arise: the isolation of strains showing MICs associated with intermediate resistance to penicillin (0.094–0.12 mg l^{-1}) without alterations in the *penA* gene (unpublished data) should be well evaluated and characterized. The existence of mechanisms other than PBP2 alterations (peptidoglycan hydrolases, permeability changes, mtrR system, etc.) might complicate the detection of resistance with molecular tools. Furthermore, attempts are being made to deploy molecular methods in the simultaneous real-time detection of resistance to penicillin and rifampicin [96].

The case of penicillin and the meningococcus provides a specific opportunity to bypass the daunting complexity of molecular susceptibility testing; and the efforts of investigators to bring useful tests to the clinical arena are likely to bear fruit in the foreseeable future.

References

1. Block, C. **2001**, Antibiotic susceptibility testing, in *Meningococcal Disease*, ed. Pollard, A. J. and Maiden, M. C., Humana Press, Totowa, N.J.
2. Vazquez, J. A., Arreaza, L., Block, C., Ehrhard, I., Gray, S. J., Heuberger, S., Hoffmann, S., Kriz, P., Nicolas, P., Olcen, P., Skoczynska, A., Spanjaard, L., Stefanelli, P., Taha, M. K., Tzanakaki, G. **2003**, Interlaboratory Comparison of agar dilution and Etest methods for determining the MICs of antibiotics used in management of *Neisseria meningitidis* infections, Antimicrob. Agents. Chemother. 47, 3430–3434.
3. Clinical and Laboratory Standards Institute **2005**, *Performance Standards For Antimicrobial Susceptibility Testing; Fifteenth Informational Supplement. CLSI/NCCLS Document M100-S15*, vol. 25, Clinical and Laboratory Standards Institute, Wayne, Pa.
4. Bolmstrom, A., Arvidson, S., Ericsson, M., Karlsson, A. **1988**, A novel technique for direct quantification of antimicrobial susceptibility of microorganisms (abstract 1209), in *Program and Abstracts of the 28th Interscience Conference on Antimicrobial Agents and Chemotherapy (Los Angeles, CA)*, American Society for Microbiology, Washington, D.C.
5. Abadi, F. J., Yakubu, D. E., Pennington, T. H. **1995**, Antimicrobial susceptibility of penicillin-sensitive and penicillin-resistant meningococci, *J. Antimicrob. Chemother*. 35, 687–690.
6. Blondeau, J. M., Yaschuk, Y. **1995**, In vitro activities of ciprofloxacin, cefotaxime, ceftriaxone, chloramphenicol, and rifampin against fully susceptible and moderately penicillin-resistant *Neisseria meningitidis*, Antimicrob. Agents Chemother. 39, 2577–2579.
7. Daher, O., Lopardo, H. A., Rubeglio, E. A. **2002**, Value of Etest penicillin V and penicillin G strips for penicillin susceptibility testing of *Neisseria meningitidis*, *Diagn. Microbiol. Infect. Dis*. 43, 119–121.
8. Gomez-Herruz, P., Gonzalez-Palacios, R., Romanyk, J., Cuadros, J. A., Ena, J. **1995**, Evaluation of the Etest for penicillin susceptibility testing of *Neisseria meningitidis*, *Diagn. Microbiol. Infect. Dis*. 21, 115–117.
9. Hughes, J. H., Biedenbach, D. J., Erwin, M. E., Jones, R. N. **1993**, E test as susceptibility test and epidemiologic tool for evaluation of *Neisseria meningitidis* isolates, *J. Clin. Microbiol*. 31, 3255–3259.
10. Perez-Trallero, E., Gomez, N., Garcia-Arenzana, J. M. **1994**, E test as susceptibility test for evaluation of *Neisseria meningitidis* isolates, *J. Clin. Microbiol*. 32, 2341–2342.
11. Marshall, S. A., Rhomberg, P. R., Jones, R. N. **1997**, Comparative evaluation of etest for susceptibility testing *Neisseria meningitidis* with eight antimicrobial agents. An investigation using U.S. Food and Drug Administration regulatory criteria, *Diagn. Microbiol. Infect. Dis*. 27, 93–97.
12. Hansman, D., Wati, S., Lawrence, A., Turnidge, J. **2004**, Have South Australian isolates of *Neisseria meningitidis* become less susceptible to penicillin, rifampicin and other drugs? A study of strains isolated over three decades, 1971–1999, *Pathology* 36, 160–165.
13. Botha, P. **1988**, Penicillin-resistant *Neisseria meningitidis* in Southern Africa, *Lancet* 1988i, 54.
14. Dillon, J. R., Pauze, M., Yeung, K.-H. **1983**, Spread of penicillinase-producing and transfer plasmids from the gonococcus to *Neisseria meningitidis*, *Lancet* 1983i, 779–781.
15. Fontanals, D., Pineda, V., Pons, I., Rojo, J. C. **1989**, Penicillin-resistant beta-lactamase producing *Neisseria meningitidis* in Spain, *Eur. J. Clin. Microbiol. Infect. Dis*. 8, 90–91.
16. Vazquez, J. A., Enriquez, A. M., De la, F. L., Berron, S., Baquero, M. **1996**, Isolation of a strain of beta-lactamase-producing *Neisseria meningitidis* in Spain, *Eur. J. Clin. Microbiol. Infect. Dis*. 15, 181–182.
17. John, C. C. **1994**, Treatment failure with use of a third-generation cephalosporin for penicillin-resistant pneumococcal meningitis: case report and review, *Clin. Infect. Dis*. 18, 188–193.

18 Bradley, J. S., Connor, J. D. **1991**, Ceftriaxone failure in meningitis caused by *Streptococcus pneumoniae* with reduced susceptibility to beta-lactam antibiotics, *Pediatr. Infect. Dis. J.* 10, 871–873.

19 Fraser, A., Gafter-Gvili, A., Paul, M., Leibovici, L. **2005**, Prophylactic use of antibiotics for prevention of meningococcal infections: systematic review and meta-analysis of randomised trials, *Eur. J. Clin. Microbiol. Infect. Dis.* 2005.

20 Fraser, A., Gafter-Gvili, A., Paul, M., Leibovici, L. **2005**, Antibiotics for preventing meningococcal infections, *Cochrane Database Syst. Rev.* CD004785

21 Carter, P. E., Abadi, F. J., Yakubu, D. E., Pennington, T. H. **1994**, Molecular characterization of rifampin-resistant *Neisseria meningitidis*, Antimicrob. *Agents Chemother.* 38, 1256–1261.

22 Nolte, O., Muller, M., Reitz, S., Ledig, S., Ehrhard, I., Sonntag, H. G. **2003**, Description of new mutations in the *rpoB* gene in rifampicin-resistant *Neisseria meningitidis* selected *in vitro* in a stepwise manner, *J. Med. Microbiol.* 52, 1077–1081.

23 Stefanelli, P., Fazio, C., La Rosa, G., Marianelli, C., Muscillo, M., Mastrantonio, P. **2001**, Rifampicin-resistant meningococci causing invasive disease: detection of point mutations in the *rpoB* gene and molecular characterization of the strains, *J. Antimicrob. Chemother.* 47, 219–222.

24 Abadi, F. J., Carter, P. E., Cash, P., Pennington, T. H. **1996**, Rifampin resistance in *Neisseria meningitidis* due to alterations in membrane permeability, Antimicrob. *Agents Chemother.* 40, 646–651.

25 Devine, L. F., Johnson, D. P., Hagerman, C. R., Pierce, W. E., Rhode, S. L., Peckinpaugh, R. O. **1970**, Rifampin levels in serum and saliva and effect on the meningococcal carrier state, *JAMA* 214, 1055–1059.

26 Weidmer, C. E., Dunkel, T. B., Pettyjohn, F. S., Smith, C. D., Leibovitz, A. **1971**, Effectiveness of rifampin in eradicating the meningococcal carrier state in a relatively closed population: emergence of resistant strains, J. Infect. Dis. 124, 172–178.

27 Guttler, R. B., Counts, G. W., Avent, C. K., Beaty, H. N. **1971**, Effect of rifampin and minocycline on meningococcal carrier rates, *J. Infect. Dis.* 124, 199–205.

28 Eickhoff, T. C. **1971**, In-vitro and in-vivo studies of resistance to rifampin in meningococci, *J. Infect. Dis.* 123, 414–420.

29 Munford, R. S., Sussuarana, D., V, Phillips, C. J., Gelli, D. S., Gorman, G. W., Risi, J. B., Feldman, R. A. **1974**, Eradication of carriage of *Neisseria meningitidis* in families: a study in Brazil, *J. Infect. Dis.* 129, 644–649.

30 Sivonen, A., Renkonen, O. V., Weckstrom, P., Koskenvuo, K., Raunio, V., Makela, P. H. **1978**, The effect of chemoprophylactic use of rifampin and minocycline on rates of carriage of *Neisseria meningitidis* in army recruits in Finland, *J. Infect. Dis.* 137, 238–244.

31 Blakebrough, I. S., Gilles, H. M. 1980, The effect of rifampicin on meningococcal carriage in family contacts in northern Nigeria, J. Infect. 2, 137–143.

32 Beaty, H. N. Rifampin and minocycline in meningococcal disease, *Rev. Infect. Dis.* 5[Suppl. 3], S451–S458.

33 Schubiger, G., Munzinger, J., Dudli, C., Wipfli, U. **1986**, Meningococcal epidemic in a boarding school: a rifampicin-resistant secondary case while under chemoprophylaxis, *Schweiz. Med. Wochenschr.* 116, 1172–1175.

34 Cooke, R. P., Riordan, T., Jones, D. M., Painter, M. J. **1989**, Secondary cases of meningococcal infection among close family and household contacts in England and Wales, 1984–7, *Br. Med. J.* 298, 555–558.

35 Chapalain, J. C., Guibourdenche, M., Perrier-Gros-Claude, J. D., Bartoli, M., Riou, J. Y. **1992**, The chemoprophylaxis of cerebrospinal meningitis using rifampin in a military population, *Pathol. Biol.* 40, 230–233.

36 Jackson, L. A., Alexander, E. R., DeBolt, C. A., Swenson, P. D., Boase, J., McDowell, M. G., Reeves, M. W., Wenger, J. D. **1996**, Evaluation of the use of mass chemoprophylaxis during a school outbreak of enzyme type 5 serogroup B meningococcal disease, *Pediatr. Infect. Dis. J.* 15, 992–998.

37 Deal, W. B., Sanders, E. **1969**, Efficacy of rifampin in treatment of meningococcal carriers, *N. Engl. J. Med.* 281, 641–645.

38 Kaiser, A. B., Hennekens, C. H., Saslaw, M. S., Hayes, P. S., Bennett, J. V. **1974**, Seroepidemiology and chemoprophylaxis disease due to sulfonamide-resistant *Neisseria meningitidis* in a civilian population, *J. Infect. Dis.* 130, 217–224.

39 Nicolle, L. E., Postl, B., Kotelewetz, E., Remillard, F., Bourgault, A. M., Albritton, W., Harding, G. K., Ronald, A. **1982**, Chemoprophylaxis for *Neisseria meningitidis* in an isolated Arctic community, *J. Infect. Dis.* 145, 103–109.

40 Pearce, M. C., Sheridan, J. W., Jones, D. M., Lawrence, G. W., Murphy, D. M., Masutti, B., McCosker, C., Douglas, V., George, D., O'Keefe, A., et al. **1995**, Control of group C meningococcal disease in Australian aboriginal children by mass rifampicin chemoprophylaxis and vaccination, *Lancet* 346, 20–23.

41 Simmons, G., Jones, N., Calder, L. **2000**, Equivalence of ceftriaxone and rifampicin in eliminating nasopharyngeal carriage of serogroup B *Neisseria meningitidis, J. Antimicrob. Chemother.* 45, 909–911.

42 Cooper, E. R., Ellison, R. T., Smith, G. S., Blaser, M. J., Reller, L. B., Paisley, J. W. **1986**, Rifampin-resistant meningococcal disease in a contact patient given prophylactic rifampin, *J. Pediatr.* 108, 93–96.

43 Berkey, P., Rolston, K., Zukiwski, A., Gooch, G., Bodey, G. P. **1988**, Rifampin-resistant meningococcal infection in a patient given rifampin chemoprophylaxis, *Am. J. Infect. Control* 16, 250–252.

44 Yagupsky, P., Ashkenazi, S., Block, C. **1993**, Rifampicin-resistant meningococci causing invasive disease and failure of chemoprophylaxis, *Lancet* 341, 1152–1153.

45 Almog, R., Block, C., Gdalevich, M., Lev, B., Wiener, M., Ashkenazi, S. **1994**, First recorded outbreaks of meningococcal disease in the Israel Defence Force: three clusters due to serogroup C and the emergence of resistance to rifampicin, *Infection* 22, 69–71.

46 Dawson, S. J., Fey, R. E., McNulty, C. A. 1999, Meningococcal disease in siblings caused by rifampicin sensitive and rifampicin resistant strains, *Commun. Dis. Public Health* 2, 215–216.

47 Tsakris, A., Trakatelli, C., Souliou, E., Sofianou, D., Ntoutsou, K., Antoniadis, A. **2001**, Failures of rifampicin and ciprofloxacin to eradicate a susceptible meningococcal isolate from a close contact of a fatal case, *Infection* 29, 293–294.

48 Khuri-Bulos, N. **1973**, Meningococcal meningitis following rifampin prophylaxis, *Am. J. Dis. Child.* 126, 689–691.

49. Cartwright, K. A., Hunt, D., Fox, A. 1995, Chemoprophylaxis fails to prevent a second case of meningococcal disease in a day nursery, *Commun. Dis. Rep. CDR Rev.* 5, R199

50 Vazquez, J. A. **2001**, The resistance of *Neisseria meningitidis* to the antimicrobial agents: an issue still in evolution, *Rev. Med. Microbiol.* 12, 39–45.

51 Centers for Disease Control and Prevention **2005**, Prevention and control of meningococcal disease recommendations of the Advisory Committee on Immunization Practices (ACIP), Morbid. Mortal. Weekly Rep. 54, 1–21.

52 Tzanakaki, G., Blackwell, C. C., Kremastinou, J., Kallergi, C., Kouppari, G., Weir, D. M. **1992**, Antibiotic sensitivities of *Neisseria meningitidis* isolates from patients and carriers in Greece, *Epidemiol. Infect.* 108, 449–455.

53 Kaczmarski, E. B., Gray, S. J., Carr, A. D., Mallard, R. H. **1999**, Antimicrobial agent susceptibility of clinical *Neisseria meningitidis* isolates from England and Wales, *Abstr. Intersci. Conf. Antimicrob. Agents Chemother.* 39, 172.

54 Casin, I., Gandry, B., Lassau, F., Janier, M., Lagrange, P., Collatz, E. **1999**, Decreased susceptibility to penicillin G (Pen), tetracyclines (Tet), and fluoroquinolones (Fq), and characterization of DNA gyrase mutations, in oropharyngeal and anogenital isolates of *Neisseria meningitidis* (Nme) in patients presenting at an STD clinic, *Abstr. Intersci. Conf. Antimicrob. Agents Chemother.* 39, 171

55 Shultz, T. R., Tapsall, J. W., White, P. A., Newton, P. J. **2000**, An invasive isolate of *Neisseria meningitidis* showing decreased

susceptibility to quinolones, *Antimicrob. Agents Chemother.* 44, 1116

56 Alcala, B., Salcedo, C., De La Fuente, L., Arreaza, L., Uria, M. J., Abad, R., Enriquez, R., Vazquez, J. A., Motge, M., de Batlle, J. **2004**, *Neisseria meningitidis* showing decreased susceptibility to ciprofloxacin: first report in Spain, *J. Antimicrob. Chemother.* 53, 409

57 Corso, A., Faccone, D., Miranda, M., Rodriguez, M., Regueira, M., Carranza, C., Vencina, C., Vazquez, J. A., Galas, M. **2005**, Emergence of *Neisseria meningitidis* with decreased susceptibility to ciprofloxacin in Argentina, *J. Antimicrob. Chemother.* 55, 596–597.

58 Shultz, T. R., White, P. A., Tapsall, J. W. **2005**, In vitro assessment of the further potential for development of fluoroquinolone resistance in *Neisseria meningitidis, Antimicrob. Agents Chemother.* 49, 1753–1760.

59 Oppenheim, B. A. **1997**, Antibiotic resistance in *Neisseria meningitidis, Clin. Infect. Dis.* 24[Suppl 1], S98–S101.

60 Drew, T. M., Altman, R., Black, K., Goldfield, M. 1976, Minocycline for prophylaxis of infection with *Neisseria meningitidis*: high rate of side effects in recipients, *J. Infect. Dis.* 133, 194–198.

61 Kamme, C., Kahlmeter, G. **1979**, Evaluation of spiramycin in meningococcal carriage, *Scand. J. Infect. Dis.* 11, 229–232.

62 Engelen, F., Vandepitte, J., Verbist, L., De Maeyer-Cleempoel, S. **1981**, Effect of spiramycin on the nasopharyngeal carriage of *Neisseria meningitidis, Chemotherapy* 27, 325–333.

63 World Health Organization **1998**, *Control of Epidemic Meningococcal Disease. WHO Practical Guidelines, 2nd edn*, WHO/EMC/BAC/98.3, World Health Organization, Geneva.

64 World Health Organization Department of Communicable Disease Surveillance and Response **2003**, *Prevention and Control of Epidemic Meningococcal Disease in Africa: Report of a WHO Technical Consultation Meeting, Burkina Faso 2002*, WHO/CDS/CSR/GAR/2003.10, World Health Organization, Geneva.

65 Kamme, C., Kahlmeter, G., Melander, A. **1978**, Evaluation of spiramycin as a therapeutic agent for elimination of nasopharyngeal pathogens. Possible use of spiramycin for middle ear infections and for gonococcal and meningococcal nasopharyngeal carriage, *Scand. J. Infect. Dis.* 10, 135–142.

66 Nicolas, P., Cavallo, J. D., Fabre, R., Martet, G. **1998**, Standardization of the *Neisseria meningitidis* antibiogram. Detection of strains relatively resistant to penicillin, Bull. *WHO* 76, 393–400.

67 Dabernat, H., Delmas, C., Lareng, M. B. **1984**, Antibiotic sensitivity of meningococci isolated from patients and carriers, *Pathol. Biol.* 32, 532–535.

68 Antignac, A., Ducos-Galand, M., Guiyoule, A., Pires, R., Alonso, J. M., Taha, M. K. **2003**, *Neisseria meningitidis* strains isolated from invasive infections in France (1999–2002): phenotypes and antibiotic susceptibility patterns, *Clin. Infect. Dis.* 37, 912–920.

69 Alonso, J. M., Taha, M. K. **2004**, Epidemiologie des pathologies invasives a *Neisseria meningitidis, Rev. Fr. Lab.* 2004, 25–28.

70 Prere, M. F., Fayet, O., Delmas, C., Lareng, M. B., Dabernat, H. **1985**, Presence of plasmids in *Neisseria meningitidis, Ann. Inst. Pasteur Microbiol.* 136A, 271–276.

71 Backmann, A., Danielsson, D., Olcen, P. **1993**, Plasmid carriage and antibiotic susceptibility of *Neisseria meningitidis* strains isolated in Sweden 1981–1990, *Eur. J. Clin. Microbiol. Infect. Dis.* 12, 683–689.

72 Miller, C. P., Bohnhoff, M. **1947**, Studies on the action of penicillin. VI Further observations on the development of penicillin resistance by meningococci *in vitro, J. Infect. Dis.* 81, 147–156.

73 Contoyiannis, P., Adamopoulos, D. A. **1974**, Penicillin-resistant *Neisseria meningitidis, Lancet* 1974i, 462

74 Turner, P. C., Southern, K. W., Spencer, N. J., Pullen, H. **1990**, Treatment failure in meningococcal meningitis, *Lancet* 335, 732–733.

75 Bardi, L., Badolati, A., Corso, A., Rossi, M. A. **1994**, Failure of the treatment with penicillin in a case of *Neisseria meningitidis* meningitis, *Medicina* 54, 427–430.

76 Casado-Flores, J., Osona, B., Domingo, P., Barquet, N. **1997**, Meningococcal meningitis during penicillin therapy for meningococcemia, *Clin. Infect. Dis.* 25, 1479

77 Luaces Cubells C., Garcia Garcia J., Roca Martinez J., Latorre Otin C. L. **1997**, Clinical data in children with meningococcal meningitis in a Spanish hospital, *Acta Paediatr. 86, 26–29.*

78 Trotter, C. L., Fox, A. J., Ramsay, M. E., Sadler, F., Gray, S. J., Mallard, R., Kaczmarski, E. B. **2002**, Fatal outcome from meningococcal disease – an association with meningococcal phenotype but not with reduced susceptibility to benzylpenicillin, *J. Med. Microbiol.* 51, 855–860.

79 Briggs, S., Ellis-Pegler, R., Roberts, S., Thomas, M., Woodhouse, A. **2004**, Short course intravenous benzylpenicillin treatment of adults with meningococcal disease, *Int. Med. J.* 34, 383–387.

80 Ellis-Pegler, R., Galler, L., Roberts, S., Thomas, M., Woodhouse, A. **2003**, Three days of intravenous benzyl penicillin treatment of meningococcal disease in adults, *Clin. Infect. Dis.* 2003, 37, 658–662.

81 Tondella, M. L., Rosenstein, N. E., Mayer, L. W., Tenover, F. C., Stocker, S. A., Reeves, M. W., Popovic, T. **2001**, Lack of evidence for chloramphenicol resistance in *Neisseria meningitidis*, Africa, *Emerg. Infect. Dis.* 7, 163–164.

82 Shultz, T. R., Tapsall, J. W., White, P. A., Ryan, C. S., Lyras, D., Rood, J. I., Binotto, E., Richardson, C. J. **2003**, Chloramphenicol-resistant *Neisseria meningitidis* containing *catP* isolated in Australia, *J. Antimicrob. Chemother.* 52, 856–859.

83 Galimand, M., Gerbaud, G., Guibourdenche, M., Riou, J. Y., Courvalin, P. **1998**, High-level chloramphenicol resistance in *Neisseria meningitidis, N. Engl. J. Med.* 339, 868–874.

84 Emele, F. E. **2000**, Etiologic spectrum and pattern of antimicrobial drug susceptibility in bacterial meningitis in Sokoto, Nigeria, *Acta Paediatr.* 89, 942–946.

85 Saez-Llorens, X., McCoig, C., Feris, J. M., Vargas, S. L., Klugman, K. P., Hussey, G. D., Frenck, R. W., Falleiros-Carvalho, L. H., Arguedas, A. G., Bradley, J., Arrieta, A. C., Wald, E. R., Pancorbo, S., McCracken, G. H., Jr., Marques, S. R. **2002**, Quinolone treatment for pediatric bacterial meningitis: a comparative study of trovafloxacin and ceftriaxone with or without vancomycin, *Pediatr. Infect. Dis. J.* 21, 14–22.

86 Girgis, N., Sultan, Y., Frenck, R. W. J., El-Gendy, A., Farid, Z., Mateczun, A. **1998**, Azithromycin compared with rifampin for eradication of nasopharyngeal colonization by *Neisseria meningitidis, Pediatr. Infect. Dis. J.* 17, 816–819.

87 Jones, R. N., Sader, H. S., Fritsche, T. R. **2005**, Antimicrobial activity of LBM415 (NVP PDF-713) tested against pathogenic Neisseria spp (*Neisseria gonorrhoeae* and *Neisseria meningitidis*), *Diagn. Microbiol. Infect. Dis.* 51, 139–141.

88 Blondeau, J. M., Castanedo, N., Gonzalez, O., Mendina, R., Silveira, E. **1999**, In vitro evaluation of G1: a novel antimicrobial compound, *Intl. J. Antimicrob. Agents* 11, 163–166.

89 Gales, A. C., Jones, R. N. **2000**, Antimicrobial activity and spectrum of the new glycylcycline, GAR-936 tested against 1,203 recent clinical bacterial isolates, *Diagn. Microbiol. Infect. Dis.* 36, 19–36.

90 Saez-Nieto, J. A., Lujan, R., Berron, S., Campos, J., Vinas, M., Fuste, C., Vazquez, J. A., Zhang, Q. Y., Bowler, L. D., Martinez-Suarez, J. V. **1992**, Epidemiology and molecular basis of penicillin-resistant *Neisseria meningitidis* in Spain: a 5-year history (1985–1989), *Clin. Infect. Dis.* 14, 394–402.

91 Spratt, B. G., Zhang, Q. Y., Jones, D. M., Hutchison, A., Brannigan, J. A., Dowson, C. G. **1989**, Recruitment of a penicillin-binding protein gene from Neisseria flavescens during the emergence of penicillin resistance in *Neisseria meningitidis, Proc. Natl Acad. Sci. USA* 86, 8988–8992.

92 Antignac, A., Boneca, I. G., Rousselle, J. C., Namane, A., Carlier, J. P., Vazquez, J. A., Fox, A., Alonso, J. M., Taha, M. K. **2003**, Correlation between alterations of the penicillin-binding protein 2 and modifications of the peptidoglycan structure in *Neisseria meningitidis* with reduced susceptibility to penicillin G, *J. Biol. Chem.* 278, 31529–31535.

93 Stefanelli, P., Carattoli, A., Neri, A., Fazio, C., Mastrantonio, P. **2003**, Prediction of decreased susceptibility to penicillin of *Neisseria meningitidis* strains by real-time PCR, *J. Clin. Microbiol. 41, 4666–4670.*

94 Antignac, A., Alonso, J. M., Taha, M. K. **2001**, Nonculture prediction of *Neisseria meningitidis* susceptibility to penicillin, Antimicrob. *Agents Chemother.* 45, 3625–3628.

95 Alcala, B., Abad, R., Arreaza, L., Enriquez, R., Salcedo, C., Uria, M. J., Vazquez, J. A. **2003**, PCR as a tool for detection of meningococcal strains with intermediate resistance to penicillin G, *Abstr. Eur. Monitor. Group Meningococci* 7, 47.

96 Stefanelli, P., Neri, A., Carattoli, A., Mastrantonio, P. **2005**, Simultaneous detection of rifampicin resistant and penicillin intermediate phenotypes in *Neisseria meningitidis* by real-time multiplex PCR (abstr. P627), *Clin. Microbiol. Infect.* 11, 176.

97 Rohner, P., Pepey, B., Hirschel, B., Auckenthaler, R. **1992**, Typing and sensitivity of meningococci isolated in Switzerland 1988–1990, *Schweiz. Med. Wochenschr.* 122,224–228.

98 Perez-Trallero, E., Aldamiz-Echeverria, L., Perez-Yarza, E. G. **1990**, Meningococci with increased resistance to penicillin, *Lancet* 335, 1096.

99 Uriz, S., Pineda, V., Grau, M., Nava, J. M., Bella, F., Morera, M. A., Fontanals, D., Font, B., Marti, C., Deulofeu, F., et al. **1991**, *Neisseria meningitidis* with reduced sensitivity to penicillin: observations in 10 children, *Scand. J. Infect. Dis.* 23, 171–174.

Part II
Genetics and Genomics of the Meningococcus

Handbook of Meningococcal Disease. Infection Biology, Vaccination, Clinical Management.
Edited by M. Frosch and M. C. J. Maiden

ISBN: 3-527-31260-9

5
Neisseria meningitidis Genome Sequencing Projects

Christoph Schoen and Heike Claus

5.1
Introduction

Neisseria meningitidis (the meningococcus) is a facultative commensal and colonises the nasopharynx of up to 30% of healthy individuals [1]. For reasons that are still mostly unknown, meningococci can enter the bloodstream and subsequently the cerebrospinal fluid, causing septicemia and meningitis, respectively. Although vaccination is an effective way to control meningococcal disease caused by serogroup A, C, W-135, and Y meningococci, currently no effective vaccine against serogroup B meningococci is available.

Since conventional technologies had failed to develop a serogroup B vaccine, genomics appeared to be a source that could lead to the development of a protein-based vaccine. In addition, genome sequencing provides an efficient tool to identify putative virulence determinants, which complete the list of meningococcal virulence factors identified in the pre-genomic era. Furthermore, comparisons of genome sequences of different meningococcal strains give the opportunity to define a common subset of genes that may be responsible for the pathogenesis of the disease. Finally, whole genome sequencing data enable the design of DNA microarrays to elucidate gene expression patterns on the transcriptional level under in vivo conditions on a genome-wide scale.

Accordingly, in the year 2000, the complete nucleotide sequences of the *N. meningitidis* serogroup A strain Z2491 and of the serogroup B strain MC58 genome were determined by random shotgun sequencing strategies and first annotations were published [2, 3]. By now, the complete but yet unpublished sequence of the *N. meningitidis* serogroup C strain FAM18, together with a first annotation, had been made available via the homepage of The Wellcome Trust Sanger Institute (http://www.sanger.ac.uk). The publication of these genome sequences had already sparked many downstream analyses, computational as well as experimental. This chapter will give a short overview over some general features of the two published meningococcal genomes and will also briefly present some data that have emerged from recent *in silico* as well as experimental analyses.

Handbook of Meningococcal Disease. Infection Biology, Vaccination, Clinical Management.
Edited by M. Frosch and M. C. J. Maiden

ISBN: 3-527-31260-9

5.2
The Genomes of *Neisseria meningitidis*

A summary of the overall features of the *N. meningitidis* Z2491 and the *N. meningitidis* MC58 genomes is given in Table 5.1. Each genome consists of a single circular chromosome. In addition, *N. meningitidis* was occasionally found to harbor cryptic plasmids encoding resistance against β-lactame antibiotics [4], sulfonamides [5], and tetracycline [6], which has raised some medical concern regarding effective antibiotic treatment of neisserial meningitis [7]. However, in contrast to many other Gram-negative pathogens, no virulence plasmids have been detected so far in *Neisseria* spp.

Both genomes are about 2.2 Mb in size and have both an average GC content of approximately 52%. The MC58 genome, however, is almost 100 kb larger than the Z2491 genome and harbors a large duplication of about 30 kb containing 36 coding sequences (CDS) (NMB1123–NMB1159: Fig. 5.1 A). Compared to the genomes of other respiratory tract pathogens, they are, for example, about half the size of the *Bordetella pertussis* genome (4.1 Mb) [8] and comparable to the *Haemophilus influenzae* genome (1.9 Mb) [9] or the *Streptococcus pneumoniae* genome (2.2 Mb) [10].

Each meningococcal genome contains four copies of a 16S-23S-5S ribosomal RNA operon and *N. meningitidis* Z2491 comes with 58 tRNA genes and *N. meningitidis* MC58 with 59, respectively. Both strains encode all of the aminoacyl transfer RNA synthetases, except for tRNAAsn which may be formed by a transamidation reaction catalyzed by a Glu-tRNAGln transamidase, leading to the formation of tRNAAsn from tRNAAsp [2].

Based on the primary annotations [2, 3], the Z2491 genome was predicted to contain 2121 putative CDS and the MC58 genome 2158 CDS, respectively, with a corresponding average CDS length of about 875 bp, resulting in a coding density of 83% in both genomes (Table 5.1). Not least due to the different computational approaches applied, these numbers might be subject to future changes in ongoing semi-automated re-annotations. For example, the numbers given for the Z2491 genome by the main genome databases like the Comprehensive Microbial Resource database (CMR) at The Institute for Genomic Research (TIGR: http://www.tigr.org), the Complete Microbial Genome database at NCBI (http://www.ncbi.nlm.nih.gov), and the Swiss-Prot HAMAP database project (http://www.expasy.org) [11], respectively, differ by over 10% compared to the primary annotation [2]. In particular, the numbers of putative CDS given for the Z2491 genome fall in the range between 2040 (HAMAP) and 2558 (TIGR-CMR) and the average CDS length accordingly between 854 bp (HAMAP) and 734 bp (TIGR-CMR). However, based on the approximately 270 genes that were found to be expressed under *in vitro* cultivation of a serogroup A meningococcus the average gene length was found to be about 1290 bp and therefore considerably longer than predicted [12]. These discrepancies have also been described for other genomes indicating that a substantial number of annotated CDS are actually not protein-coding genes [13].

Table 5.1 Comparison of the two published *N. meningitidis* genomes.

	***N. meningitidis* A Z2491**	***N. meningitidis* B MC58**
General information		
GenBank accession	AL1579 59	AE002098
Genome size (bp)	2 184 406	2 272 351
G+C content (%)	51.8	51.5
Functional RNAs [a)]		
Number of tRNAs	58	59
Number of rRNA operons	4	4
Putative coding sequences		
Primary annotation [a)]	2121	2158
TIGR-CMR [b)]	2558	2074
NCBI [c)]	2065	2079
HAMAP (Swiss-Prot) [d)]	2040	1967
Average CDS length (bp)		
Primary annotation [a)]	877	874
TIGR-CMR [b)]	734	864
NCBI [c)]	851	867
HAMAP (Swiss-Prot) [d)]	854	872
Coding area (%)		
Primary annotation [a)]	83	83
TIGR-CMR [b)]	86	79
NCBI [c]	81	79
HAMAP (Swiss-Prot) [d)]	83	79
Putative pseudogenes		
Primary annotation [a)]	≥56	n.a.
Lower estimate [e)]	≥26	≥44
Simple sequence contingency loci		
Putative phase-variable genes [f)]	68	82
Genes containing coding tandem repeats [g)]	25	26
Flexible genome pool		
Repeat sequences		
DNA uptake sequences (gccgtctgaa)	1892	1910
dRS3 (attcccnnnnnnnnngggaat)	1344	1378
Correia and Correia-related repeats [h)]	270	261
IS elements		
Primary annotation [a)]	43	51
TIGR-CMR [b]	67	53
IS Finder database [i]		
IS*3* family	1	2
IS*5* family	26	17
IS*30* family	8	14

Table 5.1 (continued)

	***N. meningitidis* A Z2491**	***N. meningitidis* B MC58**
IS*481* family	1	0
IS*630* family	3	2
IS*1016* family	23	16
Genes acquired putatively via HGT[j]	206	221
Putative genomic islands[a]	>60	IHT-A, -B, -C
Prophages and phage-like elements[k]	Pnm 1, Pnm2, Pnm3, CTXϕ-like	NeisMu1, NeisMu2, CTXϕ-like (2 copies)

a) The numbers given are based on the primary annotation as presented in [2] for *N. meningitidis* A Z2491 and in [3] for *N. meningitidis* B MC58.
b) The numbers are based on the annotations by the TIGR-CMR database available at http://www.tigr.org/tigr-scripts/CMR2/CMRHomePage.spl.
c) The numbers are according to the annotations by the NCBI complete microbial genome database available at http://www.ncbi.nlm.nih.gov/genomes/lproks.cgi.
d) The numbers are based on the annotation given by the Swiss-Prot HAMAP project [11] at http://www.expasy.org/sprot/hamap/.
e) As given in [17].
f) As given in [34].
g) As given in [35].
h) As given in [41].
i) The numbers are from the IS Finder database at http://www-is.biotoul.fr/.
j) Based on the numbers given in the Horizontal Gene Transfer DataBase (HGT-DB) [65], available via http://www.fut.es/~debb/HGT/.
k) As given in [54].

According to standard bacterial taxonomy, the genus *Neisseria* belongs to the β subdivision of the Proteobacteria. Consecutively, a sequence comparison of the *N. meningitidis* MC58 encoded proteome with that of other pathogenic bacteria stored in the TIGR-CMR database reveals that MC58 has the highest number of best hits with the *N. meningitidis* Z2491 proteome, followed by the β-proteobacterial *Burkholderia* spp, which cause life-threatening respiratory infections (Fig. 5.2). Remarkably, *N. meningitidis* MC58 has a higher number of best hits in the proteome of the γ-proteobacterium *H. influenzae* than in the proteome of other closely related β-proteobacteria like *Bordetella* spp. Although they belong to different phyletic taxa, principal component analysis of the data on the cooccurrence of genomes in the cluster of orthologous groups (COG) database also shows that *N. meningitidis* and *H. influenzae* group closely together again indicating similar functional adaptations to their life style as facultative pathogenic respiratory commensals of humans.

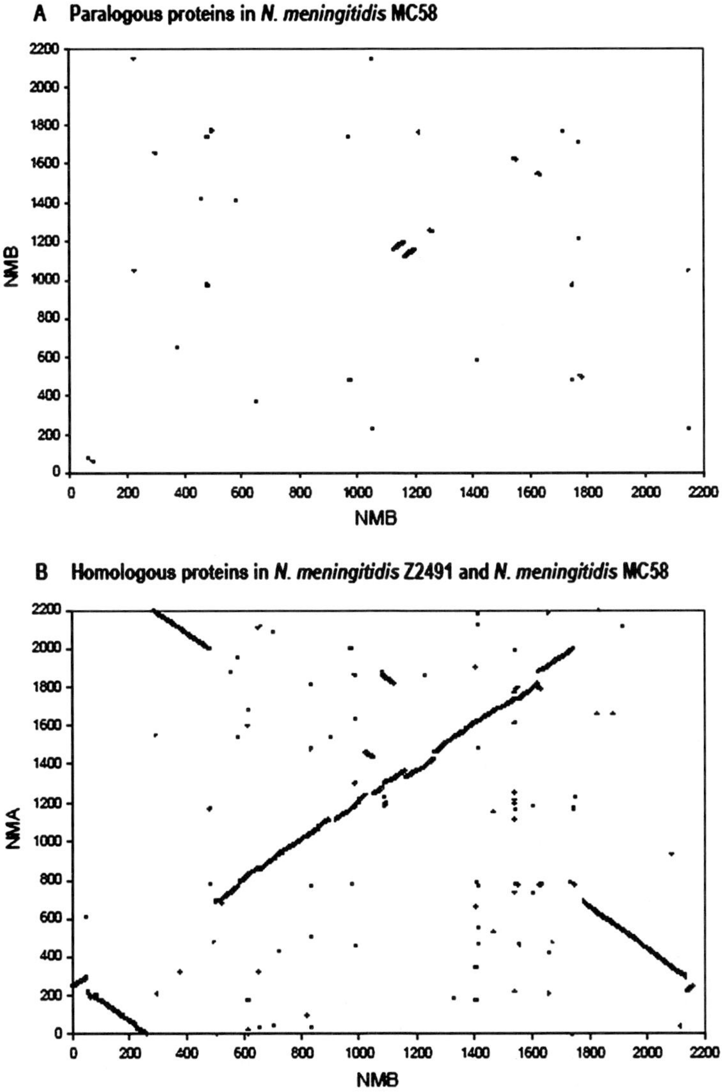

Fig. 5.1 Synteny plots showing (A) paralogous genes in the MC58 genome and (B) homologous genes in the two meningococcal genomes based on bi-directional best hit in reciprocal BLASTP analysis. The numbers of the corresponding coding sequences for *N. meningitidis* A Z2491 (NMA) and *N. meningitidis* B MC58 (NMB), respectively, are given on the x- and y-axes as indicated.

Bi-directional best hits in reciprocal BLASTP comparisons indicate that 1883 CDS may encode homologous proteins in *N. meningitidis* A Z2491 and *N. meningitidis* B MC58, respectively. As further can be seen in the synteny plots of Fig. 5.1 B, gene order is conserved over extended regions of the meningococcal genomes, although there are some rearrangements between the two chromo-

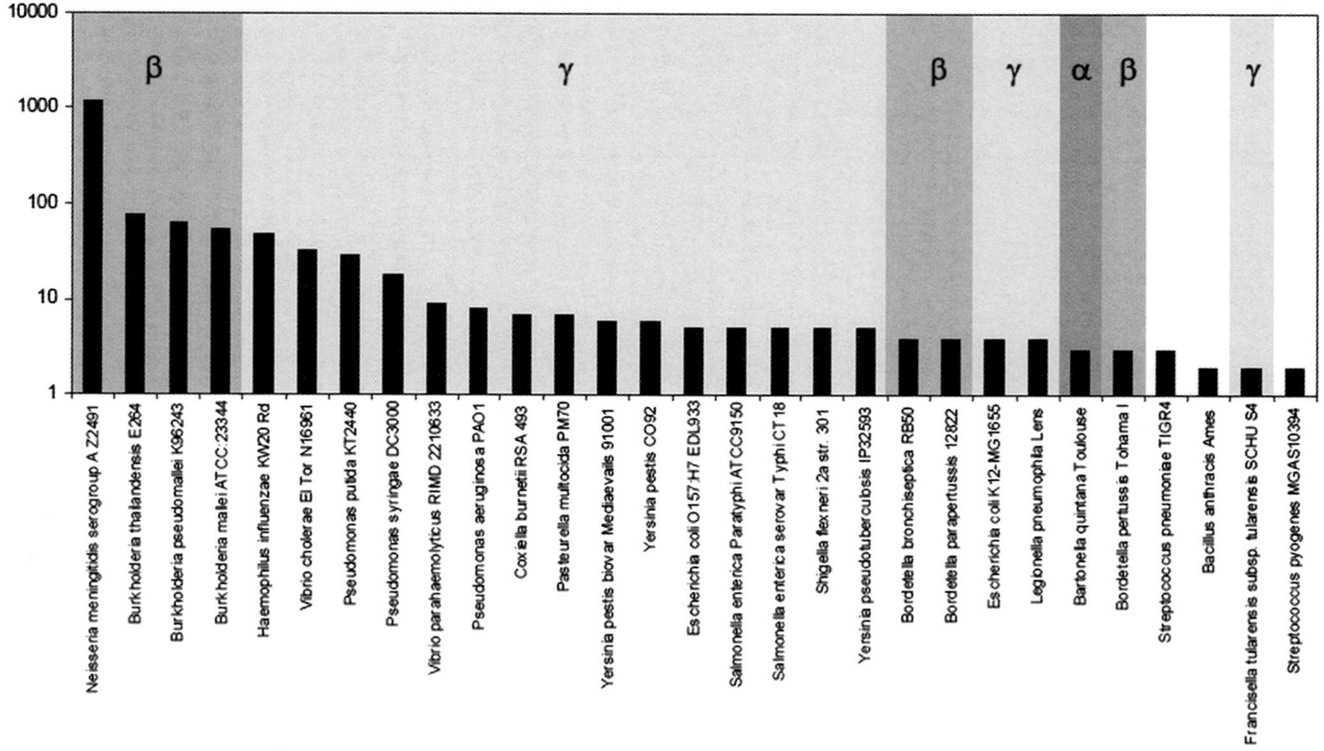

Fig. 5.2 Comparison of the *N. meningitidis* strain MC58 coding sequences to that of other completely sequenced organisms retrieved from the TIGR-CMR database. All putative CDS from *N. meningitidis* were searched against the putative CDS from all other genomes with FASTA3 and the number of *N. meningitidis* MC58 CDS whose highest similarity is to a CDS from a given species is shown (α, β, γ: α, β, γ subdivision of the Proteobacteria, respectively).

somes. In particular, relative to the MC58 chromosome, there is a large inversion of almost 1 Mb around the replication origin in the Z2491 genome which has already been identified by physical chromosomal mapping in the pre-genomic era [14, 15].

Based on the primary annotations of the encoded meningococcal proteome, biological roles could be assigned to about 60% of all CDS. According to the annotation given by NCBI, 70% of the encoded proteins could be assigned to approximately 1200 different COG, comprising 22 different functional classes (Fig. 5.3). Of these, approximately 30% belong to COG consisting of proteins with no specified function. Within the COG with functional assignment, the largest families are those involved in DNA replication and repair as well as protein and amino acid synthesis.

The fact that meningococci are fastidious bacteria being able to grow only on a restricted range of carbon sources finds its reflection in the metabolic blueprint deduced from the meningococcal genome sequences. As also confirmed by experimental proteomic approaches, *N. meningitidis* encodes the full set of enzymes of glycolysis with the exception of fructose-1-phosphate kinase and

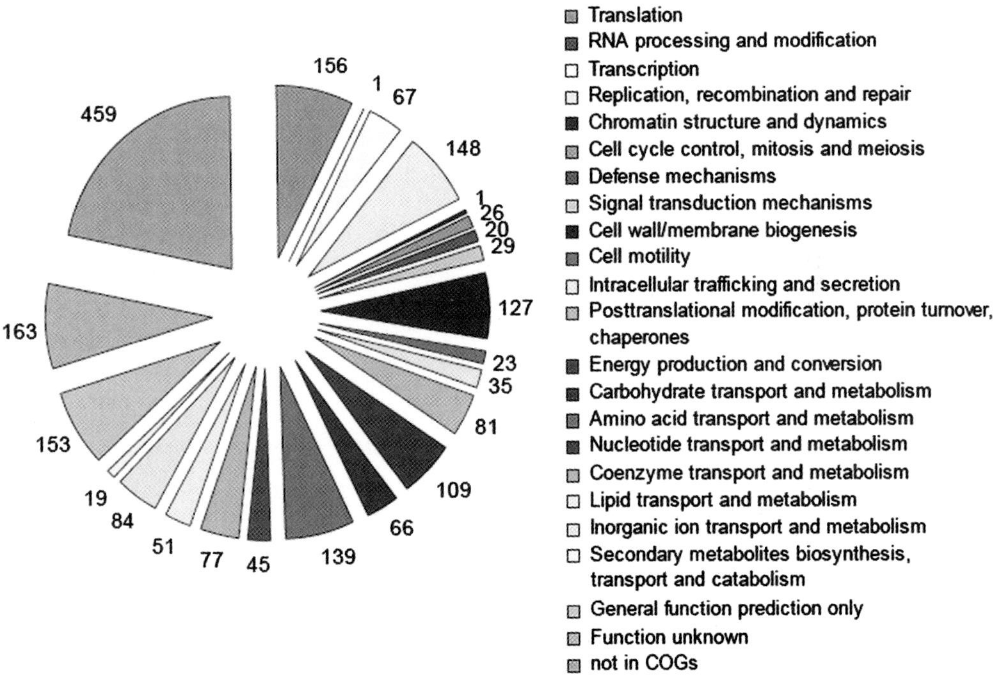

Fig. 5.3 Pie chart showing the percentage of *N. meningitidis* MC58 genes that are represented in each of the role families as indicated. The role category data shown was generated on the COG annotation of encoded proteome. (This figure also appears with the color plates.)

6-phosphofructokinase, the pyruvate dehydrogenase system, the pentose phosphate pathway, respiration, fermentation, and ATP-proton motive force. Based on the presence of homologs, *N. meningitidis* encodes all the usual citric acid cycle (CAC) enzymes. However, instead of a conventional cytoplasmic NAD-linked malate dehydrogenase the genome encodes a membrane-bound malate:quinone oxidoreductase which recycles oxaloacetate from malate [16]. In conclusion, meningococci are able to degrade glucose, the amino acids serine, proline, and glycine, and the organic acids acetate, gluconate, glutamate, lactate, malate, oxaloacetate, and pyruvate.

Genome analysis also revealed that *N. meningitidis* has a large number of ABC transporters and systems for scavenging iron, including previously recognized hemoglobin, transferrin, and lactoferrin binding proteins, as well as additional systems for iron acquisition, including siderophore acceptor and utilization homologs.

Regarding those categories that are potentially important for the pathogenesis of meningococcal disease, 9% of all functionally assigned CDS might be involved in cell wall/membrane biosynthesis, 5–6% for proteins involved in transport and binding functions and another 3% belong to the category of mobile element functions. The elucidation of the meningococcal genome sequences has also added a substantial number of novel putative virulence genes to the list of already known ones, bringing the total to 102 in strain MC58. These comprise the whole spectrum of virulence mechanisms, such as genes encoding the aforementioned iron acquisition proteins as well as genes encoding for adhesins, toxins, and proteins involved in capsule and lipopolysaccharide synthesis [3].

Besides these CDS, the genome of *N. meningitidis* also harbors a substantial number of pseudogenes. In particular, in a recent comprehensive analysis of pseudogenes in prokaryotes, among the 64 genomes compared (including 38 genomes from pathogenic species) the two *N. meningitidis* genomes had the second and third highest proportion of pseudogenes, respectively [17]. In the MC58 strain, transposase pseudogenes have been found in most of the 29 remnant insertion sequences, indicating that *N. meningitidis* strains probably undergo high selection pressure against transposases.

5.3
Repetitive DNA Sequences Abound in the Meningococcal Genomes

One of the most striking and unique characteristics of the annotated neisserial genomes is the abundance and diversity of repetitive DNA that contributes to both genome fluidity and physical variability, attesting to the adaptability of *N. meningitidis* and its potential to evade the human immune system.

5.3.1
DNA Uptake Sequences

The most obvious example is the neisserial DNA uptake sequence (DUS) involved in the recognition and uptake of DNA from the environment [18]. Briefly, there are nearly 2000 copies of the 10-bp uptake sequence in each genome which either occur alone or in inverted repeats as part of a transcriptional terminator [19]. Together with the high natural competence of the *Neisseriae*, this large number of DUS might facilitate the incorporation of foreign DNA bearing the appropriate DUS from lysed bacterial cells of the same [20–22] or related species [23, 24] via recombination into the meningococcal chromosome. This in turn results in a mosaicism of many chromosomal genes [22, 25, 26] as well as in a highly panmictic population structure [27, 28]. Remarkably, the DUS are not equally distributed over the entire genome and there is a significantly higher density of DUS within genes involved in DNA repair, recombination, restriction-modification and replication than in any other annotated gene group in these organisms [29]. This finding might reflect facilitated recovery from DNA damage after genotoxic stress caused by an adverse environment such as oxygen or modification of the pH, as occurs inside phagocytic vacuoles.

5.3.2
Simple Sequence Repeats

N. meningitidis has only a very limited number of two-component regulatory systems and other global regulators [30, 31]. However, loci termed "simple sequence contingency loci" provide an alternative mechanism of regulating gene expression, thus increasing the fitness of an organism by contributing to that organism's ability to rapidly respond to changing environmental conditions. These loci contain short tandem sequence repeats either within or 5′ to a coding region. The number of these tandemly repeated motifs can be modified during replication through slipped-strand mispairing and can consequently influence translation or transcription resulting in either a high frequency, reversible on–off switching of gene expression or an altered function and antigenicity of the encoded protein(s) (see also Chapter 6 for more details).

Early computational analyses identified 65 potentially phase variable genes in the MC58 genome sequence [32]. However, currently there is experimental evidence of phase variation for only 15 genes encoding proteins involved in the biosynthesis and modification of pili, capsular polysaccharide, lipopolysaccharide, as well as opacity proteins, hemoglobin receptors, PorA outer membrane protein, Opc outer membrane protein, ferric receptor, and a newly identified putative adhesin (*nadA*) [33]. Further computational analysis of the remaining 50 putative phase variable genes predicted that another 33 genes could be considered phase variable [33]. In a complementary approach based on a comparison of simple sequence repeats in the complete genome sequences of *N. meningitidis* strain Z2491 and *N. meningitidis* strain MC58, 68 phase-variable gene candidates

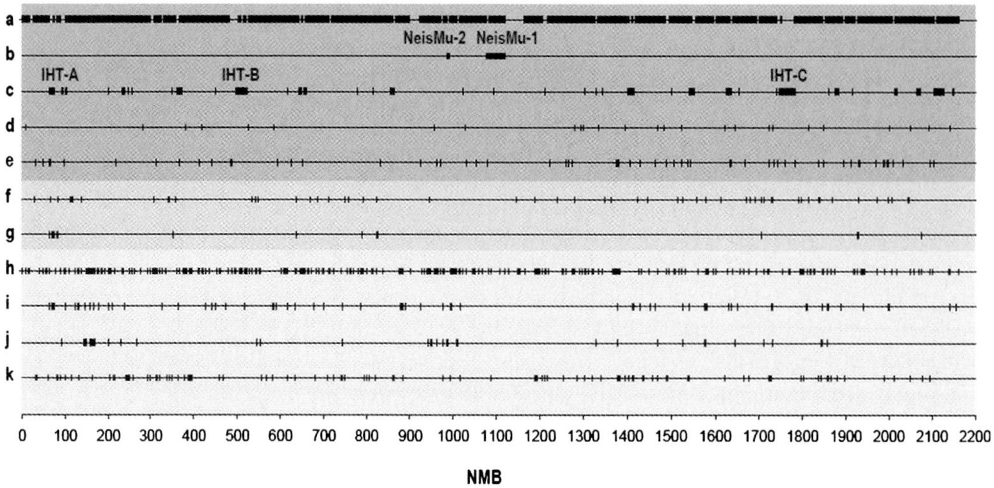

Fig. 5.4 Summary of the results of comparative and functional genomic studies using *N. meningitidis* B MC58 as model organism. Lanes a–e show the results of *in silico* analyses, lanes f and g show putative virulence proteins identified by STM, and lanes h–k show differentially regulated genes identified by DNA microarray analyses. The number of the *N. meningitidis* B MC58 CDSs (NMB1 to NMB2158) is depicted on the x-axis. Each protein is represented as a small vertical bar in lanes a–k. Proteins that have homologs based on reciprocal BLASTP comparisons in *N. meningitidis* A Z2491 are shown in lane a. Proteins encoded by the putative MC58 prophages NeisMu1 and NeisMu2 [53] are shown in lane b, and proteins putatively acquired via horizontal gene transfer in lane c [65]. Proteins containing coding tandem repeats are depicted in lane d [35] and putative phase variable ones in lane e [34]. Proteins found to be essential for bacteremia in an infant rat model as identified by STM are given in lane f [56] and those mediating resistance to complement-mediated lysis also identified by STM in lane g [57]. Adhesion to human bronchial epithelial cells [60], HeLa epithelial cells [59], and human brain microvascular endothelial cells [59] causes changes in the expression levels of genes encoding proteins as depicted in lanes h, i, and j, respectively. Finally, proteins encoded by iron-activated and -repressed Fur-dependent genes as revealed by transcriptome analysis are shown in lane k [63]. As can be seen in lanes f–k, virulence-associated proteins do not cluster in certain regions of the chromosome but rather are distributed almost randomly, indicating that virulence-associated proteins might not be encoded by pathogenicity islands.

in *N. meningitidis* strain Z2491 and 82 candidates in *N. meningitidis* strain MC58 were identified [32, 34] (Fig. 5.4, lane e). Therefore, these computationally derived numbers should not be considered as carved in stone. Irrespective of the differences in absolute numbers, the overall conclusion remains the same: *N. meningitidis* has the largest repertoire of phase variable genes described for any species so far.

In addition, in-frame changes in copy number of coding tandem repeats can also alter the function or antigenicity of the protein encoded [35]. In total, 25 and 26 candidate genes in the *N. meningitidis* Z2491 and the *N. meningitidis* MC58 genome, respectively, were identified, including known surface proteins as well as several putative lipoproteins, the Lip/H.8 antigen, AniA, and a putative adhesion (NMB0586) [35]. Remarkably, some of the genes identified encode proteins with cytoplasmic functions like sugar metabolism, DNA repair, and protein production.

Finally, *N. meningitidis* contains potentially phase-variable type III restriction-modification systems [36]. In the case of phase variation mediated by type III methyltransferases, genes may come under the influence of the methyltransferases by a few point mutations, generating a recognition site in a key position effecting transcriptional control of the gene [37].

5.3.3
IS Elements and Correia Repeats

The meningococcal genomes are also littered with insertion sequences (IS) and IS remnants. However, like the varying numbers of CDS given by the different annotations, the absolute number of putative IS elements differs due to differences in the annotation procedures. Mostly, these rely on the identification of CDS homologous to known transposases. Accordingly, a comparative analysis of the distribution of transposases among 80 bacterial genomes stored in the IS Finder database [38] reveals that *N. meningitidis* Z2491 and *N. meningitidis* MC58 have the fourth and eighth highest number of IS elements relative to the genome size [38]. For example, the genome of strain MC58 contains 22 intact and 29 remnant IS [3], which are mainly members of at least four specific families (Table 5.1) [2, 3].

Other repetitive sequence elements in the *N. meningitidis* genome are concentrated within intergenic repeat arrays of 200–2700 bp. These repeat arrays are composed of several different repeat types including larger units such as "Correia elements" (CE) which represent about 2% of the *N. meningitidis* genomes [39]. This abundance and percentage of nucleotides contained are unprecedented in other prokaryotic genomes. Correia elements are sequence indels comparable to small insertion sequences 100–155 bp in length with long terminal inverted repeats (TIR) and TA target site duplication, but in contrast to conventional IS elements, they do not encode a transposase [40–42]. They carry transcription initiation signals [43, 44] as well as functional integration host factor (IHF) binding sites [40, 45] and hence may play a role in modulating the expression of potential virulence genes [45]. Although estimates of the absolute numbers of CE again vary depending on the methodologies applied [2, 3, 41, 42] an asymmetric distribution of these elements was found among pathogenic *N. meningitidis* and nonpathogenic *Neisseria lactamica* strains, which might contribute to the distinct behaviors of each *Neisseria* species [39]. Like CE, repetitive extragenic palindromic sequences called REP2 were also found to influence the expression of a set of virulence genes, such as *pilC1* and *crgA*, which are necessary for the efficient interaction of *N. meningitidis* with host cells [46]. These elements are present at 26 copies in the Z2491 genome and contain promoter as well as ribosome binding sites [2].

5.3.4
Putative Genomic Islands

Larger entities of laterally transferred DNA called pathogenicity islands are frequently found in the genomes of many pathogenic bacteria and are generally characterized by atypical DNA composition [47]. Therefore, computational approaches like base composition analysis were performed in order to identify such regions in the meningococcal genomes. This resulted in the identification of at least 60 coding regions (nearly 5% in total) with a significantly lower G+C content when compared to the mean G+C content in the genome of strain Z2491, ranging in size from 224.0 bp to 11.3 kb and averaging 1.8 kb [2]. One-third of these regions encode proteins that are likely to be located on the surface of the cell or are responsible for the production of surface structures like the proteins of the serogroup A capsule cassette. Accordingly, three regions were identified in the MC58 genome and designated as putative islands of horizontally transferred DNA (IHTs; Fig. 5.4, lane c) coding (with the exception of IHT-A1) mostly for hypothetical proteins [3]. Similar to the situation in Z1491, IHT-A1 contains the genes for the capsule gene cluster, which is an important virulence determinant both in serogroup A and B meningococci. However, the genes for the serogroup A capsulation cluster do not generate the same IHT signature as IHT-A1 in MC58. The Z2491 genome contained only one such putative IHT that was not found to be present in the MC58 genome. Conversely, none of the MC58 IHTs could be found in the Z2491 genome. However, in striking contrast to what has been found in the Enterobacteriaceae, none of these putative islands have the typical hallmarks of canonical pathogenicity islands [47]. Although some of them code for proteins of paramount importance for neisserial pathogenicity and differ in G+C content and codon usage, almost all putative IHTs in the neisserial genomes are neither associated with tRNA loci, nor flanked by direct repeats, nor contain genes or pseudogenes coding for genetic mobility. As in the case of the *in silico* identification of putative CDS and IS elements, novel computational methods might nonetheless provide more evidence for the existence of a virulence gene pool that might be freely exchangeable between different meningococcal strains or even between *N. meningitidis* and other pathogenic bacteria via horizontal gene transfer [48, 49]. For example, using naïve Bayesian classifiers, 2% of the *N. meningitidis* genomes were classified as being of *H. influenzae* origin [50].

5.3.5
Computationally Identified Prophages

In contrast to pathogenicity islands, so far no uniform criteria have been established for the diagnosis of prophages in bacterial genome sequences [51]. Computational analyses based on the published genome sequences revealed three partially defective mosaic relatives of the Mu-like group of prophages in the genome of *N. meningitidis* Z2491, called Pnm1, Pnm2 and Pnm3, respectively

(Table 5.1). The MC58 genome contains similar prophages at the Pnm2 and Pnm3 sites, called NeisMu1 and NeisMu2, respectively (Table 5.1; Fig. 5.4, lane b); but it has no prophage at the Pnm1 integration site [52]. This type of phage integrates essentially randomly by a transposition mechanism. Thus, as the number of potential integration targets in any genome is huge, natural prophages of this type that are found at identical positions in the genomes of two independently isolated bacteria are extremely likely to be descendants of the same past phage integration event [53]. The finding that at least prophage Neis-Mu1 codes for membrane-associated antigenic proteins suggests that these proteins contribute to the variability in envelope structure and may thus influence virulence and pathogenicity [54]. In addition, a number of CTXφ-like phage genes were found in both genomes [53]. As outlined below, the existence of an integrated CTXφ-like prophage present in one (Z2491) and two (MC58) copies in the genomes of both strains could also experimentally be verified [55].

5.4
Genome-wide Mutational Analyses

The genome-wide functional analysis of N. meningitidis to identify virulence genes differs fundamentally from sequence-based methods that have been used to compile lists of pathogenicity genes, since such lists necessarily suffer from a subjective view of definitions. In search for more experimental evidence of the meningococcal virulence gene repertoire, signature-tagged mutagenesis (STM) has been used for the analysis of genes necessary for bacteremic infection in vivo [56] and mediating resistance to complement-mediated lysis in vitro [57], respectively.

Using the infant rat model, a library of 2850 insertional mutants of a clinical isolate of N. meningitidis serogroup B strain C311$^+$ were thus generated and analyzed for their capacity to cause systemic infection. In addition to eight genes encoding already known virulence factors, 65 genes were identified which have not been previously known to be involved in meningococcal pathogenesis (Fig. 5.4, lane f). Amongst others, two regulatory genes (ntrY, hfq) affecting the transcription at many loci were identified as well as two putative surface-associated ATP-binding cassette transporters. Seven mutants had insertions in genes necessary for the integrity of the cell envelope. Besides five genes encoding enzymes of the shikimate pathway, an additional six genes involved in amino acid biosynthesis were identified. Based on homology and the primary annotation, four of these 73 genes were not present in serogroup A strain Z2491: three of unknown function and the siaD gene which encodes the polysialyltransferase of the serogroup B capsular polysaccharide.

With a similar STM approach, 18 genes were identified that mediate resistance to complement-mediated lysis. In particular, four previously uncharacterized genes (NMB0065, NMB0352, NMB0638, NMB2076) involved in polysialic acid capsule production and LPS synthesis were found which, when mutated, rendered the N. meningitidis serogroup C strain used serum-sensitive [57]

(Fig. 5.4, lane g). As one might expect, all 18 genes identified were important for the synthesis of the polysialic acid capsule or the lipooligosaccharide, suggesting that these genes are likely to be the only meningococcal attributes necessary for serum resistance. However, since the authors only present the sequencing results for the first half of the library, corresponding to 2281 mutants, it may be too early still to draw definitive conclusions.

5.5
DNA Microarray Analyses

At present, several different microarrays derived from meningococcal as well as gonococcal genome sequences have been used either for genome comparisons or for the elucidation of gene expression patterns under *in vivo* conditions. Furthermore, microarray data are exploited to select antigens capable of inducing protective immunity for vaccine development.

5.5.1
Comparative Genomics

For example, DNA microarrays have already been used to analyze the genetic differences between various strains of the pathogenic *Neisseria* spp and the non-pathogenic *N. lactamica* in greater detail [58]. Comparison of eight different *N. meningitidis*, three different *N. gonorrhoeae*, and two different *N. lactamica* strains showed that 89% of the chromosome of Z2491 were shared with all other meningococcal strains, while strain-specific differences within the meningococci characterized the remaining 11% [58]. Most of the genes that were shared by all strains of *N. meningitidis* (78% of the chromosome; 1.7 Mb) were also present in all isolates of the three species and thus may correspond to the core neisserial genome. Among the *N. meningitidis*-specific sequences, only seven were >2 kb long. One of these regions corresponds to the *cps* locus specifying the production of capsular polysaccharide, which is known to be necessary for meningococcal virulence. Two other meningococcus-specific regions encode the production and secretion of the protein Frp of the RTX toxin family. One region encodes a protein with homology to proteins of the family of two-partner virulence factor secretion systems and would elaborate a 200-kDa protein with homology to the filamentous hemagglutinin of *Bordetella pertussis*. The remaining three encode a group of metabolic enzymes, a putative type I secretion system, and a disulfide oxidoreductase involved in the correct folding of secreted proteins, respectively. As the meningococcus specific regions are scattered as small islands around the chromosome dramatic differences in the pathogenic potential of the different *Neisseria* species might result from only small genetic changes [58]. In addition, many differences are strain- and not species-specific. This genomic organization therefore strongly supports the idea that *N. meningitidis* is essentially a commensal species [58].

By performing whole-genome comparisons of a greater collection of 29 invasive and 20 noninvasive meningococcal isolates, an 8-kb genetic island comprising nine CDS (corresponding to NMA1792–NMA1800 in the Z2491 genome) was found to be specific to hyperinvasive meningococcal complexes [55]. It is present in one copy in the Z2491 genome and in two copies in the MC58 genome. In support of the conception that it constitutes a genomic island, it was shown to have a low G+C content and a similarity in size and arrangement of CDS to filamentous bacteriophages, a group that includes the *Vibrio cholerae* phage CTXϕ which carries the cholera toxin. Accordingly, it encodes also a protein with homology to the CTXϕ replication protein RtsA. Sequences within a 20-bp inverted repeat called dRS3 (present several hundred times in the meningococcal chromosome [2]; Table 5.1) constitute the insertion site of the island. In support of these *in silico* findings, it was also experimentally shown that this element corresponds to an integrated phage genome which is able to excise from the chromosome and is secreted from the bacteria via the type IV pilin secretin (PilQ). As strains carrying this genetic island were significantly more likely to cause disease, it was termed "meningococcal disease associated (MDA) island". However, it is still currently unclear how this island contributes to the pathogenicity of the meningococci, since it seems not to contain genes coding for known virulence factors.

5.5.2 Transcriptomics

DNA microarrays based on the meningococcal genome sequence of strain MC58 were also used to study the transcriptome of serogroup B meningococci under different conditions. To cause meningitis, *N. meningitidis* has to interact consecutively at least with two distinct cell types: epithelial cells of the nasopharynx and cells of the blood–brain barrier. In addition, for hematogenic dissemination, meningococci have also to survive in the bloodstream. Therefore, transcriptome analyses were done after incubation of meningococci with the respective human cells [59–61] and with human serum [62]. As iron is a limiting factor for meningococcal growth in the human host, the transcriptional regulation in response to iron was also analyzed [63].

Host–cell contact of serogroup B meningococci to cultured human bronchial epithelial cells (16HBE14) induced changes in the expression of 347 genes in comparison to freely growing bacteria [60] (Fig. 5.4, line h). The upregulation of numerous genes encoding membrane proteins and transporters suggests that, upon cell contact, *N. meningitidis* undergoes substantial surface remodelling. From a selection of 12 upregulated genes, it was shown by flow cytometry that four proteins are only detectable on the bacterial surface after adhesion to the cells. The expression of five proteins increased upon interaction with host cells and three proteins were equally present on the surface of both adhering and nonadhering bacteria [60]. Furthermore, mice antisera of these 12 proteins were tested for their ability to mediate complement-dependent killing of serogroup B meningococci; and, indeed, five of the sera showed bactericidal activity.

To identify genes which are specifically regulated in pathogenic *Neisseria* upon contact with human bronchial epithelial cells, transcriptome analysis was also done with the apathogenic species *N. lactamica* [61]. Compared to 347 genes in *N. meningitidis,* 285 genes were differentially regulated in *N. lactamica.* Only 167 of the regulated genes were common to both bacteria, indicating that the different behavior of the two species most likely resides in the genes specifically regulated in meningococci and *N. lactamica,* respectively. The upregulation of transporters appeared to be more pronounced in meningococci. Especially the activation of the sulfate transport system, which is strictly linked to sulfur-containing amino acid metabolism, was the most striking difference between meningococci and *N. lactamica* after interaction with epithelial cells.

Another study investigated the transcriptome of the unencapsulated serogroup B strain MC58 in response to interaction with different cell types, i.e. during cell contact with human epithelial (HeLa) and brain microvascular endothelial cells (HBMEC), respectively [59]. Seventy-two genes were found to be differentially regulated in meningococci after contact with HeLa cells (Fig. 5.4, line i), and 48 genes were differentially regulated after contact with HBMEC (Fig. 5.4, line j), including a substantial number of well known virulence genes. Of the 13 CDS differentially regulated in both HeLa- and HBMEC-adherent meningococci, five (*rfaF, ilvI, tonB, exbD, gdhA*) were demonstrated to be essential for meningococcal pathogenesis in the infant rat model as outlined above [56]. However, only 21 of these genes were also found to be differentially regulated in the experiments with 16HBE14 bronchial epithelial cells (Fig. 5.4, lane h) [60], demonstrating the influence of the different experimental setups of these microarray studies.

In addition, transcriptome analysis of meningococci exposed to human serum in comparison to meningococci incubated in phosphate-buffered saline (PBS) revealed 279 differentially regulated genes which might therefore be important for meningococcal bacteremia [62]. These in particular included 55 genes coding for transporters and membrane proteins which might serve as antigens for the development of a novel vaccine against B meningococci. Of note, 34 of these genes were also previously shown to be essential in the infant rat model of meningococcal infection by signature-tagged mutagenesis as already described [56].

In Gram-negative bacteria, transcriptional regulation in response to iron (which is a limiting factor in the human host) is largely mediated by the ferric uptake regulator protein Fur. Therefore, DNA microarray technology was used together with computational analysis and *in vitro* binding studies to identify targets of the Fur protein in *N. meningitidis* MC58 [63]. Growth of meningococci in the presence of iron altered the expression of 235 genes in comparison to meningococci grown in iron-depleted medium (Fig. 5.4, line k). Under iron-depleted conditions, several virulence-associated genes were upregulated. Interestingly, a three-gene operon (NMB1436–NMB1438) was identified that was upregulated on iron addition. Subsequent characterization of this operon revealed its requirement for protection of serogroup B meningococci to hydrogen peroxide-mediated killing [64].

As already seen in the experimental comparisons of different neisserial genomes, the set of genes shown to be involved in pathogenesis seems to be distributed quite randomly over the entire meningococcal genome (Fig. 5.4, lanes f–k), again indicating that the concept of pathogenicity islands comprising genes responsible for the virulence might not be appropriate in the case of meningococci. In addition, many of the regulated genes encode proteins with unknown function, which highlights the limited knowledge of many genes involved in cell contact and virulence. However, although not totally identical, the results of the transcriptome analyses were in good agreement with those of the STM studies, recurrently identifying a common subset of genes comprising the already known virulence genes and some putative novel virulence gene candidates. As the results of pathogen gene expression are heavily influenced by the model system used, such results must nonetheless be interpreted with great care. In particular, expression data have limitations because mRNA levels may not reflect protein levels, and expression of a protein may not always have pathological consequences.

5.6 Conclusion

The full genome sequences of both meningococcal strains have already provided a wealth of new information about the genes potentially involved in pathogenesis. Besides the identification of a core neisserial genome, whole-genome comparisons of virulent and nonvirulent meningococci revealed a subset of common virulence-associated genes, like the aforementioned CTXϕ predominantly present in virulent lineages. In addition to these advances in the understanding of meningococcal disease, vaccine development has also already benefited from the genome projects.

References

1 Claus, H., M.C. Maiden, D.J. Wilson, N.D. McCarthy, K.A. Jolley, R. Urwin, F. Hessler, M. Frosch, U. Vogel **2005**, Genetic analysis of meningococci carried by children and young adults, *J Infect Dis* 191, 1263–1271.

2 Parkhill, J., M. Achtman, K.D. James, S.D. Bentley, C. Churcher, S.R. Klee, G. Morelli, D. Basham, D. Brown, T. Chillingworth, R.M. Davies, P. Davis, K. Devlin, T. Feltwell, N. Hamlin, S. Holroyd, K. Jagels, S. Leather, S. Moule, K. Mungall, M.A. Quail, M.A. Rajandream, K.M. Rutherford, M. Simmonds, J. Skelton, S. Whitehead, B.G. Spratt, B.G. Barrell **2000**, Complete DNA sequence of a serogroup A strain of Neisseria meningitidis Z2491, *Nature* 404, 502–506.

3 Tettelin, H., N.J. Saunders, J. Heidelberg, A.C. Jeffries, K.E. Nelson, J.A. Eisen, K.A. Ketchum, D.W. Hood, J.F. Peden, R.J. Dodson, W.C. Nelson, M.L. Gwinn, R. DeBoy, J.D. Peterson, E.K. Hickey, D.H. Haft, S.L. Salzberg, O. White, R.D. Fleischmann, B.A. Dougherty, T. Mason, A. Ciecko, D.S. Parksey, E. Blair, H. Cittone, E.B. Clark, M.D. Cotton, T.R. Utterback, H. Khouri, H.

Qin, J. Vamathevan, J. Gill, V. Scarlato, V. Masignani, M. Pizza, G. Grandi, L. Sun, H.O. Smith, C.M. Fraser, E.R. Moxon, R. Rappuoli, J.C. Venter **2000**, Complete genome sequence of Neisseria meningitidis serogroup B strain MC58, *Science* 287, 1809–1815.

4 Backman, A., P. Orvelid, J.A. Vazquez, O. Skold, P. Olcen **2000**, Complete sequence of a beta-lactamase-encoding plasmid in Neisseria meningitidis, *Antimicrob Agents Chemother* 44, 210–212.

5 Facinelli, B., P.E. Varaldo **1987**, Plasmid-mediated sulfonamide resistance in Neisseria meningitidis, *Antimicrob Agents Chemother* 31, 1642–1643.

6 Knapp, J.S., J.M. Zenilman, J.W. Biddle, G.H. Perkins, W.E. DeWitt, M.L. Thomas, S.R. Johnson, S.A. Morse **1987**, Frequency and distribution in the United States of strains of Neisseria gonorrhoeae with plasmid-mediated, high-level resistance to tetracycline, *J Infect Dis* 155, 819–822.

7 Dillon, J.A., K.H. Yeung **1989**, Beta-lactamase plasmids and chromosomally mediated antibiotic resistance in pathogenic Neisseria species, *Clin Microbiol Rev* 2[Suppl]: S125–S133.

8 Parkhill, J., M. Sebaihia, A. Preston, L.D. Murphy, N. Thomson, D.E. Harris, M.T. Holden, C.M. Churcher, S.D. Bentley, K.L. Mungall, A.M. Cerdeno-Tarraga, L. Temple, K. James, B. Harris, M.A. Quail, M. Achtman, R. Atkin, S. Baker, D. Basham, N. Bason, I. Cherevach, T. Chillingworth, M. Collins, A. Cronin, P. Davis, J. Doggett, T. Feltwell, A. Goble, N. Hamlin, H. Hauser, S. Holroyd, K. Jagels, S. Leather, S. Moule, H. Norberczak, S. O'Neil, D. Ormond, C. Price, E. Rabbinowitsch, S. Rutter, M. Sanders, D. Saunders, K. Seeger, S. Sharp, M. Simmonds, J. Skelton, R. Squares, S. Squares, K. Stevens, L. Unwin, S. Whitehead, B.G. Barrell, D.J. Maskell **2003**, Comparative analysis of the genome sequences of Bordetella pertussis, Bordetella parapertussis and Bordetella bronchiseptica, *Nat Genet* 35, 32–40.

9 Harrison, A., D.W. Dyer, A. Gillaspy, W.C. Ray, R. Mungur, M.B. Carson, H. Zhong, J. Gipson, M. Gipson, L.S. Johnson, L. Lewis, L.O. Bakaletz, R.S. Munson, Jr. **2005**, Genomic sequence of an otitis media isolate of nontypeable Haemophilus influenzae: comparative study with H. influenzae serotype d, strain KW20, *J Bacteriol* 187, 4627–4636.

10 Tettelin, H., K.E. Nelson, I.T. Paulsen, J.A. Eisen, T.D. Read, S. Peterson, J. Heidelberg, R.T. DeBoy, D.H. Haft, R.J. Dodson, A.S. Durkin, M. Gwinn, J.F. Kolonay, W.C. Nelson, J.D. Peterson, L.A. Umayam, O. White, S.L. Salzberg, M.R. Lewis, D. Radune, E. Holtzapple, H. Khouri, A.M. Wolf, T.R. Utterback, C.L. Hansen, L.A. McDonald, T.V. Feldblyum, S. Angiuoli, T. Dickinson, E.K. Hickey, I.E. Holt, B.J. Loftus, F. Yang, H.O. Smith, J.C. Venter, B.A. Dougherty, D.A. Morrison, S.K. Hollingshead, C.M. Fraser **2001**, Complete genome sequence of a virulent isolate of Streptococcus pneumoniae, *Science* 293, 498–506.

11 Gattiker, A., K. Michoud, C. Rivoire, A.H. Auchincloss, E. Coudert, T. Lima, P. Kersey, M. Pagni, C.J. Sigrist, C. Lachaize, A.L. Veuthey, E. Gasteiger, A. Bairoch **2003**, Automated annotation of microbial proteomes in SWISS-PROT, *Comput Biol Chem* 27, 49–58.

12 Bernardini, G., G. Renzone, M. Comanducci, R. Mini, S. Arena, C. D'Ambrosio, S. Bambini, L. Trabalzini, G. Grandi, P. Martelli, M. Achtman, A. Scaloni, G. Ratti, A. Santucci **2004**, Proteome analysis of Neisseria meningitidis serogroup A, *Proteomics* 4, 2893–2926.

13 Skovgaard, M., L.J. Jensen, S. Brunak, D. Ussery, A. Krogh **2001**, On the total number of genes and their length distribution in complete microbial genomes, *Trends Genet* 17, 425–428.

14 Dempsey, J.A., A.B. Wallace, J.G. Cannon **1995**, The physical map of the chromosome of a serogroup A strain of Neisseria meningitidis shows complex rearrangements relative to the chromosomes of the two mapped strains of the closely related species N. gonorrhoeae, *J Bacteriol* 177, 6390–6400.

15 Gaher, M., K. Einsiedler, T. Crass, W. Bautsch, **1996**, A physical and genetic

map of Neisseria meningitidis B1940, *Mol Microbiol* 19, 249–259.
16 Leighton, M.P., D.J. Kelly, M.P. Williamson, J.G. Shaw **2001**, An NMR and enzyme study of the carbon metabolism of Neisseria meningitidis, *Microbiology* 147, 1473–1482.
17 Liu, Y., P.M. Harrison, V. Kunin, M. Gerstein **2004**, Comprehensive analysis of pseudogenes in prokaryotes: widespread gene decay and failure of putative horizontally transferred genes, *Genome Biol* 5, R64.
18 Goodman, S.D., J.J. Scocca **1988**, Identification and arrangement of the DNA sequence recognized in specific transformation of Neisseria gonorrhoeae, *Proc Natl Acad Sci USA* 85, 6982–6986.
19 Smith, H.O., M.L. Gwinn, S.L. Salzberg **1999**, DNA uptake signal sequences in naturally transformable bacteria, *Res Microbiol* 150, 603–616.
20 Frosch, M., T.F. Meyer **1992**, Transformation-mediated exchange of virulence determinants by co-cultivation of pathogenic Neisseriae, *FEMS Microbiol Lett* 79, 345–349.
21 Linz, B., M. Schenker, P. Zhu, M. Achtman **2000**, Frequent interspecific genetic exchange between commensal Neisseriae and Neisseria meningitidis, *Mol Microbiol* 36, 1049–1058.
22 Zhou, J., L.D. Bowler, B.G. Spratt **1997**, Interspecies recombination, and phylogenetic distortions, within the glutamine synthetase and shikimate dehydrogenase genes of Neisseria meningitidis and commensal Neisseria species, *Mol Microbiol* 23, 799–812.
23 Kroll, J.S., K.E. Wilks, J.L. Farrant, P.R. Langford **1998**, Natural genetic exchange between Haemophilus and Neisseria: intergeneric transfer of chromosomal genes between major human pathogens, *Proc Natl Acad Sci USA* 95, 12381–12385.
24 Davis, J., A.L. Smith, W.R. Hughes, M. Golomb **2001**, Evolution of an autotransporter: domain shuffling and lateral transfer from pathogenic Haemophilus to Neisseria, *J Bacteriol* 183, 4626–4635.
25 Fudyk, T.C., I.W. Maclean, J.N. Simonsen, E.N. Njagi, J. Kimani, R.C. Brunham, F.A. Plummer **1999**, Genetic diversity and mosaicism at the por locus of Neisseria gonorrhoeae, *J Bacteriol* 181, 5591–5599.
26 Maiden, M.C., B. Malorny, M. Achtman **1996**, A global gene pool in the neisseriae., *Mol Microbiol* 21, 1297–1298.
27 Maiden, M.C.J. **1993**, Population genetics of a transformable bacterium: the influence of horizontal genetic exchange on the biology of Neisseria meningitidis, *FEMS Microbiol Lett* 112, 243–250.
28 Smith, J.M., N.H. Smith, M. O'Rourke, B.G. Spratt **1993**, How clonal are bacteria? *Proc Natl Acad Sci USA* 90, 4384–4388.
29 Davidsen, T., E.A. Rodland, K. Lagesen, E. Seeberg, T. Rognes, T. Tonjum **2004**, Biased distribution of DNA uptake sequences towards genome maintenance genes, *Nucleic Acids Res* 32, 1050–1058.
30 Galperin, M.Y. **2005**, A census of membrane-bound and intracellular signal transduction proteins in bacteria: Bacterial IQ, extroverts and introverts, *BMC Microbiol* 5, 35.
31 Ashby, M.K. **2004**, Survey of the number of two-component response regulator genes in the complete and annotated genome sequences of prokaryotes, *FEMS Microbiol Lett* 231, 277–281.
32 Saunders, N.J., A.C. Jeffries, J.F. Peden, D.W. Hood, H. Tettelin, R. Rappuoli, E.R. Moxon **2000**, Repeat-associated phase variable genes in the complete genome sequence of Neisseria meningitidis strain MC58, *Mol Microbiol* 37, 207–215.
33 Martin, P., T. van de Ven, N. Mouchel, A.C. Jeffries, D.W. Hood, E.R. Moxon **2003**, Experimentally revised repertoire of putative contingency loci in Neisseria meningitidis strain MC58: evidence for a novel mechanism of phase variation, *Mol Microbiol* 50, 245–257.
34 Snyder, L.A.S., S.A. Butcher, N.J. Saunders **2001**, Comparative whole-genome analyses reveal over 100 putative phase-variable genes in the pathogenic Neisseria spp, *Microbiology* 147, 2321–2332.
35 Jordan, P., L.A. Snyder, N.J. Saunders **2003**, Diversity in coding tandem repeats

in related Neisseria spp, *BMC Microbiol* 3, 23.

36 Seib, K. L., I. R. Peak, M. P. Jennings **2002**, Phase variable restriction-modification systems in Moraxella catarrhalis, *FEMS Immunol Med Microbiol* 32, 159–165.

37 Srikhanta, Y. N., T. L. Maguire, K. J. Stacey, S. M. Grimmond, M. P. Jennings **2005**, The phasevarion: a genetic system controlling coordinated, random switching of expression of multiple genes, *Proc Natl Acad Sci USA* 102, 5547–5551.

38 Mahillon, J., M. Chandler **1998**, Insertion sequences, *Microbiol Mol Biol Rev* 62, 725–774.

39 De Gregorio, E., C. Abrescia, M. S. Carlomagno, P. P. Di Nocera **2003**, Asymmetrical distribution of Neisseria miniature insertion sequence DNA repeats among pathogenic and nonpathogenic Neisseria strains, *Infect Immun* 71, 4217–4221.

40 Buisine, N., C. M. Tang, R. Chalmers **2002**, Transposon-like Correia elements: structure, distribution and genetic exchange between pathogenic Neisseria sp. *FEBS Lett* 522, 52–58.

41 Liu, S. V., N. J. Saunders, A. Jeffries, R. F. Rest **2002**, Genome analysis and strain comparison of correia repeats and correia repeat-enclosed elements in pathogenic Neisseria, *J Bacteriol* 184, 6163–6173.

42 Mazzone, M., E. De Gregorio, A. Lavitola, C. Pagliarulo, P. Alifano, P. P. Di Nocera **2001**, Whole-genome organization and functional properties of miniature DNA insertion sequences conserved in pathogenic Neisseriae, *Gene* 278, 211–222.

43 Snyder, L. A., W. M. Shafer, N. J. Saunders **2003**, Divergence and transcriptional analysis of the division cell wall (dcw) gene cluster in Neisseria spp. *Mol Microbiol* 47, 431–442.

44 Black, C., J. Fyfe, J. Davies **1995**, A promoter associated with the neisserial repeat can be used to transcribe the uvrB gene from Neisseria gonorrhoeae, *J Bacteriol* 177, 1952–1958.

45 Rouquette-Loughlin, C. E., J. T. Balthazar, S. A. Hill, W. M. Shafer **2004**, Modulation of the mtrCDE-encoded efflux pump gene complex of Neisseria meningitidis due to a Correia element insertion sequence, *Mol Microbiol* 54, 731–741.

46 Morelle, S., E. Carbonnelle, X. Nassif **2003**, The REP2 repeats of the genome of Neisseria meningitidis are associated with genes coordinately regulated during bacterial cell interaction, *J Bacteriol* 185, 2618–2627.

47 Hentschel, U., J. Hacker **2001**, Pathogenicity islands: the tip of the iceberg, *Microbes Infect* 3, 545–548.

48 Tsirigos, A., I. Rigoutsos **2005**, A sensitive, support-vector-machine method for the detection of horizontal gene transfers in viral, archaeal and bacterial genomes, *Nucleic Acids Res* 33, 3699–3707.

49 Merkl, R. **2004**, SIGI: score-based identification of genomic islands, *Bioinformatics* 5, 22.

50 Sandberg, R., G. Winberg, C. I. Branden, A. Kaske, I. Ernberg, J. Coster **2001**, Capturing whole-genome characteristics in short sequences using a naive Bayesian classifier, *Genome Res* 11, 1404–1409.

51 Canchaya, C., C. Proux, G. Fournous, A. Bruttin, H. Brussow **2003**, Prophage genomics, *Microbiol Mol Biol Rev* 67, 238–276.

52 Morgan, G. J., G. F. Hatfull, S. Casjens, R. W. Hendrix **2002**, Bacteriophage Mu genome sequence: analysis and comparison with Mu-like prophages in Haemophilus, Neisseria and Deinococcus, *J Mol Biol* 317, 337–359.

53 Casjens, S. **2003**, Prophages and bacterial genomics: what have we learned so far? *Mol Microbiol* 49, 277–300.

54 Masignani, V., M. M. Giuliani, H. Tettelin, M. Comanducci, R. Rappuoli, V. Scarlato **2001**, Mu-like prophage in serogroup B Neisseria meningitidis coding for surface-exposed antigens, *Infect Immun* 69, 2580–2588.

55 Bille, E., J. R. Zahar, A. Perrin, S. Morelle, P. Kriz, K. A. Jolley, M. C. Maiden, C. Dervin, X. Nassif, C. R. Tinsley **2005**, A chromosomally integrated bacteriophage in invasive meningococci, *J Exp Med* 201, 1905–1913.

56 Sun, Y. H., S. Bakshi, R. Chalmers, C. M. Tang **2000**, Functional genomics of Neis-

seria meningitidis pathogenesis, *Nat Med* 6, 1269–1273.

57 Geoffroy, M.C., S. Floquet, A. Metais, X. Nassif, V. Pelicic **2003**, Large-scale analysis of the meningococcus genome by gene disruption: resistance to complement-mediated lysis, *Genome Res* 13, 391–298.

58 Perrin, A., S. Bonacorsi, E. Carbonnelle, D. Talibi, P. Dessen, X. Nassif, C. Tinsley **2002**, Comparative genomics identifies the genetic islands that distinguish Neisseria meningitidis, the agent of cerebrospinal meningitis, from other Neisseria species *Infect Immun* 70, 7063–7072.

59 Dietrich, G., S. Kurz, C. Hubner, C. Aepinus, S. Theiss, M. Guckenberger, U. Panzner, J. Weber, M. Frosch **2003**, Transcriptome analysis of Neisseria meningitidis during infection, *J Bacteriol* 185, 155–164.

60 Grifantini, R., E. Bartolini, A. Muzzi, M. Draghi, E. Frigimelica, J. Berger, G. Ratti, R. Petracca, G. Galli, M. Agnusdei, M.M. Giuliani, L. Santini, B. Brunelli, H. Tettelin, R. Rappuoli, F. Randazzo, G. Grandi **2002**, Previously unrecognized vaccine candidates against group B meningococcus identified by DNA microarrays, *Nat Biotechnol* 20, 914–921.

61 Grifantini, R., E. Bartolini, A. Muzzi, M. Draghi, E. Frigimelica, J. Berger, F. Randazzo, G. Grandi **2002**, Gene expression profile in Neisseria meningitidis and Neisseria lactamica upon host-cell contact: from basic research to vaccine development, *Ann NY Acad Sci* 975, 202–216.

62 Kurz, S., C. Hubner, C. Aepinus, S. Theiss, M. Guckenberger, U. Panzner, J. Weber, M. Frosch, G. Dietrich **2003**, Transcriptome-based antigen identification for Neisseria meningitidis, *Vaccine* 21, 768–775.

63 Grifantini, R., S. Sebastian, E. Frigimelica, M. Draghi, E. Bartolini, A. Muzzi, R. Rappuoli, G. Grandi, C.A. Genco, **2003**, Identification of iron-activated and -repressed Fur-dependent genes by transcriptome analysis of Neisseria meningitidis group B, *Proc Natl Acad Sci USA* 100, 9542–9547.

64 Grifantini, R., E. Frigimelica, I. Delany, E. Bartolini, S. Giovinazzi, S. Balloni, S. Agarwal, G. Galli, C. Genco, G. Grandi **2004**, Characterization of a novel Neisseria meningitidis Fur and iron-regulated operon required for protection from oxidative stress: utility of DNA microarray in the assignment of the biological role of hypothetical genes, *Mol Microbiol* 54, 962–979.

65 Garcia-Vallve, S., E. Guzman, M.A. Montero, A. Romeu **2003**, HGT-DB: a database of putative horizontally transferred genes in prokaryotic complete genomes, *Nucleic Acids Res* 31, 187–189.

6
Phase Variation and Adaptive Strategies of *N. meningitidis*: Insights into the Biology of a Commensal and Pathogen

Peter M. Power and E. Richard Moxon

6.1
Introduction

The ability of microbes to adapt quickly to highly selective and dynamic host environments is of key importance and is well exemplified by the obligate human pathogen *Neisseria meningitidis*. In general, bacteria adapt to environments through gene regulation and gene variation. The *N. meningitidis* genome is relatively small ($\sim$2 Mb) and lacks many of the classic gene regulatory mechanisms found in other bacteria. For example, the genomes of *N. meningitidis* contain only a limited number of two-component systems and sigma factors. But, it possesses a plethora of mechanisms for promoting gene variation through mutation, including a large number of tandem single nucleotide, or short motif, repeat sequences. The hypermutability of repetitive DNA modulates the expression of genes in *Neisseria* by a process called phase variation (high frequency, reversible, on–off switching of gene expression) although other genetic switching mechanisms are also used. These hypermutable loci have been called contingency genes to emphasize their role in facilitating the exploration and adaptation of microbes to the dynamic variability and changes in the host environments, including adaptation to novel combinations of innate and acquired immune clearance mechanisms [1, 4]. Thus, a single bacterium can give rise to progeny that express a diverse range of phenotypes and from these variants, organisms of increased fitness are selected. The characterization of phase variable contingency genes is therefore critical to a better understanding of both the commensal and pathogenic behavior of *N. meningitidis*. This chapter will examine the molecular mechanisms, role and implications of phase variation in *N. meningitidis*.

Adaptive behavior in microbes has been examined in a number of reviews [1–5] and is a feature of other human bacterial pathogens, including *N. gonorrhoeae*, *Haemophilus influenzae* [6], *Heliobacter pylori* [7] and *Campylobacter jejuni* [8]. *N. meningitidis* is one of the best characterized and is a model organism for studying the biological implications of contingency genes.

Handbook of Meningococcal Disease. Infection Biology, Vaccination, Clinical Management.
Edited by M. Frosch and M.C.J. Maiden

ISBN: 3-527-31260-9

6.2
Early Studies and Genome Sequencing Identify Large Numbers of Phase-variable Genes

Changes in *N. gonorrhoeae* colony morphology were the basis of some of the first reports of phase variation in *Neisseria*. Kellogg et al. [9, 10] examined colony morphology and noted reversible changes in color, opacity and size. Sectoring of colonies (where, based on inspection by eye, there are within individual colonies segments with different phenotypic characteristics) was also observed. Subsequently, similar findings were obtained by Blake et al. [11] on *N. meningitidis* grown in candle jars at 30 °C. Importantly, colony phenotype was linked to changes in the expression of cell surface structures, such as capsule [12], pili 13], pilin glycosylation [14], Opa [15], Opc [16], LPS [17, 18] and PorA [19, 20] as phase variable structures. The molecular mechanisms of phase variation were elucidated and the importance of repetitive DNA was one of the key factors identified.

The sequencing of several neisserial genomes lead to the identification of up to 100 different simple DNA repeats having the potential to mediate phase variation of genes in the *N. meningitidis* strains MC58, Z2491 and *N. gonorrhoeae* strain FA1090 genomes [23]. These include a number of virulence factors including restriction-modification systems, metabolic proteins, bacteriocins and surface expressed proteins [21, 22]. The preponderance of cell surface exposed structures displaying phase variation is an indication of their importance in adaptation to new

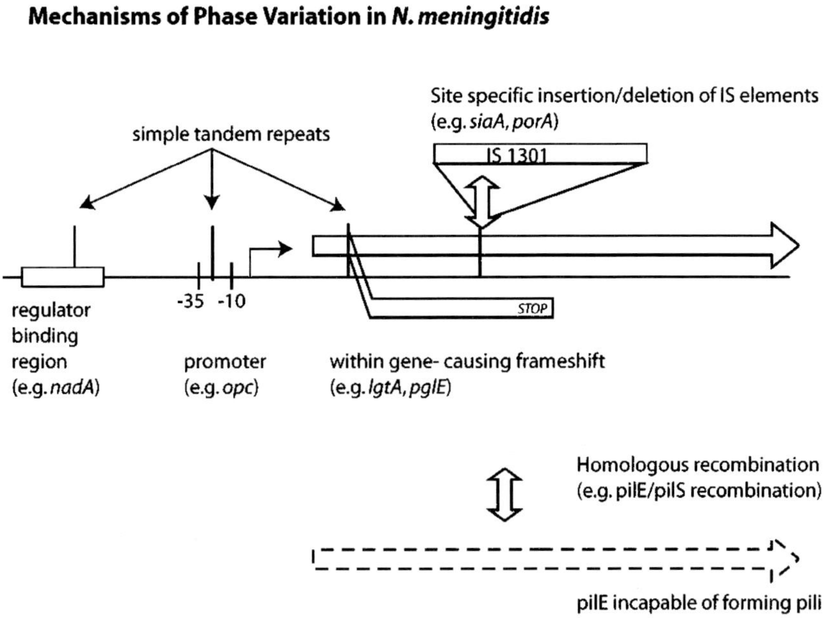

Fig. 6.1 Mechanisms of phase variation in *N. meningitidis*.

Table 6.1 Molecular mechanisms of phase variation.

Mechanism	Description	Presence (+) or absence (–) in *N. meningitidis*
Repetitive DNA-mediated	Tracts of tandemly repetitive DNA which lose or gain units at high frequency	
Homopolymeric tracts or tandem repeats	Commonly poly G or C tracts (sometimes A or T) or tandem repeats with units of 2, 4, 5, 7, 8 nt, etc.	
Within coding regions	Causing frameshifts and premature termination	+, *lgtA, pglA, pilC1, pilC2*
Outside coding regions:		
(a) Promoter	Within promoter affecting transcription	+, *opc* [16]
(b) Regulation	Within regulatory elements of ORF	+, *nadA* [24]
Homologous recombination	Site-specific homologous recombination which results in the production of non-functional proteins	+, *pilE*
Insertional sequences	IS elements which can site specifically reversibly insert into ORFs disrupting expression	+, *IS1301*
Site-specific inversion	Site-specific sequence inversions which alters the location of promoters or regulatory elements relative to the ORF	–
Dam methylation-controlled	Regulation of phase variation by a mechanism involving differential Dam methylation states	–

hosts and different environmental niches during neisserial infection. From a public health perspective, it should also be noted that these surface determinates include potential targets for innate and acquired immune system clearance mechanisms, so their intrinsic capacity for variation is a matter of great relevance to understanding *N. meningitidis* virulence and the development of vaccines to prevent the invasive diseases caused by this important pathogen.

Multiple mechanisms result in phase variation; and Fig. 6.1 and Table 6.1 summarize the mechanisms of phase variation identified to date in *N. meningitidis*.

6.3
Repetitive DNA Mediates Most Phase Variation

Most phase variation in *N. meningitidis* is mediated by tracts of repetitive DNA, but these tracts differ in sequence, length and the mechanism of mediating phase variation. Tracts of repetitive DNA are prevalent in the genomes of *N. meningitidis* and are mutational "hotspots". Through slippage-like mechanisms, loss or gain of repeat units occurs during DNA replication or repair; and these events have consequences for translation or transcription. Tracts of repetitive DNA which mediate phase variation range from short homopolymeric tracts of seven nucleotides to hepta-nucleotide repeats of several hundred base pairs. Homopolymeric tracts of guanidine (G) or cytosine (C) are the most frequent, examples being the *hmbR*, *porA* and *pglA* genes [18, 20, 25]. Tandem repeats of units of 2, 4, 5, 7, 8 nucleotides are also found upstream or within the open reading frames (ORFs) whose expression they regulate. Typically, the loss or gain of repeat units (usually a single unit) located within an ORF results in frameshifting that affects translation and results in a truncated nonfunctional protein [26]. However, repeat tracts may be located outside of the coding region, for example within the promoter region. Thus, upstream of the *porA* gene, there is a tract of guanidine residues between the –10 and –35 of the core promoter that mediates phase variation [20]. Because transcription initiation of these genes relies on precise spacing between the –35 and –10 elements, variations in the length of the repeat region can alter transcriptional activity. Another mechanism by which repetitive DNA located upstream of the reading frame can mediate phase variation is by disrupting the binding of transcriptional regulators, exemplified by NadA [24], as discussed later in this chapter.

6.4
When is a "Potentially Phase-variable Gene" Really Phase Variable?

The presence of repetitive DNA does not necessarily correlate with the capacity for phase variation. The identification of potentially phase variable genes by searching genomes for repetitive DNA, first described by Hood et al. [6] in *H. influenzae*, was applied to the neisserial genomes [21, 23] and identified 82 and 68 candidate phase variation genes in strains MC58 and Z2491 respectively, only 14 of which had been previously identified. The process of identifying potentially phase variable genes involved detection of tracts of repetitive DNA of certain lengths: homopolymeric tracts of >6 G/C, >8 A/T, dinucleotides of >3, tetranucleotide or longer tracts of >2, or shorter tracts associated with an identified frame shift. Then, the sequence context of the repeats was examined (e.g. proximity to predicted or known genes). Finally, comparison between the three genome strains was undertaken to look for polymorphisms [23]. Interstrain differences in the length of repeat tracts of 20 different potentially phase variable genes were examined in 19 genetically distinct *N. meningitidis* strains, as well as three *N. gonorrhoeae* and four *N. lactamica* strains [24]. Tracts of G or C residues longer than five bases or tracts of As or Ts longer than ten were shown to be polymorphic between strains and were therefore considered potential mediators of phase variation. Exceptions included *siaD*, in which there is a run of only seven Cs, but phase variation is known to occur. Similarly a tract of seven As in PorA was associated with phase variation [27]. Dinucleotide repeats were not associated with phase variation.

6.5 Mechanisms of Phase Variation: An Example of Convergent Evolution

6.5.1 Reversible Insertion of Insertional Elements Mediates Phase Variation in Some Genes

Two mechanisms of phase variation that do not depend on repetitive DNA are mediated by insertional elements and atypical recombination in the PilE locus. *IS1301* mediates of phase variation in *N. meningitidis* through its insertion into and excision from genes. Genes that are phase variable by this mechanism include *siaA* [28], *siaD* [29], *synA* [12], *oatWY* [30], *porA* [31] and *nadA* [32] and are responsible for capsule expression, sialic acid expression, O-acetylation of capsule and outer membrane protein expression, respectively. *IS1301* elements are found predominantly in *N. meningitidis* serogroups 29E, W135, X and Y, with 2–17 copies per genome [33], but are rarely found in serogroups A, B and C associated with epidemic meningococcal disease, *N. gonorrhoeae* and nonpathogenic species [33]. The location of most *IS1301* and other IS elements is not known and could indicate a larger repertoire of genes than has been identified to date. Interestingly, a number of the genes identified as having *IS1301* elements are genes where phase variation occurs by other mechanisms (e.g. *siaD, nadA, porA*).

6.5.2 Unidirectional Recombination of *pilE* Locus Results in Pili Phase Variation

The pili of *N. meningitidis* are important for commensal and virulence behaviour and are involved in adherence and invasion. Pili are long filamentous surface structures primarily composed of thousands of subunits encoded by *pilE*. Antigenic variation of pili is important in *N. meningitidis* and has structural, functional and immunological implications. In *pilE/pilS* antigenic variation, unidirectional RecA-dependent homologous recombination occurs between the *pilE* gene and a number of silent (nonexpressed) *pilS* genes. The outcome of these homologous recombination events is usually a change in *pilE* sequence. However, occasionally, these recombination events result in a spectrum of phenotypes ranging from absence, lesser or greater expression of pili. These variants differ in their transformability, immunogenicity and adherence [34]. In the *pilE/pilS* system, pilus expression phase varies from on → off → on via homologous recombination between *pilS* and *pilE*, although the homologous recombination system is not the major mechanism of *pilE/pilS* phase variation.

6.6
Trans-acting Genetic and Environment Factors Regulate Phase Variation

Some strains of *N. meningitidis* exhibit high rates of phase variation that are especially prevalent in disease-causing strains. Fifty-seven percent of epidemic serogroup A *N. meningitidis* strains have substantially increased mutation rates, i.e. are mutators and also have increased rates of phase variation [35]. It has been proposed that these increased phase variation rates may contribute to the fitness of the organism by increasing the probability of successful colonisation, especially in transmission between hosts [35]. In addition to mutators, it has been proposed that there may be transient mutator states, such as those purported to occur in species such as *Escherichia coli* in response to stress. *N. meningitidis* lacks an SOS response, but there are reports of transiently increased rates of phase variation by other mechanisms and there has been some progress in identifying the molecular and the environmental factors that it has been proposed may trigger increased rates of phase variation. Of the utmost importance to the interpretation of these assertions is that it is critical to distinguish increases in rates of phase variation that reflect induction (through regulated responses to external environmental factors) as opposed to selection. Investigations of *N. meningitidis* mutator states include: (a) examination of the role of candidate genes such as *mutS* and *mutL, dinB* and *dam*, (b) mutant library screening and (c) investigation of possible environmental influences of phase variation, including transformation, adherence to host cells and iron levels.

Mutations in MutS or MutL are associated with changes in phase variable switching rates of a hemoglobin receptor (HmbR) whose phase variation is mediated by a tract of G residues. These mutator strains have a concurrent, generalized (genome-wide) increase in the frequency of mutations, as indicated by increases in the rates of rifampicin or nalidixic acid resistance [36]. *mutS* inactivation increased phase variation rates on a range of different *N. meningitidis* repeats; *siaD* C_7 tract, *spr* C_{10} tract, *lgtG* C_{12} tract, but did not increase phase variation rates of *nadA* with its $[TAAA]_9$ repeat tract [37]. Mutator alleles may arise when there are strong selective pressures leading to bottlenecks, as for example during transmission from one host to another. This is because such strains have a higher probability of generating mutations that confer fitness gains. These variants rise to fixation and the mutator allele hitch-hikes with the fitness mutation. However, mutators subsequently acquire deleterious mutations at higher frequency, lose fitness and, over time, tend to be eliminated.

Polymerase IV is involved in the SOS response in *E. coli* and, in addition to effecting efficient by-pass of specific mismatches that would otherwise interfere with efficient replication, its activity as a polymerase is also relatively error-prone. *Neisseria* lacks an SOS response [38] and, although DinB overexpression in *N. meningitidis* does not result in a general mutator phenotype, it does increase *siaD* (C_7 repeat) phase variation, but has no effect on *spr* (C_{10} repeat) or *lgtG* (C_{12} repeat) tracts [39]. These findings suggest that the effects of DinB may be confined to shorter repeat tracts. Later in this chapter, we will discuss the mechanisms for phase variation mediated by homopolymeric and longer tracts and the extent to which they are influenced by *trans*-acting factors.

The DNA glycosylase MutY, of the base excision pathway, is involved in protection against oxidative stress. MutY activity was examined in lysates of mutant and wild-type *N. meningitidis*. Mutation rates were increased 60–100-fold in the mutant when compared to the wild-type and this difference reflected the role of MutY in preventing GC to AT transversions. To date, this interesting finding has not been extended to include studies on the effect of MutY on phase variation rates, but it seems likely that MutY is an antimutator and that mutations would increase phase variation rates of many contingency genes.

Random screening of a library of transposon mutants for genes which affect rates of phase variation has revealed known mediators of phase variation of the mismatch repair genes *mutS*, *mutL* and *uvrD*, as well as other genes including *pilP*, *fbpA*, *fbpB*, *NMA1233* [40]. *fbpA* and *fbpB* are involved in iron transport and utilization and seem to affect phase variation rates to different extents depending on whether phase variation rates of G8 tracts are measured by HmbR or a UROS cassette reporter [40]. The role of the intergenic regions in modulation of phase variation is unknown.

Dam methylase, a key enzyme involved in methyl-directed mismatch repair, apparently does not affect phase variation rates. Rates of phase variation determined in *dam* mutants by Richardson and Stojiljkovic [35] and Martin et al. [39] in the *siaD* (C_7) gene were similar to wild-type rates. These results are in contrast to published results where the mutant apparently had a significant effect on the phase variation rate of a *siaD* (C_7) phase variation [41]. In about two-thirds of *N. meningitidis* disease isolates, the *dam* gene is replaced by *drg* and this replacements does not change the frequency of phase variation [36, 39].

N. meningitidis is one of several naturally transformable bacterial species that can readily take up DNA from the environment. It has been reported that transformation of *N. meningitidis* with donor DNA from heterologous strains resulted in an increased rate of phase variation (24- to 73-fold change) [42]. This increase in phase variation following transformation was partially alleviated by overexpressing MutL and MutS [42].

Adherence to host cells by *N. meningitidis* requires the coordinated expression of a large number of genes, upregulates the expression of a number of genes and apparently increases the rate of phase variation [43]. One of the genes upregulated following adherence to HUVECs is XseB, a component of exonuclease VII and the methyl-directed mismatch repair pathway [43, 44]. Increased levels of XseB expression increased the rate of phase variation (as measured by the HmbR system described above), but not the rates of spontaneous mutation, transformation or recombination [43]. Mutants of XseB are also more susceptible to UV irradiation, alkylating agents and nalidixic acid. It has been suggested that the upregulation of XseB upon interaction with host cells modulates phase variation rates, so as to facilitate adaptation during this critical stage in the colonization of the host. Further work is required to confirm these observations and to pinpoint the associated environmental cues.

The meningococcus encounters iron in different forms and in different concentrations, depending on its location within the host [45]. Iron starvation is associated with increased DNA recombination and repair and phase variation of pili in *N. gonorrhoeae* [46, 47]. Iron levels regulate a large number of genes including *recN*, part of the RecBCD-dependent repair pathway, and NGO0173, which encodes a putative very short patch DNA repair endonuclease [48–50]. Thus, iron levels may be a good indicator of changed environments and stress. Importantly, the relationship between iron and phase variation may complicate experimental approaches relying on iron utilization and the manipulation of iron levels for determination of phase variation levels.

Thus, *trans*-acting factors that influence phase variation rates may fall into two categories: those that are stable heritable modulators of phase variation and those that respond dynamically to environmental or other challenges (Table 6.2). The identification of strains with intrinsically high rates of phase variation associated with disease causing lineages that include those with mutations in MutS and MutL has led to the hypothesis that high levels of phase variation may contribute to the epidemic potential of a strain [35]. However, many genes that contribute to these altered phase variation rates have not been identified; and allelic variations with altered activity, antimutator or mutator functions may add to the complexity. Presumably, under appropriate selective pressures, these

Table 6.2 *Trans*-acting factors and phase variation in *N. meningitidis*.

Gene	Description	Role in phase variation	References
dinB	Error-prone DNA polymerase IV	Affects stability of homopolymeric but not tetranucleotide tracts	39
mutS	Involved in MMR (mismatch repair)	Increased generalized mutation and phase variation	35, 36, 40
mutL	Involved in MMR	Increased generalized mutation and phase variation	35, 36, 40
dam	DNA adenine methylase	None* (Bucci saw higher levels of capsule phase variation)	36, 39, 41
pilP, fbpA, fbpB, NMA1233	Iron transport and utilisation?	Unknown	40
uvrD	Involved in MMR	Unknown	40
drg	Dam replacement gene	None	39
Transformation	Transformation of *Neisseria* with DNA	Increased phase variation	42
xseB	Exonuclease VII	Contact with host cells increases expression of XseB and increased phase variation	43

alleles may spread via homologous recombination through natural populations of meningococci.

6.7
Local Factors May Influence Rates of Phase Variation

The frequency of phase variation mediated by repetitive DNA is modulated by various factors including: the length of repeat tract, length and sequence of repeat unit, sequence of region surrounding repeats, transcription levels of region, genomic location and leading or lagging strain location of repeats (reviewed by Bayliss et al. [53]). The influence of *cis*-acting factors may be means of the further fine-tuning of a gene's rate of phase variation.

The length of repeat tracts is a critical factor in determining the rates of phase variation. The longer a repeat tract, the higher the rate of phase variation. In the poly G tract of the *hmbR* gene there is an increase in the rate of phase variation for each increase in the number of G residues in the tract (the range examined was from 7 Gs to 14 Gs) [36]. Comparison between various studies is difficult, since methods used to determine the frequency of phase variation differ widely. However, in general, a positive relationship between the length of repeat tract (regardless of repeat type) and phase variation frequency is likely to exist. The expansion of tract length is constrained where repeats are within ORF or promoter regions and the expansion of these tracts may affect protein structure, function or promoter effectiveness.

Repeat units of different length and sequence have intrinsically different rates of phase variation. Poly A/T tracts are more stable and less likely to undergo frameshifts than tracts of G/C, due to the stacking energy of these base pairs with their neighbors [51]. G/C tracts have higher rates of base pair opening and nucleotide exchange than nonhomologous tracts and tracts of A/T [52]. Base pair opening is implicated in transcription, recombination and protein interactions and partially accounts for the increase mutability of poly G/C tracts. These more mutable G/C tracts are the most frequent mediators of phase variation. Only one in eight of the homopolymeric tracts identified by Saunders et al. [21] were A/T.

Homopolymeric and longer repeat units are repaired and replicated with different fidelity by different DNA metabolism genes in *Neisseria*. MutS mutants, a cause of hypermutable strains in *N. meningitidis* [36], increased the rates of phase variation in genes with C/G homopolymeric tracts of 7–12 nucleotides in length, but not with a $[TAAA]_9$ tract [39]. The overexpression of DinB, the error-prone polymerase IV, resulted in increases in the rates of phase variation mediated by C_7 but not by C_{10} or C_{12} tracts. Further, the mismatch repair system does not impact on repeat units of greater than four nucleotides in length [53].

The context of the repeat tracts may influence the rate of its mutation and therefore the phase variation it mediates. In *E. coli* the sequence topology, G+C content or DNA secondary structure are factors which determine mutational hotspots [54]. In the regions surrounding repeats, these factors could affect the stability of repeat tracts and the fidelity of their replication. In *N. meningitidis*, recent analysis of the *pilS/pilE* antigenic variation mechanisms indicated that regions surrounding the *pilE* region affect the rates of this mechanism [47].

There does not appear to be a correlation between transcription levels of genes and frequency of phase variation. Increases (26-, 56-fold) in the transcription of *hmbR* (G_8) under the control of an ITPG inducible promoter showed no changes in phase variation rate [40]. Different transcription-coupled repair systems exist in many bacteria and may promote or diminish phase variation in highly transcribed genes, although the relationship between high rates of transcription and phase variation mediated by nonhomopolymeric tracts remains to be examined. However, a correlation between the transcription level and phase variation rate does exist when the *opa* genes (CTTCT repeats) are introduced into *E. coli* [55]. This discrepancy is puzzling and could be explained, for example, by differences in the types of mutations which are promoted by high levels of transcription [56].

The genomic location of phase-variable genes may influence the rates of phase variation. In *Salmonella enterica*, mutation rates vary with chromosomal location and are highest in the regions not at the origin or terminus [56]. An analysis of the location of the genomic location of phase variable genes shows no obvious patterns with respect to their location (unpublished observation). Replication of genomic DNA starts at the origin of replication and travels in both directions away from the origin with a strand of continuous replication (the leading strand) and a discontinuous strand of replication (lagging strand). These different methods of replication favor different types of mutations and rates of mutation [57, 58]. Leading and lagging strand biases exist in the presence of homopolymeric G tracts, mostly occurring on the leading strand (27/33 homopolymeric G tracts) [53].

6.8
Examples of Phase Variation

6.8.1
Opc: Simple Sequence Repeats, Promoter Strength and "Volume Control"

In contrast to most phase variation systems, Opc exhibits strong, intermediate and weak expression, not merely on/off switching. Changes in the length of a homopolymeric tract of cytosine residues, upstream of a −10 element of an unusual promoter sequence that lacks a −35 element, result in changes in the strength of the promoter and alteration of the level of the *opc* transcript [16]. This phenomenon, termed "volume control" [2], is a result of the relaxed specificity of the *opc* promoter. High expression occurs with 12 or 13 C residues in the tract, intermediate expression with 11 or 14 Cs and no expression with <11 or <14 C residues.

Opc, an adhesin that is important for association with and invasion of eukaryotic cells, is implicated in tissue tropism [17]. The role of Opc as an adhesin and invasin is dependent on a complex interplay between it and other surface-expressed virulence factors such as pili, capsule, Opa, sialylated LPS and host proteins [59–61]. These interactions and the modulation of levels of these factors (especially capsule expression and absence of LPS sialylation) may require compensatory changes in the level of Opc expression for effective adhesion and invasion [59, 60]. This modulation is mutational and therefore stochastic and may require multiple rounds of variation for the most advantageous phenotype to be selected.

6.8.2
NadA: Phase Variation and the Modulation of Classic Mechanisms of Gene Regulation

The expression of NadA requires an interplay between stochastic (mutational) and prescriptive (classical) mechanisms of gene regulation. Since some host environmental challenges are "predictable", they are best served by a stereotyped regulatory response; but variation through mutation can modulate the magnitude of the response.

NadA (NMB1994) is a surface-expressed protein that promotes adherence and invasion of epithelial cells and is a potential vaccine candidate [32, 62]. NadA was identified in the MC58 genome and the presence of TAAA repeats within its promoter region suggested the potential for phase variation [63]. The repeats are located upstream of the −35 and −10 regions [24]; and therefore phase variation could not be explained adequately by a mechanism implicating altered spacing within the promoter. Rather, phase variation of NadA results from altered interactions of the transcription factor IHF (integration host factor) and its DNA binding site [37].

The expression levels of NadA with different numbers of repeats shows a periodicity: ([TAAA]$_8$: high; [TAAA]$_9$: low; [TAAA]$_{10}$: high; [TAAA]$_{11}$: intermediate; [TAAA]$_{12}$: low; [TAAA]$_{13}$: high). Taken together, these findings suggested that changes in the length of repeat tract alter the relationship between the regulators bound to their target DNA and the promoter region of *nadA*. This modulation of regulator binding upstream of the core promoter of *nadA* results in fine-tuning of the response to IHF.

The phase variation of *nadA* demonstrates a conjunction between the "classic" regulation of gene expression and stochastic phase variation, thus allowing fine control of the transcriptional response of *nadA* to the activation by the IHF regulator.

6.8.3
Pili: Combinatorial Complexity of Multiple Phase-variable Genes

The examination of single phase-variable genes in isolation belies the complexity and power of phase variation as a means of adaptation. The combinatorial interplay between phase-variable genes enables the meningococcus to generate a plethora of combinations of phenotypes upon which selective pressures can act. An example of this flexibility and complexity is the combined action of a number of phase-variable genes that modulate the structure, immunogenicity and function of pili that are critically important in neisserial commensal and pathogenic behavior.

6.8.3.1 Phase Variation of Pili

Pili of pathogenic *Neisseria* are long polymeric proteins that protrude from the bacterial surface and have a crucial role in both colonization of the host and adhesion to host cells. Also, they are involved in transformation and motility [60, 64–71].

The most obvious influences of phase variation on pili are the reversible changes in the expression of the pili. Pilin, the major subunit of the pilus, displays both phase and antigenic variation (for a review, see [13]); and a byproduct of the antigenic variation of pilin is abrogation of pilus expression. Pilin antigenic variation is mediated by unidirectional recombination with DNA from several silent, nonexpressed copies of the *pilE* gene, termed *pilS*, and results in variation in adhesin function [59, 60, 68]. The outcome of these homologous recombination events is usually a change in the *pilE* sequence, although these RecA-dependent recombination events can occasionally result in a *pilE* gene which is unable to form pili (S-pilin, L-pilin). This is a reversible state and one means by which the expression of pili phase varies.

The phase variation of the expression of pilus accessory proteins, such as PilC1 and PilC2, can result in pilus phase variation as well as modulation of its structure and function. Mutants in *pilC1* and *pilC2* result in a nonpiliated phenotype in some strains [72]. The phase variation of both *pilC* alleles is mediated by a poly G tract within the 5' end of the gene within the signal peptide of the protein. The importance of the *pilC* duplication combined with phase variation is not well understood but suggests independent expression and different roles for *pilC1* and *pilC2*. These may facilitate cell and tissue tropism [73]. The independent expression of PilC1 and PilC2 may enable adaptation to different niches by modulation of pili expression and function. Additionally, *pilC1*, but not *pilC2*, is regulated by bacterial cell contact. Thus, *pilC1* expression may be conditional on cell contact, whereas the *pilC2* phase variation results in constitutive expression [72]. The phase variation of *pilC1* and *pilC2* represents a complicated phenotype which changes both the antigen expression of pili and modulation of its function.

6.8.3.2 Post-translational Modifications of Pili Modulate Their Structure and Function

A number of phase variable genes alter the post-translational modification of pilin. Pilins of pathogenic *Neisseria* are post-translationally modified by four types of modifications (for a review, see [74]). These modifications are a phosphodiester-linked glycerol [75], a covalently linked phosphorylcholine [76], a phosphate group [77] and the addition of an O-linked trisaccharide [78–80].

Warren et al. [81] identified the gene responsible for the addition of phosphorylcholine (ChoP) to pilin. The gene contains a homopolymeric tract of G residues (screening of strains revealed tracts of 8–11 Gs) within the ORF and screening colonies with an antiChoP antibody (TEPC-15) identified phase variants. Warren et al. [81] suggested that "variants expressing ChoP may be better adapted to colonization of the nasopharynx, while ChoP-negative variants may be able to avoid complement-mediated killing in serum" [81]. Phosphorylcholine is an important surface expressed structure in a number of organisms of the respiratory tract. It is an important factor for receptor binding and other host interactions and is implicated in increases in adherence and invasion [81]. Phase variation of the phosphorylcholine expression on pili may have important implications for the function of pilin.

The post-translational glycosylation of pilin requires a number of genes and is modulated by the effect of up to six phase-variable genes. Two phase-variable glycosyltransferases, *pglA* (coding a poly G tract) and *pglE* (coding a poly CAA-CAAA tract), are responsible for variation of the glycosylation structure between a mono-, di-, and trisaccharide [14, 82]. Further, PglI, an acetyltransferase, is involved in the biosynthesis of the 2,4-diacetamido-2,4,6-trideoxyhexose and its phase variation results in a modified basal sugar [83]. Two additional phase-variable glycosyltransferases, *pglG* and *pglH* (both containing coding poly G tracts), have been identified in the pilin glycosylation genetic locus in 67% of strains and could allow alternative pilin-linked structures [82]. *pglB2* is a fusion protein and an alternative allele to *pglB* in about 50% of strains and is a potentially phase-variable gene [82]. Based on a strain survey a polymorphic tract of seven or eight As was identified which is predicted to split the PglB2 protein into the two, potentially functional, proteins. The role of this phase variation is unknown but may serve to help the cellular localisation of the proteins, although its effect on pilin glycosylation is unknown [82]. Glycosylation of pilin may influence the amount of S-pilin produced and the amount of adherence mediated by pilin [80]. There has been some suggestion that the presence of the homopolymeric tract in *pglA* in *N. gonorrhoeae* correlates with the likelihood of that strain causing disseminated gonococcal disease [84].

Changes in the glycosylation and phosphorylcholine phenotypes may have distal effects on the action of other structures: for example the different glycosylations of pilin may effect the topology and display of PilC proteins [73]. Differential glycosylation affects both the ability of the TEPC-15 to recognise the pilin-linked ChoP epitope and the adherence to epithelial cells (M. Warren, unpublished data) and may modulate the function of ChoP and affect host interactions.

Pili expression is controlled in a complex manner by a large number of phase-variable genes. The on–off switching of pili and accessory protein expression, and alterations in the type of pili expressed and changes in the post-translational modifications of the pilin (with or without phosphorylcholine and the expression of a mono-, di- or trisaccharide and modification of the sugar composition of the pilin-linked glycan) are all controlled by phase variation and all vary

Table 6.3 Phase variation and pili.

Pili phase variation		References
	pilE/pilS homologous recombination	13
	pilC1/pilC2 Poly G tract	19, 69, 85–87
Pilin post-translational modification phase variation		
Glycosylation	*pglA*, coding poly G	14
	pglE, coding $[CAACAA]_{25}$	82
	pglG [a)], H [a)] coding poly G	82
	pglI, coding poly G	83
	pglB2, coding poly A	82
Phosphorylcholine	*pptA*, coding poly G	81

a) Potential pilin glycosylation genes.

independently of each other. The diversity of pili-related phenotypes that can be expressed by a single strain and combined with the antigenic variation of pilin [13] indicate the polymorphic nature of the pilus structure in *Neisseria*. The mechanisms used to create this diversity have the benefit of not "losing information"; and thus a complex array of phenotypes is available to any strain and serves as a repository of possible phenotypes which may allow survival in unpredictable and challenging environments (Table 6.3).

6.9
Conclusion: *N. meningitidis* is Adapted to Adapt

N. meningitidis is under constant host immune and environmental selective pressure; and one major means of adaptation to these pressures is to generate offspring that are phenotypically diverse, from which fitter variants can be selected. Phase variation is a means of creating biologically useful, but reversible phenotypic variation.

N. meningitidis is an obligate human pathogen and, as a result of bottlenecks during transmission, the size and heterogeneity of the founder population at the inception of infection is likely to be constrained. Phase variation enables a single bacterium to carry with it the information required for rapidly generating diversity. This mechanism avoids the loss of "information" that is characteristic of high rates of random mutations, as in mutators.

An unproven and controversial feature of phase variation is the possibility that its rates may be influenced by environmental factors via classic regulatory mechanisms acting through genes of DNA metabolism. It has been proposed that such systems occur in other species, e.g. increases in general mutation in *E. coli* through the SOS response. Recent work in *N. meningitidis* has identified some potential environmental factors that may influence the rate of phase variation [89, 91, 92]. For example, it has been proposed that increased rates of phase variation occur in response to adherence to cultured cells, high levels of DNA transformation and iron levels. Adherence may be critical to the fitness of *N. meningitidis* in adapting to new host environments and a number of determinants, such as PilC1/2 and Opc, are implicated in tissue tropism where variable expression may facilitate receptor-mediated adherence.

N. meningitidis must trade-off successful replication (fitness) against excessive pathogenicity that overwhelms and kills its host. However, *N. meningitidis* is predominately a commensal organism and as such its adaptive mechanisms have evolved to facilitate the commensal state, not disease. The latter is an evolutionarily dead end and therefore phase variation must be considered as an adaptation which facilitates the commensal state, either by increased transmissibility between humans or increased fitness for residency within individuals. A number of microbial determinants must be expressed or not expressed to achieve fitness. *Neisseria* has evolved multiple mechanisms for diversifying its phenotype, while minimizing the costs of multiple and complex regulatory systems. However, pathogenicity offers only a short-term advantage to the microbe; indeed, it is ultimately self-defeating, since organisms involved in invasive disease do not enable transmission to a new host and persistence is usually incompatible with host survival [90].

This mechanism of adaptation used by *Neisseria* might be considered analogous to the "brute force" methods used to solve mathematical problems, involving the enumeration of many potential solutions to a problem until an appropriate one is found. Refinements of the "brute force" methods in cryptology and mathematics often focus on limiting the number of combinations that need to be tried, for example using words from a dictionary when trying to guess a password. Phase variation at contingency loci has the potential to generate a myriad of phenotypic combinations, some of which may enhance fitness and be selected. Localized hypermutation predominantly affects microbial determinants on the microbial cell surface, a strategy in which the trade-off between enhanced rather than diminished fitness is rendered relatively advantageous as compared to genome-wide hypermutability. Further, mutations are reversible at high frequency, so that the genetic information and its corresponding phenotype is not lost. Mathematical models suggest that phase variation may minimize growth rate variance and the probability of extinction, even though it may not maximize the growth rate in any condition. They also suggest that phase variation may be the best strategy for coping with abrupt environmental change but that it may not be the best strategy for promoting adaptation in different spatial compartments, although this analysis assumes an initial population heterogeneity. Thus, it is proposed that phase variation is an efficient survival strategy for time-variable selection applied to a whole population (e.g. change to a new host) and not time-invariant changes to different compartments within the same host [88].

The ability of phase variation to produce combinations of phenotypes that facilitates commensal infection in an adverse environment may also be one of the critical factors resulting in pathogenic behavior. The generation of diverse phenotypes increases the probability of fit (rapidly proliferating) variants and their subsequent dissemination within the blood stream and translocation across the blood–meningeal barrier.

References

1 Moxon, E.R., et al. **1994**, Adaptive evolution of highly mutable loci in pathogenic bacteria, Curr Biol 4, 24–33.
2 Henderson, I.R., P. Owen, J.P. Nataro **1999**, Molecular switches–the ON and OFF of bacterial phase variation, Mol Microbiol 33, 919–932.
3 van der Woude, M.W., A.J. Baumler **2004**, Phase and antigenic variation in bacteria, Clin Microbiol Rev 17, 581–611.
4 Bayliss, C.D., D. Field, E.R. Moxon **2001**, The simple sequence contingency loci of Haemophilus influenzae and Neisseria meningitidis, J Clin Invest 107, 657–662.
5 Hallet, B. **2001**, Playing Dr Jekyll and Mr Hyde: combined mechanisms of phase variation in bacteria, Curr Opin Microbiol 4, 570–581.
6 Hood, D.W., et al. **1996**, DNA repeats identify novel virulence genes in Haemophilus influenzae, Proc Natl Acad Sci USA 93, 11121–11125.
7 Tomb, J.F., et al. **1997**, The complete genome sequence of the gastric pathogen Helicobacter pylori, Nature 388, 539–547.
8 Parkhill, J., et al. **2000**, The genome sequence of the food-borne pathogen Campylobacter jejuni reveals hypervariable sequences, Nature 403, 665–668.
9 Kellogg, D.S., Jr., et al. **1963**, Neisseria gonorrhoeae. I. Virulence genetically linked to clonal variation, J Bacteriol 85, 1274–1279.
10 Kellogg, D.S., Jr., et al. **1968**, Neisseria gonorrhoeae. II. Colonial variation and pathogenicity during 35 months in vitro, J Bacteriol 96, 596–605.
11 Blake, M.S., C.M. MacDonald, K.P. Klugman **1989**, Colony morphology of piliated Neisseria meningitidis, J Exp Med 170, 1727–1736.
12 Hammerschmidt, S., et al. **1996**, Capsule phase variation in Neisseria meningitidis serogroup B by slipped-strand mispairing in the polysialyltransferase gene (siaD): correlation with bacterial invasion and the outbreak of meningococcal disease, Mol Microbiol 20, 1211–1220.
13 Seifert, H.S. **1996**, Questions about gonococcal pilus phase- and antigenic variation, Mol Microbiol 21, 433–440.
14 Jennings, M.P., et al. **1998**, Identification of a novel gene involved in pilin glycosylation in Neisseria meningitidis, Mol Microbiol 29, 975–984.
15 Stern, A., T.F. Meyer, Common mechanism controlling phase and antigenic variation in pathogenic neisseriae, Mol Microbiol 1, 5–12.
16 Sarkari, J., et al. **1994**, Variable expression of the Opc outer membrane protein in Neisseria meningitidis is caused by size variation of a promoter containing polycytidine, Mol Microbiol 13, 207–217.
17 de Vries, F.P., et al. **1996**, Invasion of primary nasopharyngeal epithelial cells by Neisseria meningitidis is controlled by phase variation of multiple surface antigens, Infect Immun 64, 2998–3006.
18 Jennings, M.P., et al. **1999**, The genetic basis of the phase variation repertoire of lipopolysaccharide immunotypes in Neisseria meningitidis, Microbiology 145, 3013–3021.
19 van der Ende, A., et al. **1995**, Variable expression of class 1 outer membrane protein in Neisseria meningitidis is caused by variation in the spacing between the −10 and −35 regions of the promoter, J Bacteriol 177, 2475–2480.
20 van der Ende, A., C.T. Hopman, J. Dankert **2000**, Multiple mechanisms of phase variation of PorA in Neisseria meningitidis, Infect Immun 68, 6685–6690.
21 Saunders, N.J., et al. **2000**, Repeat-associated phase variable genes in the complete genome sequence of Neisseria me-

ningitidis strain MC58, *Mol Microbiol* 37, 207–215.

22 Snyder, L. A., W. M. Shafer, N. J. Saunders **2003**, Divergence and transcriptional analysis of the division cell wall (dcw) gene cluster in *Neisseria* spp, *Mol Microbiol* 47, 431–442.

23 Snyder, L. A., S. A. Butcher, N. J. Saunders **2001**, Comparative whole-genome analyses reveal over 100 putative phase-variable genes in the pathogenic *Neisseria* spp, *Microbiology* 147, 2321–2332.

24 Martin, P., et al. **2003**, Experimentally revised repertoire of putative contingency loci in *Neisseria meningitidis* strain MC58: evidence for a novel mechanism of phase variation, *Mol Microbiol* 50, 245–257.

25 Richardson, A. R., I. Stojiljkovic **1999**, HmbR, a hemoglobin-binding outer membrane protein of *Neisseria meningitidis*, undergoes phase variation, *J Bacteriol* 181, 2067–2074.

26 Moxon, E. R., et al. **1994**, Adaptive evolution of highly mutable loci in pathogenic bacteria, *Curr Biol* 4, 24–33.

27 Alcala, B., et al. **2004**, Antigenic and/or phase variation of PorA protein in non-subtypable *Neisseria meningitidis* strains isolated in Spain, *J Med Microbiol* 53, 515–518.

28 Hilse, R., et al. **1996**, Site-specific insertion of *IS1301* and distribution in *Neisseria meningitidis* strains, *J Bacteriol* 178, 2527–2532.

29 Sadler, F., et al. **2003**, Genetic analysis of capsular status of meningococcal carrier isolates, Epidemiol Infect 130, 59–70.

30. Claus, H., et al. **2004**, Genetics of capsule O-acetylation in serogroup C, W-135 and Y meningococci, *Mol Microbiol* 51, 227–239.

31 Newcombe, J., et al. **1998**, Naturally occurring insertional inactivation of the *porA* gene of *Neisseria meningitidis* by integration of *IS1301*, *Mol Microbiol* 30, 453–454.

32 Comanducci, M., et al. **2002**, NadA, a novel vaccine candidate of *Neisseria meningitidis*, *J Exp Med* 195, 1445–1454.

33 Hilse, R., et al. **2000**, Distribution of the meningococcal insertion sequence *IS1301* in clonal lineages of *Neisseria meningitidis*, *Epidemiol Infect* 124, 337–340.

34 Long, C. D., R. N. Madraswala, H. S. Seifert **1998**, Comparisons between colony phase variation of *Neisseria gonorrhoeae* FA1090 and pilus, pilin, and S-pilin expression, *Infect Immun* 66, 1918–1927.

35 Richardson, A. R., et al. **2002**, Mutator clones of *Neisseria meningitidis* in epidemic serogroup A disease, *Proc Natl Acad Sci USA* 99, 6103–6107.

36 Tapsall, J. W., et al. **2001**, Surveillance of antibiotic resistance in invasive isolates of *Neisseria meningitidis* in Australia 1994–**1999**, *Pathology* 33, 359–361.

37 Martin, P., et al. **2005**, Microsatellite instability regulates transcription factor binding and gene expression, *Proc Natl Acad Sci USA* 102, 3800–3804.

38 Black, C. G., J. A. Fyfe, J. K. Davies **1998**, Absence of an SOS-like system in *Neisseria gonorrhoeae*, *Gene* 208, 61–66.

39 Martin, P., et al. **2004**, Involvement of genes of genome maintenance in the regulation of phase variation frequencies in *Neisseria meningitidis*, *Microbiology* 150, 3001–3012.

40 Alexander, H. I., A. W. Rasmussen, I. Stojiljkovic **2004**, Identification of *Neisseria meningitidis* genetic loci involved in the modulation of phase variation frequencies, *Infect Immun* 72, 6743–6747.

41 Bucci, C., et al. **1999**, Hypermutation in pathogenic bacteria: frequent phase variation in meningococci is a phenotypic trait of a specialized mutator biotype, *Mol Cell* 3, 435–445.

42 Alexander, H. L., A. R. Richardson, I. Stojiljkovic **2004**, Natural transformation and phase variation modulation in *Neisseria meningitidis*, *Mol Microbiol* 52, 771–783.

43 Morelle, S., et al. **2005**, Contact with host cells induces a DNA repair system in pathogenic *Neisseriae*, *Mol Microbiol* 55, 853–861.

44 Morelle, S., E. Carbonnelle, X. Nassif **2003**, The REP2 repeats of the genome of *Neisseria meningitidis* are associated with genes coordinately regulated during bacterial cell interaction, *J Bacteriol* 185, 2618–2627.

45 Schryvers, A. B., I. Stojiljkovic **1999**, Iron acquisition systems in the pathogenic *Neisseria*, *Mol Microbiol* 32, 1117–1123.

46 Serkin, C. D., H. S. Seifert **2000**, Iron availability regulates DNA recombination in *Neisseria* gonorrhoeae, *Mol Microbiol* 37, 1075–1086.

47 Sechman, E. V., M. S. Rohrer, H. S. Seifert 2005, A genetic screen identifies genes and sites involved in pilin antigenic variation in *Neisseria* gonorrhoeae, *Mol Microbiol* 57, 468–483.

48 Grifantini, R., et al. **2002**, Gene expression profile in *Neisseria meningitidis* and *Neisseria* lactamica upon host-cell contact: from basic research to vaccine development, *Ann NY Acad Sci* 975, 202–216.

49 Skaar, E. P., M. P. Lazio, H. S. Seifert **2002**, Roles of the recJ and *recN* genes in homologous recombination and DNA repair pathways of *Neisseria* gonorrhoeae, *J Bacteriol* 184, 919–927.

50 Ducey, T. F., et al. **2005**, Identification of the iron-responsive genes of *Neisseria* gonorrhoeae by microarray analysis in defined medium, *J Bacteriol* 187, 4865–4874.

51 Warmlander, S., et al. **2002**, The influence of the thymine C5 methyl group on spontaneous base pair breathing in DNA, J Biol Chem 277, 28491–28497.

52 Dornberger, U., M. Leijon, H. Fritzsche **1999**, High base pair opening rates in tracts of GC base pairs, *J Biol Chem* 274, 6957–6962.

53 Bayliss, C. D., K. M. Dixon, E. R. Moxon **2004**, Simple sequence repeats (microsatellites): mutational mechanisms and contributions to bacterial pathogenesis. A meeting review, *FEMS Immunol Med Microbiol* 40, 11–19.

54 Rogozin, I. B., Y.I. Pavlov **2003**, Theoretical analysis of mutation hotspots and their DNA sequence context specificity, *Mutat Res* 544, 65–85.

55 Belland, R. J., et al. **1997**, Promoter strength influences phase variation of neisserial opa genes, *Mol Microbiol* 23, 123–135.

56 Hudson, R. E., et al. **2002**, Effect of chromosome location on bacterial mutation rates, *Mol Biol Evol* 19, 85–92.

57 Fijalkowska, I. J., et al. 1998, Unequal fidelity of leading strand and lagging strand DNA replication on the *Escherichia coli* chromosome, *Proc Natl Acad Sci USA* 95, 10020–10025.

58 Gawel, D., et al. **2002**, Asymmetry of frameshift mutagenesis during leading and lagging-strand replication in *Escherichia coli*, *Mutat Res* 501, 129–136.

59 Virji, M., et al. **1993**, Pilus-facilitated adherence of *Neisseria meningitidis* to human epithelial and endothelial cells: modulation of adherence phenotype occurs concurrently with changes in primary amino acid sequence and the glycosylation status of pilin, *Mol Microbiol* 10, 1013–1028.

60 Virji, M., et al. **1992**, Variations in the expression of pili: the effect on adherence of *Neisseria meningitidis* to human epithelial and endothelial cells, *Mol Microbiol* 6, 1271–1279.

61 Virji, M., et al. **1995**, Opc- and pilus-dependent interactions of meningococci with human endothelial cells: molecular mechanisms and modulation by surface polysaccharides, *Mol Microbiol* 18, 741–754.

62 Capecchi, B., et al. **2005**, *Neisseria meningitidis* NadA is a new invasin which promotes bacterial adhesion to and penetration into human epithelial cells, *Mol Microbiol* 55, 687–698.

63 Jordan, P., L.A. Snyder, N.J. Saunders **2003**, Diversity in coding tandem repeats in related *Neisseria* spp, *BMC Microbiol* 3, 23.

64 McGee, Z.A., D.S. Stephens **1984**, Common pathways of invasion of mucosal barriers by *Neisseria* gonorrhoeae and *Neisseria meningitidis*, *Surv Synth Pathol Res* 3, 1–10.

65 Merz, A.J., et al. **1996**, Traversal of a polarized epithelium by pathogenic *Neisseriae*: facilitation by type IV pili and maintenance of epithelial barrier function, *Mol Med* 2, 745–754.

66 Merz, A.J., M. So, M.P. Sheetz **2000**, Pilus retraction powers bacterial twitching motility, *Nature* 407, 98–102.

67 Tonjum, T., M. Koomey **1997**, The pilus colonization factor of pathogenic neisserial species: organelle biogenesis and

structure/function relationships – a review, *Gene* 192, 155–163.
68 Nassif, X., et al. **1993**, Antigenic variation of pilin regulates adhesion of *Neisseria meningitidis* to human epithelial cells, *Mol Microbiol* 8, 719–725.
69 Nassif, X., et al. **1994**, Roles of pilin and PilC in adhesion of *Neisseria meningitidis* to human epithelial and endothelial cells, *Proc Natl Acad Sci USA* 91, 3769–3773.
70 Nassif, X., et al. **1997**, Type-4 pili and meningococcal adhesiveness, *Gene* 192, 149–153.
71 Virji, M., et al. 1991, The role of pili in the interactions of pathogenic *Neisseria* with cultured human endothelial cells, *Mol Microbiol* 5, 1831–1841.
72 Morand, P. C., et al. **2004**, Type IV pilus retraction in pathogenic *Neisseria* is regulated by the PilC proteins, *EMBO J* 23, 2009–2017.
73 Kirchner, M., T. F. Meyer **2005**, The PilC adhesin of the *Neisseria* type IV pilus-binding specificities and new insights into the nature of the host cell receptor, *Mol Microbiol* 56, 945–957.
74 Virji, M. **1997**, Post-translational modifications of meningococcal pili. Identification of common substituents: glycans and alpha-glycerophosphate – a review, Gene 192, 141–147.
75 Stimson, E., et al. **1996**, Discovery of a novel protein modification: alpha-glycerophosphate is a substituent of meningococcal pilin, *Biochem J* 316, 29–33.
76 Weiser, J. N., et al. **1998**, The phosphorylcholine epitope undergoes phase variation on a 43-kilodalton protein in Pseudomonas aeruginosa and on pili of *Neisseria meningitidis* and *Neisseria* gonorrhoeae, *Infect Immun* 66, 4263–4267.
77 Forest, K. T., et al. **1999**, Crystallographic structure reveals phosphorylated pilin from *Neisseria*: phosphoserine sites modify type IV pilus surface chemistry and fibre morphology, *Mol Microbiol* 31, 743–752.
78 Parge, H. E., et al. **1995**, Structure of the fibre-forming protein pilin at 2.6 Å resolution, *Nature* 378, 32–38.
79 Stimson, E., et al. **1995**, Meningococcal pilin: a glycoprotein substituted with digalactosyl 2,4-diacetamido-2,4,6-trideoxyhexose, *Mol Microbiol* 17, 1201–1214.
80 Marceau, M., et al. **1998**, Consequences of the loss of O-linked glycosylation of meningococcal type IV pilin on piliation and pilus-mediated adhesion, *Mol Microbiol* 27, 705–715.
81 Warren, M. J., M. P. Jennings **2003**, Identification and characterization of pptA: a gene involved in the phase-variable expression of phosphorylcholine on pili of *Neisseria meningitidis*, *Infect Immun* 71, 6892–6898.
82 Power, P. M., et al. **2003**, Genetic characterization of pilin glycosylation and phase variation in *Neisseria meningitidis*, *Mol Microbiol* 49, 833–847.
83 Warren, M. J., et al. **2004**, Analysis of the role of pglI in pilin glycosylation of *Neisseria meningitidis*, *FEMS Immunol Med Microbiol* 41, 43–50.
84 Banerjee, A., et al. **2002**, Implications of phase variation of a gene (pgtA) encoding a pilin galactosyl transferase in gonococcal pathogenesis, *J Exp Med* 196, 147–162.
85 Jonsson, A. B., G. Nyberg, S. Normark **1991**, Phase variation of gonococcal pili by frameshift mutation in *pilC*, a novel gene for pilus assembly, *EMBO J* 10, 477–488.
86 Ryll, R. R., et al. **1997**, PilC of *Neisseria meningitidis* is involved in class II pilus formation and restores pilus assembly, natural transformation competence and adherence to epithelial cells in PilC-deficient gonococci, *Mol Microbiol* 23, 879–892.
87 Taha, M. K., et al. **1998**, Pilus-mediated adhesion of *Neisseria meningitidis*: the essential role of cell contact-dependent transcriptional upregulation of the PilC1 protein, *Mol Microbiol* 28, 1153–1163.
88 Wolf, D. M., V. V. Vazirani, A. P. Arkin **2005**, Diversity in times of adversity: probabilistic strategies in microbial survival games, *J Theor Biol* 234, 227–253.
89 Wolf, D. M., V. V. Vazirani, A. P. Arkin **2005**, A microbial modified prisoner's dilemma game: how frequency-dependent selection can lead to random phase variation, *J Theor Biol* 234, 255–262.

90 Levin, B. R., J. J. Bull **1994**, Short-sighted evolution and the virulence of pathogenic microorganisms, *Trends Microbiol* 2, 76–81.

91 Jolley, K. A., et al. **2005**, The influence of mutation, recombination, population history, and selection on patterns of genetic diversity in *Neisseria meningitidis*, Mol Biol Evol 22, 562–569.

92 Davidsen, T, et al. **2005**, Antimutator role of DNA glycosylase MutY in pathogenic neisseria species, *J Bacteriol* 187, 2801–2809.

7
Meningococcal Transformation and DNA Repair

Tonje Davidsen, Ole Herman Ambur and Tone Tønjum

7.1
Introduction

In addition to abundant horizontal gene transfer dominated by transformation and subsequent recombination events, exogenous and endogenous stress induces DNA damage in the meningococcal genome that must be repaired. In this chapter, we first describe the neisserial transformation process. We then discuss mechanisms of meningococcal genome instability that contribute to high genome fluidity, elucidating the consequent need for DNA repair. Finally, we consider the meningococcal DNA repair profile, as contrasted to that of *Escherichia coli*. Although more experiments generally have been performed on the gonococcus than the meningococcus, these species are very closely related, and the neisserial genome sequences indicate that findings on the gonocococcus is relevant for the meningococcus.

7.2
Meningococcal Transformation

7.2.1
Role of Transformation in Horizontal Gene Transfer

Bacteria use three major genetic mechanisms for genetic exchange: transformation, conjugation and transduction. Transformation is the predominant source of new genetic information integrated into the genome in the pathogenic *Neisseria* [1, 2]; and the relative contribution of transformation to horizontal gene transfer in nature has often been under-rated. Also, a number of conjugative neisserial plasmids have been described [3].

Handbook of Meningococcal Disease. Infection Biology, Vaccination, Clinical Management.
Edited by M. Frosch and M. C. J. Maiden

ISBN: 3-527-31260-9

7.2.2 The Transformation Process

Transformation is the binding and uptake of exogenous DNA by a bacterial cell and the subsequent incorporation of this nascent DNA into the chromosome by homologous recombination [4–6]. *Neisseria meningitidis* is one of nearly 50 known species that are naturally competent for transformation [6, 7]. The pathogenic *Neisseria* are different from other species in that they do not regulate competence like many naturally competent bacteria, such as *Bacillus subtilis, Streptococcus pneumoniae* and *Haemophilus influenzae,* rather, the *Neisseria* sp. are competent throughout their entire life cycle [1]. Efficient neisserial transformation is dependent on the presence of the 10-bp DNA uptake sequence (DUS) in the exogenous DNA, type IV pilus (or pilin) expression and homologous recombination mediated by RecA [8–11].

Transporting DNA from the extracellular milieu into the cytosolic compartment is a complex task. The incoming DNA must cross the neisserial outer membrane, the peptidoglycan layer, the periplasm and the cytoplasmic membrane. During the early phase of the transformation process, DNA binding and uptake occur. DNA uptake in this context is operationally defined as the conversion of exogenous, DNase-sensitive DNA into a DNase-protected state. In the *Neisseriae,* this protection can be achieved by crossing the outer membrane. Only one strand of the DNA molecule is effectively transported into the cytoplasm, while the other strand is degraded.

7.2.2.1 The Neisserial DNA Uptake Sequence

By far the most frequent repeat sequence element in the meningococcal genomes is the genus-specific neisserial DNA uptake sequence (DUS). This is a 10-bp sequence, 5′-GCCGTCTGAA-3′, required for efficient natural transformation of meningococci and gonococci, and was first described by Goodman and Scocca in 1988 [12]. Approximately 1900 copies of the DUS are present in the genomes of both meningococci and gonococci [12–16]. Transformation of DNA between meningococcal and gonococcal piliated strains occurs at a frequency of 10^{-1} to 10^{-3} per cell. However, as demonstrated by transformation studies, the pathogenic *Neisseria* rarely take up DNA from bacterial species other than those in its own genus. One exception is the introduction of the gene that encodes *H. influenzae* superoxide dismutase (SodC) into the meningococcus by a horizontal gene transfer event [17]. Specific DUS receptors on the bacterial surface have not yet been identified. The putative receptor presumably recognizes the DUS and might trigger the uptake process – the transport of DNA across the outer membrane – into either the periplasmic space or specialized vesicle structures (transformasomes) that have been described in *H. influenzae* [18]. Originally found as parts of inverted repeats downstream of genes, DUS have been postulated to function as transcriptional regulators [12]. However, the complete genome sequences of meningococcal strains MC58 and Z2491 show that DUS are distributed throughout the genomes, both in intergenic and intragenic regions, and that many of them are present as single copies [13, 14]. When exposed to a mixture of homologous and foreign DNAs, the *Neisseriae* show preferential uptake of DUS-containing DNA [19]. It is, however, not yet clear if DUS act in DNA binding and/or uptake or has other functions, for instance in recombination; thus, the exact function of DUS remains unknown. However, an over-representation of DUS inside genes encoding DNA repair, recombination, replication and restriction/modification components has been identified [15]. A similar bias of the DNA uptake signal sequences (USS; 5′-AAGTGCGGT-3′) towards genome maintenance genes was found in genomes of the distantly related Pasteurellaceae (e.g. *Haemophilus influenzae*) [15]. These results imply that the high frequency of DUS/USS in genome maintenance genes is conserved among phylogenetically divergent species and thus are of significant biological importance. Increased DUS density is expected to enhance DNA uptake; and the over-representation of DUS in genome maintenance genes might reflect facilitated recovery of genome preserving functions (see below).

7.2.2.2 **The Type IV Pilus**

A consistent theme in genetic transformation is the involvement of type IV pili or components related to the type IV pilus biogenesis machinery in the initial events of DNA recognition and uptake (Fig. 7.1) [20]. Type IV pili are long, thin appendages that are present on the surface of many Gram-negative microorganisms. Type IV pili function in bacterial cell-to-cell interactions, adhesion to host cells and twitching motility – a form of locomotion that is powered by extension and retraction of the pilus filament [21, 22]. Owing to their importance as a prerequisite for adherence and colonization, type IV pili have been studied in detail (see Chapter 12). The main structural constituent of the pilus is the type IV pilin subunit (PilE), which is assembled to form the pilus fiber, while a few minor pilins (such as PilV and PilX) participate in the biogenesis process [38, 52]. Type IV pilins are small proteins (usually <20 kDa), which are made as precursors (prepilins) that comprise a short, positively charged amino-terminal leader peptide, a hydrophobic stretch and a carboxy-terminal domain. The N-terminal leader peptide and hydrophobic region sequences are relatively conserved, whereas the C-terminal region is hypervariable. The single *pilE* expression locus is changed by unidirectional donation of coding sequences from multiple silent partial *pilS* genes in a process similar to gene conversion (Fig. 7.2) [23–25].

7.2.2.3 **Type IV Pilus Biogenesis**

Type IV pilus biogenesis requires a complex machinery, to which the enigmatic processes involved in neisserial transformation also are coupled [20]. The pilus biogenesis apparatus is homologous to the type II secretion system, also known as the secreton or main terminal branch of the general secretory pathway, which mediates the translocation of macromolecules from the periplasm across the

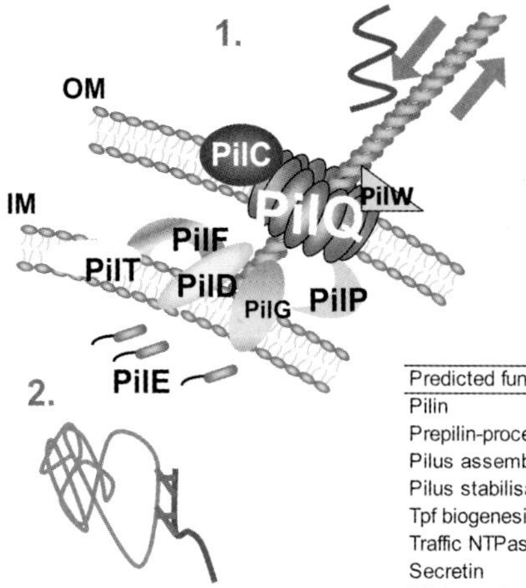

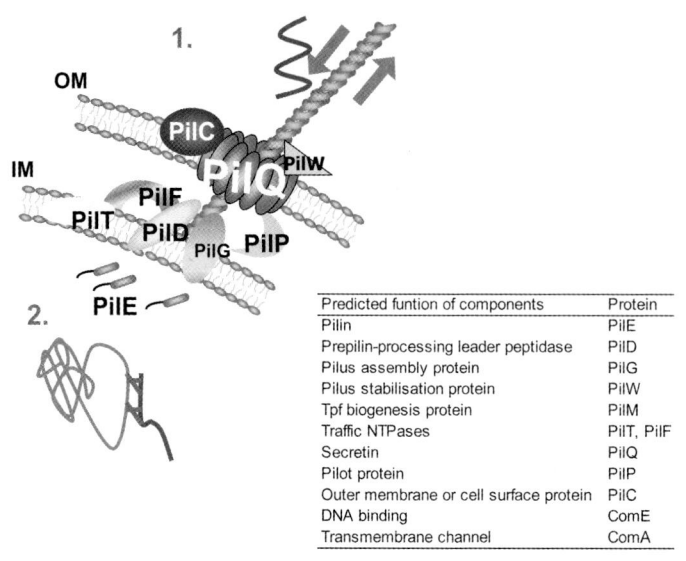

Predicted funtion of components	Protein
Pilin	PilE
Prepilin-processing leader peptidase	PilD
Pilus assembly protein	PilG
Pilus stabilisation protein	PilW
Tpf biogenesis protein	PilM
Traffic NTPases	PilT, PilF
Secretin	PilQ
Pilot protein	PilP
Outer membrane or cell surface protein	PilC
DNA binding	ComE
Transmembrane channel	ComA

Fig. 7.1 Horizontal gene transfer through transformation of exogenous DNA. 1. A schematic model for type IV pilus formation and competence, based on the *Neisseria meningitidis* pilus. The major pilin (PilE) and minor pilins are processed by the prepilin peptidase (PilD) and assembled into the pilus fibre. The polytopic membrane protein (PilG) and the traffic NTPase (PilF) participate in this process. The outer membrane/tip-located protein (PilC) stabilizes the assembled filament. The pilus crosses the outer membrane through a channel that is formed by the secretin (PilQ), with the assistance of its pilot protein (PilP). DNA present in the environment is entangled by retracting pili and introduced into the meningococcal cell through the outer membrane (OM) and inner membrane (IM). The incoming DNA is transported across the outer membrane through a channel that is formed by the secretin (PilQ), with the assistance of its pilot protein (PilP). 2. One strand of the DNA enters the cytosol; the other is degraded and the degradation products are released into the periplasmic space. In the cytoplasm the incoming DNA (blue) is integrated into the genome (gray) by homologous recombination [145]. (This figure also appears with the color plates.)

outer membrane of Gram-negative bacteria [26, 27]. Several, if not all, proteins that participate in pilus assembly are known, but the biogenesis process itself is not yet clearly understood [28]. The prepilins are found associated with the cytoplasmic membrane through their hydrophobic domains. They are processed by a specific enzyme that resides in the cytoplasmic membrane – the prepilin peptidase (PilD), an aspartic acid protease that cleaves the leader peptide and *N*-methylates the new N-terminal residue of the mature pilin [29]. After processing by PilD, which probably facilitates the translocation of mature pilins across the membrane [30], the pilins are assembled into the pilus filament, which protrudes from the membrane. As it is assembled, the pilus filament extends outwards from the cytoplasmic membrane, across the peptidoglycan layer and periplasmic space, and crosses the outer membrane through a channel formed by the secretin (PilQ) [31, 32], assisted by its pilot protein (PilP) [33]. An ATPase

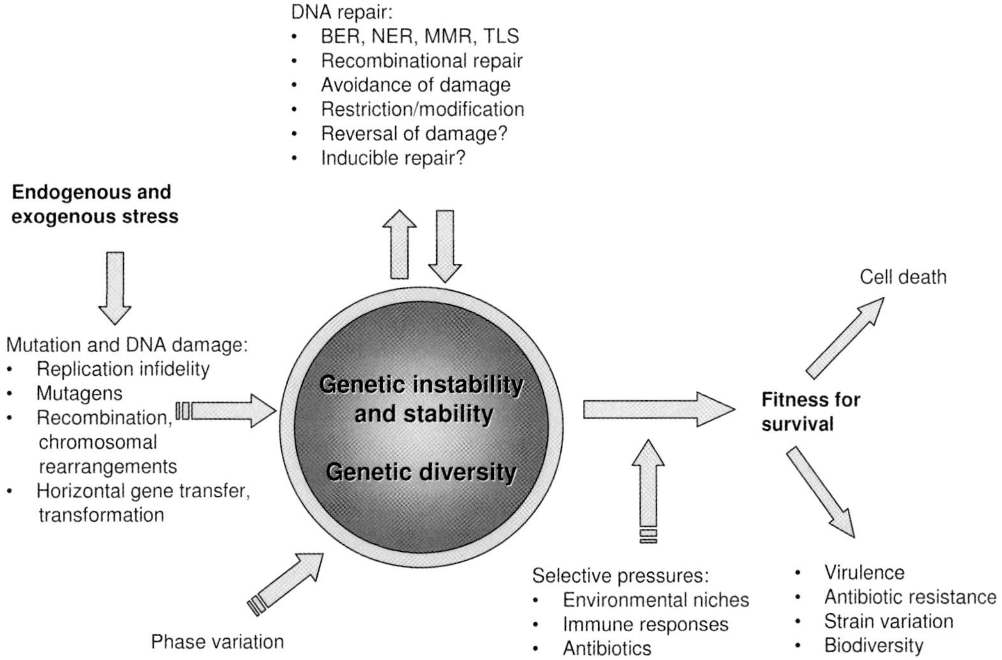

Fig. 7.2 Genome instability/maintenance and genetic variability. The balance between sources of genetic variation, DNA repair and selective pressures defines the genetic diversity and fitness of the resulting microbial population. Endogenous and exogenous stress leads to mutations and DNA damage. Recombination and horizontal gene transfer also allow variation to occur, together with phase and antigenic variation that contribute to the vast amount of different antigens in the important membrane-associated virulence factors. DNA repair pathways counteract deleterious DNA damaging events and at the same time, the infidelity of these mechanisms allows variation and together with selective pressures determine the net outcome of nucleotide change. BER – base excision repair, MMR – mismatch repair, NER – nucleotide excision repair, TLS – translesion synthesis. Adapted from Tønjum and Seeberg [101].

(PilT) is needed for twitching motility – which is caused by retraction of the pilus filament – but is dispensable for pilus assembly [34]. The NTPases PilF and PilT are closely related and belong to a large family of proteins that are involved in several transport systems, called the traffic NTPases. A tip-located adhesin (PilC) seems to stabilize the pilus filament and can also be found associated with the outer membrane [35].

Among the pilus biogenesis components, at least four proteins are essential for DNA uptake: PilQ [36], PilP [33], ComP (which shares homology with PilE) [37–39] and PilT [21]. Secretins, such as PilQ, are outer-membrane proteins that are involved in the extrusion of type IV pili and filamentous phages, type II and type III secretion, and transformation in Gram-negative microorganisms. The meningococcal secretins form stable multimeric ring structures with 12 subunits [40–42], whose correct assembly and insertion into the outer membrane requires the presence of the pilot lipoprotein PilP [33]. Electron microscopy shows that meningococcal secretins form doughnut-like structures with a diameter of the central cavity of approximately 6.5 nm [40–42]. Direct interaction of PilQ with its substrate, the polymerized pilus, has been demonstrated; and this interaction has been shown to induce a conformational change in the PilQ complex [36]. The central cavity in the PilQ 12-mer fits to accommodate the proposed pilus fibre model (~6 nm diam.) [33, 40–43] and could easily also accommodate the DNA double helix (~2.4 nm), either by itself or in a nucleoprotein complex. DNA uptake in *N. meningitidis* requires the presence of a DUS, so the putative DUS receptor could potentially participate in signaling the opening of the PilQ channel during transformation; and the pilus itself might also be involved. Direct evidence that DNA binds to the inner part of the meningococcal secretin channel in a nonspecific manner has recently been demonstrated (Assalkhou and Tønjum, personal communication). Intriguingly, single-stranded DNA generally interacts more strongly with PilQ than double-stranded DNA. Although transforming DNA is thought to bind to the cell as double-stranded molecules [44], substantial amounts of single-stranded DNA is formed during transformation and this conversion primarily occurs in the cytoplasm [45].

7.2.2.4 **Required for Transformation: Pili or Pilus-like Structures?**

N. meningitidis DUS-specific binding of DNA to the cell depends on the presence of the major pilin (PilE) and can be modulated by the expression of different minor pilins [37–39]. Thus, in *Neisseria*, there is a correlation between the presence of pili and competence [46, 47]. However, it is unclear whether pili themselves play a direct role in transformation or not. No interaction between DNA and the pilus or pilins has so far been detected [48]. The models for pilus structure show a cavity in the middle of the filament, but its narrow diameter (1.2 nm) and hydrophobicity argue against its role as a conduit for DNA. Although there is evidence that assembled pili are not necessary for transformation in *N. meningitidis*, the expression of pilin might be absolutely required [32, 49, 50].

If it is the assembled type IV pilus which is involved in transformation, it could exert this function by unspecifically entangle the negatively charged DNA and after, or during retraction, present the DNA to DNA-binding components, such as the secretin PilQ and also to the putative DUS receptor (Fig. 7.1). Normally, a large surplus of type IV pili is expressed compared to what is required for transformation, since a 10-fold reduction in piliation does not reduce competence [32]. Alternatively, a competence “pseudopilus” might exist, a structure similar to but distinct from type IV pili, that participates in the transport of DNA during transformation [5, 49]. Such a competence “pseudopilus” could be assembled using the same components as the type IV pilus, thereby linking competence and piliation. Various observations indicate that the presence of functional type IV pili and the ability to take up DNA have different requirements, for instance, transformation can be supported by the presence of pilin variants that cannot assemble efficiently into a pilus fibre and the requirement of minor pilins for competence but not for type IV pilus formation [37]. However, competence is linked to a colony morphology that can only be associated with the expression of type IV pili [46, 51]. The major pilin should be a structural component of both type IV pili and the competence pseudopilus; and the minor pilins could for instance be important in determining which structure is formed. Supporting this hypothesis, two minor pilins have been found to have antagonistic effects in competence in *N. gonorrhoeae*: the expression of PilV inhibits transformation [52], whereas transformation is enhanced by ComP [37, 49]. How would they participate in DNA uptake? As mentioned, a direct interaction between DNA and pilins or pseudopilins has so far not been detected. However, in organisms with type IV pili, the traffic NTPase that mediates pilus retraction (PilT) is required for DNA uptake [34, 53], which indicates that a pseudopilus could retract and pull DNA into the cell, facilitating the interaction of the incoming DNA with its DUS-specific receptor (Fig. 7.1). In the meningococcus, the retraction of pili, or the pseudopilus, could very likely mediate passage of the DNA through the PilQ channel (Fig. 7.1).

7.2.3 Periplasmic Interactions

The periplasmic component ComE is required for DNA uptake in *Neisseria*; and the protein binds DNA without DUS-specificity [54]. The role of neisserial ComE in DNA transport has not been clearly established. However, as described above, DNA uptake in this organism is dependent on the presence of the DUS. ComE might be a secondary DNA receptor in *Neisseria* and could therefore bind to DNA molecules that have already been selected by the presence of the DUS [5]. The putative DUS receptor might recognize DUS-containing DNA and trigger the opening of the secretin channel, thereby allowing the passage of DNA – which could be mediated by ComE. In this way, ComE could link the pilus or putative competence pseudopilus (which participates in DNA uptake) with the transport machinery at the inner membrane.

Mutations in the neisserial genes *comA*, *comL* and *tpc* also diminish natural transformation. The competence lipoprotein ComL and Tpc are associated with the murein layer and is thought to be involved in puncturing the peptidoglycan layer for incoming DNA entry [55–57]. ComA is predicted to be an inner membrane protein involved in DNA transport into the cytosol, since mutants that lack ComA retain the incoming DNA as a double-stranded molecule in the periplasmic space [56].

7.2.3.1 **Inner Membrane Transport of DNA**

A nuclease activity might be coupled to the transport of DNA across the inner membrane, so that the transforming DNA can enter the cytoplasm as a single strand, while the other strand is degraded. A link between DNA transport to the cytoplasm and degradation was observed in *N. gonorrhoeae*, as no nucleolytic processing of DNA after uptake was observed in a strain that lacked the putative channel protein ComA [56]. However, low levels of single-stranded DNA are formed during transformation of *N. gonorrhoeae*, regardless of the presence of ComA [45].

7.2.4
DNA Integration

Incoming single-stranded DNA can be integrated into the meningococcal chromosome by a RecA-dependent process that requires sequence homology between the incoming DNA and the bacterial chromosome [23, 25]. The interaction of the incoming DNA with cytoplasmic proteins protects it from degradation and is essential for transformation. A number of other *rec* genes have been shown to participate in neisserial recombinational pathways (for a review, see Kline et al. 2003 [58]). Recombination during transformation also displayed partial requirement for RecBCD, RecN, RecX and a homolog of Rep – an *E. coli* ATP-dependent helicase [59–61].

7.2.5
Sources of Exogenous DNA: Autolysis and Type IV Secretion

Most species are thought to donate DNA for subsequent transformation by autolysis. However, *N. gonorrhoeae* can also donate DNA for transformation by type IV secretion [62, 63]. The type IV secretion system is a multicomponent secretion system utilized by Gram-negative bacteria to secrete macromolecular substrates across the cell envelope. The process of DNA donation for the natural transformation of bacteria is poorly understood and has been assumed to involve bacterial cell death. In *N. gonorrhoeae*, mutations in three genes in the gonococcal genetic island (GGI) reduced the ability of a strain to act as a donor in transformation and to release DNA into the culture. The GGI has characteristics of a horizontally acquired genomic island and encodes homologues of type IV secretion system proteins. The GGI is likely to be acquired and integrated into the neisserial chromosome by site-specific recombination and may be lost by site-specific recombination or natural transformation. It is still not known if most gonococcal strains with the GGI contain all the genes essential for type IV secretion of DNA.

7.2.6
Effect of Transforming DNA in the Cell

Transforming DNA has traditionally been perceived as generating genetic variability and conferring change, such as antibiotic resistance [64]. However, our hypothesis is that transforming DNA also restores genes that are damaged after genotoxic stress. Indirect evidence for this possibility comes from findings that DUS are overrepresented within DNA repair and metabolism genes in phylogenetically different species, as discussed above [15]. Neisserial DUS and Pasteurellaceae USS required for transformation both exhibit a biased distribution towards genome maintenance genes, possibly ensuring their uptake through transformation if irrepairably damaged or lost. The need for the DUS uptake pathway is evident by the fact that mismatch repair (MMR) genes such as *mutS* and *mutL* are frequently deteriorated by mutation and recombination events [65, 66]. Such a deterioration creates mutators [66], but also generates a demand for gene restoration; and in this context it is significant that neisserial MMR genes have a particularly high DUS density, facilitating the uptake of these genes [15]. In this context, questions to be answered include the following: Does DNA uptake act as a signal for repair/recombination? Is DNA uptake predominantly a source for genetic change or is it a mechanism for conservation and DNA repair? What is the contribution of recombination and transforming DNA to mutator activity?

7.3
Mechanisms of Meningococcal Genome Instability

Meningococcal genomes possess several important characteristics that differ from *E. coli* (Table 7.1). Not only do the genome sizes and numbers of genes differ, but also the gene contents and genome dynamics are disparate. In order to adapt to changing local environments, it is beneficial to the meningococcus to possess a fluid genome. In contrast to *E. coli*, meningococcal adaptation is dominated by random mutational events and not by regulated responses. For example, the *E. coli* genome harbors many genes involved in sensing environmental changes, such as seven sigma factors and approximately 30 two-component regulatory systems [67]. By comparison, meningococcal genomes contain only three sigma factors and five putative two-component regulatory systems, possibly with redundant functions; and only a few neisserial global regulatory components have been identified [68]. Thus, compared with *E. coli*, meningococci have very few genes encoding regulatory response elements [13, 14].

Meningococcal genome fluidity is promoted by spontaneous mutational mechanisms that originate from local genomic changes caused by repeat sequences, phase and antigenic variation, recombination and horizontal gene transfer, or globally from mutator alleles. These simultaneous events all contribute to the polyphyletic nature of meningococcal genomes [64, 69]. Phase and

Table 7.1 Meningococcal adaptation is dominated by random mutational events – and not by regulated mechanisms.

Adaptation/parameters	Number of genes involved	
	Escherichia coli K12 [67]	*Neisseria meningitidis* Z2491 [13]
Genetic adaptation: phase and antigenic variation	<10	~100
Physiological adaptation:		
Sigma factors	7	3
Two-component regulatory systems	62	<10
Regulatory proteins (specific, global)	~110	~44
Genome size (Mb)	4.6	2.2
Total number of genes	4288	2065

antigenic variation alone involves close to 100 genes [13, 14, 70, 71], while in *E. coli* less than ten genes are subject to phase variation (Table 7.1) [67]. Consequently, rather than sensing and responding to the environment, meningococcal cells seem to generate a surplus of genetic variants, a prerequisite for natural selection [72, 73]. The features permitting the meningococcus to generate this abundance of variants optimize the chances of survival but also represent a potential risk by creating a highly unstable genome (Fig. 7.2).

7.3.1
Repeat Sequence Elements

The neisserial genome sequencing projects [13, 14] have revealed the presence of abundant repetitive DNA sequences with the associated intrinsic potential for genetic instability. Hundreds of repetitive DNA elements ranging from short repeats to insertion sequences and gene duplications of 1 kb or more are found. Repetitive DNA elements are major organisational components of the genome [74]. Repeats facilitate the duplication or deletion of regions of the genome as well as recombination and thereby establish small and large alterations that may be either beneficial or detrimental. The most frequent neisserial repeat element, the DUS, has been described above. Additionally, high numbers of tandem repeats ranging from homopolymeric tracts of G or C nucleotides to di-, tetra- and penta-nucleotide repeats have been identified, facilitating DNA slippage events [13, 14, 70]. Recently, Jordan and coworkers showed that, in the meningococcus, repeat length variation also exists in genes not typically associated with phase variation, including the DNA metabolism component transcription-repair coupling factor, *mfd* [75]. Furthermore, the gene encoding the meningococcal outer membrane secretin PilQ harbors 4–7 copies of a 24-nucleotide repeat, while gonococcal strains only have 2–3 copies [32]. Changes in the copy number of tandem repeats will necessarily change the structure and antigenicity of these components and may therefore represent a significant but largely unexplored mechanism of generating meningococcal diversity.

Other repeat sequences with incompletely determined functions such as Correia elements [76–78], neisserial intergenic mosaic elements (NIMEs), large insertion elements, AT-rich repeats (ATR) [13] and REP2 [79] are also present in meningococcal genomes. These repeats are all suggested to play a role in genome organization, function and evolution [74].

7.3.2 Phase Variation

Bacteria have evolved mechanisms to produce high mutation rates in specific regions of their genomes, i.e. localized hypermutation (see Chapter 9). High mutation rates in specific loci result in the rapid generation of variants, which increases the diversity of a population and might have a positive effect on fitness. The elements causing localized hypermutation are short repeat sequences consisting of multiple copies of the same sequence (tandem repeats). Tandem repeats are widespread in bacteria such as *Neisseria* and *Haemophilus* [72, 80]; and when they occur within the coding sequence, the promoter region, or close to the promoter region, they may change the transcriptional and translational state of the gene, leading to an on/off switching of the gene product called phase variation. More than 100 putative phase-variable meningococcal genes have been identified in which phase variation is used to alter virulence-associated surface-exposed molecules like outer membrane proteins PorA, Opc, opacity proteins, pili and specific adhesions, as well as lipooligosaccharide and capsule [35, 70, 71, 81–87]. Recently, mismatch repair and other DNA repair pathways and metabolic components have been implicated in the control of phase variation [88].

7.3.3 Antigenic Variation

Antigenic variation refers to the expression of functionally conserved moieties that are antigenically distinct within a clonal population [89]. Only one variant is expressed at any given time, though the cell contains the genetic information to produce a whole range of antigenic variants. In the pathogenic *Neisseria*, antigenic variation occurs in a number of surface components, including type IV pili and Opa proteins [23, 90–95]. The best characterized system is the expression of type IV pili, which involves RecA-dependent recombination similar to gene conversion (Fig. 7.3) [35, 94, 96].

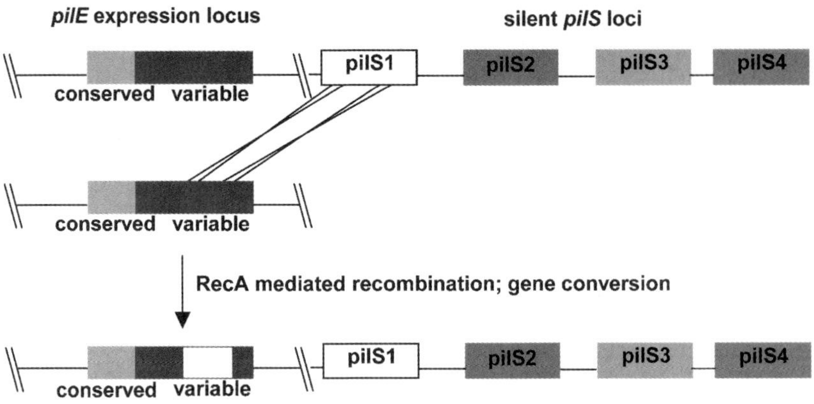

Fig. 7.3 Meningococcal antigenic variation by gene conversion. Meningococcal pilin antigenic variation is mediated by RecA-dependent gene conversion. Pili consist of thousands of pilin (PilE) subunits polymerized into long fibers. The PilE protein contains a highly conserved N-terminal domain and a variable C-terminal domain, the latter determining the antigenicity of the pili. The variable region is the result of a nonreciprocal transfer of DNA from one of a number of silent partial *pilS* loci to the single *pilE* expression locus. The silent loci, sometimes present several hundred basepairs away from the *pilE* expression locus, may donate a stretch of nucleotides, on the basis of short sequence homology. The genetic mechanism proceeds through a form of gene conversion requiring RecA and multiple crossover events during recombination that results in a unidirectional transfer of a *pilS* segment to the *pilE* variable region. (This figure also appears with the color plates.)

7.4
Meningococcal DNA Repair Profile

Both endogenous and exogenous insults can be harmful and result in DNA damage [97]. The repair machinery that protects against these DNA lesions has been extensively studied in both prokaryotes and eukaryotes [98–100] and the pathways that operate in *E. coli* serve as a model for DNA repair systems in other microorganisms. According to the *E. coli* paradigm, excision repair pathways include base excision repair (BER), mismatch repair (MMR) and nucleotide excision repair (NER), while other repair strategies encompass recombinational repair, reversal of DNA damage and tolerance of DNA damage (Fig. 7.4) [101]. Only limited experimental information about meningococcal DNA repair systems is currently available (Table 7.2). However, a comparison of the three completed meningococcal genome sequences and one gonococcal genome sequence with *E. coli* has disclosed interesting findings concerning the occurrence of DNA repair genes (Table 7.2) [13, 14].

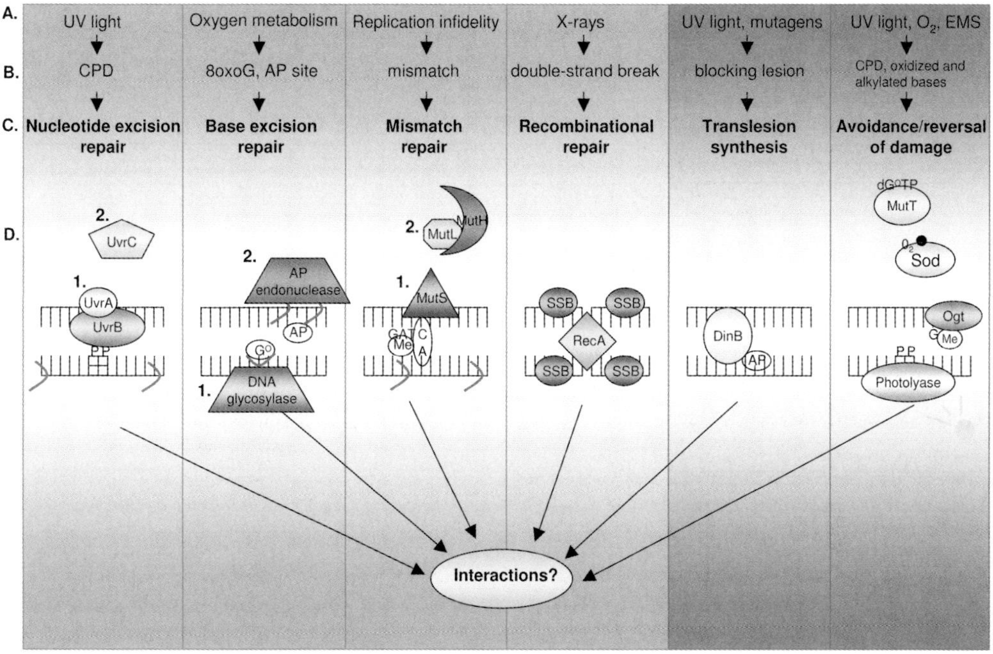

Fig. 7.4 Major DNA repair pathways. A number of repair pathways exist in organisms to manage the cytotoxic and mutagenic effect of DNA damage that can arise through endogenous and exogenous stress. A. Some examples of DNA-damaging agents. EMS – ethanemethyl sulfonate. B. DNA damage typically induced by the agent. CPD – cyclobutane pyrimidine photodimer, 8oxoG (G^O) – 7,8-dihydro-8oxo-2′-deoxyguanosine, AP site – abasic site. C. The DNA repair pathway often involved in removing the DNA lesion. Blue-colored pathways represent true repair, green pathways represent avoidance or reversal of a damage or a manner of bypassing a lesion. D. Important components participating in the repair pathway in *E. coli*. Red arrows indicate cleaved DNA strand. Please note that this figure does not show the detailed steps or every component involved in each repair pathway. P – pyrimidine, Me – methyl group, SSB – single-stranded binding protein, $O_2^{\bullet}$ – oxygen radical, SOD – superoxide dismutase. (This figure also appears with the color plates.)

7.4.1
Base Excision Repair

As meningococcal cells are likely to be exposed to high loads of oxidative stress, defense against oxidative DNA damages may be particularly important to this organism. One of the most frequent forms of oxidative DNA damage is the oxidation product of guanine, 7,8-dihydro-8-oxo-2′-deoxyguanosine (8oxoG) [102], which results in base mispairing during replication. The BER pathway is probably the cell's major line of defense against the deleterious effects of such DNA damage [103, 104]. BER involves the release of modified base residues from DNA by DNA glycosylases that leave abasic (AP) sites in the DNA (Fig. 7.4).

Table 7.2 DNA repair pathway characteristics in *Neisseria meningitidis* based on MC58 and Z2491 genome sequences as well as experiments conducted in *Neisseria gonorrhoeae.*

DNA repair pathway	+/–	Comments and special features
Avoidance of damage	+	Catalase, SodB, SodC, Glutathione peroxidase and a Sco homologue together with other components, participate in the defence against oxygen radicals. MutT family and Dut homologs for keeping dGTP pool clean and dUTP pool low
Direct repair/damage reversal		
Photoreactivation	–	Phr homolog identified (authentic frameshift) [130]
Alkylation reversal	?	No *alkB* homolog but sequence homology identified to *ogt/ada* [a)]
Excision repair		
1. Base excision repair (BER)	+	Homologs identified to all known steps of pathway
Ung (uracil glycosylase)		Homolog identified
Mug (T:G, T:U glycosylase)		Putative homolog
MutY (A/G DNA glycosylase)		Homolog identified [105]
Nth (excises oxidized pyrimidines)		Homolog identified
Fpg (excises 8-oxoG, FaPy-lesions)		Homolog identified [107]
Nei (excises oxidized pyrimidines)		No homolog identified
Tag (3-methyladenine DNA glycosylase)		Homolog identified
AlkA (3-methyladenine DNA glycosylase)		No homolog identified
Xth (5′ AP endonuclease)		Homolog identified
Nfo (5′ AP endonuclease)		No homolog identified
2. Nucleotide excision repair (NER)	+	Homologs identified to all known steps of pathway: UvrA, UvrB, UvrC, UvrD [118]
3. Mismatch excision repair (MMR)	+	Homologs identified to part of pathway[b]: *mutS* and *mutL* identified but apparent lack of *mutH* [114]
Recombinational repair	+	Components of RecBCD, RecF and branch migration/resolution pathways identified [59]
RecA (recombinase)		Involved in DNA transformation, pilin antigenic variation and DNA repair [59, 125]
Translesion synthesis	+	Only one DNA translesion polymerase, DinB
SOS response	–	No homologs of *lexA* or SOS boxes; and absence of an SOS-like system [123]

a) The C-terminal part of NMB1528 (MC58)/NMA1728 (Z2491) protein, methylated DNA–protein cysteine methyltransferase, shows similarity to both *E. coli ada* and *ogt*.

b) Additional components normally associated with MMR missing in one of the sequenced meningococcal genomes are *vsr* (identified in Z2491 but not in MC58) and *dam* (identified in MC58 but not in Z2491). *dcm* is found in both Z2491 and MC58.

The AP site is cleaved by the AP-lyase activity of many DNA glycosylases or by an AP-endonuclease, leaving a strand break, which is in turn repaired by enzymes that include a DNA polymerase and a DNA ligase.

The meningococcal genome sequences reveal that homologs of all steps in the BER pathway are present, although homologs of the DNA glycosylases *nei* and *alkA* and the endonuclease *nfo* are missing (Table 7.2). The only meningococcal DNA repair component fully characterized to date is the DNA glycosylase MutY, which participates in BER [105]. MutY is an atypical glycosylase in that it removes a normal base, adenine, from DNA when it is mispaired with 8oxoG, thereby preventing GC to TA transversions [106]. Interestingly, neisserial *mutY* mutants show high spontaneous mutation rates. Thus, the DNA glycosylase MutY exerts a prominent role in neisserial DNA repair. Another significant feature of meningococcal DNA repair is the combination of the particularly strong synergy between the DNA glycosylases MutY and Fpg of BER (Davidsen and Tønjum, personal communication) with a relative abundance of antioxidants such as SodC [107–109].

7.4.2 Mismatch Repair

Mismatch repair (MMR) recognizes base–base mismatches and insertion/deletion nucleotide loops that result from DNA polymerase errors during replication [110]. In *E. coli* MMR, MutS mismatch recognition [111, 112] is followed by MutL recruitment [113]. Together, these enzymes activate MutH, an endonuclease that directs the strand specificity of the repair machinery (Fig. 7.4). The meningococcus has homologs of the genes that encode MMR enzymes MutS and MutL, but it lacks the MutH endonuclease, as do humans. It is possible that another meningococcal component carries out the MutH strand-specificity function found in *E. coli*, or that the meningococcus does not need this function. Stojiljkovic and coworkers have hypothesized that defects in MMR might influence neisserial virulence and demonstrated that *mutS* mutants had a significantly increased frequency of phase variation and moderate increases in the rate of missense mutations [114, 115]. However, the majority of meningococcal mutators examined could not be complemented by *mutS* or *mutL*, indicating that other mechanisms influence meningococcal mutability.

7.4.3 Nucleotide Excision Repair and the SOS Response

The NER pathway repairs bulky lesions caused by exogenous damage such as UV light or polycyclic aromatic hydrocarbons that interfere with normal base-pairing, thereby impairing transcription and replication [116]. In *E. coli*, NER is executed by the UvrABC complex, which removes a stretch of nucleotides including the lesion (Fig. 7.4) [116, 117]. A gonococcal nucleotide excision repair system that functions on pyrimidine dimers has been identified [118]; and the gonococcus has been shown to express functional *uvrA* and *uvrB* genes [119, 120]. In contrast to *E. coli* NER genes, gonococcal *uvrA* and *uvrB* do not contain LexA binding sites or SOS boxes, the general hallmarks of an active SOS response. In *E. coli*, the SOS response allows increased repair and the restoration of replication by inducing the expression of more than 40 genes when large amounts of genomic DNA damage are present [121, 122]. The lack of a functional gonococcal SOS response has been experimentally confirmed by Davies and coworkers, who demonstrated that exposure to the mutagen methyl methanesulfonate (MMS) and UV radiation did not cause an increase in the gonococcal *uvrA* and *uvrB* transcripts [123]. The authors concluded that, in *Neisseria*, the prime effector of the SOS response, the RecA protein, has evolved for recombination purposes only. Although several homologues of genes known to be SOS-inducible are present in the Neisseriae, no homolog of the gene encoding LexA or SOS boxes has so far been identified [13, 14, 124].

7.4.4
Recombinational Repair

Due to the absence of an SOS response, it is hypothesized that recombination pathways are very important for the pathogenic *Neisseria* as a prime response to double-strand breaks in DNA (Fig. 7.4). RecA has an important role in most meningococcal repeat-associated events, including those associated with homologous recombination, antigenic variation and transformation [59]. Gonococcal RecA was first identified by complementation studies in *E. coli* [10]. Later, the function of *E. coli* RecA in the gonococcus was examined; and it was shown that species-specific interactions were important for RecA-dependent DNA repair functions but not for homologous recombination [60]. A number of other *rec* genes participate in neisserial recombinational pathways (for a review, see Kline et al. 2003 [59]). Although a *recF* homologue in the pathogenic *Neisseria* is absent, the RecF- and RecBCD-like pathways are present and involved in recombinational repair [59] and gonococcal RecA acts in both pathways [58, 59, 125]. Recombination during transformation also displayed a partial requirement for RecBCD, RecN, RecX and an *E. coli* ATP-dependent helicase Rep homolog [59, 61, 126], while recombination associated with antigenic variation was supported by RecF family members RecO, RecQ and RecJ, as well as RecX and Rep [59, 61, 126, 127]. Interestingly, meningococcal strains belonging to the hypervirulent lineage ET-37 have multiple missense mutations in the gene encoding RecB, which confers a UV-sensitive phenotype, increased mutagenicity and also increased pilin antigenic variation [128].

7.4.5
Other DNA Repair Strategies

In addition to the excision repair and recombinational pathways, other strategies are available to the meningococcus to avoid the mutagenic and cytotoxic effects of DNA damage (Fig. 7.4). In *E. coli*, translesion synthesis (TLS) is performed by three translesion DNA polymerases that allow replication past blocking lesions with the risk of generating mutations [129]. Interestingly, only a single translesion DNA polymerase homologue is present in the meningococcus (*dinB* homolog). Additionally, the neisserial genomes exhibit a number of putative gene products involved in neutralizing DNA-damaging agents before they can harm the DNA (Table 7.2), such as oxygen radical scavengers like catalase and SodC. In addition to the SOS response, the only mode of DNA repair that seems to be completely absent in the meningococcus is direct repair of DNA damage, or damage reversal. In 1979, Campbell demonstrated that gonococcal and meningococcal strains exposed to photoreactivating light (UV radiation) showed no difference in survival compared with strains not receiving this radiation [130]. Meningococcal genome sequences later confirmed the absence of such an enzymatic property in strain MC58, since the gene encoding the meningococcal Phr photolyase contains an authentic frameshift [4, 14]. Intriguingly, also all major alkylation repair genes except 3-methyladenine DNA glycosylase I (Tag) are absent in the meningococcus. In *E. coli*, the "suicide" action of methyltransferases (Ada, Ogt) or iron-dependent dioxygenases (AlkB) removes the added methylgroup only, or alkylated bases are excised by BER 3-methyladenine DNA glycosylases (Tag, AlkA) [131]. The lack of *alkB* and other alkylation repair genes in *Neisseria* is a significant deviation, suggesting that alkylation repair might not be in demand in the meningococcal habitat, that other repair pathways may exert this function, or that Tag is sufficient for the repair of aberrantly alkylated DNA.

7.4.6
Meningococcal DNA Repair Profile Adjusted to its Habitat

As described above, homologs of *E. coli* genes encoding components of the major DNA repair pathways base excision, mismatch repair, nucleotide excision and recombinational repair are present in the meningococcus, although the complexity of genes participating in each pathway is somewhat reduced (Table 7.2). Only one homolog of *fpg/nei* (BER) and only a single gene encoding a translesion DNA polymerase are present (Table 7.1) [58]. In contrast, *Mycobacterium tuberculosis* contains four homologs of *fpg/nei*, while *E. coli* harbors three translesion DNA polymerases, as previously mentioned. This incapacity could possibly reflect both a strategy for saving genome space and "habitat" preferences. The meningococcus resides relatively protected in human oral mucosal surfaces. In this rather limited habitat, the environmental challenges and opportunities consist of fluctuations in nutrients, pH, gas exchange (oxygen/carbon dioxide) and the competing normal flora in addition to the host responses. Conversely, *E. coli* with its more than twice as large genome (Table 7.1) has a much broader repertoire of tools for responding and adapting to external stimuli and can therefore survive in a myriad of environments.

7.5
Mutator Alleles and Fitness for Survival

Mutations in MMR genes usually result in a global increase in the rate of genetic variation and generate a mutator phenotype. Mutators may have an advantage in situations where there is an environmental flux and/or selective pressure, but any hypermutation also imposes a cost on the organism. Strains with increased mutation rates form variants more rapidly than strains with a low mutation rate, ultimately increasing the fitness of the population. However, bacteria with high mutation rates over time have an increased accumulation of deleterious mutations, generating reduced fitness or nonviable genomes [132]. Mutators in various bacterial species have been associated with increased survival rates [133, 134], overexpression of virulence factors [135], outbreaks of epidemic disease [115] and increased occurrence of antibiotic resistance [136, 137], yet a general link between invasive disease and mutator phenotypes has not been clearly established.

The negative fitness impact associated with meningococcal DNA repair defects may be compensated for and balanced *in vivo* by an enhanced capability to create variants. This is emphasized by the establishment of the participation of MMR components in controlling phase variation in disease-associated meningococcal isolates. MMR *mutS, mutL* and *uvrD*-defective strains show enhanced phase variation [88, 114, 115, 138], while conflicting evidence exists on the association of DNA adenine methyl-transferase variants causing hypermutable neisserial strains with enhanced phase-variable capsule-switching [139, 140]. Bacterial MMR-deficient mutants, exhibiting high mutation and homologous recombination rates, are frequently found in natural populations. The sequence mosaicism of MMR genes may be a hallmark of a mechanism of adaptive evolution that involves modulation of mutation and recombination rates by recurrent losses and reacquisitions of MMR gene functions [65].

The intricate paradox of genome stability versus instability is most evident under stress, where repair of lethal DNA lesions is absolutely required, while perfect restoration of original genetic information is not [141]. Stress is a condition meningococci are more or less exposed to at all times when residing in the human host. Multiple studies predict or modulate scenarios of adaptive mutations and evolution, both in experimental populations as well as in the natural host; and DNA repair pathways have been found to play a crucial role in controlling such events [142, 143]. Recently, results showed that meningococcal contact with host cells induces a DNA repair system: the upregulation of an open reading frame encoding a homolog to the *E. coli* exonuclease XseB enhanced meningococcal ability to repair DNA and increased the phase variation frequency. This finding emphasizes the significance of DNA repair systems when the meningococcus adapts to its niches during colonization of a new host [144], thus implicating a pivotal role for DNA repair pathways in the fitness and survival of this organism. In this context, it is interesting that the gene encoding the DNA glycosylase MutY is the most DUS-dense of all neisserial DNA repair genes, while *mutS* and *uvrA* each contain four DUS [15, 145]. A transient and beneficial increase in genome instability might therefore be allowed during colonization and pathogenesis simply through the inactivation and/or loss of antimutator genes, since these DUS-containing sequences might be preferentially recovered.

7.6
Concluding Remarks

Horizontal gene transfer together with DNA repair and recombination functions provide the principal means for creating diversity in prokaryotes. The genomic alterations and polymorphisms ensuing from these processes have profound consequences for the way in which the meningococcus interacts with its human host by leading to increased fitness and antibiotic resistance as well as structural and antigenic changes in critical surface components [64]. Basic knowledge as to how DNA transfer events might be integrated or linked to subsequent repair and recombination processes is virtually nonexistent.

Understanding genome dynamics in detail, including horizontal gene transfer mechanisms, recombination and DNA repair, requires a combined multidisciplinary approach. Importantly, much can be learned by recognition of the structural and functional relationships between systems for genetic transformation and DNA repair. However, many components specific for these processes remain to be identified and their interactions are elusive. We need a better understanding of the entire DNA metabolism machinery in bacterial organisms, as a prerequisite to combat the explosive occurrence of infectious diseases. In this context, the meningococcus is a most relevant model organism.

References

1 M. Koomey **1988**, Competence for natural transformation in *Neisseria gonorrhoeae*: a model system for studies of horizontal gene transfer, *APMIS Suppl.* 84, 56–61.

2 M. Fussenegger, T. Rudel, R. Barten, R. Ryll, T. F. Meyer **1997**, Transformation competence and type-4 pilus biogenesis in *Neisseria gonorrhoeae* – a review, *Gene* 192, 125–134.

3 M. C. Roberts **1989**, Plasmids of *Neisseria gonorrhoeae* and other *Neisseria* species, *Clin. Microbiol. Rev.* 2, S18–S23.

4 T. Davidsen, T. Tønjum **2006**, Meningococcal genome dynamics, *Nat. Rev. Microbiol.* 4, 11–22.

5 I. Chen, D. Dubnau **2004**, DNA uptake during bacterial transformation, *Nat. Rev. Microbiol.* 2, 241–249.

6 M. G. Lorenz, W. Wackernagel **1994**, Bacterial gene transfer by natural genetic transformation in the environment, *Microbiol. Rev.* 58, 563–602.

7 T. Tønjum, K. Bøvre, E. Juni **1995**, Fastidious Gram-negative bacteria: Meeting the diagnostic challenge with nucleic acid analysis, *APMIS* 103, 609–627.

8 G. D. Biswas, T. Sox, E. Blackman, P. F. Sparling **1977**, Factors affecting genetic transformation of *Neisseria gonorrhoeae*, *J. Bacteriol.* 129, 983–992.

9 J. F. Graves, G. D. Biswas, P. F. Sparling **1982**, Sequence-specific DNA uptake in

transformation of *Neisseria gonorrhoeae*, *J. Bacteriol.* 152, 1071–1077.

10 J.M. Koomey, S. Falkow **1987**, Cloning of the *recA* gene of *Neisseria gonorrhoeae* and construction of gonococcal *recA* mutants, *J. Bacteriol.* 169, 790–795.

11 L.S. Mathis, J.J. Scocca **1982**, *Haemophilus influenzae* and *Neisseria gonorrhoeae* recognize different specificity determinants in the DNA uptake step of genetic transformation, *J. Gen. Microbiol.* 128, 1159–1161.

12 S.D. Goodman, J.J. Scocca **1988**, Identification and arrangement of the DNA sequence recognized in specific transformation of *Neisseria gonorrhoeae*, *Proc. Natl Acad. Sci. USA* 85, 6982–6986.

13 J. Parkhill, et al. **2000**, Complete DNA sequence of a serogroup A strain of *Neisseria meningitidis* Z2491, *Nature* 404, 502–506.

14 H. Tettelin, et al. **2000**, Complete genome sequence of *Neisseria meningitidis* serogroup B strain MC58, *Science* 287, 1809–1815.

15 T. Davidsen, et al. **2004**, Biased distribution of DNA uptake sequences towards genome maintenance genes, *Nucleic Acids Res.* 32, 1050–1058.

16 G.O. Smith, M.L. Gwinn, S.L. Salzberg **1999**, DNA uptake signal sequences in naturally transformable bacteria, *Res. Microbiol.* 150, 603–616.

17 J.S. Kroll, K.E. Wilks, J.L. Farrant, P.R. Langford **1998**, Natural genetic exchange between *Haemophilus* and *Neisseria*: intergeneric transfer of chromosomal genes between major human pathogens, *Proc. Natl Acad. Sci. USA* 95, 12381–12385.

18 M.E. Kahn, F. Barany, H.O. Smith **1983**, Transformasomes: specialized membranous structures that protect DNA during *Haemophilus* transformation. *Proc. Natl Acad. Sci. USA* 80, 6927–6931.

19 C. Elkins, C.E. Thomas, H.S. Seifert, P.F. **1991**, Sparling, Species-specific uptake of DNA by gonococci is mediated by a 10-base-pair sequence, *J. Bacteriol.* 173, 3911–3913.

20 T. Tønjum, M. Koomey **1997**, The pilus colonization factor of pathogenic neisserial species: organelle biogenesis and structure/function relationships – a review, *Gene* 192, 155–163.

21 A.J. Merz, M. So, M.M.P. Sheetz **2000**, Pilus retraction powers bacterial twitching motility, *Nature 407, 98–102*

22 J.M. Skerker, H.C. Berg **2001**, Direct observation of extension and retraction of type IV pili, *Proc. Natl Acad. Sci. USA* 98, 6901–6904

23 J. Swanson et al. **1986**, Gene conversion involving the pilin structural gene correlates with pilus+ in equilibrium with pilus– changes in *Neisseria gonorrhoeae*. *Cell*, 47, 267–276.

24 C.P. Gibbs, et al. **1989**, Reassortment of pilin genes in *Neisseria gonorrhoeae* occurs by two distinct mechanisms, *Nature* 338, 651–652.

25 A.C. Perry, I.J. Nicolson, J.R. Saunders **1988**, *Neisseria meningitidis* C114 contains silent, truncated pilin genes that are homologous to *Neisseria gonorrhoeae* pil sequences, *J. Bacteriol.* 170, 1691–1697.

26 M. Russel **1998**, Macromolecular assembly and secretion across the bacterial cell envelope: type II protein secretion systems, *J. Mol. Biol.* 279, 485–499.

27 M. Sandkvist **2001**, Biology of type II secretion, *Mol. Microbiol.* 40, 271–283.

28 J.S. Mattick **2002**, Type IV pili and twitching motility, *Annu. Rev. Microbiol.* 56, 289–314.

29 C.F. LaPointe, R.K. Taylor **2000**, The type 4 prepilin peptidases comprise a novel family of aspartic acid proteases, *J. Biol. Chem.* 275, 1502–1510.

30 D. Nunn **1999**, Bacterial type II protein export and pilus biogenesis: more than just homologies? *Trends Cell Biol.* 9, 402–408.

31 S.L. Drake, M. Koomey **1995**, The product of the *pilQ* gene is essential for the biogenesis of type IV pili in *Neisseria gonorrhoeae*, *Mol. Microbiol.* 18, 975–986.

32 T. Tønjum, D.A. Caugant, S.A. Dunham, M. Koomey **1998**, Structure and function of repetitive sequence elements associated with a highly polymorphic domain of the *Neisseria meningitidis* PilQ protein, *Mol. Microbiol.* 29, 111–124.

33 S.L. Drake, S.A. Sandstedt, M. Koomey **1997**, PilP, a pilus biogenesis lipoprotein in *Neisseria gonorrhoeae*, affects expression of PilQ as a high-molecular-mass multimer, *Mol. Microbiol.* 23, 657–668.

34 M. Wolfgang, et al. **1998**, PilT mutations lead to simultaneous defects in competence for natural transformation and twitching motility in piliated *Neisseria gonorrhoeae*, *Mol. Microbiol.* 29, 321–330.

35 T. Rudel, et al. **1995**, Role of pili and the phase-variable PilC protein in natural competence for transformation of *Neisseria gonorrhoeae*, *Proc. Natl Acad. Sci. USA* 92, 7986–7990.

36 R.F. Collins et al. **2005**, Interaction with type IV pili induces structural changes in the bacterial outer membrane secretin PilQ, *J. Biol. Chem.* 280, 18923–18930

37 M. Wolfgang, J.P. van Putten, S.F. Hayes, M. Koomey **1999**, The *comP* locus of *Neisseria gonorrhoeae* encodes a type IV prepilin that is dispensable for pilus biogenesis but essential for natural transformation, *Mol. Microbiol.* 31, 1345–1357.

38 F.E. Aas, C. Lovold, M. Koomey **2002**, An inhibitor of DNA binding and uptake events dictates the proficiency of genetic transformation in *Neisseria gonorrhoeae*: mechanism of action and links to type IV pilus expression, *Mol. Microbiol.* 46, 1441–1450.

39 F.E. Aas, M. Wolfgang, S. Frye, S. Dunham, C. Lovold, M. Koomey **2002**, Competence for natural transformation in *Neisseria gonorrhoeae*: components of DNA binding and uptake linked to type IV pilus expression. *Mol. Microbiol.* 46, 749760

40 R.F. Collins, L. Davidsen, J.P. Derrick, R.C. Ford, T. Tønjum **2001**, Analysis of the PilQ secretin from *Neisseria meningitidis* by transmission electron microscopy reveals a dodecameric quaternary structure, *J. Bacteriol.* 183, 3825–3832.

41 R.F. Collins, et al. **2003**, Three-dimensional structure of the *Neisseria meningitidis* secretin PilQ determined from negative stain transmission electron microscopy, *J. Bacteriol.* 185, 2611–2617.

42 R.F. Collins, et al. **2004**, Structure of the *Neisseria meningitidis* outer membrane PilQ secretin complex at 12 Å resolution, *J. Biol. Chem.* 279, 39750–39756.

43 H.E. Parge, et al. **1995**, Structure of the fibre-forming protein pilin at 2.6 Å resolution, *Nature* 378, 32–38.

44 G.D. Hill **1981**, Entry of double-stranded deoxyribonucleic acid during transformation of *Neisseria gonorrhoeae*, *J. Bacteriol.* 145, 638–640.

45 M.S. Chaussee, S.A. Hill **1998**, Formation of single-stranded DNA during DNA transformation of *Neisseria gonorrhoeae*, *J. Bacteriol.* 180, 5117–5122.

46 K. Jyssum, S. Lie **1965**, Genetic factors determining competence in transformation of *Neisseria meningitidis*. 1. A permanent loss of competence, *Acta Pathol. Microbiol. Scand.* 63, 306–316.

47 P.F. Sparling **1966**, Genetic transformation of *Neisseria gonorrhoeae* to streptomycin resistance, *J. Bacteriol.* 92, 1364–1371.

48 L.S. Mathis, J.J. Scocca **1984**, On the role of pili in transformation of *Neisseria gonorrhoeae*, *J. Gen. Microbiol.* 130, 3165–3173.

49 M. Wolfgang, J.P. van Putten, S.F. Hayes, D. Dorward, M. Koomey **2000**, Components and dynamics of fiber formation define a ubiquitous biogenesis pathway for bacterial pili, *EMBO J.* 19, 6408–6418.

50 C.D. Long, D.M. Tobiason, M.P. Lazio, K.A. Kline, H.S. Seifert **2003**, Low-level pilin expression allows for substantial DNA transformation competence in *Neisseria gonorrhoeae*, *Infect. Immun.* 71, 6279–6291.

51 J. Swanson, O. Barrera **1983**, Gonococcal pilus subunit size heterogeneity correlates with transitions in colony piliation phenotype, not with changes in colony opacity, *J. Exp. Med.* 158, 1459–1472.

52 H.C. Winther-Larsen, et al. **2001**, *Neisseria gonorrhoeae* PilV, a type IV pilus-associated protein essential to human epithelial cell adherence, *Proc. Natl Acad. Sci. USA* 98, 15276–15281.

53 M. Wolfgang, H.S. Park, S.F. Hayes, J.P. van Putten, M. Koomey **1998**, Suppression of an absolute defect in type IV pilus biogenesis by loss-of-function mutations in *pilT*, a twitching motility gene in *Neisseria gonorrhoeae*, *Proc. Natl Acad. Sci. USA* 95, 14973–14978.

54 I. Chen, E.C. Gotschlich **2001**, ComE, a competence protein from *Neisseria gonorrhoeae* with DNA-binding activity, *J. Bacteriol.* 183, 3160–3168.

55 D. Facius, T.F. Meyer **1993**, A novel determinant (*comA*) essential for natural transformation competence in *Neisseria gonorrhoeae, Mol. Microbiol.* 10, 699–712.

56 D. Facius, M. Fussenegger, T.F. Meyer **1996**, Sequential action of factors involved in natural competence for transformation of *Neisseria gonorrhoeae, FEMS Microbiol. Lett.* 137, 159–164.

57 S.B. Graupner, W. Wackernagel **2001**, Identification and characterization of novel competence genes *comA* and *exbB* involved in natural genetic transformation of *Pseudomonas stutzeri, Res. Microbiol.* 152, 451–460.

58 K.A. Kline, E.V. Sechman, E.P. Skaar, H.S. Seifert **2003**, Recombination, repair and replication in the pathogenic *Neisseriae*: the 3 Rs of molecular genetics of two human-specific bacterial pathogens, *Mol. Microbiol.* 50, 3–13.

59 I.J. Mehr, H.S. Seifert **1998**, Differential roles of homologous recombination pathways in *Neisseria gonorrhoeae* pilin antigenic variation, DNA transformation and DNA repair, *Mol. Microbiol.* 30, 697–710.

60 E.A. Stohl, L. Blount, H.S. Seifert **2002**, Differential cross-complementation patterns of *Escherichia coli* and *Neisseria gonorrhoeae* RecA proteins, *Microbiology* 148, 1821–1831.

61 E.P. Skaar, M.P. Lazio, H.S. Seifert **2002**, Roles of the *recJ* and *recN* genes in homologous recombination and DNA repair pathways of *Neisseria gonorrhoeae, J. Bacteriol.* 184, 919–927.

62 H.L. Hamilton, K.J. Schwartz, J.P. Dillard **2001**, Insertion-duplication mutagenesis of neisseria: use in characterization of DNA transfer genes in the gonococcal genetic island, *J. Bacteriol.* 183, 4718–4726.

63 H.L. Hamilton, N.M. Domingue, K.J. Schwartz, K.T. Hackett, J.P. Dillard **2005**, *Neisseria gonorrhoeae* secretes chromosomal DNA via a novel type IV secretion system, *Mol. Microbiol.* 55, 1704–1721.

64 B.G. Spratt, L.D. Bowler, Q.Y. Zhang, J. Zhou, J.M. Smith **1992**, Role of interspecies transfer of chromosomal genes in the evolution of penicillin resistance in pathogenic and commensal *Neisseria* species, *J. Mol. Evol.* 34, 115–125.

65 E. Denamur, et al. **2000**, Evolutionary implications of the frequent horizontal transfer of mismatch repair genes, *Cell* 103, 711–721.

66 I. Bjedov et al. **2003**, Stress-induced mutagenesis in bacteria, *Science* 300, 1404–1409.

67 F.R. Blattner, et al. **1997**, The complete genome sequence of *Escherichia coli* K-12, *Science* 277, 1453–1474.

68 The Sanger Institute, **2005**, http://www.sanger.ac.uk/Projects/N_meningitidis/.

69 K.A. Jolley, D.J. Wilson, P. Kriz, G. McVean, M.C. Maiden **2005**, The influence of mutation, recombination, population history, and selection on patterns of genetic diversity in *Neisseria meningitidis, Mol. Biol. Evol.* 22, 562–569.

70 L.A. Snyder, S.A. Butcher, N.J. Saunders **2001**, Comparative whole-genome analyses reveal over 100 putative phase-variable genes in the pathogenic *Neisseria* spp, *Microbiology* 147, 2321–2332.

71 P. Martin, et al. **2003**, Experimentally revised repertoire of putative contingency loci in *Neisseria meningitidis* strain MC58: evidence for a novel mechanism of phase variation, *Mol. Microbiol.* 50, 245–257.

72 E.R. Moxon, R.E. Lenski, P.B. Rainey **1998**, Adaptive evolution of highly mutable loci in pathogenic bacteria, *Perspect. Biol. Med.* 42, 154–155.

73 E.J. Feil, B.G. Spratt **2001**, Recombination and the population structures of bacterial pathogens, *Annu. Rev. Microbiol.* 55, 561–590.

74 J.A. Shapiro **2002**, Repetitive DNA, genome system architecture and genome reorganization, *Res. Microbiol.* 153, 447–453.

75 P. Jordan, L.A. Snyder, N.J. Saunders **2003**, Diversity in coding tandem repeats in related Neisseria spp, *BMC Microbiol.* 3, 23.

76 F. F. Correia, S. Inouye, M. Inouye **1988**, A family of small repeated elements with some transposon-like properties in the genome of *Neisseria gonorrhoeae, J. Biol. Chem.* 263, 12194–12198.

77 F. F. Correia, S. Inouye, M. Inouye **1986**, A 26-base-pair repetitive sequence specific for *Neisseria gonorrhoeae* and *Neisseria meningitidis* genomic DNA, *J. Bacteriol.* 167, 1009–1015.

78 M. Mazzone, et al. **2001**, Whole-genome organization and functional properties of miniature DNA insertion sequences conserved in pathogenic *Neisseriae, Gene* 278, 211–222.

79 S. Morelle, E. Carbonnelle, X. Nassif **2003**, The REP2 repeats of the genome of *Neisseria meningitidis* are associated with genes coordinately regulated during bacterial cell interaction, *J. Bacteriol.* 185, 2618–2627.

80 C. D. Bayliss, D. Field, E. R. Moxon **2001**, The simple sequence contigency loci of *Haemophilus influenzae* and *Neisseria meningitidis, J. Clin. Invest.* 107, 657–662.

81 G. L. Murphy, T. D. Connell, D. S. Barritt, M. Koomey, J. G. Cannon **1989**, Phase variation of gonococcal protein II: regulation of gene expression by slipped-strand mispairing of a repetitive DNA sequence, *Cell* 56, 539–547.

82 T. H. Kawula, E. L. Aho, D. S. Barritt, D. G. Klapper, J. G. Cannon **1988**, Reversible phase variation of expression of *Neisseria meningitidis* class 5 outer membrane proteins and their relationship to gonococcal proteins II, *Infect. Immun.* 56, 380–386.

83 J. Sarkari, N. Pandit, E. R. Moxon, M. Achtman **1994**, Variable expression of the Opc outer membrane protein in *Neisseria meningitidis* is caused by size variation of a promoter containing polycytidine, *Mol. Microbiol.* 13, 207–217.

84 S. Hammerschmidt, et al. **1996**, Capsule phase variation in *Neisseria meningitidis* serogroup B by slipped-strand mispairing in the polysialyltransferase gene (*siaD*): correlation with bacterial invasion and the outbreak of meningococcal disease, *Mol. Microbiol.* 20, 1211–1220.

85 A. Rytkonen, et al. **2004**, *Neisseria meningitidis* undergoes PilC phase variation and PilE sequence variation during invasive disease, *J. Infect. Dis.* 189, 402–409.

86 M. P. Jennings, et al. **1999**, The genetic basis of the phase variation repertoire of lipopolysaccharide immunotypes in *Neisseria meningitidis, Microbiology* 145, 3013–3021.

87 A. W. Berrington, et al. **2002**, Phase variation in meningococcal lipooligosaccharide biosynthesis genes, *FEMS Immunol. Med. Microbiol.* 34, 267–275.

88 P. Martin, L. Sun, D. W. Hood, E. R. Moxon **2004**, Involvement of genes of genome maintenance in the regulation of phase variation frequencies in *Neisseria meningitidis, Microbiology* 150, 3001–3012.

89 P. Borst **1991**, Molecular genetics of antigenic variation, *Immunol. Today* 12, A29–A33.

90 T. D. Connell, D. Shaffer, J. G. Cannon **1990**, Characterization of the repertoire of hypervariable regions in the Protein II (opa) gene family of *Neisseria gonorrhoeae, Mol. Microbiol.* 4, 439–449.

91 K. S. Bhat, et al. **1991**, The opacity proteins of *Neisseria gonorrhoeae* strain MS11 are encoded by a family of 11 complete genes, *Mol. Microbiol.* 5, 1889–1901.

92 E. L. Aho, J. A. Dempsey, M. M. Hobbs, D. G. Klapper, J. G. Cannon **1991**, Characterization of the *opa* (class 5) gene family of *Neisseria meningitidis, Mol. Microbiol.* 5, 1429–1437.

93 J. A. Vazquez, et al. **1995**, Interspecies recombination in nature: a meningococcus that has acquired a gonococcal PIB porin, *Mol. Microbiol.* 15, 1001–1007.

94 P. Hagblom, E. Segal, E. Billyard, M. So **1985**, Intragenic recombination leads to pilus antigenic variation in *Neisseria gonorrhoeae, Nature* 315, 156–158.

95 A. Stern, M. Brown, P. Nickel, T. F. Meyer **1986**, Opacity genes in *Neisseria gonorrhoeae*: control of phase and antigenic variation, *Cell* 47, 61–71.

96 Q. Y. Zhang, D. DeRyckere, P. Lauer, M. Koomey **1992**, Gene conversion in *Neisseria gonorrhoeae*: evidence for its role in pilus antigenic variation, *Proc. Natl Acad. Sci. USA* 89, 5366–5370.

97 T. Lindahl **1993**, Instability and decay of the primary structure of DNA, *Nature* 362, 709–715.

98 J.A. Eisen, P.C. Hanawalt **1999**, A phylogenomic study of DNA repair genes, proteins, and processes, *Mutat. Res.* 435, 171–213.

99 J.H. Hoeijmakers **2001**, Genome maintenance mechanisms for preventing cancer, *Nature* 411, 366–374.

100 E.C. Friedberg, L.D. McDaniel, R.A. Schultz **2004**, The role of endogenous and exogenous DNA damage and mutagenesis, *Curr. Opin. Genet. Dev.* 14, 5–10.

101 T. Tønjum, E. Seeberg **2001**, Microbial fitness and genome dynamics, *Trends Microbiol.* 9, 356–358.

102 B. Demple, L. Harrison **1994**, Repair of oxidative damage to DNA: enzymology and biology, *Annu. Rev. Biochem.* 63, 915–948.

103 E. Seeberg, L. Eide, M. Bjøras **1995**, The base excision repair pathway, *Trends Biochem. Sci.* 20, 391–397.

104 G. Slupphaug, B. Kavli, H.E. Krokan **2003**, The interacting pathways for prevention and repair of oxidative DNA damage, *Mutat. Res.* 531, 231–251.

105 T. Davidsen, M. Bjøras, E.C. Seeberg, T. Tønjum **2005**, Antimutator role of DNA glycosylase MutY in pathogenic *Neisseria* species, *J. Bacteriol.* 187, 2801–2809.

106 Y. Nghiem, M. Cabrera, C.G. Cupples, J.H. Miller **1988**, The *mutY* gene: a mutator locus in *Escherichia coli* that generates G.C-T.A transversions, *Proc. Natl Acad. Sci. USA* 85, 2709–2713.

107 T. Davidsen **2005**, Genome instability and maintenance in *Neisseria meningitidis*, Ph.D. thesis, ISBN 82-8072-636-5.

108 R.G. Fowler, et al. **2003**, Interactions among the *Escherichia coli mutT, mutM*, and *mutY* damage prevention pathways, *DNA Repair* 2, 159–173.

109 M.L. Michaels, C. Cruz, A.P. Grollman, J.H. Miller **1992**, Evidence that MutY and MutM combine to prevent mutations by an oxidatively damaged form of guanine in DNA, *Proc. Natl Acad. Sci. USA* 89, 7022–7025.

110 M.J. Schofield, P. Hsieh **2003**, DNA mismatch repair: molecular mechanisms and biological function, *Annu. Rev. Microbiol.* 57, 579–608.

111 M.H. Lamers, et al. **2000**, The crystal structure of DNA mismatch repair protein MutS binding to a G × T mismatch, *Nature* 407, 711–717.

112 G. Obmolova, C. Ban, P. Hsieh, W. Yang **2000**, Crystal structures of mismatch repair protein MutS and its complex with a substrate DNA, *Nature* 407, 703–710.

113 C. Ban, M. Junop, W. Yang **1999**, Transformation of MutL by ATP binding and hydrolysis: a switch in DNA mismatch repair, *Cell* 97, 85–97.

114 A.R. Richardson, I. Stojiljkovic **2001**, Mismatch repair and the regulation of phase variation in *Neisseria meningitidis, Mol. Microbiol.* 40, 645–655.

115 A.R. Richardson, Z. Yu, T. Popovic, I. Stojiljkovic **2002**, Mutator clones of *Neisseria meningitidis* in epidemic serogroup A disease, *Proc. Natl Acad. Sci. USA* 99, 6103–6107.

116 P.C. Hanawalt **2002**, Subpathways of nucleotide excision repair and their regulation, *Oncogene* 21, 8949–8956.

117 E. Seeberg **1978**, Reconstitution of an *Escherichia coli* repair endonuclease activity from the separated *uvrA*+ and *uvrB+/uvrC+* gene products, *Proc. Natl Acad. Sci. USA* 75, 2569–2573.

118 L. A. Campbell, R.E. Yasbin **1984**, A DNA excision repair system for *Neisseria gonorrhoeae, Mol. Gen. Genet.* 193, 561–563.

119 C.G. Black, J. A. Fyfe, J.K. Davies **1997**, Cloning, nucleotide sequence and transcriptional analysis of the *uvrA* gene from *Neisseria gonorrhoeae, Mol. Gen. Genet.* 254, 479–485.

120 C.G. Black, J.A. Fyfe, J.K. Davies **1995**, A promoter associated with the neisserial repeat can be used to transcribe the *uvrB* gene from *Neisseria gonorrhoeae, J. Bacteriol.* 177, 1952–1958.

121 J. Courcelle, A. Khodursky, B. Peter, P.O. Brown, P.C. Hanawalt **2001**, Comparative gene expression profiles following UV exposure in wild-type and SOS-deficient *Escherichia coli, Genetics* 158, 41–64.

122 E.C. Freidberg, G.C. Walker, W. Siede **1995**, *DNA Repair and Mutagenesis*, American Society for Microbiology, Washington, D.C.

123 C.G. Black, J.A. Fyfe, J.K. Davies **1998**, Absence of an SOS-like system in *Neisseria gonorrhoeae*, *Gene* 208, 61–66.

124 P.O. Falnes, T. Rognes **2003**, DNA repair by bacterial AlkB proteins, *Res. Microbiol.* 154, 531–538.

125 M. Koomey, E.C. Gotschlich, K. Robbins, S. Bergstrom, J. Swanson **1987**, Effects of recA mutations on pilus antigenic variation and phase transitions in *Neisseria gonorrhoeae*, *Genetics* 117, 391–398.

126 K.A. Kline, H.S. Seifert **2005**, Role of the Rep helicase gene in homologous recombination in *Neisseria gonorrhoeae*, *J. Bacteriol.* 187, 2903–2907.

127 S.A. Hill **2000**, *Neisseria gonorrhoeae recJ* mutants show defects in recombinational repair of alkylated bases and UV-induced pyrimidine dimers, *Mol. Gen. Genet.* 264, 268–275.

128 P. Salvatore, et al. **2002**, Phenotypes of a naturally defective *recB* allele in *Neisseria meningitidis* clinical isolates, *Infect. Immun.* 70, 4185–4195.

129 R. Napolitano, R. Janel-Bintz, J. Wagner, R.P. Fuchs **2000**, All three SOS-inducible DNA polymerases (Pol II, Pol IV and Pol V) are involved in induced mutagenesis, *EMBO J.* 19, 6259–6265.

130 L.A. Campbell, R.E. Yasbin **1979**, Deoxyribonucleic acid repair capacities of *Neisseria gonorrhoeae*: absence of photoreactivation, *J. Bacteriol.* 140, 1109–1111.

131 B. Sedgwick, T. Lindahl **2002**, Recent progress on the Ada response for inducible repair of DNA alkylation damage, *Oncogene* 21, 8886–8894.

132 P. Funchain, et al. **2000**, The consequences of growth of a mutator strain of *Escherichia coli* as measured by loss of function among multiple gene targets and loss of fitness, *Genetics* 154, 959–970.

133 P.D. Sniegowski, P.J. Gerrish, R.E. Lenski **1997**, Evolution of high mutation rates in experimental populations of *E. coli*, *Nature* 387, 703–705.

134 L. Notley-McRobb, S. Seeto, T. Ferenci **2002**, Enrichment and elimination of *mutY* mutators in *Escherichia coli* populations, *Genetics* 162, 1055–1062.

135 S.L. Harris, et al. **1990**, Isolation and characterization of mutants with lesions affecting pellicle formation and erythrocyte agglutination by type 1 piliated *Escherichia coli*, *J. Bacteriol.* 172, 6411–6418.

136 A. Oliver, R. Canton, P. Campo, F. Baquero, J. Blazquez **2000**, High frequency of hypermutable *Pseudomonas aeruginosa* in cystic fibrosis lung infection, *Science* 288, 1251–1254.

137 M.E. Rad, et al. **2003**, Mutations in putative mutator genes of *Mycobacterium tuberculosis* strains of the W-Beijing family, *Emerg. Infect. Dis.* 9, 838–845.

138 H.L. Alexander, A.W. Rasmussen, I. Stojiljkovic **2004**, Identification of *Neisseria meningitidis* genetic loci involved in the modulation of phase variation frequencies, *Infect. Immun.* 72, 6743–6747.

139 K.A. Jolley, L. Sun, E.R. Moxon, M.C. Maiden **2004**, Dam inactivation in *Neisseria meningitidis*: prevalence among diverse hyperinvasive lineages, *BMC Microbiol.* 4, 34.

140 C. Bucci, et al. **1999**, Hypermutation in pathogenic bacteria: frequent phase variation in meningococci is a phenotypic trait of a specialized mutator biotype, *Mol. Cell* 3, 435–445.

141 I. Matic, F. Taddei, M. Radman **2004**, Survival versus maintenance of genetic stability: a conflict of priorities during stress, *Res. Microbiol.* 155, 337–341.

142 S.M. Rosenberg, P.J. Hastings **2003**, Microbiology and evolution. Modulating mutation rates in the wild, *Science* 300, 1382–1383.

143 B.E. Wright **2004**, Stress-directed adaptive mutations and evolution, *Mol. Microbiol.* 52, 643–650.

144 S. Morelle, E. Carbonnelle, I. Matic, X. Nassif **2005**, Contact with host cells induces a DNA repair system in pathogenic *Neisseriae*, *Mol. Microbiol.* 55, 853–861.

145 T. Tønjum, L.S. Håvarstein, M. Koomey, E. Seeberg **2004**, Transformation and DNA repair: linkage by DNA recombination, *Trends Microbiol.* 12, 1–4.

8
Structure and Genetics of the Meningococcal Capsule

Matthias Frosch and Ulrich Vogel

8.1
Introduction

Many bacterial species, especially those causing invasive infections, are surrounded by polysaccharides that are attached to the cell by covalent linkage to phospholipids or lipid A molecules. These outermost polysaccharide layers of a bacterial cell, termed the capsule, may interfere in a first line with the environment and may mediate a variety of biological processes relevant to the pathogenesis of invasive bacterial infections [1]. As highly hydrated structures with more than 95% water content [2] bacterial polysaccharide capsules may prevent desiccation and thus might provide the basis for transmission and maintenance of the bacterial species in their populations. While it is not clear whether this aspect of capsule formation is relevant for the spread of meningococci in the human population, since only prolonged and close contacts are considered to be permissive for transmission [3], encapsulation of the meningococcus definitively is a central prerequisite for the survival of the bacteria during systemic spread. The interaction of meningococci with the innate and adaptive immune system and the critical role of the capsular polysaccharide for resistance to complement-mediated bacteriolysis and phagocytosis as well as the problems in induction of a humoral immune response against capsular polysaccharide antigens have been addressed in great detail in other chapters of this book (see Chapters 14, 15, 17). This chapter will focus on the structural diversity of the meningococcal capsules and the genetic and biochemical basis for the formation of one of the key virulence determinants of meningococci.

8.2
Chemical Structure of Meningococcal Capsular Polysaccharides

According to their biochemical and genetic attributes, meningococcal capsular polysaccharides belong to the group II capsule antigens, which are characterized by a high charge density, by expression at temperatures above 20 °C and, in sev-

Handbook of Meningococcal Disease. Infection Biology, Vaccination, Clinical Management.
Edited by M. Frosch and M. C. J. Maiden

ISBN: 3-527-31260-9

eral instances by substitution with phospholipids at the reducing end of the polysaccharide chain, which may anchor the polysaccharides in the outer membrane. The genes encoding group II capsules are similarly organized in different bacterial species and share significant homologies (for a review, see [4]).

As in other bacterial species, there is a great variety of capsular antigens, which were originally defined by serological means. The antigenic diversity of capsular polysaccharides in meningococci led to the definition of serogroups for the serological characterization of meningococci at a primary level (see Chapter 3). There are 13 different serogroups, but of these only the polysaccharide capsules that define the serogroups A, B, C, W-135 and Y usually cause invasive disease [5].

In the 1970s and 1980s, nuclear magnetic resonance spectroscopy greatly improved the analytical procedures to elucidate the chemical composition of purified capsular polysaccharides [6–8]. With the exception of serogroup D, for which neither structural nor genetic information are available, structural data of meningococcal capsular polysaccharides have been accumulated by several groups.

Most of the serogroups frequently found in meningococcal disease, i.e. B, C, W-135 and Y, contain 5-*N*-acetyl-neuraminic acid (Neu5Ac, sialic acid) as a key component of the polysaccharide [9, 10] (see Table 8.1). The α(2–8) linked sialic acid homopolymer characteristic of serogroup B is also found as a modification of the mammalian neural cell adhesion molecule (NCAM), which is involved in axonal growth and synaptic plasticity (for a review, see [11]). The mammalian expression of α(2–8) linked polysialic acid on NCAM is responsible for the poor mammalian immune response against this structure. The serogroup B polysaccharide is highly related to the serogroup C polysaccharide [10]. The serological differentiation arises from the different linkage between sialic acid monomers, i.e. α(2–9) in the case of serogroup C meningococci. This structure is highly immunogenic, especially if applied as a conjugated vaccine [12]. The structural similarities of group B and C polysaccharides are not surprising, considering the related amino acid sequences of serogroup B and C polysialyltransferases [13, 14], which catalyze the polymerization and formation of polysaccharide chains composed of more than 200 Neu5Ac residues. Four to five α(2–9) linked sialic acid residues are sufficient to block serogroup C specific antibodies [15], whereas up to 10-mer oligosaccharides are needed in the case of serogroup B, suggesting that the α(2–8) linked oligosaccharides display conformational epitopes or a less ordered structure due to a higher flexibility [16–18]. Using the monoclonal IgG 2a antibody 735 specific to α(2-8) polysialic acid [19], crystallographic and thermodynamic evidence has been compiled confirming the binding of oligosaccharides of at least eight residues in length in a helical conformation [20].

Escherichia coli K1 expresses a polysaccharide capsule chemically similar to the capsule of serogroup B meningococci. However, phase-variable expression of an O-acetyltransferase is characteristic to *E. coli* K1 [21], in contrast to serogroup B meningococci, which have never been reported to be O-acetylated. The

Table 8.1 Summary of biochemical and genetic information concerning meningococcal capsule polysaccharides. Information about O-acetylation is provided in the text.

Serogroup	Structure	Genes	References
A	→ 6)-α-D-Man*p*NAc-(1 → OPO_3 →	*mynA–mynD* (Syn: *sacA–sacD*)	28, 29
B	→ 8)-α-D-Neu*p*5Ac-(2 →	*siaA–siaD*$_B$ [a]	10, 44
C	→ 9)-α-D-Neu*p*5Ac-(2 →	*siaA–siaD*$_C$ [a]	10, 14
D	Unknown		
29E	→ 3)-α-D-Gal*p*NAc-(1 → 7)-β-D-KDO*p*-(2 →	*cap29eA–H* [b]	37
H	→ 4)-α-D-Gal*p*-(1 → 2)-Gro-(-3 → OPO_3 →		38
I	→ 4)-α-L-Gul*p*NAcA-(1 → 3)-β-D-Man*p*NAcA(→		43
K	→ 3)-β-D-Man*p*NAcA-(1 → 4)-β-D-Man*p*NAcA-(1 →		42
L	→ 3)-β-D-Glc*p*NAc-(1 → 3)-β-D-Glc*p*NAc-(1 → 3)-α-D-Glc*p*NAc-(1 → OPO_3 →	*lcbA–lcbC* [c]	34
W-135	→ 4)-α-D-Neu*p*5Ac-α-(2 → 6)-α-D-Gal-(1 →	*siaA–siaD*$_{W\text{-}135}$ [a]	9, 13, 25
X	→ 4)-α-D-Glc*p*NAc-(1 → OPO_3 →	*xcbA–C*	26–28, 30
Y	→ 4)-α-D-Neu*p*5Ac-α-(2 → 6)-α-D-Glc-(1 →	*siaA–siaD*$_Y$ [a]	9, 13
Z	→ 3)-α-D-Gal*p*NAc-(1 → 1)-Gro-(3 → OPO_3 →	*capZA–D* [d]	36

a) Alternatively, the *sia* genes are termed *syn*; i.e. *siaD*$_B$, *siaD*$_C$, *siaD*$_{W\text{-}135}$, *siaD*$_Y$ are referred to as *synD*, *synE*, *synG*, *synF*, respectively.
b) GenBank accession no. AJ576117.
c) AF112478.
d) AJ744766.

serogroup C polysaccharide may be O-acetylated at positions 7 and 8 [7]. It has been shown that freshly isolated polysaccharide contains predominantly O-acetyl groups at position 8 [22]. During storage of the polysaccharide, migration of O-acetyl groups to position 7 occurs. While the genetic basis for O-acetylation in meningococci has been elucidated [23], the biological function of O-acetylation in meningococcal group C carriage and disease is unclear. However, the de-O-acetylated polysaccharide has been shown to be more immunogenic than the O-acetylated one [24], but it is unclear at the moment whether these differences have an effect on the virulence of group C meningococci.

To a varying proportion, O-acetylation has also been identified in sialic acid heteropolymers, first in serogroup Y [7] and later also in W-135 meningococci [25]. These highly related serogroups comprise disaccharide repeating units of → 4)-α-D-Neu*p*5Ac-α-(2 → 6)-α-D-Gal-(1 → in the case of serogroup W-135 and → 4)-α-D-Neu*p*5Ac-α-(2 → 6)-α-D-Glc-(1 → in the case of serogroup Y. Thus, the serological differentiation of the group W-135 and Y polysaccharides is based on the configuration of a single hydroxyl group.

All meningococcal polysaccharides appear to be linear and acidic; and, with the exception of serogroup H, they contain acetamido groups (for a review, see

[8]). Besides the before-mentioned relationships of the capsules containing sialic acid, there are further relationships in the other serogroups. Serogroup A [→6)-α-D-Man*p*NAc-(1→OPO_3→] is closely related to serogroup X [→4)-α-D-Glc*p*NAc-(1→OPO_3→] [26–28]. Accordingly, the putative polysaccharide polymerases of serogroup A and X, i.e. MynB and XcbA, share significant homology at the amino acid level [29, 30]. The serogroup A polysaccharide is O-acetylated, which is a prerequisite for its immunogenicity [31], and the O-acetyltransferase gene has been identified [32]. The components of the serogroup L polysaccharide, which was identified in an isolate from a healthy carrier [33], is identical to that of serogroup X, although linkage and molar ratios of N-acetyl-glucosamine and phosphate differ [34]. Not surprisingly, the deduced amino acid sequence of the *lcbA* gene located within the capsule synthesis region of serogroup L meningococci (AF112478) displays significant homology to the abovementioned XcbA.

Immunological cross reactivity of the serogroups 29E and Z is the reason for the former assignment Z′ for 29E [35]. The capsule synthesis regions of both serogroups have not been published yet, but our own sequence data show that, despite the structural homology, the genomic capsule synthesis regions of both serogroups developed independently (GenBank accession numbers AJ744766, AJ576117). Both serogroups contain N-acetyl-galactosamine, linked with either 3-deoxy-D-manno-2-octulosonic acid (KDO) in the case of 29E, or glycerol-3-phosphate in the case of serogroup Z [36, 37]. In serogroup 29E, our own yet unpublished data suggest that the genes for KDO synthesis in the genomic capsule synthesis island are dispensable, probably due to complementation of lipopolysaccharide-KDO synthesis genes located elsewhere on the genome. It should be noted that serogroup Z together with serogroups A and X belongs to those serogroups which exhibit a phosphate–diester bond. Furthermore, the serogroup Z polysaccharide is related to that of serogroup H, which is the only structure lacking an acetamido group [38]. Instead of an N-acetyl-galactosamine residue, serogroup H harbors a partially O-acetylated D-galactose residue. It is structurally and immunologically related to capsular polysaccharides from *Pasteurella hemolytica* serotype T15 and *Escherichia coli* K62 [39, 40].

Along with serogroup H, serogroups I and K were first identified by Ding et al. [41]; and 56 strains of these three serogroups were isolated from healthy carriers in 12 Chinese provinces. Serogroups I and K contain N-acetyl-D-mannuronic acid (Man*p*NAcA) [42]. The serogroup I polysaccharide is a heteropolymer containing also 2-acetamido-2-deoxy-L-guluronic acid [43]. Both polysaccharides are O-acetylated. In the case of the group I polysaccharide, O-acetylation was indispensable for agglutination with a rabbit anti-group I antiserum. Genetic information about the capsule synthesis regions of serogroups H, I and K is not available.

8.3
Genetics of Capsule Expression

Our current understanding of the molecular mechanisms of capsular polysaccharide synthesis, a process that takes place in the cytoplasm, and the subsequent translocation of the polysaccharide chains to the cell surface evolved mainly from the detailed biochemical analysis and studies of the capsule genetics, including the availability of genetic tools for the inactivation of capsule genes and biochemical analysis of the phenotype in isogenic capsule mutants.

As in other group II polysaccharide-producing bacteria, the genes involved in polysaccharide biosynthesis and cell surface translocation are clustered at a single chromosomal locus, termed *cps* [44]. Functional analysis of the *cps* locus indicated that the genes required for capsule expression can be assigned to three regions, i.e. A, B and C (Fig. 8.1), where genes of region A encode enzymes for the biosynthesis of the capsular polysaccharide and regions B and C are involved in the translocation of the high molecular weight polysaccharides to the cell surface. However, in contrast to the *E. coli* capsule gene clusters, where all genes for biosynthesis and transport are closely linked [45–47], the meningococcal *cps* cluster is interrupted by genes involved in LPS biosynthesis (regions D, D′) [48], a methyltransferase gene and a gene homologous to the *tex* gene of *Bordetella pertussis* (region E) [49], respectively, whose function is still unknown (Fig. 8.1). This indicates that acquisition of the capsule genes by meningococci was accompanied by genomic rearrangement events. This recombination process is still going on within the *cps* locus, as we have learned from the genome analysis of a couple of meningococcal strains.

The order of the regions of *cps* was first determined using the invasive serogroup B strain B1940 [44]. Consecutively, the genome sequences of strains MC58 (serogroup B, ST-32 complex [50]), Z2491 (serogroup A, ST-4 [51]) and FAM18 (serogroup C, ST-11; unpublished data) revealed a different organization, in which region B was located adjacent to region D′ instead of region D (Fig. 8.1). Theoretically, this phenomenon can be explained by chromosomal inversion via indirect repeats. Indeed, regions D and D′ differ only with regard to a 5′ truncation of the *galE* gene. We therefore analyzed the possibility that a B1940-like organization might also occur in strains of the ST-32 complex. Of 14 genetically related ST-32 isolates obtained during a carriage study in Bavaria, Germany [52], seven exhibited a B1940-like organization of the *cps*, whereas seven isolates resembled the organization elucidated by the MC58 genome sequencing project (Claus et al., unpublished data). These results suggest that both organisations of the *cps* can occur in genetically related strains. However, the inversion frequency in single isolates remains to be determined as well as the biological implication this process might have.

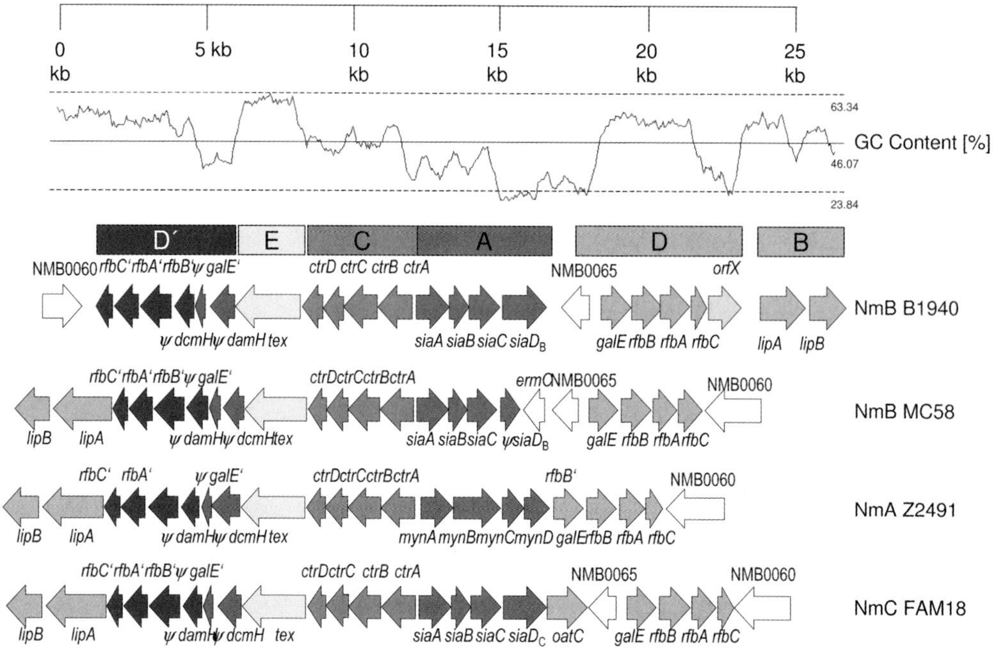

Fig. 8.1 The genetic organization of *cps* locus in serogroup B strains B1940 and MC58, serogroup A strain Z2491 and serogroup C strain FAM18. The plot demonstrates the GC content and the boxes indicating the functional regions A–E refer to strain B1940. Homologous genes in the *cps* locus are indicated by the same colors. The genome sequences of MC58, Z2491 and FAM18 were obtained, respectively, from TIGR (http://www.tigr.org/tigr-scripts/CMR2/GenomePage3.spl?database=gnm) and the Sanger Centre (http://www.sanger.ac.uk/Projects/N_meningitidis/; for references see text). The MC58 derivative subjected to genome sequencing by TIGR carried an inactivated version of the *siaD* gene. (This figure also appears with the color plates.)

8.4 Biochemistry and Genetics of Capsule Biosynthesis

Although the genetics of capsule expression share many common principals in all serogroups, much has been learned from the capsule genetics and biochemical analysis of serogroup B meningococci, to which we will refer primarily, but we will also discuss special aspects for the other serogroups.

Region A of the *cps* locus contains the genes required for the biosynthesis of the capsular polysaccharide. In the *cps* loci of serogroup B, C, W-135 and Y meningococci, region A comprises the *siaA*, *siaB*, *siaC* and *siaD* genes [13, 14, 44]. These genes constitute a transcriptional unit, which allows their coordinate regulation and expression. In addition, we could recently show that, in serogroup C, W-135 and Y meningococci, O-acetyltransferase genes are part of this transcriptional unit [23]. All region A encoded *sia* genes show an unusual high AT content of 60–70%, indicative for the acquisition of the *sia* genes by horizontal gene transfer (Fig. 8.1). The *siaA*, *siaB* and *siaC* genes are highly conserved in all these serogroups, as they exhibit the same function, i.e. the synthesis of monomeric sialic acid and its activation to form CMP-sialic acid [13].

As a first step in polysialic acid biosynthesis, ManNAc-6-phosphate is generated by isomerization of GlcNAc-6-phosphate [53, 54]. This enzymatic reaction is performed by the *siaA* gene product (Fig. 8.2). In the next step, catalyzed by SiaC, Neu5Ac is generated by condensation of ManNAc and phosphoenolpyruvate [55, 56]. Since SiaC (the Neu5Ac-condensing enzyme) utilizes ManNAc but not ManNAc-6-phosphate, a phosphatase may be required for dephosphorylation before Neu5Ac condensation can proceed. However, a specific phosphatase is not encoded by a gene of the *cps* locus and therefore ubiquitous phosphatases in the meningococcal cytoplasm may catalyze the dephosphorylation reaction. It is important to note that a *siaA* homologous gene of the *E. coli* K1 capsule locus, termed *neuC*, catalyzes the epimerization of GlcNAc to form ManNAc [57]. Therefore, in *E. coli* K1 there is no need for dephosphorylation before the subsequent condensation reaction. As the meningococcal SiaA and NeuC from *E. coli* share only 25% identity, the differences in the enzymatic activities in both species can be explained. The third step in polysialic acid biosynthesis is the activation of Neu5Ac to form CMP-Neu5Ac. The CMP-Neu5Ac synthetase is encoded by the *siaB* gene [55, 58]. CMP-Neu5Ac is the substrate for the polysialyltransferase encoded by *siaD*, which directs the polymerization of the CMP-sialic acid monomers [59, 60].

The *siaD* genes are the only capsule biosynthesis genes with functional and nucleotide sequence specificity for the four serogroups B, C, W-135 and Y. The *siaD* genes of serogroup B (*siaD*$_B$) and serogroup C (*siaD*$_C$) meningococci share only 64.4% identity and are completely unrelated to the *siaD* genes of serogroup W-135 and Y meningococci. The W-135 and Y polysialyltransferases are highly related, with a sequence identity to each other of more than 98% [13]. There is one polymorphic region, between nucleotides 885 and 1029 of the 3114-bp *siaD* genes, which distinguishes the *siaD*$_{W\text{-}135}$ and *siaD*$_Y$ genes. The polymorphisms

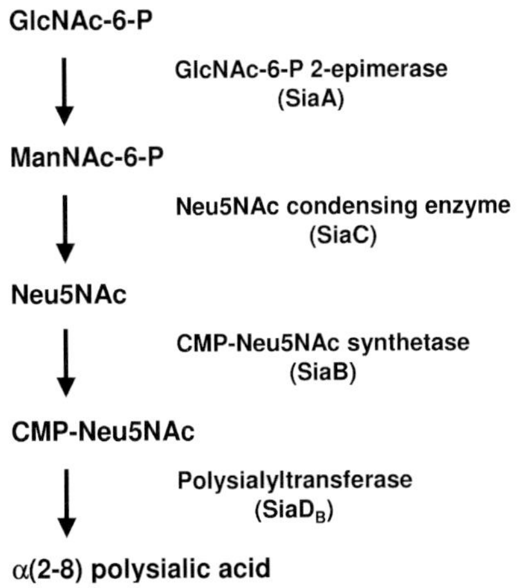

Fig. 8.2 Biosynthetic steps of polysialic acid synthesis in serogroup B meningococci.

in this short gene region are serogroup-specific and can be used to differentiate serogroup W-135 and Y meningococci at a molecular level [61]. Both genes, *siaD*$_{W\text{-}135}$ and *siaD*$_Y$, are probably the result of a gene fusion event, with the glycosyltransferase moiety located at the N-terminus of the holoenzyme (Claus and Vogel, unpublished data).

It has long been a matter of debate how the initiation of the polymerization reaction may occur. For *E. coli* K1 and K5, it has been hypothesized that undecaprenol phosphate (UP) substituted with KDO may act as an acceptor for the subsequent polysialic acid polymerisation [62, 63] or, alternatively, that UP alone is sufficient as an acceptor for capsule polymerization. As the capsular polysaccharide chains inserted in the outer membrane are substituted with diacylglycerol at the reducing end of the polymer and no KDO can be detected [64], the high molecular weight polymers therefore need the replacement of UP-KDO or UP before translocation to the cell surface. Interestingly, Tzeng et al. [65] identified two genes involved in KDO synthesis outside the *cps* locus as critical determinants for capsular polysaccharide biosynthesis in all meningococcal serogroups. Meningococcal mutants in *kspF* (encoding arabinose-5-phosphate isomerase, the first enzyme in KDO biosynthesis) and *kdsB* (encoding CMP-KDO synthetase) expressed significantly reduced amounts of capsule polymers, suggesting that KDO may function in capsule assembly as (part of) an acceptor for initiation of capsule polymerization.

8.5
Genetics of O-Acetylation

As figured out above, the sialic acid residues in the polysaccharide molecules only of serogroups C, W-135 and Y can be substituted with O-acetyl groups. O-acetylation depends on the presence of the genes OatC and OatWY, which are located downstream of *siaD* and are cotranscribed together with the *sia* operon. According to sequence homologies, the O-acetyltransferases of serogroups W-135 and Y belong to the NodL-LacS-CysE family of O-acetyltransferases [23]. However, no sequence homology could be described for OatC. As stated above, the immunogenicity of the serogroup A polysaccharide depends on O-acetylation [31], and the O-acetyltransferase gene has been recently identified to be the *mynC* gene of region A of the *cps* [32].

8.6
Molecular Mechanisms of Capsular Polysaccharide Transport

The genes of regions B and C (Fig. 8.1) share a high degree of homology in all serogroups, independent of the chemical composition of the capsular polysaccharide; and homologous genes are present even in the genome of other group II capsule-expressing bacterial species [4]. Functional analysis of region B and C genes and gene products clearly indicated their participation in the transport process of the polysaccharide chains to the cell surface, although several details of the transport mechanism await further investigations.

Clear evidence has accumulated that the export of group II capsular polysaccharide to the cell surface is an ATP-dependent process requiring the action of an ATP-binding cassette (ABC) transporter system [4]. Members of the ABC transporter superfamily couple the energy released from ATP hydrolysis with the transport of a large variety of substrates into or out of the cells. ABC transporters are characterized by a common organization, each consisting of four domains or subunits, two hydrophobic integral membrane proteins (which are thought to form the channel across the membrane) and two hydrophilic membrane-associated ATP-binding proteins (for a review, see [66]). Among the numerous substrates of ABC transporters are the capsular polysaccharides. According to homologies to other ABC transporters, the *ctrD* gene encodes the ATP-binding protein of the transporter complex. This also includes the presence of the characteristic Walker A and B motifs and the ABC signature [60]. Further functional evidence was provided by the analysis of a protein of the *E. coli* K1 capsular polysaccharide transport system, KpsT, with significant homology to the meningococcal CtrD, as KpsT was characterized as an ATP-hydrolyzing enzyme by site-directed mutagenesis and ATP-binding [67]. Together with the CtrC protein as an integral membrane protein with six transmembrane segments, CtrD is thought to form the ABC transporter for export of the capsular polysaccharide through the inner membrane.

Two further auxiliary proteins are coexpressed together with the ABC transporters CtrC and CtrD. CtrB is an inner membrane protein with two transmembrane-spanning segments at the N- and C-termini, with a central loop being localized in the periplasm. CtrA could be identified as a protein of the outer membrane [60, 68]. The N-terminal part of CtrA forms a β-barrel typical of other channels of the outer membrane, followed by a periplasmic domain. Polysaccharide transport based on ABC transporters together with two auxiliary proteins of the inner and outer membranes is termed a type 4 polysaccharide export system [69]. However, an exact function of the auxiliary proteins has not been described so far.

Interestingly, there are remarkable similarities between the type 4 polysaccharide export system and the bacterial type I secretion system for polypeptides, which in addition to the ABC transporters also requires two further accessory proteins. As in the *ctr* locus, genes of the type I secretion system are in many instances located in a single operon [70]. The *E. coli* hemolysin transporter is a paradigm for type I secretion systems. In this transport system, the outer membrane protein TolC forms a channel that spans both the outer membrane and the periplasm [71, 72] and interacts with a further hydrophobic inner membrane protein, termed HlyD [73]. The role of this accessory protein is to link the ABC transporter to the outer membrane channel and to stabilize this assembly. Although no exact functional and structural data are available for the type 4 polysaccharide export system, CtrB and CtrA could function in a similar way as

TolC and HlyD (Fig. 8.3). The periplasmic domain of CtrA putatively would then connect the outer membrane via CtrB to the ABC transporter, resulting in a tightly coupled transport of the meningococcal capsular polysaccharide through the inner and outer membranes. In accordance with this is the observation that, in the absence of CtrA, the capsular polysaccharide remains in the cytoplasm and is anchored in the inner membrane by phospholipids at the reducing end of the polysaccharide chains [74]. However, the extrapolation of the assembly of capsule transporter proteins to the type I secretion systems awaits further support from structural and functional data of the Ctr proteins.

In type I secretion systems, the ABC transporter and auxiliary inner membrane proteins have been implicated in substrate recognition [66]. For capsular polysaccharide export, the recognition signal is unknown, but considering the high homology of the *ctr* genes in antigenetically different meningococcal serogroups, it is conceivable that recognition does not occur via (part of) the polysaccharide chain itself, but that the phospholipid anchor plays a crucial role in substrate recognition and transport by the CtrABCD complex. However, it is still a matter of debate at which step in polysaccharide biosynthesis and by which enzymes phospholipid substitution occurs. Previous data suggested that the proteins LipA and LipB encoded by region B of the *cps* locus direct phospholipid substitution at the reducing end of the full-length polysaccharide chain [74]. These observations were in accordance to data obtained from analysis of the *E. coli* capsule system. Mutations within the *kpsC* or *kpsS* genes, which encode proteins homologous to the meningococcal LipA and LipB, resulted in cytoplasmic accumulation of the polysaccharides which completely lacked phospholipids and KDO [75, 76]. In contrast to these observations, a recent report demonstrated

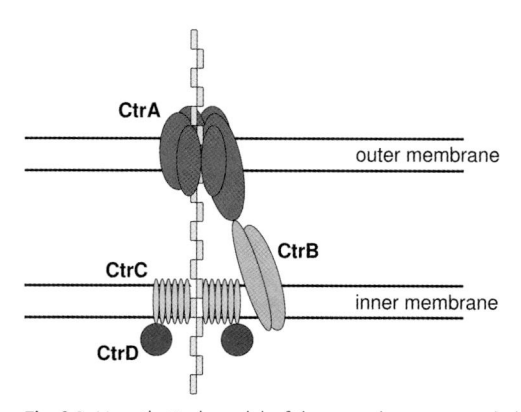

Fig. 8.3 Hypothetical model of the capsular polysaccharide transport system. The ABC transporter proteins CtrC and CtrD direct the translocation of the polysaccharide (yellow chain) through the inner membrane. Transport of the polysaccharide through the inner and outer membranes is tightly coupled. Translocation through the outer membrane is enabled by the auxiliary protein CtrA, which forms a β-barrel structure. The translocation zones of the inner and outer membrane are stabilized through CtrB, which links CtrA to the inner membrane. (This figure also appears with the color plates.)

phospholipids at the reducing end of the group B meningococcal polysaccharides in *lipA* and *lipB* mutants [77]. However, these data were obtained in a different genetic background and it is unclear whether other genes within the meningococcal genome can complement LipAB functions. Therefore, the exact function of LipAB awaits further elucidation.

The molecular principles of capsule formation are common to all encapsulated gram-negative bacteria which express group II capsules [4, 60]. Genes homologous to *ctrABCD* and *lipAB* have been described in other bacterial species, like *E. coli*, *Haemophilus influenzae* and *Actinobacillus pleuropneumoniae*, which indicates a common evolutionary origin of group II capsule expression. However, some differences between the capsule gene clusters in these species have evolved, which limits the extrapolation of the mechanisms of meningococcal capsule expression in other gram-negative bacteria. Compared to meningococci and *H. influenzae*, the *E. coli* capsule locus contains several additional genes. In contrast, *E. coli* lacks a CtrA homologous outer membrane protein, but expresses a periplasmic protein, KpsD, which is part of the polysaccharide export process in *E. coli*, but not in meningococci and *H. influenzae*. For a deeper review of the capsule export mechanisms in *E. coli* and the common principles of capsule expression in gram-negative bacteria, we refer to the excellent review by Ian Roberts [4].

8.7
Genetics of Capsule Expression in Serogroup A and Other Rare Serogroups

The two different organisations of the functional regions within the *cps* locus discussed above (Fig. 8.1) can be found in all meningococcal serogroups analyzed so far. Whereas the gene content and the homology of genes within regions B and C are almost identical, the genes of region A vary considerably and show no sequence homologies to each other and to region A genes of the sialic acid-containing serogroups B, C, W-135 and Y. This reflects the different chemical composition and immunological properties of the nonB/C/W-135/Y serogroups.

The region A genes of serogroup A meningococci, termed *mynA*, *mynB*, *mynC* and *mynD*, encode the synthesis of the $a(2–6)$ linked N-acetyl-D-mannosamine-1-phosphate polymer. The function of these genes awaits further characterization, but on the basis of sequence identity, *mynA* seems to encode the UDP-N-acetyl-D-glucosamine (UDP-GlcNAc) 2-epimerase, which may be responsible for the conversion of UDP-GlcNAc into UDP-N-acetyl-D-mannosamine as the first biosynthetic step of capsular polysaccharide formation in serogroup A meningococci. *mynB* is thought to encode the polymerase linking individual UDP-ManNAc monomers together [29]. Recently, the *mynC* gene product was characterized and found to exhibit acetyltransferase activity responsible for O-acetylation at O-3 and O-4 [32].

Region A of serogroup X meningococci has also been analyzed in great detail [30]. The capsule biosynthesis region consists of three cotranscribed genes *xcbA*, *xcbB* and *xcbC* [30]. Upstream of *xcbA*, an insertion sequence was identified (IS*1016*). The deduced amino acid sequence of the *xcbA* gene showed significant homology to MynB, the putative serogroup A capsule polymerase, and LcbA of serogroup L meningococci, which is in line with the observed structural homologies of the three serogroups and which further suggests that XcbA is a capsule polymerase.

The capsule biosynthesis regions of serogroups 29E and Z have not been published yet, but our laboratory has submitted the nucleotide sequences to GenBank (Table 8.1). Compared to region A of all other serogroups, region A of serogroup 29E is very large, with eight genes on an 8.7-kb DNA fragment. Sequence comparison suggests that the first half of region A contains glycosyltransferases, whereas two genes are involved in KDO synthesis. Preliminary gene knockout analysis suggested that these genes are functionally complemented by KDO synthesis genes outside *cps* (Claus et al., unpublished data).

Region A in serogroup Z comprises four genes. The encoded proteins of *cpaZA*, *cpaZB* and *capZC*, respectively, are surprisingly homologous to proteins harbored in the capsule synthesis regions from *Actinobacillus pleuropneumoniae* (Claus et al., unpublished data). This particular finding touches the interesting question about the evolutionary origin of the capsule synthesis genes, whose aberrant DNA compositions are indicative of DNA acquisition by horizontal gene transfer from unrelated bacterial genera. In the exceptional case of serogroup Z, the high homology to genes of the etiological agent of porcine pleuropneumonia either points to a member of the *Pasteurellaceae* as a source, or suggests that both *Actinobacillus* and *Neisseria* acquired the DNA from the same source.

8.8
Adaptation, Phase Variation

A characteristic feature of the meningococcus is the ability to modulate the expression of surface molecules. Especially those structures that play a role in the interaction with the host undergo antigenic variation and/or off–on switching with high frequency (see also Chapter 9). Strong experimental evidence suggests that the capsule inhibits binding to and invasion of epithelial and endothelial cells [78–80]. In contrast, the capsule is required for protection against the innate immune system and therefore is a prerequisite for systemic infection. Thus, modulation of capsule expression and phase variation between the capsular and acapsular state are important events required for the colonization and invasion of the infected human host.

Several mechanisms have been described for phase variation and the control of capsule expression. One mechanism is based on the reversible inactivation of the *siaA* gene by insertion and exact excision of a naturally occurring insertion sequence element, termed IS*1301* [78, 81]. Interestingly, IS*1301*, which is present also in other serogroups, can reversibly inactivate the O-acetyltransferase genes *oatWY* in serogroup W135 and Y strains, thus resulting in modification of the capsular polysaccharide in these serogroups [23]. A further mechanism of capsular polysaccharide phase variation results from reversible changes in the number of dC residues within an oligo-(dC) stretch at the 5' region of the *siaD* gene, a mechanism termed slipped-strand mispairing [82]. These frameshift mutations result in premature arrest of translation and Rho-dependent transcriptional termination [83]. Phase variation by slipped-strand mispairing has been described for several other virulence associated genes and is described in detail in Chapter 6. In the context of phase-variable capsule expression, it is remarkable that O-acetylation of the capsular polysaccharide in serogroup C meningococci is controlled by slipped-strand mispairing in two homopolymeric tracts of the *oatC* gene [23]. The relevance of phase variation in O-acetylation for the immunogenicity of the capsular polysaccharide and the virulence of meningococci await further investigations.

The requirement of an acapsulate state for intimate adhesion of meningococci to epithelial and endothelial cells suggests that capsule expression is regulated upon contact with target cells. Deghmane et al. [84] identified a LysR-type transcriptional regulator, CrgA, which controls a number of meningococcal genes during intimate adhesion. Among those genes that are negatively regulated by CrgA are the *sia* genes of the *cps* locus [85]. Thus, transcriptional control of capsule expression is part of the complex events of attachment and invasion of host cells, which are reviewed in Chapter 13 of this book.

A further strategy of the meningococcus to adapt to its host is antigenic variation of surface antigens. Several mechanisms of antigenic variation have been evolved and are discussed in Chapters 13–15. Among these mechanisms is the allelic exchange of genes or gene fragments as a result of transformation and horizontal DNA transfer. The identical genetic organisation of the *cps* locus with a central, serogroup-specific region (region A, see Fig. 8.1), which is flanked by conserved regions (regions B, C, D) present in all serogroups favors the allelic replacement of the biosynthesis genes by homologous recombination. Indeed, such replacements have been observed *in vitro* and *in vivo*, resulting in serogroup switching [14, 86, 87]. Capsule switching is regarded as an important virulence mechanism, which enables meningococci to escape vaccine-induced or natural protective immunity.

Acknowledgements

We are indebted to Heike Claus and Christoph Schoen for critical discussions and help with the manuscript and figures. The Institute for Genomic Research and the Sanger Centre are gratefully acknowledged for generously sharing genome sequence information with the scientific community via the internet.

References

1 Kroll, S., Moxon, E. R. **1990**, The role of bacterial polysaccharide capsules as virulence factors, *Curr. Top. Microbiol. Immunol.* 150, 65–85.

2 Costerton, J. W., Irvin, R. T., Cheng, K. J. **1981**, The bacterial glycocalyx in nature and disease, *Annu. Rev. Microbiol.* 35, 299–324.

3 Musher, D. M. **2003**, How contagious are common respiratory tract infections? *N. Engl. J. Med.* 348, 1256–1266.

4 Roberts, I. S. **1996**, The biochemistry and genetics of capsular polysaccharide production in bacteria, *Annu. Rev. Microbiol.* 50, 285–315.

5 Rosenstein, N. E., Perkins, B. A., Stephens, D. S., Popovic, T., Hughes, J. M. **2001**, Meningococcal disease, *N. Engl. J. Med.* 344, 1378–1388.

6 Jones, C., Lemercinier, X. **2002**, Use and validation of NMR assays for the identity and O-acetyl content of capsular polysaccharides from *Neisseria meningitidis* used in vaccine manufacture, *J. Pharm. Biomed. Anal.* 30, 1233–1247.

7 Jennings, H. J., Bhattacharjee, A. K., Bundle, D. R., Kenny, C. P., Martin, A., Smith, I. C. **1977**, Structures of the capsular polysaccharides of *Neisseria meningitidis* as determined by ^{13}C-nuclear magnetic resonance spectroscopy, *J. Infect. Dis.* 136[Suppl.], S78–S83.

8 Jennings, H. J. **1983**, Capsular polysaccharides as human vaccines, *Adv. Carbohydr. Chem. Biochem.* 41, 155–208.

9 Bhattacharjee, A. K., Jennings, H. J., Kenny, C. P., Martin, A., Smith, I. C. **1976**, Structural determination of the polysaccharide antigens of *Neisseria meningitidis* serogroups Y, W-135, and BO1, *Can. J. Biochem.* 54, 1–8.

10 Bhattacharjee, A. K., Jennings, H. J., Kenny, C. P., Martin, A., Smith, I. C. P. **1975**, Structural determination of the sialic acid polysaccharide antigens of *Neisseria meningitidis* serogroups B and C with carbon 13 nuclear magnetic resonance, *J. Biol. Chem.* 250, 1926–1932.

11 Mühlenhoff, M., Eckhardt, M., Gerardy-Schahn, R. **1998**, Polysialic acid: three-dimensional structure, biosynthesis and function, *Curr. Opin. Struct. Biol.* 8, 558–564.

12 Fairley, C. K., Begg, N., Borrow, R., Fox, A. J., Jones, D. M., Cartwright, K. **1996**, Conjugate meningococcal serogroup A and C vaccine: reactogenicity and immunogenicity in United Kingdom infants, *J. Infect. Dis.* 174, 1360–1363.

13 Claus, H., Vogel, U., Mühlenhoff, M., Gerardy-Schahn, R., Frosch, M. **1997**, Molecular divergence of the sia locus in different serogroups of *Neisseria meningitidis* expressing polysialic acid capsules, *Mol. Gen. Genet.* 257, 28–34.

14 Swartley, J. S., Marfin, A. A., Edupuganti, S., Liu, L. J., Cieslak, P., Perkins, B., Wenger, J. D., and Stephens, D. S. **1997**, Capsule switching of *Neisseria meningitidis*, *Proc. Natl Acad. Sci. USA* 94, 271–276.

15 Jennings, H. J., Roy, R., Michon, F. **1985**, Determinant specificities of the groups B and C polysaccharides of *Neisseria meningitidis*, *J. Immunol.* 134, 2651–2657.

16 Yamasaki, R., Bacon, B. **1991**, Three-dimensional structural analysis of the group B polysaccharide of *Neisseria meningitidis* 6275 by two-dimensional NMR: the polysaccharide is suggested to exist in helical conformations in solution, *Biochemistry* 30, 851–857.

17 Michon, F., Brisson, J. R., Jennings, H. J. **1987**, Conformational differences between linear alpha (2→8)-linked homosialooligosaccharides and the epitope of the group B meningococcal polysaccharide, *Biochemistry* 26, 8399–8405.

18 Brisson, J. R., Jennings, H. J. **2001**, NMR and molecular modeling of complex carbohydrates and carbohydrate–protein interactions. Applications to anti-bacteria vaccines, *Adv. Exp. Med. Biol.* 491, 543–550.

19 Frosch, M., Gorgen, I., Boulnois, G. J., Timmis, K. N., Bitter-Suermann, D. **1985**, NZB mouse system for production of monoclonal antibodies to weak bacterial antigens: isolation of an IgG antibody to the polysaccharide capsules of *Escherichia coli* K1 and group B menin-

gococci, *Proc. Natl Acad. Sci. USA* 82, 1194–1198.
20 Evans, S.V., Sigurskjold, B.W., Jennings, H.J., Brisson, J.R., To, R., Tse, W.C., Altman, E., Frosch, M., Weisgerber, C., Kratzin, H.D., et al. **1995**, Evidence for the extended helical nature of polysaccharide epitopes. The 2.8 Å resolution structure and thermodynamics of ligand binding of an antigen binding fragment specific for alpha-(2 → 8)-polysialic acid, *Biochemistry* 34, 6737–6744.
21 Orskov, F., Orskov, I., Sutton, A., Schneerson, R., Lin, W., Egan, W., Hoff, G.E., Robbins, J.B. **1979**, Form variation in *Escherichia coli* K1: determined by O-acetylation of the capsular polysaccharide, *J. Exp. Med.* 149, 669–685.
22 Michon, F., Huang, C.H., Farley, E.K., Hronowski, L., Di, J., Fusco, P.C. **2000**, Structure activity studies on group C meningococcal polysaccharide–protein conjugate vaccines: effect of O-acetylation on the nature of the protective epitope, *Dev. Biol.* 103, 151–160.
23 Claus, H., Borrow, R., Achtman, M., Morelli, G., Kantelberg, C., Longworth, E., Frosch, M., Vogel, U. **2004**, Genetics of capsule O-acetylation in serogroup C, W-135 and Y meningococci, *Mol. Microbiol.* 51, 227–239.
24 Richmond, P., Borrow, R., Goldblatt, D., Findlow, J., Martin, S., Morris, R., Cartwright, K., Miller, E. **2001**, Ability of 3 different meningococcal C conjugate vaccines to induce immunologic memory after a single dose in UK toddlers, *J. Infect. Dis.* 183, 160–163.
25 Lemercinier, X., Jones, C. **1996**, Full 1H NMR assignment and detailed O-acetylation patterns of capsular polysaccharides from *Neisseria meningitidis* used in vaccine production, *Carbohydr. Res.* 296, 83–96.
26 Bundle, D.R., Jennings, H.J., Kenny, C.P. **1973**, An improved procedure for the isolation of meningococcal polysaccharide antigens and the structural determination of the antigen from serogroup X, *Carbohydr. Res.* 26, 268–270.
27 Bundle, D.R., Jennings, H.J., Kenny, C.P. **1974**, Studies on the group-specific polysaccharide of *Neisseria meningitidis* serogroup X and an improved procedure for its isolation, *J. Biol. Chem.* 249, 4797–4801.
28 Bundle, D.R., Smith, I.C., Jennings, H.J. **1974**, Determination of the structure and conformation of bacterial polysaccharides by carbon 13 nuclear magnetic resonance. Studies on the group-specific antigens of *Neisseria meningitidis* serogroups A and X, *J. Biol. Chem.* 249, 2275–2281.
29 Swartley, J.S., Liu, L.J., Miller, Y.K., Martin, L.E., Edupuganti, S., Stephens, D.S. **1998**, Characterization of the gene cassette required for biosynthesis of the (alpha 1 → 6)-linked *N*-acetyl-D-mannosamine-1-phosphate capsule of serogroup A *Neisseria meningitidis*, *J. Bacteriol.* 180, 1533–1539.
30 Tzeng, Y.L., Noble, C., Stephens, D.S. **2003**, Genetic basis for biosynthesis of the (alpha 1 → 4)-linked *N*-acetyl-D-glucosamine-1-phosphate capsule of *Neisseria meningitidis* serogroup X, *Infect. Immun.* 71, 6712–6720.
31 Berry, D.S., Lynn, F., Lee, C.H., Frasch, C.E., Bash, M.C. **2002**, Effect of O acetylation of *Neisseria meningitidis* serogroup A capsular polysaccharide on development of functional immune responses, *Infect. Immun.* 70, 3707–3713.
32 Gudlavalleti, S.K., Datta, A.K., Tzeng, Y.L., Noble, C., Carlson, R.W., Stephens, D.S. **2004**, The *Neisseria meningitidis* serogroup A capsular polysaccharide O-3 and O-4 acetyltransferase, *J. Biol. Chem.* 279, 42765–42773.
33 Ashton, F.E., Ryan, A., Diena, B., Jennings, H.J. **1983**, A new serogroup (L) of *Neisseria meningitidis*, *J. Clin. Microbiol.* 17, 722–727.
34 Jennings, H.J., Lugowski, C.W., Ashton, F.E., Ryan, J.A. **1983**, The structure of the capsular polysaccharide obtained from a new serogroup (L) of *Neisseria meningitidis*, *Carbohydr. Res.* 112, 105–111.
35 Griffiss, J.M., Brandt, B.L. **1983**, Immunological relationship between the capsular polysaccharides of *Neisseria meningitidis* serogroups Z and 29E, *J. Gen. Microbiol.* 129, 447–452.

36 Jennings, H.J., Rosell, K.-G., Kenny, C.P. **1979**, Structural elucidation of the capsular polysaccharide antigen of *Neisseria meningitidis* serogroup Z using ^{13}C nuclear magnetic resonance, *Can. J. Chem.* 57, 2902–2907.

37 Bhattacharjee, A.K., Jennings, H.J., Kenny, C.P. **1978**, Structural elucidation of the 3-deoxy-D-manno-octulosonic acid containing meningococcal 29-e capsular polysaccharide antigen using carbon-13 nuclear magnetic resonance, *Biochemistry* 17, 645–651.

38 Van der Kaaden A., van Doorn-van Wakeren JI, Kamerling, J.P., Vliegenthart, J.F., Tiesjema, R.H. **1984**, Structure of the capsular antigen of *Neisseria meningitidis* serogroup H, *Eur. J. Biochem.* 141, 513–519.

39 Adlam, C., Knights, J.M., Mugridge, A., Lindon, J.C., Williams, J.M., Beesley, J.E. **1985**, Purification, characterization and immunological properties of the capsular polysaccharide of Pasteurella haemolytica serotype T15: its identity with the K62 (K2ab) capsular polysaccharide of *Escherichia coli* and the capsular polysaccharide of *Neisseria meningitidis* serogroup H, *J. Gen. Microbiol.* 131, 1963–1972.

40 Beynon, L.M., Richards, J.C., Perry, M.B. **1992**, Nuclear magnetic resonance analysis of the capsular antigen of Actinobacillus pleuropneumoniae serotype 9. Its identity with the capsular antigen of *Escherichia coli* K62 (K2ab), *Neisseria meningitidis* serogroup H and *Pasteurella haemolytica* serotype T15, *Eur. J. Biochem.* 210, 119–124.

41 Ding, S.Q., Ye, R.B., Zhang, H.C. **1981**, Three new serogroups of *Neisseria meningitidis, J. Biol. Stand.* 9, 307–315.

42 Van der Kaaden A., Gerwig, G.J., Kamerling, J.P., Vliegenthart, J.F., Tiesjema, R.H. **1985**, Structure of the capsular antigen of *Neisseria meningitidis* serogroup K, *Eur. J. Biochem.* 152, 663–668.

43 Michon, F., Brisson, J.R., Roy, R., Ashton, F.E., Jennings, H.J. **1985**, Structural determination of the capsular polysaccharide of *Neisseria meningitidis* group I: a two-dimensional NMR analysis, *Biochemistry* 24, 5592–5598.

44 Frosch, M., Weisgerber, C., Meyer, T.F. **1989**, Molecular characterization and expression in *Escherichia coli* of the gene complex encoding the polysaccharide capsule of *Neisseria meningitidis* group B, *Proc. Natl Acad. Sci. USA* 86, 1669–1673.

45 Boulnois, G.J., Roberts, I.S., Hodge, R., Hardy, K.R., Jann, K.B., Timmis, K.N. **1987**, Analysis of the K1 capsule biosynthesis genes of *Escherichia coli*: definition of three functional regions for capsule production, *Mol. Gen. Genet.* 208, 242–246.

46 Boulnois, G.J., Roberts, I.S. **1990**, Genetics of capsular polysaccharide production in bacteria, *Curr. Topics Microbiol. Immunol.* 150, 1–18.

47 Roberts, I.S., Mountford, R., Hodge, R., Jann, K.B., Boulnois, G.J. **1988**, Common organization of gene clusters for production of different capsular polysaccharides (K antigens) in *Escherichia coli, J. Bacteriol.* 170, 1305–1310.

48 Hammerschmidt, S., Birkholz, C., Zähringer, U., Robertson, B.D., van Putten, J., Ebeling, O., Frosch, M. **1994**, Contribution of genes from the capsule gene complex (cps) to lipooligosaccharide biosynthesis and serum resistance in *Neisseria meningitidis, Mol. Microbiol.* 11, 885–896.

49 Petering, H., Hammerschmidt, S., Frosch, M., van Putten, J.P., Ison, C.A., Robertson, B.D. **1996**, Genes associated with meningococcal capsule complex are also found in *Neisseria gonorrhoeae, J. Bacteriol.* 178, 3342–3345.

50 Tettelin, H., Saunders, N.J., Heidelberg, J., et al. **2000**, Complete genome sequence of *Neisseria meningitidis* serogroup B strain MC58, *Science* 287, 1809–1815.

51 Parkhill, J., Achtman, M., James, K.D., et al. **2000**, TI Complete DNA sequence of a serogroup A strain of *Neisseria meningitidis* Z2491, *Nature* 404, 502–506.

52 Claus, H., Maiden, M.C., Wilson, D.J., McCarthy, N.D., Jolley, K.A., Urwin, R., Hessler, F., Frosch, M., Vogel, U. **2005**, Genetic analysis of meningococci carried by children and young adults, *J. Infect. Dis.* 191, 1263–1271.

53 Ghosh, S., Roseman, S. **1965**, The sialic acids. IV. *N*-acyl-D-glucosamine 6-phosphate 2-epimerase, *J. Biol. Chem.* 240, 1525–1530.

54 Petersen, M., Fessner, W., Frosch, M., Lüneberg, E. **2000**, The *siaA* gene involved in capsule polysaccharide biosynthesis of *Neisseria meningitidis* B codes for *N*-acylglucosamine-6-phosphate 2-epimerase activity, *FEMS Microbiol. Lett.* 184, 161–164.

55 Edwards, U., Muller, A., Hammerschmidt, S., Gerardy Schahn, R., Frosch, M. **1994**, Molecular analysis of the biosynthesis pathway of the alpha-2, 8 polysialic acid capsule by *Neisseria meningitidis* serogroup B, *Mol. Microbiol.* 14, 141–149.

56 Warren, L., Blacklow, R. S. **1962**, The biosynthesis of cytidine 5′-monophospho-*N*-acetylneuraminic acid by an enzyme from *Neisseria meningitidis*, *J. Biol. Chem.* 237, 3527–3534.

57 Ringenberg, M. A., Steenbergen, S. M., Vimr, E. R. **2003**, The first committed step in the biosynthesis of sialic acid by *Escherichia coli* K1 does not involve a phosphorylated *N*-acetylmannosamine intermediate, *Mol. Microbiol.* 50, 961–975.

58 Edwards, U., Frosch, M. **1992**, Sequence and functional analysis of the cloned *Neisseria meningitidis* CMP-NeuNAc synthetase, *FEMS Microbiol. Lett.* 75, 161–166.

59 Troy, F. A. **1979**, The chemistry and biosynthesis of selected bacterial capsular polymers, *Annu. Rev. Microbiol.* 33, 519–560.

60 Frosch, M., Edwards, U., Bousset, K., Krausse, B., Weisgerber, C. **1991**, Evidence for a common molecular origin of the capsule gene loci in gram-negative bacteria expressing group II capsular polysaccharides, *Mol. Microbiol.* 5, 1251–1263.

61 Borrow, R., Claus, H., Chaudhry, U., Guiver, M., Kaczmarski, E. B., Frosch, M., Fox, A. J. **1998**, *siaD* PCR ELISA for confirmation and identification of serogroup Y and W135 meningococcal infections, *FEMS Microbiol. Lett.* 159, 209–214.

62 Finke, A., Jann, B., Jann, K. **1990**, CMP-KDO-synthetase activity in *Escherichia coli* expressing capsular polysaccharides, *FEMS Microbiol. Lett.* 57, 129–133.

63 Finke, A., Bronner, D., Nikolaev, A. V., Jann, B., Jann, K. **1991**, Biosynthesis of the *Escherichia coli* K5 polysaccharide, a representative of group II capsular polysaccharides: polymerization in vitro and characterization of the product, *J. Bacteriol.* 173, 4088–4094.

64 Gotschlich, E. C., Fraser, B. A., Nishimura, O., Robbins, J. B., Liu, T. Y. **1981**, Lipid on capsular polysaccharides of gram-negative bacteria, *J. Biol. Chem.* 256, 8915–8921.

65 Tzeng, Y. L., Datta, A., Strole, C., Kolli, V. S., Birck, M. R., Taylor, W. P., Carlson, R. W., Woodard, R. W., Stephens, D. S. **2002**, KpsF is the arabinose-5-phosphate isomerase required for 3-deoxy-D-manno-octulosonic acid biosynthesis and for both lipooligosaccharide assembly and capsular polysaccharide expression in *Neisseria meningitidis*, *J. Biol. Chem.* 277, 24103–24113.

66 Davidson, A. L., Chen, J. **2004**, ATP-binding cassette transporters in bacteria, *Annu. Rev. Biochem.* 73, 241–268.

67 Pavelka, M. S. Jr., Hayes, S. F., Silver, R. P. **1994**, Characterization of KpsT, the ATP-binding component of the ABC-transporter involved with the export of capsular polysialic acid in *Escherichia coli* K1, *J. Biol. Chem.* 269, 20149–20158.

68 Frosch, M., Müller, D., Bousset, K., Müller, A. **1992**, Conserved outer membrane protein of *Neisseria meningitidis* involved in capsule expression, *Infect. Immun.* 60, 798–803.

69 Paulsen, I. T., Beness, A. M., Saier, M. H. Jr. **1997**, Computer-based analyses of the protein constituents of transport systems catalysing export of complex carbohydrates in bacteria, *Microbiology* 143, 2685–2699.

70 Andersen, C. **2003**, Channel-tunnels: outer membrane components of type I secretion systems and multidrug efflux pumps of Gram-negative bacteria, *Rev. Physiol. Biochem. Pharmacol.* 147, 122–165.

71 Koronakis, V., Sharff, A., Koronakis, E., Luisi, B., Hughes, C. **2000**, Crystal structure of the bacterial membrane protein TolC central to multidrug efflux and protein export, *Nature* 405, 914–919.
72 Andersen, C., Koronakis, E., Bokma, E., Eswaran, J., Humphreys, D., Hughes, C., Koronakis, V. **2002**, Transition to the open state of the TolC periplasmic tunnel entrance, *Proc. Natl Acad. Sci. USA* 99, 11103–11108.
73 Dinh, T., Paulsen, I.T., Saier, M.H. Jr. **1994**, A family of extracytoplasmic proteins that allow transport of large molecules across the outer membranes of gram-negative bacteria, *J. Bacteriol.* 176, 3825–3831.
74 Frosch, M., Müller, A. **1993**, Phospholipid substitution of capsular polysaccharides and mechanisms of capsule formation in *Neisseria meningitidis, Mol. Microbiol.* 8, 483–493.
75 Bronner, D., Sieberth, V., Pazzani, C., Smith, A., Boulnois, G., Roberts, I., Jann, B., Jann, K. **1993**, Synthesis of the K5 (group II) capsular polysaccharide in transport-deficient recombinant *Escherichia coli, FEMS Microbiol. Lett.* 113, 279–284.
76 Bronner, D., Sieberth, V., Pazzani, C., Roberts, I.S., Boulnois, G.J., Jann, B., Jann, K. **1993**, Expression of the capsular K5 polysaccharide of *Escherichia coli*: biochemical and electron microscopic analyses of mutants with defects in region 1 of the K5 gene cluster, *J. Bacteriol.* 175, 5984–5992.
77 Tzeng, Y.L., Datta, A.K., Strole, C.A., Lobritz, M.A., Carlson, R.W., Stephens, D.S. **2005**, Translocation and surface expression of lipidated serogroup B capsular Polysaccharide in *Neisseria meningitidis, Infect. Immun.* 73, 1491–1505.
78 Hammerschmidt, S., Hilse, R., van Putten, J.P., Gerardy-Schahn, R., Unkmeir, A., Frosch, M. **1996**, Modulation of cell surface sialic acid expression in *Neisseria meningitidis* via a transposable genetic element, *EMBO J.* 15, 192–198.
79 Virji, M., Makepeace, K., Ferguson, D.J., Achtman, M., Sarkari, J., Moxon, E.R. **1992**, Expression of the Opc protein correlates with invasion of epithelial and endothelial cells by *Neisseria meningitidis, Mol. Microbiol.* 6, 2785–2795.
80 Virji, M., Makepeace, K., Ferguson, D.J., Achtman, M., Moxon, E.R. **1993**, Meningococcal Opa and Opc proteins: their role in colonization and invasion of human epithelial and endothelial cells, *Mol. Microbiol.*, 10, 499–510.
81 Hilse, R., Hammerschmidt, S., Bautsch, W., Frosch, M. **1996**, Site-specific insertion of IS1301 and distribution in *Neisseria meningitidis* strains, *J. Bacteriol.* 178, 2527–2532.
82 Hammerschmidt, S., Muller, A., Sillmann, H., Mühlenhoff, M., Borrow, R., Fox, A., van Putten, J., Zollinger, W.D., Gerardy-Schahn, R., Frosch, M. **1996**, Capsule phase variation in *Neisseria meningitidis* serogroup B by slipped strand mispairing in the polysialyltransferase gene (siaD): correlation with bacterial invasion and the outbreak of meningococcal disease, *Mol. Microbiol.* 20, 1211–1220.
83 Lavitola, A., Bucci, C., Salvatore, P., Maresca, G., Bruni, C.B., Alifano, P. **1999**, Intracistronic transcription termination in polysialyltransferase gene (*siaD*) affects phase variation in *Neisseria meningitidis, Mol. Microbiol.* 33, 119–127.
84 Deghmane, A.E., Petit, S., Topilko, A., Pereira, Y., Giorgini, D., Larribe, M., Taha, M.K. **2000**, Intimate adhesion of *Neisseria meningitidis* to human epithelial cells is under the control of the *crgA* gene, a novel *LysR*-type transcriptional regulator, *EMBO J.* 19, 1068–1078.
85 Deghmane, A.E., Giorgini, D., Larribe, M., Alonso, J.M., Taha, M.K. **2002**, Down-regulation of pili and capsule of *Neisseria meningitidis* upon contact with epithelial cells is mediated by CrgA regulatory protein, *Mol. Microbiol.* 43, 1555–1564.
86 Frosch, M., Meyer, T.F. **1992**, Transformation-mediated exchange of virulence determinants by co-cultivation of pathogenic Neisseriae, *FEMS Microbiol. Lett.* 79, 345–349.
87 Vogel, U., Claus, H., Frosch, M. **2000**, Rapid serogroup switching in *Neisseria meningitidis* [letter], *N. Engl. J. Med.* 342, 219–220.

Genetics, Structure and Function of Lipopolysaccharide

J. Claire Wright, Joyce S. Plested and E. Richard Moxon

9.1
Introduction

The lipopolysaccharide (LPS) of *Neisseria meningitidis* is an amphipathic glycolipid with a molecular mass of around 4.8 kDa, the most abundant antigenic component of the *N. meningitidis* cell envelope. It consists of two genetically and structurally distinct regions: a lipophilic portion termed lipid A and the core oligosaccharide. The lipid A backbone consists of a β-$(1' \rightarrow 6)$ linked disaccharide and carries two phosphate groups at positions 4' and 1, both of which are often substituted, anchored in the membrane by acyl chains. Lipid A, an endotoxin, is linked to a heterogenous surface exposed core oligosaccharide composed mainly of neutral sugars. The structures of the core regions vary greatly from strain to strain but also, through phase variation, among progeny derived from any one individual strain. Because the core LPS of *N. meningitidis* lacks the highly repetitive sugar side-chains, for example those characteristic of the O antigens of enterobacteriaceae, many refer to the truncated or rough *N. meningitidis* LPS as lipooligosaccharide (LOS), but we prefer to retain the traditional LPS designation [5, 6]. Twelve structural variations (immunotypes) have been described [7] and this variation affects the role of *N. meningitidis* LPS in commensal and virulence behavior. *N. meningitidis* LPS mimics human glycosphingolipids, such as paraglobuside and sialylparagloboside, precursors of the glycolipid antigens of human erythrocytes, suggesting that molecular mimicry may be a factor in the evasion of host clearance mechanisms [8]. Given the important role that LPS plays in determining the physiological functions of Gram-negative bacteria, it came as a major surprise when it was discovered that viable meningococci can be completely deficient in LPS when cultured in the laboratory on artificial media [9]. Nonetheless, meningococcal LPS has a critical role in the pathogenesis of colonization, invasion, bloodstream dissemination and damage to host tissues. The inter- and intrastrain diversity of glycoforms characteristic of *N. meningitidis* LPS likely results in part from these multifunctional roles and the dynamic interactions with the innate and acquired components of the

Handbook of Meningococcal Disease. Infection Biology, Vaccination, Clinical Management.
Edited by M. Frosch and M. C. J. Maiden
Copyright © 2006 WILEY-VCH Verlag GmbH & Co. KGaA, Weinheim
ISBN: 3-527-31260-9

Lipid A Structure

The lipid A structure of N. meningitidis is based upon a β-D-glucosaminyl-(1'→6)-D-glucosamine disaccharide backbone which can be variably substituted at positions 4' and 1 (Fig. 9.1). In LPS, the 6' hydroxyl group is substituted by the oligosaccharide chain. The fatty acids anchoring the lipid A into the outer membrane have been identified as dodecanoic acid (C12:0), 3-hydroxy dodecanoic acid (3-OH C12:0) and 3-hydroxytetradecanoic acid (3-OH C14:0). Kulshin et al. [1] found that three lipid A species could be distinguished, although there was a predominance of a hexaacyl component with minor species representing a pentaacyl and tetraacyl lipid A. In the hexaacyl form, C12:0 is bound to the hydroxyl groups at positions 3 and 3' and 3-OH C14:0 is linked to the amino groups at positions 2 and 2', with the hydroxyl groups being acylated by C12:0 in turn. The symmetric acylation pattern of N. meningitidis lipid A was first encountered in *Chromobacterium violaceum* and is therefore referred to as a *C. violaceum*-type lipid A. The phosphate groups at positions 1 and 4' on the diglucos-

Fig. 9.1 Structure of lipid A in N. meningitidis (adapted from Kulshin et al. [1]): the phosphate groups at the 4' and 1 positions of the diglucosamine backbone have been found to be substituted with a variety of moieties leading to the term "phosphoforms". The substitutions have been found to include an extra phosphate or phosphoethanolamine (as shown above) or pyrophosphoethanolamine. These substitutions have been found to be non-stoichiometric and seem to vary between strains.

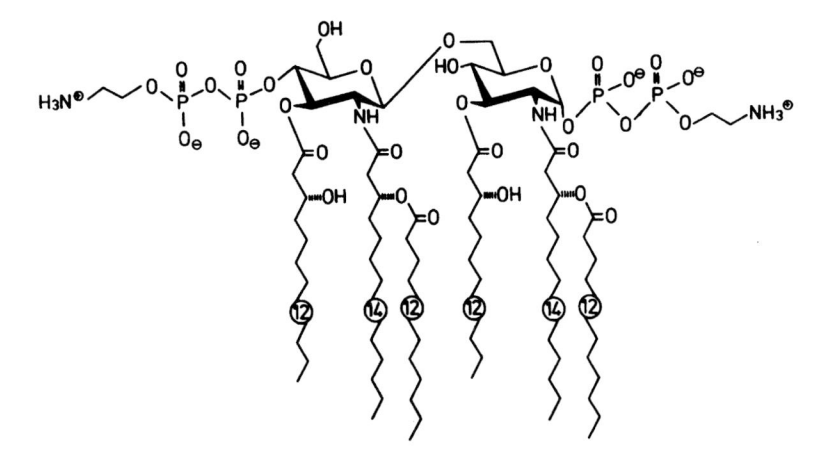

amine backbone can both be substituted by an extra phosphate, phosphoethanolamine or pyrophosphoethanolamine, substitutions that are nonstoichiometric.

9.3
Core Oligosaccharide Structure

N. meningitidis LPS has been classified into 12 distinct immunotypes (L1–L12) originally defined by monoclonal antibody (mAb) activity [7], the basis of which has been further defined by structural analysis: L1 and L6 [10, 11], L2 [12], L3 [13], L4 and L7 [14], L5 [15], L9 [16]. The oligosaccharide portion of the LPS is divided into the relatively conserved inner core region and the more heterogenous outer core region. Figure 9.2 shows the structures of the different immunotypes and details the specific linkages between the sugars.

The inner core region of the LPS is based on a diheptose backbone which is attached via one of the two 3-deoxy-D-*manno*-2-octulosonic acid (KDO) molecules to the lipid A portion. Additions occur to the first heptose (Hep I); and extension past the proximal glucose (Glc) is referred to as the outer core. The second heptose (Hep II) is invariably substituted at the 2-position by an N-acetyl glucosamine (GlcNAc); and in some structures Glc is present at the 3-position. Phosphoethanolamine (PEtn) additions can occur at the 3-, 6- and possibly the 7-position of Hep II. The presence of Glc and position of PEtn on Hep II, coupled with the outer core structure, gives the immunotype classification. The L5 immunotype is the only structure where PEtn is absent. In the L1, L3, L7, L8 and L10 structures, PEtn is present at the 3-position on Hep II. In the remaining immunotypes, L2, L4 and L6, PEtn is found at either the 6- or perhaps the 7-position. In some strains, PEtn has been found at either position [10, 12, 17], whereas in others it has only ever been found at the 6-position [3, 14].

In all the immunotypes except L5 and L10, the first sugar in the outer core region is a galactose (Gal). In the L5 and L10 structures, a Glc is present. The outer core extension, consisting of the lacto-N-neotetraose structure (Gal-GlcNAc-Gal), is present in six of the 12 immunotypes (L2, L3, L4, L5, L7, L9). Antibodies recognizing specific inner core structures have been raised and used to screen collections of strains, including carriage and disease isolates. This has identified strains that give nontypical patterns of reactivity with these antibodies and structural analysis of the LPS produced by these strains has revealed two structures not covered in the 12 immunotype structures [4]. The first of these structures is one where two PEtn molecules are added to Hep II at the 3- and 6-positions [18]. This structure has been found in only a small number of strains and the addition of PEtn at these two positions appears to be stoichiometric in some strains and nonstoichiometric in others. The two genes encoding the transferases responsible for these additions have both been identified and screening for a full-length copy of each gene in collections of strains has shown both genes to be present in over one-third of all the strains tested [3, 19]. This suggests that a di-PEtn structure may be present in far more strains than

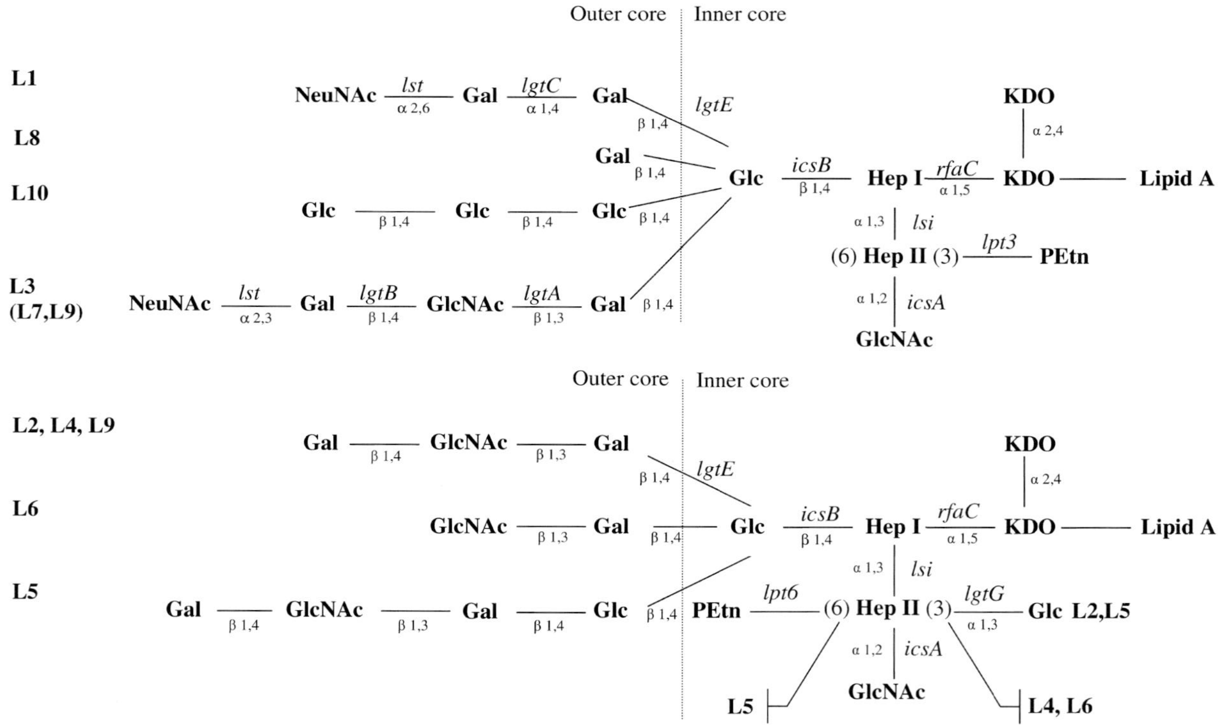

Fig. 9.2 LPS oligosaccharide structure found in immunotypes L1–L12 of *N. meningitidis*. The position of PEtn in immunotype L9 is unknown. Genes encoding the transferases responsible for addition of the individual sugars are indicated, together with the specific linkages. The genes *icsA* and *icsB* are also known as *rfaK* and *lgtF* respectively, whilst *lsi* is also known as *rfaF*. KDO – 3-Deoxy-D-*manno*-2-octulosonic acid, Hep – heptose, Glc – glucose, Gal – galactose, GlcNAc – N-acetyl glucosamine, PEtn – phosphoethanolamine, NeuNAc – sialic acid.

previously thought, although there may be a predominance of PEtn at one position, effectively masking the minor di-PEtn glycoform. The second nonimmunotype structure was shown to possess two Glc residues on Hep I, with the second Glc having a $\beta 1 \rightarrow 2$ linkage [20]. This structure seems to be very rare and to date has only been found in three strains. The transferase responsible for this addition has not yet been identified.

Other species that are found decorating the LPS of some strains of *N. meningitidis* are O-acetyl groups and the amino acid glycine. Partial, but substantial O-acetylation has been found in the L2, L4 and L5 immunotypes [12, 14, 15]. The O-acetyl group is attached to the GlcNAc on Hep II and has been found at either the O-3 or O-7 position [14, 21]. LPS in its native form may show a higher degree of O-acetylation, but the mild acid hydrolysis treatment required to obtain oligosaccharide from the LPS would effect their removal. A glycine residue has also been found in the inner core oligosaccharide in the immunotype L3 and L4 strains, where it is located at the 7-position on Hep II [21]. The mechanism of this substitution is unknown.

Sialylation of the LPS can occur when the extension from Hep I contains the minimum structure of a trisaccharide terminating in a Gal residue, such as in the L1 and L3 immunotypes. The extension from Hep I in the L8 immunotype consists of the disaccharide Gal-Glc and this is unable to serve as an acceptor for sialylation, probably due to the steric hindrance from components of the inner core region of the LPS [22]. Serogroup B, C, Y and W-135 *N. meningitidis*, which synthesize CMP-N-acetylneuraminic acid (CMP-NeuNAc) as a substrate for capsule synthesis, can endogenously sialylate LPS. Exogenous CMP-NeuNAc from the host environment can also be synthesized and used to sialylate LPS.

9.4 Genetics

The genes required for the biosynthesis of the lipid A portion of the LPS are discussed in detail in a review by Kahler and Stephens [23]. The biosynthesis of Lipid A has been investigated extensively in *Escherichia coli* and many of the genes involved have subsequently been identified in *N. meningitidis*. UDP-N-acetylglucosamine is the basic building block of both peptidoglycan and lipid A. The UDP-GlcNAc acyltransferase, LpxA, transfers the acyl chain from R-3 hydroxydodecanoyl acyl carrier protein to the hexose 3-OH of UDP-GlcNAc. De-acetylation by LpxC occurs before the N-linked R-3-hydroxydodecanoate is attached by LpxD to produce UDP-2,3-diacylglucosamine. Lipid X is formed by the release of UMP from UDP-2,3-diacylglucosamine. The disaccharide 1-phosphate backbone of lipid A (Lipid IV_A) is produced by the lipid A dissacharide synthase, LpxB condensing one molecule of lipid X with one molecule of UDP-2,3-diacylglucosamine. In *E. coli*, *lpxA* is an essential gene, but inactivation of the gene in *N. meningitidis* results in a viable strain possessing an outer membrane with nondetectable LPS [9]. KDO_2-lipid A is formed by the addition of two KDO sugars and two acyl chains to lipid IV_A. The transferase encoded by *kdtA* is a bifunctional enzyme that catalyzes the addition of both KDO residues. The synthesis of lipid A is completed by the substitution of dodecanoic acid to the acyl chains at positions 2 and 2′ of KDO_2-lipid IV_A by the acyl transferase HtrB. The diheptose backbone of the oligosaccharide portion of the LPS is formed by two heptosyltransferases. The gene product of *rfaC* adds Hep I to the lipid A-KDO_2 structure, whilst the *lsi* or *rfaF* [24] product is responsible for the addition of Hep II to Hep I.

During the past decade, most of the genes responsible for the additions of the sugars in the *N. meningitidis* oligosaccharide portion of the LPS have been identified, many by homology to LPS genes in other Gram-negative bacteria. The majority of LPS genes are clustered together in three regions of the genome, termed Lgt-1, Lgt-2 and Lgt-3, as described by Zhu et al. [2]. In individual strains, however, different combinations of the genes within the regions are present, leading to the formation of different LPS structures. The genes encoding the specific transferases are shown in Fig. 9.2 and the chromosomal arrangements of Lgt-1, -2 and -3 are shown in Fig. 9.3.

Lgt-1, first identified in *N. gonorrhoeae* [25] and subsequently found also in *N. meningitidis* [26], may contain up to five genes (*lgtA, lgtB, lgtC, lgtD, lgtE*) that encode glycosyl transferases responsible for additions to the outer core region of the LPS. The transferase responsible for the addition of the first sugar is encoded by *lgtE* or *lgtH*. This addition is usually a Gal residue, but in the L5 and L10 immunotypes, a Glc is added with the same linkage. When the translated amino acid sequences of the *lgtE* gene from a number of strains are aligned, then it can be seen that there is a single amino acid change from threonine to methionine, present in all strains where Glc is added instead of the usual Gal. This same amino acid change has also been noted in LPS glycosyl transferases present in *Haemophilus influenzae,* where it has been shown experimentally that this single amino acid change is responsible for the addition of Gal or Glc to the LPS (M.E. Deadman, personal communication). The amino acid sequences of the translated products of *lgtE* and *lgtH* show a 77% similarity and 73% identity to each other; and both transferases encoded by these genes demonstrate homologous function. No strain has been found to contain the *lgtE* and *lgtH* gene, leading to the suggestion that these are allelic variants of the same gene. The genes, *lgtB* and *lgtC* encode Gal transferases, whilst the transferase encoded by *lgtA* is responsible for the addition of GlcNAc. The products of the three genes *lgtA, lgtB* and *lgtE* are all required for the formation of the lacto-N-neotetraose structure. *N. gonorrhoeae,* unlike *N. meningitidis,* is able to add N-acetylgalactosamine (GalNAc) to the outer core structure, resulting in an extension of GalNAc-Gal-GlcNAc-Gal; and the gene *lgtD* encodes the transferase responsible for this addition.

Sequencing studies have shown recombination to occur within this region, due to the sequence similarity of the *lgtB* and *lgtE* genes, with "hybrids" such as *lgtZ* being formed and resulting in partial copies of *lgtA* and *lgtC* being present. The open reading frame *lgtZ* has arisen due to a 1.5-kb deletion removing the

3′ end of the *lgtA* gene and fusing it with the 3′ end of the *lgtB* gene. Zhu et al. [2] identified eight different combinations of genes to be present in the Lgt-1 region of pathogenic and nonpathogenic *Neisseria* species, as shown in Fig. 9.3 a, which are termed types I to VIII. The type I arrangement is unique to, but found in all, *N. gonorrhoeae* strains studied, whilst types III to VIII are found in different *N. meningitidis* strains. The type II arrangement is found only in the commensal species *N. subflava* and *N. lactamica*. This suggests that *N. meningitidis* is capable of greater variation in the structure of the outer core region of the LPS than other *Neisseria* species.

The genes *lgtA*, *lgtC* and *lgtD* all demonstrate phase variation, allowing the switching "on or off" of gene expression by means of a homopolymeric tract of guanines. The process of phase variation occurs by slippage of the repeat tracts, resulting in the translated product being brought in or out of frame with the relevant initiation codon (see Chapter 6). The number of guanines in the repeat tracts has been found to vary between strains from 5 to 14 for *lgtA* and from 10 to 13 for *lgtC*. The *lgtD* gene has only been found in one *N. meningitidis* strain, where sequencing has revealed that the homopolymeric tract contains eight guanines, which would result in an out of frame translation product. No *N. meningitidis* strain to date has been found to present GalNAc as the terminal residue on the outer core region of the LPS. This mechanism of phase variation enables an individual bacterium to have the potential to display a repertoire of different LPS structures.

Lgt-2 is an operon of two genes: *lgtF* [27] or *icsB* [28] and *rfaK* [29] or *icsA* [28] that encode the glycosyl transferases required for chain elongation from the lipid A-$(KDO)_2$-Hep_2 basal structure (Fig. 9.3 b). The product of *icsA* is responsible for the addition of GlcNAc to Hep II; and subsequently the product of *icsB* is able to add Glc to Hep I. These additions must both occur before the outer core structures can be added. The Lgt-2 locus has been found to be invariably present in all *N. meningitidis* strains studied to date.

The Lgt-3 region contains two known LPS genes: *lgtG* [30] and *lpt6* [3], and potentially a third gene which shows homology to acetyl transferase genes. The transferase encoded by *lgtG* is responsible for the addition of Glc to the 3-position of Hep II. Like *lgtA* and *lgtC*, the *lgtG* gene contains a homopolymeric tract allowing phase variation to occur; and individual strains have been found to have from 10 to 14 cytosines present. The transferase encoded by *lpt6* has been shown to be responsible for the addition of PEtn at the 6- and 7-position of Hep II [3, 17]. The presence/absence of the genes in the Lgt-3 region has been shown to vary between strains and, to date, five different combinations, termed type I–V have been identified [2, 3] (Fig. 9.3 c).

The remaining two genes required for the formation of the LPS structure are found in regions of the genome not associated with other LPS-related genes, i.e. *lst* and *lpt3*.

The addition of PEtn to Hep II in part defines the immunotype to which the LPS structure is designated. *N. meningitidis* has been shown to possess three LPS PEtn transferase genes. *lpt6*, as discussed previously, is present in the Lgt-3

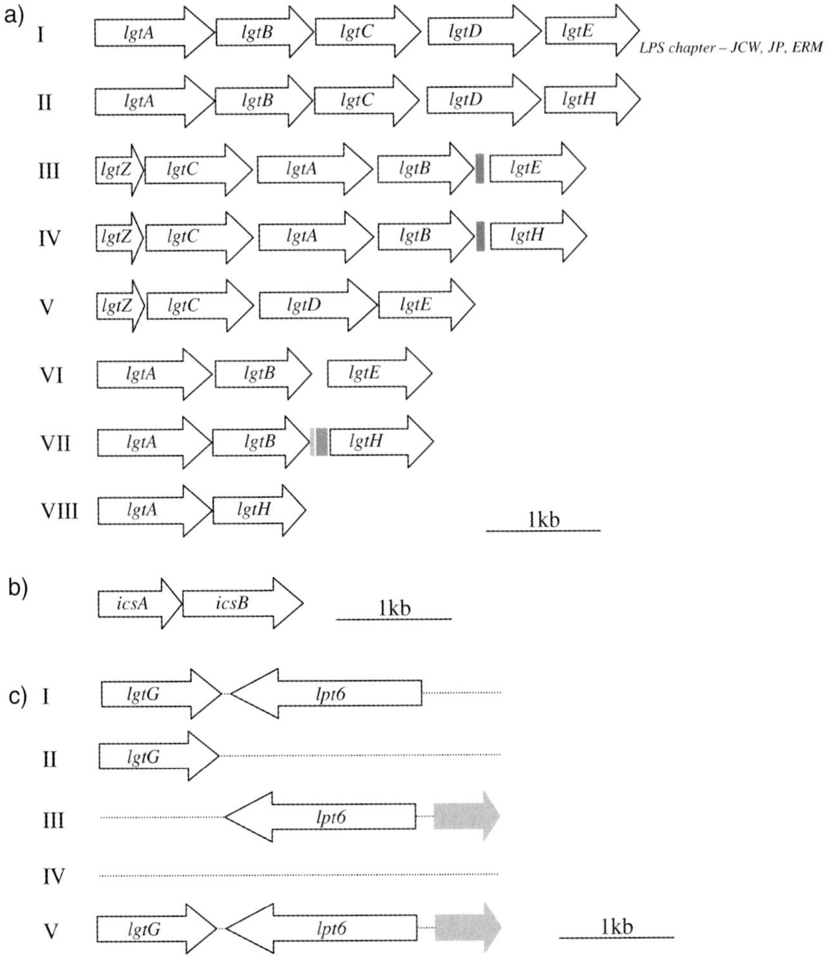

Fig. 9.3 (a) Lgt-1 region (adapted from Zhu et al. [2]). This region contains the genes encoding glycosyltransferases responsible for the outer core extension of the LPS oligosaccharide and may contain up to five genes. Genes in this region show high levels of homology, particularly between *lgtB* and *lgtE*, leading to recombination and the formation of new open reading frames such as *lgtZ*, a hybrid of *lgtA* and *lgtB*, and also leaving partial copies of duplicated genes (shown as gray boxes). Screening of collections of pathogenic and nonpathogenic strains has shown that eight possible combinations of genes may be present and these arrangements have been termed types I–VIII. The type I arrangement has been found only in *N. gonorrhoeae* strains, whilst type II has been found only in the commensals *N. lactamica* and *N. subflava. The genes lgtE* and *lgtH* show high levels of homology and have been hypothesized to be allelic variants of the same gene. The genes *lgtA*, *lgtC* and *lgtD* all contain homopolymeric tracts and are capable of exhibiting phase variation. (b) Lgt-2 region. This locus invariably contains two genes, *icsA* and *icsB* (also known as *rfaK* and *lgtF*), encoding glycosyl transferases responsible for the addition of GlcNAc to Hep II and Glc to Hep I, respectively. These additions must occur before the outer core region can be assembled. (c) Lgt-3 region (adapted from Wright et al. [3]). This region contains two

region and is required for the addition of PEtn at the 6-position of Hep II. The gene product of *lpt3* shows 43% similarity to that of *lpt6* and is required for addition of PEtn to the 3-position of Hep II [19]. In some strains, a copy of the *lpt3* gene is present with a 280-bp deletion in the central portion of the gene, rendering the gene product nonfunctional. The third transferase, encoded by *lptA*, shows 41% similarity to *lpt6* and is responsible for the addition of PEtn to the lipid A moiety [31]. When a collection of strains including carriage and disease isolates was screened for the presence of full-length copies of these three PEtn transferase genes, the results were as follows: the *lptA* gene was present in all strains, the *lpt6* gene alone was present in 12% of strains, the *lpt3* gene alone was present in 50% of strains and both the *lpt3* and *lpt6* genes were present in 36% of strains. Only one strain lacked both *lpt3* and *lpt6* [3].

Homology searching through the genome sequence databases of many Gram-negative bacteria has shown these three *N. meningitidis* genes to belong to a large, previously unidentified family of genes [31], encoding transferases for PEtn and the related species phosphocholine [32], allowing the decoration of surface structures of the bacteria, such as LPS and pili.

The *lpt3* and the phase-variable *lgtG* genes both encode transferases that add residues to the 3-position of Hep II. When both genes are present and *lgtG* is in-frame, enabling a functional transferase to be produced, then a Glc residue is added to Hep II in preference to PEtn. The PEtn residue is only incorporated into the LPS at this position if the *lgtG* gene product is out of frame and consequently not translated [19].

The final LPS specific gene to be discussed here is *lst*, encoding the sialyltransferase responsible for the addition of CMP-NeuNAc to those LPS structures where the outer core extension from Hep I consists of the minimum structure of a trisaccharide terminating with a Gal residue [22]. The Lst enzyme was first identified as an α-2,3-sialyltransferase in a strain expressing the L3 immunotype, where the terminal Gal possesses a $\beta 1 \rightarrow 3$ linkage [33]. However, sialylation of the LPS was also observed when the structure of a strain expressing the L1 immunotype was determined [11]. In the L1 immunotype structure, the terminal Gal residue possesses an $\alpha 1 \rightarrow 4$ linkage, which had been previously considered as unable to act as an acceptor for CMP-NeuNAc. On further investigation into the function of Lst, the transferase was found to have a relaxed acceptor specificity, being able to use synthetic acceptors presenting terminal N-acetyllactosamine, lactose or Gal [33]. The Lst transferase from the L1 strain has been shown to make both the $\alpha 2 \rightarrow 3$ and $\alpha 2 \rightarrow 6$ linkages *in vitro*, but

known LPS genes, *lgtG* and *lpt6*. The transferase encoded by the phase variable *lgtG* gene is responsible for the addition of Glc to Hep II at the 3-position and the product of *lpt6* allows the addition of PEtn to Hep II at the 6-position. The open reading frame in gray shows homology to acetyl transferases. Screening of collections of strains has shown five possible combinations of these three genes exist, ranging from all three genes being present to none at all; and these are termed types I–V.

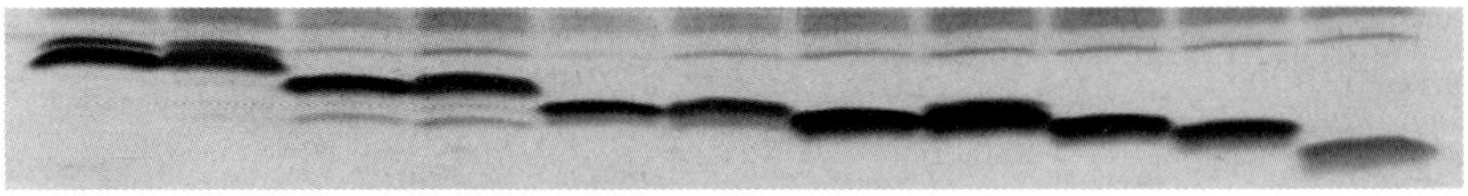
WT
lpt3
lgtB
lgtB-lpt3
lgtA
lgtA-lpt3
lgtE
galE
icsB
icsA
lsi

Fig. 9.4 LPS profiles: individual LPS genes in the strain MC58 (L3 immunotype), have been disrupted by insertion of an antibiotic resistance cassette. Whole-cell lysates have been separated by electrophoresis and stained with silver in order to compare the LPS profiles produced by the different mutations. The reduction in size by one sugar can clearly be seen as a change in the molecular mass of the band. However, the removal of phosphoethanolamine (*lpt3*) from the inner core region of the LPS does not result in a change of band size, rather a change in the quality of staining.

only the $\alpha 2 \rightarrow 6$ has been seen *in vivo* [34]. A comparison of the amino acid sequences of the L3 Lst and L1 Lst transferases revealed only six differences. Site-directed mutagenesis of the L3 *lst* gene showed that a single amino acid change from glycine to isoleucine was responsible for the bifunctional nature of this transferase, resulting in sialylation of the L3 strain with an $\alpha 2 \rightarrow 6$ linkage [34].

The gene *galE*, although not directly an LPS gene, is often disrupted to give bacteria that are only capable of producing inner core LPS structures [35]. GalE is a UDP-glucose 4-epimerase which catalyzes the final step in the Leloir pathway of galactose metabolism, interconverting UDP-galactose and UDP-glucose. When *galE* is disrupted, the bacterium is unable to provide activated Gal for incorporation into the LPS, therefore producing a structure which extends from Hep I no further than the Glc residue. The gene *galU*, which encodes the UTP-glucose-1-phosphate uridyltransferase, an enzyme which is also involved in the Leloir pathway, was recently shown when disrupted to prevent the incorporation of Glc in the LPS structure [3].

The LPS profiles produced by individual strains can be viewed by separating whole-cell lysates by electrophoresis, followed by staining with silver. The LPS genes have all been individually interrupted, usually by the insertion of an antibiotic resistance cassette and the profiles viewed as described (Fig. 9.4). As the genes encoding the glycosyl transferases adding the distal to the proximal sugar are in turn disrupted, the profile of the LPS can be seen to be reduced in size. Interestingly, the two PEtn transferase genes, when disrupted do not cause a change in the banding profile, but instead lead to a difference in the quality of staining.

9.5
LPS and the Biology of Commensal and Virulence Behavior

Colonization of the human respiratory tract has been studied, predominantly using *in vitro* cultured cell lines. LPS, in conjunction with pili, outer membrane proteins and capsule, has been found to play a role in the adherence and invasion of *N. meningitidis*. The effects of different LPS structures were examined in variants expressing either sialylated (L3 immunotype) or truncated nonsialylated (L8 immunotype) LPS. Pili were found to be essential for the adherence of sialylated meningococci (immunotype L3) to HUVECs, whether encapsulated or not [36]. This essential role of LPS to the adherence functions mediated by pili is apparently independent of pilus fiber formation and twitching motility [37]. Further, adherence to epithelial cells can be mediated through defensin-like molecules, but not in the absence of LPS [38]. In terms of the invasiveness of *N. meningitidis*, an LPS-deficient mutant did not enter into or pass through host cells. Jones et al. [39] found an association between certain LPS immunotypes and invasive disease: 97% of case isolates expressed the L3, 7, 9 immunotype, whereas the immunotypes associated with carriage were heterogenous. Isolates possessing the L3, 7, 9 immunotype produced greater nasal colonization of mice and were more invasive in mice than strains of immunotype L1,8,10. Further, an *in vivo* switch from an inoculum of L1,8,10 organisms to those having L3, 7, 9 immunotype recovered from blood was observed [40]. In studies on human nasopharyngeal tissue in organ culture, meningococci result in a marked reduction in ciliary activity, but this was not apparently mediated by LPS [23]. Thus, LPS and variations in its structure are likely to modulate the adherence and invasion of *N. meningitidis* from the upper respiratory tract through properties that affect the susceptibility of *N. meningitidis* to immune clearance, as well as by modulating the functions of many outer membrane adhesins [41].

Sialylation of neisserial LPS and its contribution to serum resistance was first demonstrated in *N. gonorrhoeae* and is characteristic of bacteria grown *in vivo*, although this phenotype may be lost on *in vitro* culture [42]. Serum resistance is important in the pathogenesis of invasive disease but is also a potential factor when there is local inflammation at mucosal sites. This modification occurs through exposure to host cytidine 5′-monophospho-N-acetyl neuraminic acid and affects many aspects of *N. gonorrhoeae* pathogenicity [43, 44]. Exogenous LPS sialylation also occurs in *N. meningitidis*, but may occur endogenously [45]; but the contribution to *N. meningitidis* pathogenicity is not as profound as for *N. gonorrhoeae* because of the primacy of *N. meningitidis* capsular polysaccharides in virulence. The distinct contributions of capsulation and sialylation of LPS have been difficult to disentangle, but sialylation appears to exert its major effect in strains lacking capsule. This may be important, in that a substantial proportion of natural isolates from *N. meningitidis* carriage lack capsule [40, 46–48]. In summary, the contribution of LPS sialylation to serum resistance is modest, although a fully extended lacto-N-tetraose molecule that is sialylated hinders C3b insertion and assembly of the membrane attack complex. In *N. meningitidis*, the role of LPS, if any, in affecting factor H binding is uncertain.

Plasma concentrations of *N. meningitidis* LPS correlate closely with disease manifestations and outcome. Indeed, fulminant *N. meningitidis* sepsis is considered the prototypical Gram-negative sepsis and there is compelling evidence that the major determinant of proinflammatory cytokine production is through the endotoxic properties of *N. meningitidis* LPS [38, 47, 49]. The role of LPS in *N. meningitidis* sepsis requires an understanding of the processes of recognition by host cells through LPS-dependent interactions of *N. meningitidis* with CD-14 and Toll-like receptor 4 (TLR4) and its co-factor MD2, the resultant triggering of the cascade of pro- and counter-inflammatory cytokines and subsequent endothelial damage [50]. In an LPS-deficient mutant, 10- to 100-fold higher concentrations of *N. meningitidis* bacteria are required to elicit the same level of TNFα, interleukin (IL)-1B and IL-6 as compared to a wild-type strain [51]. There is also evidence that strain-to-strain variations in lipid A structure are responsible for differences in TLR-4/MD2 signaling. Patients with persistent septic shock and multiple organ failure have very high levels of endotoxin in plasma [38]. Mortality increases from 0% to >80% commensurate with a 10-fold increase in plasma LPS and a corresponding increase from 10 units/ml to 100 units/ml of limulus lysate endotoxin. Vascular damage is the major factor in the pathology of *N. meningitidis* sepsis and this depends upon the migration and binding of host inflammatory cells to endothelium which, in turn, is influenced by the induction of adhesion molecules [52]. Both LPS and capsule modulate the induction of adhesion, following which injury to endothelial cells occurs through upregulation of tissue factor and the induction of coagulation, together with inhibition of fibrinolysis by plasminogen activator inhibitor 1.

9.6
LPS as a Vaccine Candidate

Polyclonal and monoclonal antibodies to LPS have been shown to be protective *in vitro* and *in vivo* against meningococci. Evidence for their potential relevance has been demonstrated in convalescent sera from children following invasive meningococcal disease [53–55]. Zollinger et al. [56] observed that naturally acquired bactericidal antibodies in sera from Chilean children could be specifically inhibited by L3, 7, 9 LPS. However, antibodies induced in volunteers by LPS-containing OMP vesicle vaccines in Norwegian serogroup B vaccine trials were not bactericidal [57, 58].

The candidacy of LPS as a vaccine must take into account the toxicity of lipid A [59] as well as its propensity for molecular mimicry [60] and the phase variation [61] of outer core structures. The toxicity of LPS can be substantially lessened by removing or altering the O- and/or N-acylation [62]. Other approaches employed to detoxify LPS include the use of liposomes. Petrov and co-workers found native LPS presented within liposomes had reduced toxicity and was moderately immunogenic in animals [63]. Zollinger et al. [64] prepared soluble noncovalent complexes of alkaline detoxified LPS (L3, 7, 9) bound to purified OMP in liposomes that were safe and immunogenic in Phase I trials of human volunteers. The other possibilities to avoid toxicity are to use peptide mimics of LPS structures identified using phage display libraries and LPS mAbs. Using this approach, mice immunized with peptides conjugated to diphtheria toxoid, identified using L3, 7, 9 immunotyping mAb 9-2-L379, elicited increased IgG$_1$ LPS-specific antibodies [65]. However, it should be noted that similar approaches using monoclonal antibodies reactive with the serogroup B capsular polysaccharide resulted in poorly immunogenic mimetics that failed to elicit anticapsular antibodies in mice [66].

Conserved inner core LPS structures (Fig. 9.5) could be exploited to elicit cross-protective antibodies, while lessening the risk of autoimmunity to epitopes of the outer core and immune-escape mediated by phase variation. The availability of complete genome sequences has facilitated a comprehensive identification of the genes involved in the biosynthesis of N. meningitidis LPS. Using mutants, structural analysis and immunobiological assays, it is feasible to identify conserved and accessible inner core LPS epitopes and to investigate the potential of antibodies to these inner core structures to elicit a protective immune response. A set of three mAbs to inner core LPS epitopes reacted with almost all (97/102) of a collection of meningococcal strains representative of the genetic diversity of disease-causing isolates [4]. One of these mAbs, designated B5, provides a limited proof in concept of the candidacy of inner core LPS as a vaccine, in that it is bactericidal and protective in vivo against some but not all meningococcal strains [67, 68]. However, inner core LPS glycoforms are poorly immunogenic; and, to elicit a strong and long-lived IgG immune response, conjugation to a carrier protein is required. However, the chemistry used to make conjugates must ideally avoid changes to the conformation of target epitope(s) [69–71]. There are two functional groups available in the N. meningitidis LPS inner core for coupling to free carboxyl, amino or sulfhydryl groups of a carrier protein: linkage either by the free amino group of PEtn, or by the carboxylic acid group of one of the KDO moieties. The carboxyl group of the terminal KDO was used to introduce an ethane thiol function in the core oligosaccharide and this group was coupled to bromoacetylated proteins. Core oligosaccharide conjugates of immunotypes L2 and L3, 7, 9, prepared using tetanus toxoid (TT) or meningococcal outer membrane proteins, were highly immunogenic in rabbits and mice (high titers of IgG), but were not bactericidal [70], suggesting that the KDO backbone and linkage to lipid A is important for appropriate presentation of the inner core LPS epitopes. Gu and Tsai [71] used O-deacylated LPS and the spacer, adipic hydrazide (ADH), with conjugation through the carboxyl group of one of the KDO moieties to prepare L8 LPS-TT conjugates that were able to induce bactericidal antibodies in rabbits that reacted with L3, 7, 9 by ELISA. The presence of PEtn and its position in the inner core have been shown to be an important factor in immunogenicity [69, 70, 72].

Other studies have attempted to identify cross-reactive LPS epitopes that do not contain the lacto-N-neotetraose group but are able to elicit bactericidal antibodies against L3, 7, 9 LPS. Estabrook et al. [73] identified a 3.6-kDa epitope that bound the monoclonal antibody D6A but was inhibited by human immune sera, using a HIM-ELISA. Using oligosaccharide conjugates, Verheul et al. [72] used synthetic conjugates prepared from oligosaccharides representative of the partial structures of the common inner core and found that a β-Glc substituted diheptosyl oligosaccharide (representative of inner core with α chain substitution) was the minimal structural unit required for induction of a cross-reactive

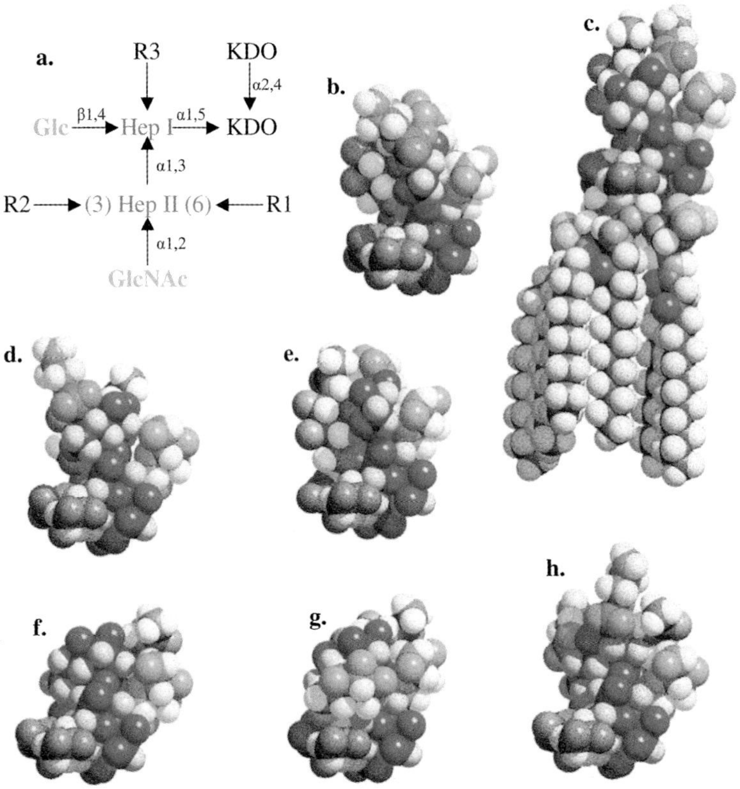

Fig. 9.5 Conserved structures within the inner core LPS region (adapted from Gidney et al. [4]). Seven structural variants are found within the inner core region of *N. meningitidis* LPS. (a) Structural representation of the inner core LPS. Substitutions to the second heptose (Hep II) can occur at the 3- and/or 6-position. (b–h) Three-dimensional space-filling molecular models of the seven LPS inner core structural variants are color-coded as follows: phosphoethanolamine (PEtn, orange), glucose (Glc, green), N-acetyl glucosamine (GlcNAc, pale blue), heptose (Hep, red), 3-deoxy-D-*manno*-2-octulosonic acid (KDO, dark gray), lipid A (pale gray). Molecular models were constructed using a Metropolis Monte-Carlo approach and are drawn with the same orientation for the KDO residue. The lipid A moiety is shown in panel (c) only, (b) immunotype L2 (R1 PEtn, R2 Glc-*α*1,3), (c) immunotype L3 (R2 PEtn), (d) immunotype L4 (R1 PEtn), (e) immunotype L5 (R2 Glc-*α*1,3), (f) an *lpt3* mutant of an L3 immunotype (no substitutions), (g) strain 1000 (R3 Glc-*α*1,2), (h) strain 2220Y (R1 PEtn, R2 PEtn). (This figure also appears with the color plates.)

response to L1, L2 and L3, 7, 9, but this approach failed to induce bactericidal or protective antibodies.

In more recent work, a limited number of *N. meningitidis* inner core LPS structural variants have been identified [67, 74]. These comprise PEtn at the 3-position, the 6- or 7-position of HepII, or the absence of PEtn [68]. Functional studies using monoclonal, polyclonal antibodies and O-deacylated immunotype

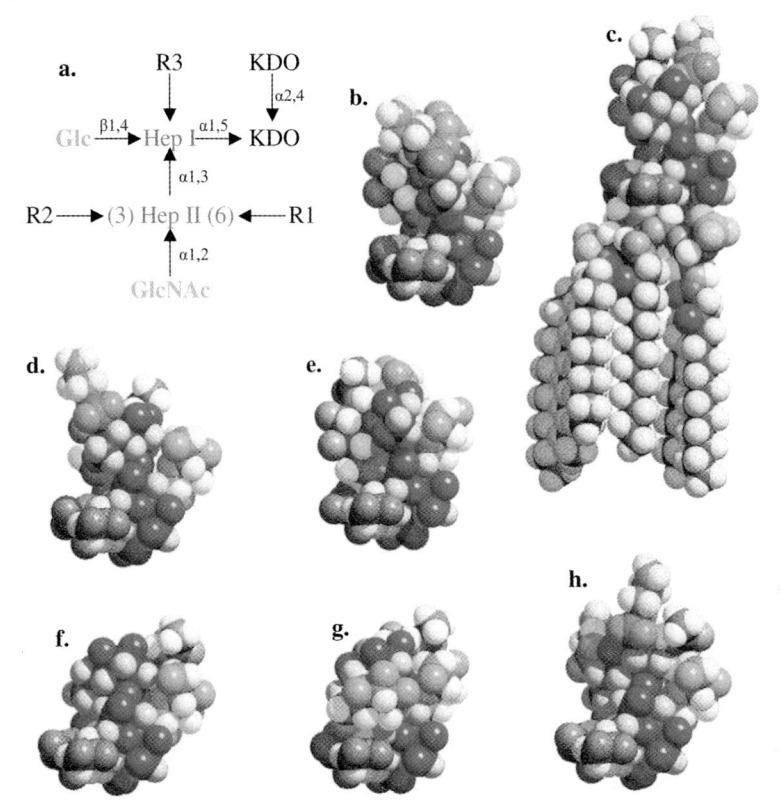

L3 conjugates have shown that antibodies to inner core structures can be bactericidal, opsonophagocytic and can passively protect against challenge with virulent *N. meningitidis* organisms in an infant rat model [

24 Jennings, M. P., Bisercic, M., Dunn, K. L., Virji, M., Martin, A., Wilks, K. E., Richards, J. C., Moxon, E. R. **1995**, *Microb Pathog* 19, 391–407.

25 Gotschlich, E. C. **1994**, *J Exp Med* 180, 2181–2190.

26 Jennings, M. P., Hood, D. W., Peak, I. R., Virji, M., Moxon, E. R. **1995**, *Mol Microbiol* 18, 729–740.

27 Kahler, C. M., Carlson, R. W., Rahman, M. M., Martin, L. E., Stephens, D. S. **1996**, *J Bacteriol* 178, 6677–6684.

28 van der Ley, P., Kramer, M., Martin, A., Richards, J. C., Poolman, J. T. **1997**, *FEMS Microbiol Lett* 146, 247–253.

29 Kahler, C. M., Carlson, R. W., Rahman, M. M., Martin, L. E., Stephens, D. S. **1996**, *J Bacteriol* 178, 1265–1273.

30 Banerjee, A., Wang, R., Uljon, S. N., Rice, P. A., Gotschlich, E. C., Stein, D. C. **1998**, *Proc Natl Acad Sci USA* 95, 10872–10877.

31 Cox, A. D., Wright, J. C., Li, J., Hood, D. W., Moxon, E. R., Richards, J. C. **2003**, *J Bacteriol* 185, 3270–3277.

32 Warren, M. J., Jennings, M. P. **2003**, *Infect Immun* 71, 6892–6898.

33 Gilbert, M., Watson, D. C., Cunningham, A. M., Jennings, M. P., Young, N. M., Wakarchuk, W. W. **1996**, *J Biol Chem* 271, 28271–28276.

34 Wakarchuk, W. W., Watson, D., St Michael, F., Li, J., Wu, Y., Brisson, J. R., Young, N. M., Gilbert, M. **2001**, *J Biol Chem* 276, 12785–12790.

35 Jennings, M. P., van der Ley, P., Wilks, K. E., Maskell, D. J., Poolman, J. T., Moxon, E. R. **1993**, *Mol Microbiol* 10, 361–369.

36 Virji, M., Makepeace, K., Peak, I. R., Ferguson, D. J., Jennings, M. P., Moxon, E. R. **1995**, *Mol Microbiol* 18, 741–754.

37 Albiger, B., Johansson, L., Jonsson, A. B. **2003**, *Infect Immun* 71, 155–162.

38 Brandtzaeg, P. **2003**, *Expert Rev Anti Infect Ther* 1, 589–596.

39 Jones, D. M., Borrow, R., Fox, A. J., Gray, S., Cartwright, K. A., Poolman, J. T. **1992**, *Microb Pathog* 13, 219–224.

40 Mackinnon, F. G., Borrow, R., Gorringe, A. R., Fox, A. J., Jones, D. M., Robinson, A. **1993**, *Microb Pathog* 15, 359–366.

41 Virji, M., Hill, D. J. **2003**, *Methods Mol Med* 71, 297–314.

42 Smith, H., Parsons, N. J., Cole, J. A. **1995**, *Microb Pathog* 19, 365–377.

43 Parsons, N. J., Constantinidou, C., Cole, J. A., Smith, H. **1994**, *Microb Pathog* 16, 413–421.

44 Apicella, M. A., Mandrell, R. E., Shero, M., Wilson, M. E., Griffiss, J. M., Brooks, G. F., Lammel, C., Breen, J. F., Rice, P. A. **1990**, *J Infect Dis* 162, 506–512.

45 Mandrell, R. E., Kim, J. J., John, C. M., Gibson, B. W., Sugai, J. V., Apicella, M. A., Griffiss, J. M., Yamasaki, R. **1991**, *J Bacteriol* 173, 2823–2832.

46 Virji, M., Makepeace, K., Ferguson, D. J., Achtman, M., Moxon, E. R. **1993**, *Mol Microbiol* 10, 499–510.

47 Brandtzaeg, P., Bjerre, A., Ovstebo, R., Brusletto, B., Joo, G. B., Kierulf, P. **2001**, *J Endotoxin Res* 7, 401–420.

48 Estabrook, M. M., Griffiss, J. M., Jarvis, G. A. **1997**, *Infect Immun* 65, 4436–4444.

49 Brandtzaeg, P., van Deuren, M. **2002**, *Curr Opin Infect Dis* 15, 247–252.

50 de Kleijn, E. D., Hazelzet, J. A., Kornelisse, R. F., de Groot, R. **1998**, *Eur J Pediatr* 157, 869–880.

51 van der Ley, P., Steeghs, L. **2003**, *J Endotoxin Res* 9, 124–128.

52 Dixon, G. L., Heyderman, R. S., Kotovicz, K., Jack, D. L., Andersen, S. R., Vogel, U., Frosch, M., Klein, N. **1999**, *Infect Immun* 67, 5626–5633.

53 Griffiss, J. M., Brandt, B. L., Broud, D. D., Goroff, D. K., Baker, C. J. **1984**, *J Infect Dis* 150, 71–79.

54 Plested, J. S., Gidney, M. A., Coull, P. A., Griffiths, H. G., Herbert, M. A., Bird, A. G., Richards, J. C., Moxon, E. R. **2000**, *J Immunol Methods* 237, 73–84.

55 Saukkonen, K., Leinonen, M., Kayhty, H., Abdillahi, H., Poolman, J. T. **1988**, *J Infect Dis* 158, 209–212.

56 Zollinger, W. D., Moran, E. E., Devi, S. J., Frasch, C. E. **1997**, *Infect Immun* 65, 1053–1060.

57 Rosenqvist, E., Hoiby, E. A., Wedege, E., Bryn, K., Kolberg, J., Klem, A., Ronnild, E., Bjune, G., Nokleby, H. **1995**, *Infect Immun* 63, 4642–4652.

58 Rosenqvist, E., Hoiby, E.A., Wedege, E., Kusecek, B., Achtman, M. **1993**, *J Infect Dis* 167, 1065–1073.

59 Poolman, J.T. **1990**, in *Bacterial Vaccines*, ed. Mizrahi, A., John Wiley and Sons, New York, p. 57–86.

60 Tsai, C.M., Civin, C.I. **1991**, *Infect Immun* 59, 3604–3609.

61 Jennings, M.P., Srikhanta, Y.N., Moxon, E.R., Kramer, M., Poolman, J.T., Kuipers, B., van der Ley, P. **1999**, *Microbiology* 145, 3013–3021.

62 Verheul, A.F., Snippe, H., Poolman, J.T. **1993**, *Microbiol Rev* 57, 34–49.

63 Petrov, A.B., Semenov, B.F., Vartanyan, Y.P., Zakirov, M.M., Torchilin, V.P., Trubetskoy, V.S., Koshkina, N.V., L'Vov, V.L., Verner, I.K., Lopyrev, I.V., et al. **1992**, *Infect Immun* 60, 3897–3903.

64 Zollinger, W.D., Moran, E.E., Ray, J., McClain, B. **1991**, *Frontiers in Vaccine Research*, Hanasaari, Helsinki.

65 Charalambous, B.M., Feavers, I.M. **2000**, *FEMS Microbiol Lett* 191, 45–50.

66 Moe, G.R., Tan, S., Granoff, D.M. **1999**, *FEMS Immunol Med Microbiol* 26, 209–226.

67 Plested, J.S., Ferry, B.L., Coull, P.A., Makepeace, K., Lehmann, A.K., MacKinnon, F.G., Griffiths, H.G., Herbert, M.A., Richards, J.C., Moxon, E.R. **2001**, *Infect Immun* 69, 3203–3213.

68 Plested, J.S., Makepeace, K., Jennings, M.P., Gidney, M.A., Lacelle, S., Brisson, J., Cox, A.D., Martin, A., Bird, A.G., Tang, C.M., Mackinnon, F.M., Richards, J.C., Moxon, E.R. **1999**, *Infect Immun* 67, 5417–5426.

69 Jennings, H.J., Lugowski, C., Ashton, F.E. **1984**, *Infect Immun* 43, 407–412.

70 Verheul, A.F., Van Gaans, J.A., Wiertz, E.J., Snippe, H., Verhoef, J., Poolman, J.T. **1993**, *Infect Immun* 61, 187–196.

71 Gu, X.X., Tsai, C.M. **1993**, *Infect Immun* 61, 1873–1880.

72 Verheul, A.F., Braat, A.K., Leenhouts, J.M., Hoogerhout, P., Poolman, J.T., Snippe, H., Verhoef, J. **1991**, *Infect Immun* 59, 843–851.

73 Estabrook, M.M., Baker, C.J., Griffiss, J.M. **1993**, *J Infect Dis* 167, 966–970.

74 Plested, J.S., Harris, S.L., Wright, J.C., Coull, P.A., Makepeace, K., Gidney, M.A., Brisson, J.R., Richards, J.C., Granoff, D.M., Moxon, E.R. **2003**, *J Infect Dis* 187, 1223–1234.

75 Pavliak, V., Fortuna-Nevin, M., Monteiro, M., Mason, K., Zhu, D. **2004**, *Int Pathog Neisseria Conf* 14.

10
Major Outer Membrane Proteins of Meningococci

Jeremy Derrick, John E. Heckels and Mumtaz Virji

10.1
Introduction

Neisseria meningitidis have the typical triple-layered cell envelope characteristic of Gram-negative bacteria: the cytoplasmic membrane is protected by a peptidoglycan layer and itself is covered by a second or outer membrane (OM). As the outermost layer of the cell, the outer membrane plays a critical role in the interactions of meningococci with the outside world. These include meningococcal–host cell interactions that are responsible for colonization and invasion, interaction with the immune system responsible for the development of immunity to infection and for the serological differences between strains that have formed the basis of epidemiological studies. In addition, the outer membrane has been the major focus for the development of vaccines against serogroup B meningococcal infection, both those currently undergoing human trials and those in further laboratory development.

In addition to lipids and lipopolysaccharide (LPS, see Chapter 9), the outer membrane contains a restricted number of major proteins which have been the subject of considerable interest because of their potential roles in the key biological processes outlined above. In early studies, Frasch and colleagues identified five structural classes of OM proteins, based on relative mobility on SDS-polyacrylamide gel electrophoresis, and designated them Class 1–5 proteins [1]. Subsequent studies revealed that the Class 2 and 3 proteins corresponded to one protein, now designated PorB, which is encoded by two different alleles of a single gene, *porB*. Similarly, the Class 1, 4 and 5 proteins are now designated PorA, Rmp and Opa/Opc respectively [2].

This chapter will describe in detail some of the major outer membrane proteins (MOMPs) whose functions, properties and three-dimensional structures have been extensively investigated. The chapter is presented in two sections: the first deals with the expression, biological properties and immunochemistry of the major proteins, including the porins, iron-regulated proteins and Class 5 adhesins. We cite examples of their interplay with other surface structures, includ-

Handbook of Meningococcal Disease. Infection Biology, Vaccination, Clinical Management.
Edited by M. Frosch and M.C.J. Maiden

ISBN: 3-527-31260-9

ing capsule, surface sialic acids and pili. In addition, other relatively recently discovered OM proteins are described briefly. Although not regarded as major proteins, these may play important functional roles *in vivo* and/or represent potential targets for vaccine development. The second section describes the three-dimensional structures of some of these proteins.

10.2
Mechanisms of Expression, Biological and Immunochemical Properties of Meningococcal MOMPs

10.2.1
The Porin Proteins

The porin proteins (PorA, PorB) are amongst the most abundant proteins produced by meningococci and are the predominant proteins present on the bacterial surface. Like other bacterial porins, they assemble as trimers within the outer membrane and function as pores, through which small hydrophilic nutrients can diffuse into the cell, showing a preference for cations or anions, respectively [3, 4]. The PorA protein varies in molecular mass between strains in the range 44–47 kDa, whereas PorB is present as one of two mutually exclusive forms PorB2 (formerly Class 2 protein, typically 40–42 kDa) or PorB3 (Class 3, 37–39 kDa) [5]. The vast majority of meningococcal strains produce both PorA and PorB, although some isolates exhibit lower expression of PorA due to variation in the number of residues in the promoter region of the *porA* gene, caused by slipped strand mispairing within a polyguanidine stretch [6]. As the major proteins on the meningococcal surface, the porins are also the most immunogenic, with the result that early attempts to produce antisera for serological differentiation of meningococci were dominated by the presence of antibodies to PorA and PorB. Subsequent analysis showed that the PorB protein was responsible for serotype specificity and that PorA was responsible for serosubtype specificity [5].

10.2.1.1 Structure and Immunological Properties
The cloning and sequencing of *porA* and *porB* genes has revealed considerable structural homology between the two proteins and also to the equivalent porins from other *Neisseria* species. Further, these studies have led to the development of a model [7] that has provided insight into the structural basis of the immunological properties of the proteins. PorA and PorB are predicted to adopt a structure in which a series of β-sheets traverse the outer membrane to form eight surface exposed hydrophilic loops, a model that has been supported by X-ray crystallographic studies of porins from other species (see Section 10.3.4). Variations between the proteins are largely confined to the loops, with loops 1 and 4 being significantly longer in PorA compared with PorB. Within each porin

class, the variations are even more restricted. With PorA, major differences between strains are confined to the apices of predicted loops 1 and 4, designated variable regions 1 and 2 (VR1 and VR2), respectively, with minor variations occurring in loops 5 and 6, designated as semivariable (SV) regions 1 and 2 [8]. This restricted structural diversity is responsible for the subtype specificity of the PorA protein. Epitope mapping experiments with subtype-specific monoclonal antibodies showed that most recognise short linear peptides corresponding to amino acid sequences located at the apex of either loop 1 or loop 4. Thus, a subtype 7-specific antibody recognized the sequence ASGQVKV at the apex of loop 1 of strain H44/76, while a subtype 16-specific antibody recognized the sequence KDTNNN at the apex of loop 4 [9]. The antigenic independence of the two variable regions explained previous observations that strains could express two independent serosubtypes, with strain H44/76 being designated subtype P1.7,16. In addition, sequence analysis enabled the identification of new subtypes for which serological reagents were not available. Subsequent analysis of PorA sequences from strains showed that further minor variations occurred within the subtype-specific regions that did not influence reactivity with subtyping antibodies but provided further differentiation between strains [8]. In contrast, an isolate obtained from a cluster of cases that showed only a single amino acid difference from the prototype P1.7,16 strain, failed to react with a subtype 16-specific monoclonal antibody. The substitution of an aspartic acid by asparagine in VR2 abolished reactivity with the antibody [8]. As a consequence of these and other studies, subtype definition of strains for epidemiological purposes is now based on sequence analysis of the VR1 and VR2 regions [10], providing much greater discrimination between strains, with a sequence database accessible via the World Wide Web (http://neisseria.org/nm/typing/pora). Surprisingly, given the similarity between the proteins and the success of epitope mapping with PorA, it has not been possible to use similar techniques to identify linear epitopes responsible for serotype specificity in PorB. Variation between strains occurs in loops 1, 4, 6 and 7; and it is likely that subtypes are defined by conformational or discontinuous epitopes which may involve more than one variable loop [11]. Nevertheless, as with PorA, sequence information identifies novel serotypes and provides additional epidemiological discrimination [12]. Indeed, the combination of *porA* and *porB* sequencing, combined with sequencing of housekeeping genes (MLST), provides a powerful tool for investigating outbreaks of meningococcal disease [13].

In addition to their importance as serological markers, the porin proteins, particularly PorA, provide potential targets for a protective immune response. Monoclonal antibodies directed against both PorA and PorB activate complement-mediated killing of meningococci, the accepted correlate of potential protection against infection; and the antibodies directed against PorA were shown to be the most effective in preventing infection in an infant rat model of meningococcal disease [14, 15]. The production of a bactericidal response following meningococcal infection has also been correlated with presence of antibodies directed against PorA [16, 17], as has the development of bactericidal activity following nasopharyngeal colonization by meningococci [18, 19]. The bactericidal activity of antibodies directed against outer membrane proteins has led to the development of experimental vaccines against serogroup B meningococci, which contain outer membranes that have been depleted of the toxic LPS component. Such outer membrane vesicle vaccines (OMV) have undergone phase III trials in humans, have been shown to induce bactericidal activity and to provide some degree of protection against infection [20, 21]. Analysis of sera from vaccine trials has revealed that the protective effect correlates with the presence of antibodies directed against PorA [17, 22–24]. In contrast, although immunization with OMV also induces antibodies directed against PorB, no evidence for a bactericidal response could be identified in immunised individuals [25]. It has been suggested that the reduced size of the surface exposed loops, particularly in PorB3, compared with PorA, make it less accessible to the immune system [26]. However, monoclonal antibodies directed against PorB induce bactericidal activity [14], as does immunization with purified PorB3 protein refolded by incorporation into liposomes [27]. It is possible that the use of purified protein, produced by recombinant DNA technology, may overcome problems caused by steric interference from other molecules present in OMV preparations.

These studies have identified PorA as currently the most promising antigen for incorporation into vaccines designed to prevent infection with serogroup B meningococci. However, such vaccines have the limitation that they induce serosubtype-specific immunity. One possibility to circumvent this problem is the use of multivalent vaccines. Experimental OMV vaccines have been produced from meningococci genetically engineered to express multiple PorA proteins [28] and the resulting hexavalent vaccine contains PorA subtypes that cover over 80% of the strains found in Europe. Phase I and II trials demonstrated induction of bactericidal activity against each of the constituent subtypes [29, 30]. Similarly, immunization of mice with liposomes containing purified refolded recombinant proteins from four different strains induced bactericidal activity against each strain [31]. A situation where PorA-based vaccines may be particularly effective is the targeting of epidemics caused by a single subtype. Such a vaccine of this type has recently been licensed for use in New Zealand, where an epidemic of meningococcal disease dominated by a single serosubtype (P1.7-2,4) has continued unabated for several years since 1991 [32].

10.2.1.2 Roles in Cellular Interactions and Immunomodulation

As the major proteins present on the meningococcal surface, the porin proteins have been shown to participate in a number of interactions with host cells that may play important roles in the pathogenesis of meningococcal disease. Porins from both meningococci and gonococci have been shown to spontaneously transfer from the outer membrane into artificial membranes, creating ion-permeable channels, whereas the porin from the nonpathogenic *Neisseria sicca* did not transfer [33]. Studies with gonococci have shown that the equivalent porins are also transferred to eukaryotic cell membranes [34] and that invasion is related to the type of porin expressed [35]. It is therefore possible that meningococcal porins insert into the cell membrane at sites of close contact and contribute to invasive ability by interference with membrane potential and cell Ca^{2+} signaling [36]. PorB has also been shown to interact with the mitochondrial membrane of eukaryotic cells through the mitochondrial VDAC porin [37]. As a result, the mitochondrial membrane was stabilized and the cells protected from apoptosis, an effect that would be expected to contribute to pathogenesis by prolonging intracellular survival and permitting multiplication of the bacteria. Meningococcal porins also have immunomodulating properties and have been used as adjuvants in vaccine formulation, both in the form of outer membrane proteosomes [37] and as purified recombinant PorB [38]. The adjuvant properties of PorB have been associated with its ability to induce proliferation of B cells [39] and enhanced B/T cell interactions [40]. Similarly PorA has been shown to induce monocyte-derived dendritic cell maturation, augment their ability to activate T cells and direct T-cell differentiation towards the Th2 type response required for generating the antibody responses required for protective immunity [41].

10.2.2
Rmp Protein

The initial studies of Frasch and colleagues identified a protein of apparent molecular mass 33 kDa, designated as class 4 protein, as one of the five structural classes of major outer membrane proteins [1]. An equivalent protein, designated PIII, was identified in gonococci [42] and both proteins were subsequently redesignated as Rmp (reduction-modifiable protein) because they undergo a shift in apparent molecular mass after reduction [2]. Despite its early identification, there is limited information on the structure and particularly the function of the Rmp protein. The amino acid sequences of Rmp from meningococci (sometimes designated RmpM) and gonococci have a high degree of homology and also show similarity with the C-terminal portion of the *E. coli* OmpA porin protein [43]. However, Rmp lacks the equivalent portion of the N-terminus of OmpA that is associated with porin function. Rmp occurs in the outer membrane in close association both with the PorA and PorB porins [44] and with the iron-regulated outer membrane proteins LbpA, TbpA and FrpB [45]. This suggests that a major physiological role of Rmp may be the stabilization of oligomeric protein clusters in the outer membrane, although mutants lacking Rmp appear fully viable at least in *in vitro* culture [43].

At least one study reported that the *rmp* gene is confined to the pathogenic *Neisseria* species, suggesting a specific role in pathogenesis [46]. However, more recent studies have detected an equivalent gene in both *N. sicca* and *N. lactamica*, and expression of a 31-kDa protein that shows immunological cross-reactivity with Rmp from meningococci [47]. Studies with gonococci have revealed that one intriguing immunological property of antibodies directed against Rmp is the ability to inhibit the normal bactericidal activity of other antibodies. Purified human IgG antibodies directed against Rmp have been shown to inhibit or block the bactericidal activity of normal human sera for gonococci [48]. Further, anti-Rmp monoclonal antibodies blocked the bactericidal activity of both normal serum and monoclonal antibodies directed against both porin and LPS [49]. In addition, the presence of anti-Rmp antibodies in human sera has been associated with increased susceptibility to gonococcal infection [50]. Although most evidence of the blocking effect of anti-Rmp antibodies has involved studies with gonococci, a similar blocking effect of a monoclonal anti-Rmp antibody has been demonstrated on the bactericidal activities against meningococci of both anti-PorA antibodies and normal human serum [51]. To avoid the possibility that such "blocking antibodies" might be induced by immunization, it has therefore been suggested that OMV vaccines based on PorA should be constructed from strains in which the *rmp* gene has been deleted [43]. In the case of the multivalent OMV vaccine, the *rmp* gene has been replaced by an additional *porA* gene [52]. However, in studies of vaccinees immunised with OMV vaccines containing Rmp, no evidence has been found for the induction of blocking antibodies, suggesting that, at least with meningococci, the potential blocking effect may not be a problem in practice [53].

10.2.3 Iron-regulated Proteins

Iron is an essential element for meningococci acting as a cofactor in several key metabolic processes. However, there is virtually zero free iron available in the host, the majority being complexed to high-affinity iron binding proteins such as transferrin (in serum), lactoferrin (on mucosal surfaces) and hemoglobin. Therefore, a major determinant in pathogenesis is the ability of meningococci to scavenge for iron under the iron-restricted conditions that they encounter *in vivo*. When growing under conditions where iron is limiting, meningococci express a number of outer membrane proteins (under negative regulation by Fur protein) that are involved in iron acquisition from transferrin, lactoferrin and hemoglobin. These receptors function by removing iron from these iron-storage proteins and then transporting the mineral across the outer membrane in a process that is coupled to the periplasmic/inner membrane protein TonB, which is involved in supplying the energy for the process from the proton gradient across the inner membrane. In addition, the FetA (formerly FrpB) protein has the ability to scavenge iron complexed with siderophores produced by other bacteria as part of their iron acquisition mechanisms [54]. For a detailed description of the physiological role of the iron-regulated OM proteins, see Chapter 11.

Because of their importance in virulence, the iron-regulated proteins have received attention as potential vaccine candidates. The transferrin and lactoferrin receptors have received the greatest attention, as they are constitutively expressed under conditions of iron restriction, while expression of the hemoglobin receptors HmbR and HpuAB are subject to phase variation with high-frequency switching to non-expression [55]. The transferrin receptor is a complex of two proteins, TbpA and TbpB, of approximately 98 kDa and 80 kDa respectively, with TbpB showing greater heterogeneity in molecular mass. Antibodies raised against the more conserved TbpA do not show bactericidal activity [56], although they have been reported to protect against experimental infection in a mouse model of meningococcal infection [57]. In contrast, antibodies directed against the more heterogeneous TbpB do show bactericidal activity but have restricted cross-reactivity between strains [56]. However, it is possible that a limited number of Tbp2 species might be expected to provide protection against a wider number of strains [58]. Less information is available on the immunological properties of the lactoferrin receptor which is also a complex of two proteins, LbpA and LbpB [59]. However, studies of the human immune response to LbpA suggest that it does not induce a cross-reactive immune response [60] and sequence analysis of LbpB has revealed significant sequence variability between strains [61]. An alternative strategy for the incorporation of an iron-regulated protein into vaccine design has been suggested from studies of the diversity of the *fetA* gene encoding the 7-kDa FetA protein [62] together with knowledge of the known protective effect of antibodies directed against PorA. Antibodies directed against FetA are bactericidal, although the protein displays structural and antigenic diversity between strains [63]. However, the extent of this variability is limited; and sequence analysis of a panel of hyperinvasive strains suggested that an OM-based vaccine containing five FetA variants combined with six PorA sequences could potentially provide protection against all 78 isolates studied [62].

10.2.4 The Major Adhesins

Adhesion to respiratory epithelium is regarded as the primary and principal event in colonisation of the nasopharynx by *N. meningitidis* and as such also represents the first step in pathogenesis of this largely commensal bacterium. As with many other mucosal bacteria, *Neisseria meningitidis* has evolved numerous surface-expressed adhesive structures (ligands) that facilitate interactions with the host. Target molecules range from nutrients, e.g. iron, to serum/secreted proteins and surface-located adhesion receptors. Host-specificity of the bacterium resides in the structural specificity of several meningococcal ligands for accessible human molecules.

As reflected in *in vitro* studies, the mechanisms of meningococcal adhesion are multifactorial, dynamic and carefully orchestrated, displaying temporal changes during the course of tissue invasion. Complexities of targeting schemes are rooted in the immune evasion mechanisms which include structural (antigenic) and phase variation of meningococcal OMPs. Elaboration of multiple adhesins compensates for phase variation and may lead to altered tissue tropism. Several adhesins may also be present simultaneously and often cooperate to increase the avidity of binding, a common prerequisite for internalization into host cells. The latter may in itself be another strategy for immune evasion and access to a new source of nutrients. The consequence of such plasticity of adhesins may suggest their unsuitability as vaccine candidates. However, frequency of expression, abundance, as well as functional conservation (and therefore degree of structural conservation) within families of adhesins such as Opa proteins argue in favor of their potential as vaccine candidates. These reasons have led to in-depth studies on their structure/function relationship and mechanisms of receptor targeting, with a view to identifying intervention strategies to prevent infection (further discussed below).

10.2.4.1 **Interplay Between Surface Ligands**

The major adhesive proteins of *N. meningitidis* are the outer membrane opacity proteins, Opa and Opc as well as pili (fully described in Chapter 12). Pili traverse the capsule, the outermost layer of the bacterium, and are generally regarded as the most important adhesins in capsulate bacteria and/or in bacteria with sialylated LPS, whereas the integral OM adhesins Opa and Opc are partly or totally masked by the surface capsule and LPS sialic acids, resulting in their reduced functional efficacy. However, there is recent evidence that, under some conditions, these OMPs may function effectively in capsulate/sialylated bacteria [64–67]. Notably, pili often act to synergize the functional efficacy of MOMPs. For example, they have been shown to increase invasion of endothelial cells mediated by Opc [68] (Fig. 10.1 A, B) and adhesion to meningioma cells [64], as well as both adhesion and invasion of various human epithelial cells mediated by Opa proteins (Rowe, Bradley, Virji, unpublished data).

Fig. 10.1 Antigenic and phase variation of *N. meningitidis* adhesins and synergism in cellular interactions. (A) Adhesion to human endothelial cells of fully capsulate bacteria mediated primarily by pili. No cellular invasion is apparent despite the presence of Opa and Opc, whose functions are impaired significantly in the presence of capsule and sialylated LPS. (B) In acapsulate bacteria, the expression of Opc results in cellular invasion which is significantly enhanced (as seen here) when pili are additionally expressed (68). (C) A proposed mechanism of the translational control of phase variation of Opa proteins. The number of coding repeats CTCTT within the open reading frame determines whether the gene is in or out of frame. DNA regions containing nucleotide repeats have a tendency to form single stranded structures and are susceptible to cleavage by nucleases. Subsequent reannealing may result in misalignment of the CRs leading to increase or decrease in their number during repair and replication. This may lead to different numbers of CRs in the daughter nuclei as depicted (adapted from [72–74, 173]). (D) Transcriptional control of Opc expression is directed by a poly C tract in the promoter region of the gene and determines the efficiency of RNA polymerase binding. (E) Western blot showing Opc (developed using anti-Opc monoclonal antibody B306) and pilin expression (developed using anti-pilin antibody SM1) in variants of serogroup B strain MC58. Variants used were piliated Opc– (lane 1), piliated Opc+++ (lane 2, variant also shown in B above), non-piliated, with intermediate levels of Opc expression (lanes 4–6) and Pil– Opc– (lane 7). In each case, Opc expression (%), as determined by densitometric analysis, is shown in addition to the levels of bacterial adhesion to human endothelial cells (Adh, $\times 10^6$ per monolayer; adapted from [68]).

10.2.4.2 **The Opacity Genes and Modulation of Their Expression**

The outer membrane opacity proteins Opa and Opc, are so called since they impart opacity to colonies of bacteria expressing the proteins. However, the opacities are generally not clearly discernible in colonies of capsulate or LPS sialylated phenotypes. The Opa proteins (initially termed PII or Class 5 proteins [2]) are expressed both by the pathogenic *Neisseria* spp, *N. meningitidis* and *N. gonorrhoeae,* as well as by some commensal *Neisseria* strains [46, 69]. Opa are structurally highly variable proteins and are encoded by a family of genes of which there are three or four in *N. meningitidis* isolates [70, 71]. In the closely-related *N. gonorrhoeae,* up to 12 homologous *opa* genes may be present. Distinct Opa proteins are characterized by variant extracellular domains. Of the four domains

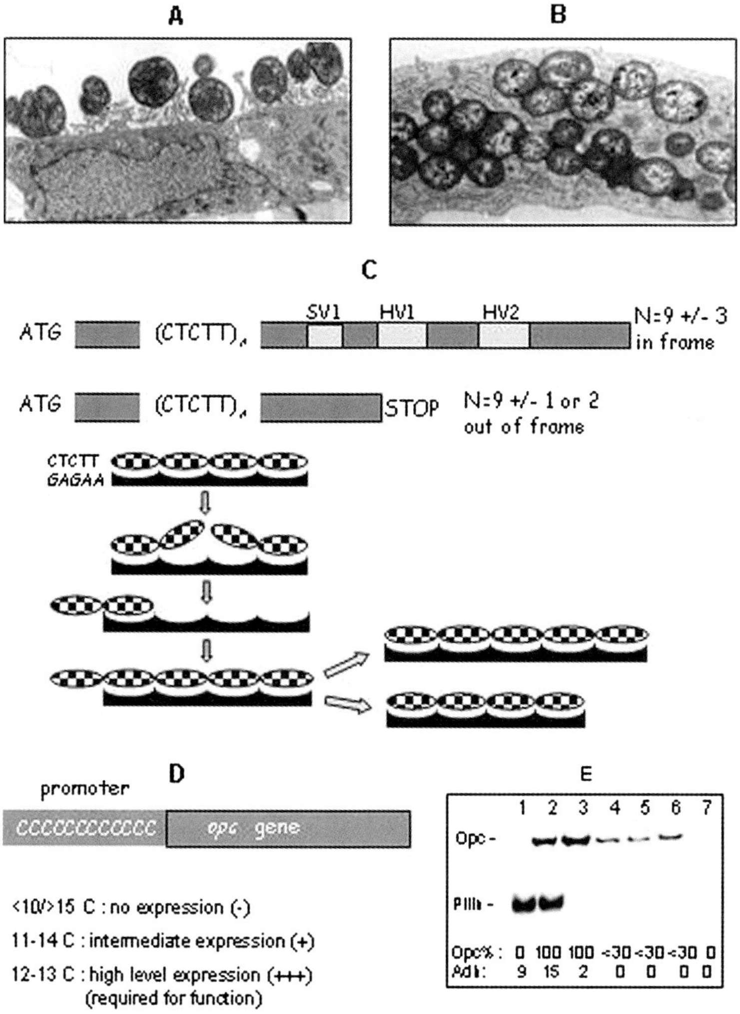

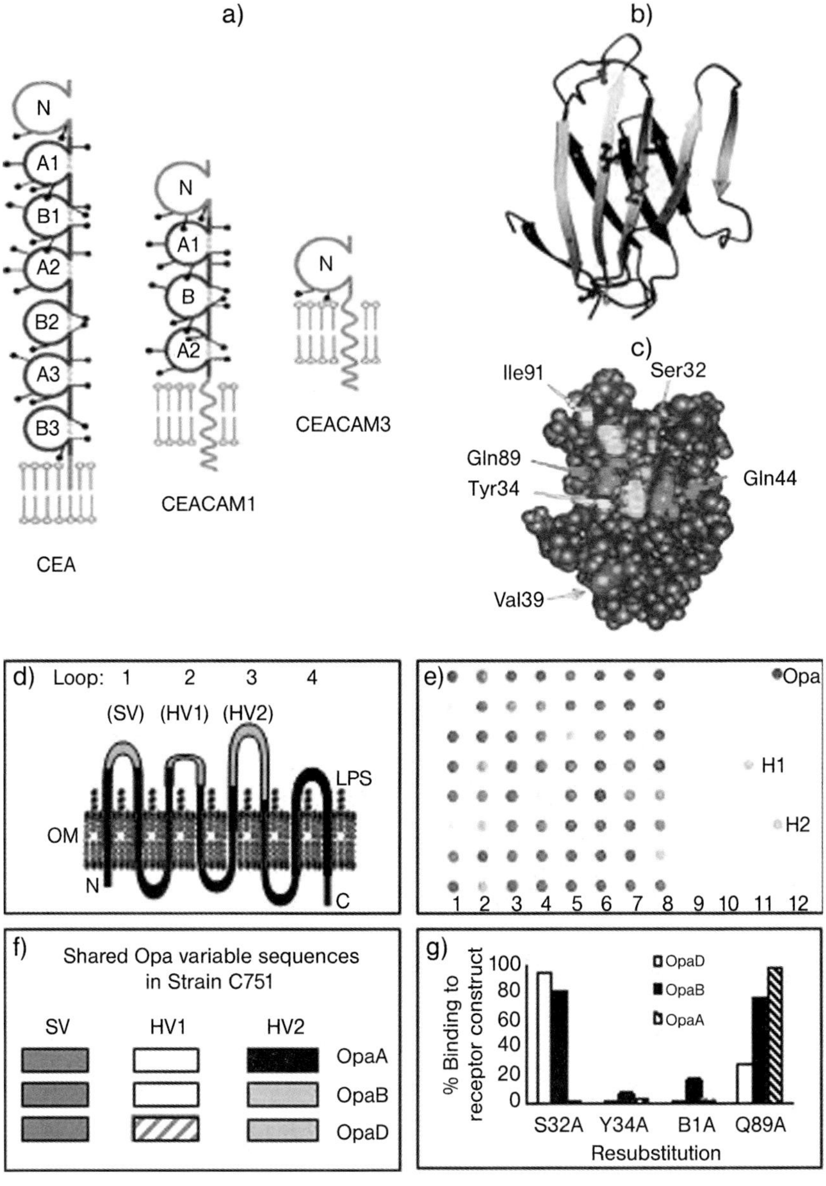

Fig. 10.2 Structures of CEACAMs, the principal receptors for Opa adhesins and their binding site on the receptor. (A) CEA and CEACAM1, the epithelial receptors and CEACAM3, the granulocyte-specific receptor, each contains a highly homologous N-terminal domain targeted by Opa proteins. Glycosylation sites are depicted by ball and stick representations. CEACAM1 and CEACAM3 contain immunoreceptor tyrosine-based inhibitory (ITIM) and activation (ITAM) motifs respectively in their cytoplasmic regions whilst CEA, the largest member of the family is a GPI-anchored molecule (adapted from CEA website; http://cea.klinikum.uni-muenchen.de). (B) Ribbon diagram showing the arrangement of eight beta strands that make up the N-terminal domain. Residues of

(loops 1–4) predicted to be exposed on the bacterial surface, only loop 4 (the most proximal to the C terminus) is conserved. Loop 1 maintains some structural similarities between Opa proteins and is termed semivariable (SV), whereas loops 2 and 3 are hypervariable (HV1 and HV2 [71]; Figs. 10.1 C, 10.2 D). Opa proteins undergo antigenic and phase variation at a high frequency (ca. 10^{-3} to 10^{-4} per cell per generation). The two events are linked since the random on/off switching of each *opa* gene gives rise to the variation of expression from none to several Opa proteins. One mechanism for such switching involves variation in the CTCTT coding repeats (CRs) that is generated during DNA replication arising from slipped strand mispairing common to DNA regions containing nucleotide repeats (Fig. 10.1 C). Further increase in Opa structural variation may arise as a result of homologous recombination [72–74].

Unlike the Opa proteins, Opc is antigenically relatively invariant and is encoded by a single gene [75, 76]. The Opc protein (initially termed Class 5c) was discovered as a result of the analysis of Opa protein expression in the serogroup A *N. meningitidis* strains that caused epidemics in the "Meningitis Belt" in Africa and China [77, 78]. Opc shares a number of physicochemical properties with Opa proteins, which initially led to its classification as a Class 5 protein. For example, both proteins were regarded as able to form trimers, could be heat-modified, are of a similar size (24–35 kDa) and basic in nature, have similar amino acid composition and are phase variable. However, they are structurally distinct. Interestingly, in African isolates, the Opa/Class 5 proteins (designated 5 a, 5 b, 5 d–5 h) were confined to particular clonal groups, whereas Class 5 c was widely distributed and was detected in diverse *N. meningitidis* of serogroups A, 29E and W135 [76]. In later clonal analysis, *opc* gene was shown to be absent from certain *N. meningitidis* clonal lineages [79].

The distinction between Opa and Opc became apparent on cloning of the *opc* gene [75], revealing limited homology with the *opa* genes and a lack of the CTCTT repeats that regulate Opa expression. In addition, whilst Opa proteins

importance for Opa targeting on the CFG face of the N-domain are shown. (C) Van der Waals surface representation of the N-domain model showing these residues in color, the key amino acids being shown in red (based on [92]). (D) Two-dimensional arrangement of the semivariable and hypervariable loops of Opa proteins [71]. (E) Whole cell lysates of pathogenic neisseria isolates (columns 1–8) and other mucosal isolates including *P. aeruginosa, E. coli, H. influenzae* were overlaid with a soluble receptor construct containing the N-terminal domain of CEACAM1 linked to human Fc. Receptor binding was detected using anti-Fc alkaline phosphatase conjugate. Binding of the majority of pathogenic Opa-expressing bacteria to the receptor can be seen in addition to two *H. influenzae* strains (H1, H2) as well as purified Opa protein [65]. (F) *N. meningitidis* Strain C751 Opa derivatives contain three different combinations of HV1 and HV2 (OpaA and B share HV1, OpaB and D share HV2, whereas HV1 of Opa D and HV2 of OpaA are unique). (G) Receptor-binding properties of the C751 Opa proteins using single amino acid substituted N-domain constructs show the primary importance of Y34 and I91 and the influence of HV1 and HV2 in adhesion to the receptor with S32A and Q89A substitutions (adapted from [92]). (This figure also appears with the color plates.)

are subject to on–off variation, the Opc expression was quantitatively variable. Further studies also revealed little antigenic similarity between Opa and Opc. These distinctions led to a separate classification of the product of the *opc* gene which was subsequently named Opc [80] in accordance with the recommended nomenclature for genes and proteins of pathogenic *Neisseria* [2].

opc expression is controlled at the transcriptional level and is determined by a track of a variable number of contiguous cytidine residues in the promoter region of *opc*. The number of nucleotide repeats determines the promoter strength and the binding efficiency of RNA polymerase, and therefore the transcription of *opc* (Fig. 10.1 D, E). The number of the repeats changes as a result of SSM described for Opa proteins [81].

N. meningitidis and *N. gonorrhoeae* contain two paralogous *opc* genes, the transcribed *opc* gene (termed *opcA*) and a pseudogene (psi *opcB*). Their predicted products differ extensively in four of the five surface-exposed loops. Gonococcal *opc* was expressed weakly under *in vitro* conditions, no information is available whether it can be expressed at high levels under any conditions. Apparently, *opcA* and *opcB* are located on DNA islands probably acquired from unrelated bacteria [82]. An *opcA* gene with 93% homology with *N. gonorrhoeae opcA* was also found in *N. polysaccharea*, although *opc* genes are absent from *N. lactamica* and other commensal *Neisseria* species that have been investigated [82, 83]. The 3-D structure of Opc is described in Section 10.3.1.

10.2.4.3 Adhesion Targets

ECM and Integrins Both Opa and Opc can bind to extracellular matrix (ECM) components and serum proteins. By interacting with Arg-Gly-Asp (RGD) sequence-bearing serum proteins such as vitronectin and fibronectin, bacteria bind to their cognate receptor integrins $a v \beta 3$ (vitronectin receptor, VNR) and/or $a 5 \beta 1$ (fibronectin receptor, FNR). RGD-dependent binding of Opc-expressing meningococci appears to be the major mode of interaction with polarized human endothelial cells. Interestingly, VNR appears to be the principal receptor targeted on human umbilical vein endothelial cells, whilst FNR is principally targeted on human brain microvascular endothelial cells (HBMECs) [66, 68, 84]. This interaction is significantly more effective in mediating cellular invasion compared with Opa interactions with unstimulated endothelial cells [84].

In addition to utilizing the integrin ligands, further factors may be involved in the interactions via the vitronectin receptor, since Opc expression in heterologous strains (*E. coli*) does not support adhesion of *E. coli* to endothelial cell integrins [80]. It is known that integrins often interact with proteins and glycans simultaneously via distinct binding domains. The complement receptor 3 (CR3, $am\beta 2$ integrin) is a good example, since it interacts simultaneously with C3bi-coated particles and with microbial glycolipids at distinct sites [85]. The vitronectin receptor also exhibits binding sites for ganglioside GD2 [86] and thus possibly LPS with similar structural characteristics. It is possible that Opc binding to integrins also requires the participation of N. meningitidis LPS. However, it is also possible that the level of Opc expressed by E. coli is not optimum since efficient interactions of N. meningitidis via Opc require the protein to be expressed at a high density on the bacterial surface [68].

Recent studies on HBMECs have shown that Opc-mediated binding of N. meningitidis leads to phosphorylation and activation of c-Jun N-terminal kinases (JNK1, JNK2), leading to downstream signaling important for meningococcal uptake. Inhibition of the kinases reduced the N. meningitidis uptake but not adhesion. The studies also indicated the importance of protein tyrosine kinases in general for N. meningitidis-induced cellular responses [87].

ECM and Proteoglycans Studies on several bacterial adhesins that bind to ECM proteins have shown that such targeting may also bring into play proteoglycans (PGs), since many ECM proteins bind to heparin or heparan sulfate proteoglycans (HSPGs). Besides their presence in ECM, PGs decorate a wide range of mammalian cells. Transmembrane PGs, the syndecans, are decorated with heparan sulfate or chondroitin sulfate glycosaminoglycans (GAG). For targeting of GAGs by GAG-binding proteins, including bacterial ligands, a defined clustered sequence of basic amino acids appears to be required [88]. Such structural features are predicted to be present in Opc; and both Opc and certain Opa proteins of N. meningitidis and N. gonorrhoeae bind to heparin and HSPGs. In addition, since interactions of bacteria with PGs may be of low affinity, coligation of secondary receptors may also be required for uptake of microbes [89–93].

The mechanisms of Opa-HSPG interactions have been studied in greater detail in N. gonorrhoeae and it has been reported that the over-expression of Syndecan-4 in HeLa cells increases vitronectin-triggered uptake of the Opa expressing bacteria, whereas in the absence of vitronectin, only basal levels of invasion occur. Thus secondary recruitment of vitronectin and fibronectin by Opa-expressing N. gonorrhoeae triggers efficient uptake in an integrin-dependent manner. In addition, N. gonorrhoeae porins may facilitate cellular invasion following Opa-HSPG interactions [94–96]. Mutational studies have implicated the HV1 region in binding to HSPGs, although apparently several domains rich in basic amino acids are present in Opa proteins [97].

Lectin-like interactions of Opa proteins with terminal glycans of the LPS lacto-N-neotetraose (LNnT) have also been reported for gonococci [98]. This ability of Opa proteins also allows gonococci to interact with the structures present on host gangliosides. The binding of Opa protein to LNnT is also akin to binding of LNnT-type structures to certain host receptors. For example a 70-kDa protein on HepG2 cells binds LNnT of LPS and shares antigenic properties with Opa proteins [98–100].

Lectin-like characteristics of meningococcal Opa and Opc were explored in recent studies, demonstrating that both proteins of strain C751 bind to soluble saccharides. Opc exhibited high-affinity binding to sialic acid and complex saccharides with terminal sialic acids. This property may be the molecular basis for the inhibition of Opc-dependent interactions with cellular receptors mediated by LPS sialylation. Opa proteins of C751 also bound sialic acid and mannose and the binding involved tyrosine residues at the base of the HV2 loop. Soluble sialic acid and mannose partly inhibited meningococcal interaction to epithelial cells via the Opc and Opa proteins, respectively [101].

CEACAMs, Cell-expressed Receptors The majority of Opa proteins of N. meningitidis and N. gonorrhoeae target a family of cell-expressed receptors, termed CEACAMs, belonging to the immunoglobulin superfamily [65, 92, 94, 102–106]. CEACAMs [Carcinoembryonic antigen (CEA)-related cell adhesion molecules] belong to the CEA family, which includes clinically important tumor markers such as the carcinoembryonic antigen [107].

CEACAMs characteristically contain highly homologous N-terminal domains and, in addition, may contain none to several IgC2-like extracellular domains (Fig. 10.2 A, domains A1, B1, etc.). A single Opa protein may bind to several CEACAMs via protein–protein interactions at the N-terminal domain. In addition, despite the large repertoire of surface-exposed variable loops, the majority of pathogenic neisserial Opa proteins can bind CEACAM1 (Fig. 10.2 E) [65], which is widely expressed on human epithelial and endothelial cells as well as lymphocytes.

The amino acid residues targeted by distinct Opa proteins are located on the exposed glycan-free CFG face of the N-domain (Fig. 10.2 B, C). Site-directed mutants of surface-exposed residues of this domain have helped to identify a number of critical amino acids (Tyr34, Ile91) required for Opa attachment. Other targeted residues are scattered on the C/F/G strands and loops of the N-domain but form a continuous adhesiotope in the three-dimensional model (Fig. 10.2 C) and determine the efficiency of interaction of distinct Opa proteins. Studies from three laboratories have confirmed the critical binding regions of neisserial Opa proteins on CEACAM receptors [92, 108, 109].

Many studies have examined the contribution of the SV and HV loops in receptor interactions. For N. meningitidis, studies conducted using Opa variants of strain C751 that share some variable sequences (Fig. 10.2 F) demonstrated that the three C751Opa proteins bound equally well to CEA-transfected cells but exhibited distinct tropism for CEACAM3- and CEACAM6-expressing cells, implying that these Opa proteins make up distinct structures via combinations of their HV domains, and that the HV1 and HV2 regions appeared to be involved in tropism for the distinct CEACAMs [92]. A striking influence of HV1 and HV2 regions on receptor-targeting could also be seen using the N-terminal mutants of the receptor. For example, the mutant receptor with alanine substitution at Ser32 on the beta strand "C" was not recognized by an OpaA variant with a distinct HV2 but OpaD and OpaB bound to the mutant receptor efficiently. Also, Gln89 mutation on the "F" strand resulted in significant reduction in binding particularly of OpaD which has a distinct HV1 region (Fig. 10.2 G) [92].

Overall, it appears that specific conserved residues in the N-domains of distinct CEACAM family members determine the primary receptor specificity of the majority of Opa proteins. The tropism is determined by further less conserved residues arranged around the primary binding site. The data suggest that Opa proteins have evolved to generate a variety of hyper-variable domains that may not only help avoid the host immune response but retain receptor binding capacity in such a way that they compensate for the heterogeneity in their target receptor family, thus increasing their host tissue range.

10.2.4.4 Potential Outcomes of CEACAM Targeting

Interactions with Immune Cells Interactions of *N. meningitidis*, which could occur readily between acapsulate phenotypes and granulocytes via one or more of the several CEACAMs expressed on them (CEACAM1, CEACAM6, CEACAM3, CEACAM8) [107], leads to bacterial elimination, a counter-productive strategy of interaction. However, it has been suggested that non-opsonic interactions of *N. gonorrhoeae* Opa with granulocytes may lead to bacterial localisation in an intracellular niche that may allow prolonged survival [110]. Although this remains to be demonstrated, it is possible that bacteria able to survive for a relatively short period within the cells may be carried from site to site in a "Trojan horse" manner. Signalling via Opa/CEACAM interactions in professional phagocytes may be dependent on the ability of the expressed Opa to bind to inhibitory (CEACAM1) or stimulatory (CEACAM3) signaling molecules [94]. It often appears to involve Src kinases, Rac1, PAK and Jun terminal kinase. The pathway differs from the opsonic pathway of internalization via FcγR, which results in activation of cellular killing mechanisms. It is suggested that signaling via the ITIM (immunoreceptor tyrosine-based inhibitory motif) motifs present, e.g. in the CEACAM1 cytoplasmic domain, may improve the chances of gonococcal survival within the phagocyte [94, 110].

Two separate lines of evidence suggest that gonococcal interactions with CEACAM1 results in suppression of immune responses. Interactions with B cells may lead to CEACAM1-dependent cell death and thus inhibition of antibody production. The signaling cascade in this case does not involve the inhibitory signals of SHP1 phosphatases [111]. In addition, gonococcal interaction with T cells leads to the inhibition of T cell proliferation; and the inhibition depends on the activation status of the CD4+ T cells. The studies demonstrate that, after ligation with *N. gonorrhoeae*, CEACAM1 associates with the tyrosine phosphatases SHP-1 and SHP-2, implicating the ITIM of the protein in T cell inhibition [112].

Epithelial Interactions Human epithelial cells may commonly express CEACAM1 and CEA and may also express CEACAM6 and CEACAM7 [107]. Interestingly, it has been suggested that molecules such as CEA may have evolved to reduce the burden of microbes on the mucosa. Late evolutionary development of the GPI-anchored members, apical location and shedding/secretion of large amounts of CEA in the gut suggest the possibility that CEA, which is targeted by enteric pathogens, may have developed as an arm of innate immunity [107,

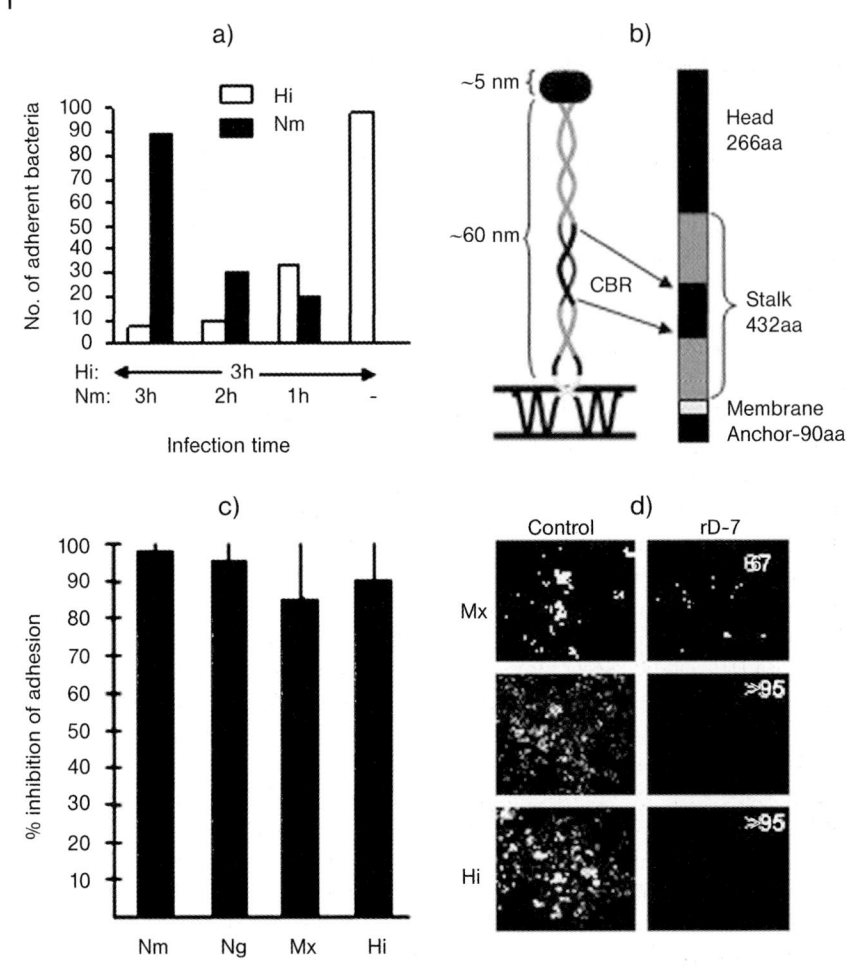

Fig. 10.3 CEACAM1 targeting by mucosal pathogens and competition for the receptor. (A) Competition between *N. meningitidis* (Nm) and *H. influenzae* (Hi) strains for occupancy of the receptor on Chinese hamster ovary cells transfected with human CEACAM1. Coinfection of the two pathogens was carried out for the periods shown such that Hi was present for the 3 h duration of the experiment whereas Nm was added at different intervals. As shown, Nm progressively occupied more binding sites on target cells compared with the Hi strain (adapted from [116]). (B) *M. catarrhalis* (Mx) also interacts with human CEACAM1 and does so via the UspA1 protein, a homologue of *Yersinia* YadA and *N. meningitidis* NadA. The CEACAM1-binding region (CBR) lies in the coiled coil section of UspA1 as shown. (C) A recombinant CEACAM-binding polypeptide (rD-7; corresponding to a partial sequence of UspA1) inhibits receptor interactions of multiple strains of CEACAM-binding species shown. In each case, mean inhibition is shown (%, plus range) of the binding of ten strains in the presence of rD-7, compared to a control peptide. (D) Binding of representative strains of *M. catarrhalis*, *N. meningitidis* and *H. influenzae* to confluent monolayers of the lung epithelial cell line A549 in the presence of a control peptide or rD-7. Bacteria were labeled with TRITC-conjugated antibodies. Numbers represent inhibition of binding (%; adapted from [117]).

113]. Studies of the interactions of meningococci and gonococci with distinct CEACAMs have predominantly used transfected HeLa cells revealing distinct outcomes which depended on the receptor expressed. In general, targeting of the transmembrane CEACAM1 correlated with greater invasion than GPI-anchored CEA and CEACAM6 [92, 114].

Targeting of transmembrane CEACAMs would also be expected to lead to the manipulation of host signaling mechanisms, which could result in either transcytosis or paracytosis; and, by either mechanism, bacteria may traverse the epithelial barriers. CEACAM-mediated traversal of colonic epithelial cells by a gonococcal strain has been reported. In studies of the potential of other mucosal pathogens to target CEACAMs, two other upper respiratory tract bacteria, *Haemophilus influenzae* and *Moraxella catarrhalis*, were shown also to bind to CEACAMs, with CEACAM1 being the major target [115, 116]. This indicates the potential of these bacteria to compete with each other for receptor engagement in their common respiratory niche. Indeed, this can be demonstrated *in vitro* [116] (Fig. 10.3 A). In addition, a recombinant protein homologous to the binding region of the *M. catarrhalis* CEACAM-binding ligand UspA1 has been shown to inhibit the interactions of a wide range of mucosal pathogens that target CEACAMs, including *N. meningitidis* (Fig. 10.3 B–D) [117].

CEACAM Density-dependent Interactions of Capsulate Phenotypes CEACAMs are usually expressed at low levels but are subject to upregulation in response to inflammatory cytokines [118–120]. Receptor levels on target cells may be pivotal in determining the fate of adherent bacteria. For example, increased strength of ligand–receptor ligation, which may be achieved when receptors are expressed at high levels, could lead to increased invasion of cells by adherent bacteria [121]. This may be a key event that may determine increased host susceptibility to some bacterial infections. An important observation in favor of this argument is that, even in capsulate bacteria, certain Opa proteins with a high affinity for CEACAM1 may effectively bind to host cells expressing large numbers of these receptors and bring forth an invasion by virulent capsulate phenotypes [65, 67]. Thus, targeting of cell adhesion molecules on mucosal epithelial cells, which are upregulated during inflammation, may be critical to bacterial pathogenesis and may shift the balance from a carrier state to dissemination. A low-level constitutive expression of the receptor on epithelial cells may favor attachment without invasion. Viral infections or other conditions, during which cytokines may be upregulated, could result in increased expression of signaling receptors targeted by bacteria and thereby increase their potential to enter both mucosal epithelial cells as well as phagocytic cells. Massive invasion of epithelial cells could be injurious to the host, while that of phagocytic cells could result in incomplete elimination of bacteria and the possibility of transmission within them.

10.2.4.5 MBL Interactions

MBL, a mannose-binding lectin, is an innate defense protein, which acts by complement activation or opsonization in the absence of specific antibody. MBL has been shown to bind to the polysaccharide capsule of serogroup B and C meningococci. In addition, it has been shown to bind both to *N. meningitidis* Opa proteins and to PorB. In this case, the lectin binds to the two non-glycosylated proteins via protein–protein interactions. Binding of MBL to PorB inhibits factor H interactions with the porin [122]. The implications of such competition between the mechanisms of complement activation (MBL binding) and serum resistance (factor H binding) remain to be investigated. In addition, binding of MBL to Opa and PorB may also affect their targeting of cellular receptors.

10.2.4.6 Immunogenicity of the Opacity Proteins

Although Opa proteins induce bactericidal antibodies in humans [123], they characteristically give rise to type-specific antibodies, limiting their efficacy as cross-protective antigens. However, if antibodies that block Opa–receptor interactions could be elicited, they could prove effective in reducing mucosal colonization and thus the disease burden. Purified Opa proteins were shown to elicit antibodies that inhibited Opa–CEACAM interactions but no significant bactericidal or opsonic response was observed [124]. In another study, immunization of CEA transgenic and normal mice with CEA-binding and non-binding Opa of meningococci gave rise to mucosal anti-Opa antibody response. Interestingly, only the CEA non-binding Opa could induce serum bactericidal antibodies which were type-specific [125]. In these studies, meningococcal LPS used as an adjuvant was required for serum antibody responses.

In contrast, Opc, with its limited antigenic diversity, might be expected to induce cross-protective antibodies. Indeed, Opc is highly immunogenic in humans and elicits serum bactericidal and opsonic antibodies [126–128]. Whilst cross-reactive anti-Opc monoclonal antibodies have been generated [76] recent studies have shown limitations of Opc as a vaccine candidate. Recombinant Opc protein was shown to induce serum bactericidal antibodies highly effective against homologous strain but not against heterologous strains expressing Opc with limited sequence variations. In addition, the magnitude of the bactericidal effect was strongly influenced by the level of expression of the Opc protein [129].

10.2.5 Recently Identified Proteins

Availability of neisserial genome sequences has enabled identification of novel surface antigens, which have been sought primarily with the aim to identifying novel cross-protective antigens against *N. meningitidis* [130]. These OMPs have previously not been detected because either they are normally expressed at low levels or they are specifically induced by certain environmental conditions that may be encountered *in vivo*. The importance of surface proteins other than the MOMPs has been noted both in protection and in cellular interactions. For example, potential heterologous protection via antibodies other than those cross-reacting with the serogroup B capsule, LPS, PorA, PorB, Rmp, Opa, Opc or pilin was implicated in studies on a cohort of university students [19]. In addition, involvement of adhesins other than Opa and Opc in intimate cellular interactions has been implicated in several studies [131, 132].

NspA (neisserial surface protein A), a basic protein of ca. 18 kDa, is a widely expressed antigen [133] common both to *N. meningitidis* and *N. gonorrhoeae* and is highly conserved. However, it is present in relatively low copy numbers [134]. It is a member of the β-barrel family of transmembrane proteins and a homolog of Opa proteins [135]. Its structure is described in Section 10.3.2. Recombinant NspA elicited bactericidal antibodies but with limited efficacy in some capsulate bacteria [136]. However, sequential immunization of animals using outer membrane vesicles from three strains with heterologous PorA, PorB and capsule was shown to elicit broadly cross-protective responses directed against NspA (in addition to other antigens) [137]. There is evidence for the requirement for natural conformation of the protein for a protective response [138, 139].

Of the novel surface antigens, NadA (Neisserial adhesin A) has received considerable recent attention. It is a protein of 38 kDa and has the propensity to form oligomers, common to the Oca (oligomeric coiled coil) family of autotransporter proteins, of which YadA of *Yersiniae* and UspA of *M. catarrhalis* are key examples (Fig. 10.3 B). TAAA repeats in the promoter region of *nadA* control the level of protein expression [140]. NadA is expressed by several *N. meningitidis* virulent lineages but not by lineage III. It is absent from *N. gonorrhoeae* and *N. lactamica* [141]. Bactericidal antibodies to NadA can be elicited and, whilst healthy adults have antibodies to the protein, healthy infants lack such antibodies, since childhood carriage of *N. meningitidis* is rare. Thus, despite its limitation as a cross-protective vaccine candidate due to limited and variable expression, it has been proposed as a vaccine component for immunizing children [142]. NadA confers adhesion and invasion properties to recombinant *E. coli* expressing the protein. It mediates binding to Chang conjunctiva cells but not to human umbilical vein endothelial cells. Unlike the UspA protein, whose binding region to the epithelial receptor CEACAM1 is located in the coiled coil region (Fig. 10.3 B) [117], the NadA binding site is located in its "head" domain [143].

In addition to the above, other autotransporter-like molecules have been described in Neisseriae and include NhhA (ca. 57 kDa), which is similar to *H. influenzae* Hsf/Hia adhesins, and App (ca. 160 kDa), which bears resemblance to *H. influenzae* Hap adhesin. Both elicit bactericidal antibodies. App contains serine protease activity in its N-terminal domain and binding activity in its C-terminal region. The protein mediates binding to human epithelial cells [144–146].

10.3
The Three-dimensional Structures of Meningococcal Outer Membrane Proteins

Since the determination of the first crystal structures of porin proteins in the early 1990s, a good deal of structural information on outer membrane proteins (OMPs) has appeared from a variety of Gram-negative bacteria (reviewed by Wimley [147]). Determination of the 3-D structure of a protein is a key step in understanding its mechanism; and this has certainly turned out to be the case for OMPs. OMPs mediate a variety of different functions, from pore formation for the passage of low molecular weight solutes, to complex secretion processes such as pilus formation. Despite the successes in OMP structure determination in recent years, there are still many classes of OMP for which there is no crystal structure. It is not the function of this article to review all aspects of OMP structure and function, but rather to focus on the current structural information for particular OMPs from *Neisseria* for which structures are known, or for which reliable structural models can be built by homology modeling. We are therefore taking the first faltering steps towards a structural description of the full complement of *Neisseria* OMPs at the atomic level.

The determination of the 3-D structure of a membrane protein by X-ray crystallography, NMR or electron microscopy presents certain technical challenges which do not pertain to their soluble counterparts. One of the most serious obstacles is the isolation of milligram quantities of pure, correctly folded protein. In the case of OMPs, there are generally two approaches to this problem. Direct solubilization of the protein from the outer membrane is frequently employed; and the choice of detergent and solubilization conditions can be critical in ensuring efficient extraction [76, 148]. The solubilized OMP can then be purified by standard methods. The principal disadvantage of such an approach is that OMPs which are not naturally abundant in the outer membrane can be difficult to obtain in quantities sufficient for structural analysis. Fortunately, a variety of methods have been established for the refolding of OMPs [149]. A second approach, therefore, involves expression of the OMP without a signal sequence, so that it forms inclusion bodies which can then be solubilized and refolded. This approach has been applied to a number of OMPs from *Neisseria*, including PorA [44], Opc [148] and the Opa proteins [124].

The formation of crystals of membrane proteins which diffract to high resolution has long been acknowledged as a challenging task. All OMPs whose structures have been determined to date adopt a β-barrel structure distinct from the transmembrane α-helices which characterize most other membrane proteins. It seems that this architecture is more conducive to the formation of high quality crystals, given the relatively high proportion of OMPs within the database of integral membrane protein structures. Recent technical developments in NMR have led to the determination of the first solution state structures of OMPs, for example the PagP protein from *E. coli* [150]. There is no reason in principle why these methods could not be extended to neisserial OMPs. For much larger membrane proteins, electron microscopy offers an alternative approach, either through the formation of 2-D crystals, or single particle averaging (SPA) methods. Although electron microscopy is generally unable to provide structural information at the atomic level for biological macromolecules, determination of a lower resolution 3-D reconstruction can be valuable in providing information about the overall conformation of the molecule and any structural changes which might occur on association with other proteins. SPA methods generally require much less protein than other structural methods, making them ideal in circumstances where protein supply is limited.

10.3.1 Adhesin Opc

Achtman et al. [76] showed that the adhesin Opc could be purified to homogeneity by extraction with the detergent zwittergent and purification by ion exchange and size exclusion chromatography. Crystals of Opc were initially obtained from the detergent β-D-octyl glucoside, but their diffraction was poor (3.5 Å at best) and anisotropic (Derrick, unpublished data). Much better quality crystals were obtained from the polyoxyethylene detergent C_8E_5, in the presence of PEG 6000 and Zn^{2+} [148]. Crystals were initially obtained from native Opc, isolated directly from meningococci; and, for convenience, a protocol was developed for the refolding of recombinant, insoluble Opc from the haotrope. Purification, crystallization and data collection from crystals of the recombinant protein showed the crystals of the recombinant protein were essentially identical to those obtained from native material. Opc contains no methionine, outside of the initiator residue, which limited the application of selenomethione/MAD-based phasing methods. The structure was solved using MIR phases, in combination with multi-crystal averaging applied to a second crystal form, which could be produced by soaking the crystals in Cd^{2+} [93]. The final resolution of the structure was 2.0 Å. Opc forms a 10-stranded β-barrel structure (Fig. 4a): the loop regions on the external face of the protein are much longer than those at the periplasmic side, a feature which Opc has in common with other small OMPs, such as OmpA and OmpX [147]. At least three Zn^{2+} ions were identified within the structure, two associated with the outer face and the third located inside the barrel. No Zn^{2+} ions were present during the refolding and purification stages, so the ion presumably diffuses into the barrel during crystallization. The barrel is flattened in cross-section (Fig. 10.4a), with the longest loop, loop 2, closing over the end of the barrel. Solvent accessibility calculations indicated that loop 2 effectively closes off the end of the barrel, preventing passage of water molecules through the protein; and it seems unlikely that Opc could function effectively as a pore-forming protein.

Crystals were not formed in the absence of Zn^{2+}; and it appears that these ions play a critical part in mediating crystal contacts between the loop regions. In common with other OMP structures, the external loop regions are highly mobile: a plot of the temperature factors, which provide an indication of atomic mobilities within the crystal, shows a wide variation, with the lower values cor-

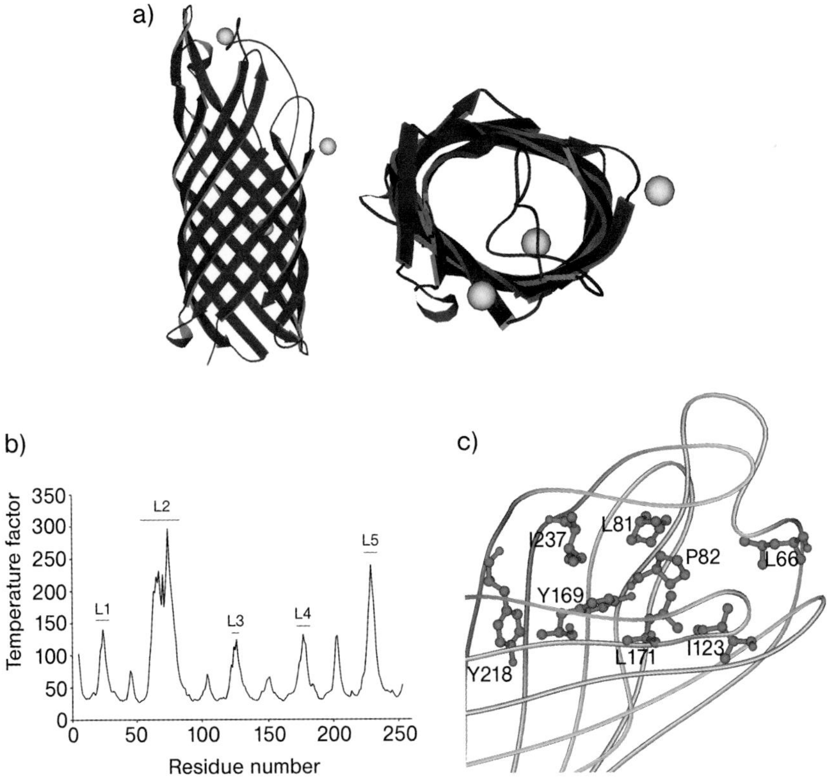

Fig. 10.4 The Opc adhesin. (a) Side and top views, shown as ribbon plots, of the overall structure. Loop 2 is indicated with an arrow. (b) Mainchain temperature factors of Opc. The approximate location of the external loop regions, L1–L5, are indicated. (c) View of selected residues within the external loop regions of Opc. Individual residues are shown as ball-and-stick models, superimposed on a wireframe trace of the Opc polypeptide backbone. Structures were plotted using MOLSCRIPT [174].

responding to the barrel residues and the highest values coming from loops 2 and 5 (Fig. 10.4b). To a good approximation, Opc can be thought of as a relatively rigid cylinder-like structure, with much more mobile regions appended to one end.

An interesting feature of the structure of the external loop regions is their mode of interaction. Loops 2–5 are in direct contact with each other, forming a compact unit: these contacts are mediated by interactions between hydrophobic residues within the loops (Fig. 10.1c). This effectively forms a hydrophobic core, somewhat similar to those found in soluble globular proteins. This is in contrast to the β-barrel, which forms an "inverse micelle" structure, characterized by hydrophobic residues on the external surface, which interact with the membrane, and hydrophilic residues within the interior of the barrel.

Given the involvement of Opc in adhesion to epithelial and endothelial cells, the structure was examined for clues to suggest how this function might be mediated. A notable feature in the external surface of the protein is the cleft formed between loops 2–5 on the one side, and loop 1 on the other. It was noted by Prince et al. [93] that this cleft contained a high proportion of basic residues which could contribute to the binding of the negatively charged heparin and heparan sulfate ligands. This proposal remains conjectural at present, however.

10.3.2
NspA Protein

NspA of *N. meningitidis* and *N. gonorrhoeae* exhibits a high degree of sequence conservation and antibodies against NspA are protective and bactericidal against a variety of meningococcal strains. The principal interest behind the determination of the crystal structure of NspA was therefore to obtain more detailed information about the structure of epitopes within the protein which would be recognised by antibody. A secondary reason for interest in NspA was the homology which it shares with the Opa, or opacity, family of proteins. A wide body of evidence has established the involvement of Opa proteins in adhesion to the human carcinoembryonic antigen proteins and to proteoglycan receptors [151]. Although the Opa proteins are larger than NspA, there are significant levels of sequence homology within the predicted transmembrane–strand regions. The structure of NspA was therefore of additional interest as the basis for a model for Opa structure.

As for Opc, NspA was expressed without a signal sequence into inclusion bodies, before being refolded, purified and crystallized [135]. NspA has a monomeric molecular mass of 18 kDa and is therefore significantly smaller than Opc. The overall fold of the protein was an 8-stranded, rather than 10-stranded, β-barrel and with shorter external loop regions than Opc (Fig. 10.5 a). The precise function of NspA is unclear, although it may function as an adhesin in a similar fashion to the Opa proteins. A notable feature of the crystal structure of NspA was the formation of a long hydrophobic groove at the external face of the protein. The groove is formed between the L2 and L3 loops on the one side, and L1 and L4 on the other. Electron density for a ligand was apparent within the groove; and a single $C_{10}E_5$ detergent molecule built into the site (Fig. 10.5 b). The highly hydrophobic nature of the groove is unusual for OMPs of this size and may reflect the chemical character of the natural ligand. It is likely that the Opa proteins will retain the same structure for the β-barrel, but the more extensive loop regions will probably form different binding sites for the carcinoembryonic antigen and proteoglycan ligands.

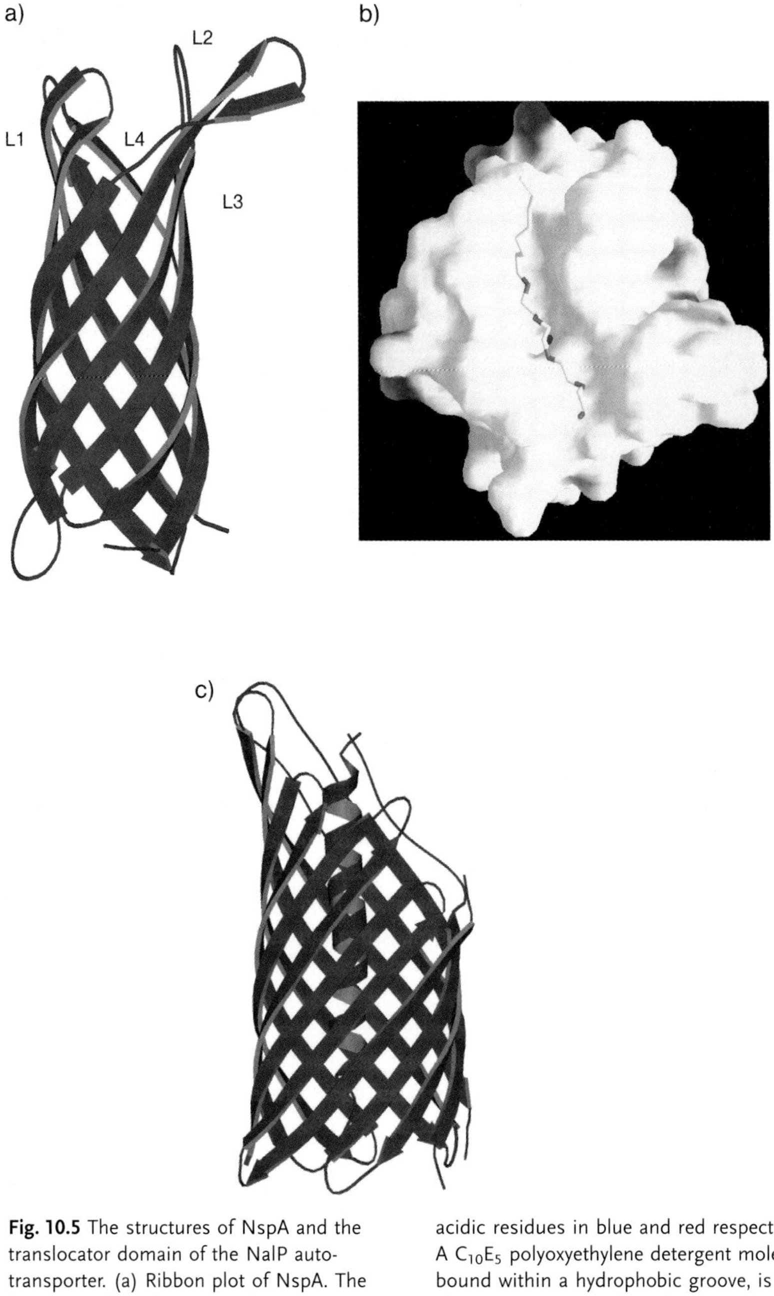

Fig. 10.5 The structures of NspA and the translocator domain of the NalP autotransporter. (a) Ribbon plot of NspA. The locations of the four external loop regions are indicated. The structure was plotted using MOLSCRIPT [174]. (b) Surface representation of NspA viewed from the top, prepared using GRASP [175], with basic and acidic residues in blue and red respectively. A $C_{10}E_5$ polyoxyethylene detergent molecule, bound within a hydrophobic groove, is shown superimposed on the structure. (c) Ribbon plot of the translocator domain of the NalP autotransporter. The structure was plotted using MOLSCRIPT [174]. (This figure also appears with the color plates.)

10.3.3
The Translocator Domain of the NalP Autotransporter

Autotransporter proteins are produced by a variety of Gram-negative pathogens and are known in many cases to contribute to virulence. Each autotransporter consists of a signal sequence, the secreted functional domain and a translocator domain at the C-terminus. The translocator domain adopts a β-structure and has been shown to be required for transport of the functional domain through the outer membrane. The details of this transport process are obscure, however. Oomen et al. [152] have described the determination of the crystal structure of the translocator domain from the meningococcal autotransporter NalP. The structure reveals a remarkable variation on the transmembrane β-barrel structure: a 12-stranded barrel which is filled by an N-terminal α-helix (Fig. 10.5 c). The interior of the β-barrel is lined with hydrophilic residues which make specific interactions with residues in the α-helix. The packing of the helix leaves a small channel which runs from the periplasmic side to the external side of the outer membrane. Conductivity measurements confirmed the existence of pores mediated by the NalP translocator domain. An antibiotic sensitivity assay was used to show that removal of the α-helix produced an increase in diffusion of various antibiotics through the pore. The structure raised some important questions about the mechanism of translocation of the functional domain across the outer membrane. Even without the α-helix, the pore through the 12-stranded β-barrel is too small to accommodate even a small, folded protein. And yet a "threading" model, which proposes passage of the functional domain in an unfolded state, would require specific targeting of the N-terminus to the pore and it is not apparent how this would occur. The structure therefore prompted a re-evaluation of potential transport mechanisms for autotransporters, and the authors propose the involvement of the Omp85 complex, which has been shown to affect autotransporter secretion.

10.3.4
Porins

The major role that the porin proteins PorA and PorB have played in the development of meningococcal vaccines has meant that there has been particular interest in their 3-D structures. Conditions for expression and refolding of both proteins have been reported but, to date, there has been no report of the determination of their crystal structures. The structure and function of porin proteins are probably better understood than any other group of OMPs (reviewed by Nikaido [153]) and hence it has been possible to use information gleaned from work on porins from other organisms to make predictions about PorA and PorB structure. Both proteins, which are highly related in sequence, are predicted to adopt the 16-stranded β-barrel fold that is characteristic of porins of this type [154, 155]. The best current model for the 3-D structures of PorA and PorB is Omp32, an anion-selective porin from *Comamonas acidovorans* [156]

Fig. 10.6 Structures of neisserial OMP orthologues. (a) Side and top views of the structure of Omp32 from *Comamonas acidovorans*. (b) Side and top views of the *E.coli* ferric citrate transporter. The figures were produced using MOLSCRIPT [174].

(Fig. 10.6a). Even in this case, the levels of sequence identity between Omp32 and the *Neisseria* porins are only around 24–25%; and regions of sequence divergence occur particularly within the external loop regions whose conformations are consequently poorly predicted by the homology modeling process. Nevertheless, some features of the Omp32 structure are likely to pertain to PorA and PorB: in common with other porins, the pore is constricted by the third external loop, L3, which folds back into the β-barrel. A feature peculiar to Omp32 is a β-bulge motif within a second β-strand, which folds inwards and narrows the channel to relatively small dimensions of 5 Å by 7 Å. There is a high preponderance of positively charged side-chains lining the pore; and this feature, along with the lack of acidic residues lining the constriction, provides an explanation

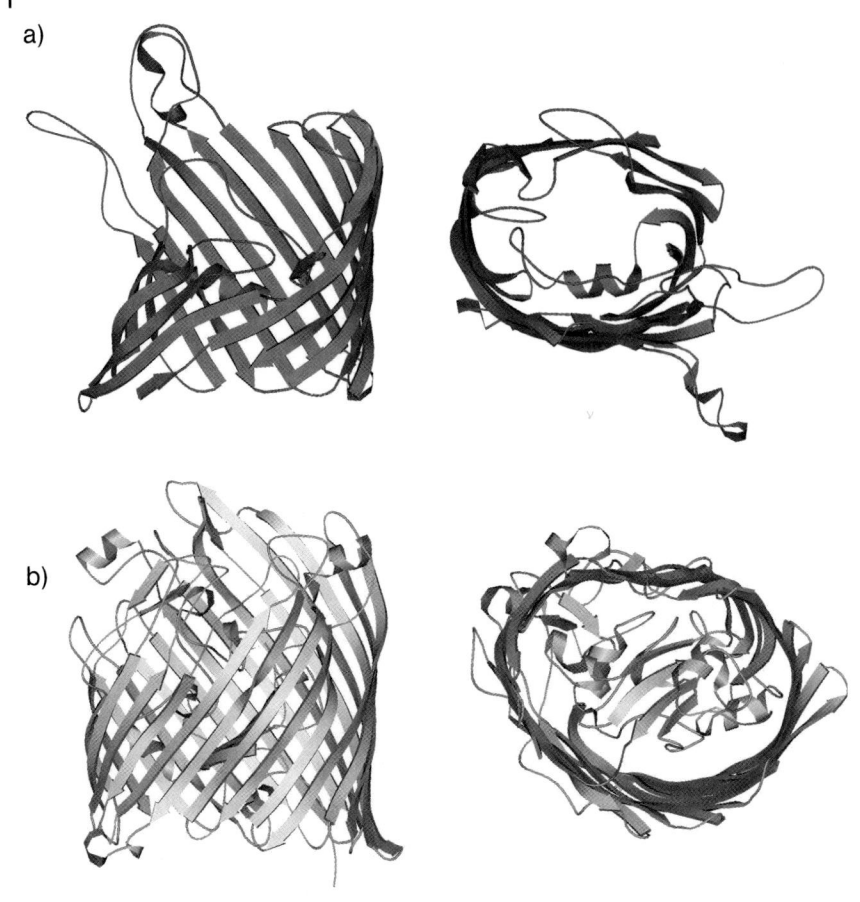

for the strong anion selectivity of the porin. It is noteworthy that many of the basic residues involved in lining the pore are also conserved in the *Neisseria* porins [156]. The Omp32 monomers are apparently stabilised by a low molecular weight peptide which binds in a 1:1 stoichiometry on the periplasmic side of the protein, close to the 3-fold rotational symmetry axis. The authors also observe that residues within β-turns 1 and 7 are highly conserved with the *Neisseria* porins, suggested that they are also involved in stabilizing trimer formation.

The length (and sequence divergence from Omp32) of the VR1 and VR2 hypervariable regions makes prediction of their 3-D structures unreliable by standard homology modeling procedures. Some structural information on this part of PorA has been obtained by determination of the crystal structures of antibody Fab fragments in complex with short synthetic peptide antigens. Both the VR2 serosubtype variants P1.16 [157, 158] and P1.2 [159] as well as the VR1 variant P1.7 [160] adopt β-hairpin-like structures in complex with their respective Fab fragments. Information on the contribution of particular residues within the antigen to immune recognition (Asp-182 in the P1.16 variant for example) has led to a better understanding of the structural basis for antigenic variation with the VR1 and VR2 regions.

10.3.5
The Iron-regulated, TonB-dependent Receptors

At the time of writing, there are no crystal structures reported for any of the TonB-dependent, iron-regulated proteins involved in iron uptake by *Neisseria*. However, sequence similarities and other evidence suggests that they are likely to adopt a similar fold to the iron siderophores from *E. coli*, whose structures have been determined [161]. An example is shown in Fig. 10.6b of the structure of the ferric citrate transporter: it has a 22-stranded β-barrel with extensive loop regions and, at the N-terminal end, a "plug" structure which fills the barrel. Recognition of the iron–siderophore complex is mediated by residues from the barrel and plug regions and binding of the transported substrate appears to propagate subtle structural changes through the protein to signal occupancy of the binding site to TonB. In the case of the HmbR hemoglobin receptor, the processes of hem extraction from hemoglobin and its subsequent transport across the outer membrane have been shown, by mutagenesis, to be separable events [162]. The neisserial receptors are therefore, to some degree, rather more complex than the iron–siderophore complexes in *E. coli*; and the dispositions of the external loop regions are likely to play an important role in the early stages of iron or hem acquisition from donor proteins, before transport across the outer membrane.

10.3.6
PilQ Secretin

The PilQ secretin plays a central role in the biogenesis of type IV pili in meningococci. It has a subunit molecular mass of 82 kDa, is located in the outer membrane and its expression is mandatory for the formation of type IV pili. Type IV pilus biogenesis requires the involvement of at least 12 different proteins [163]. PilQ is the only integral outer membrane protein directly involved in pilus biogenesis and is therefore believed to play a role in mediating the transport of pili across the outer membrane. Pilus formation is a staged process [164], initially involving secretion of the prepilin protein PilE across the inner membrane and cleavage of the signal peptide by the protease PilD. The PilE subunits are then assembled into a nascent pilus fiber and must be transferred across the outer membrane. There is some evidence to suggest that pilus formation occurs in the periplasm: a double mutation in PilQ and the pilus retraction protein PilT leads to the production of pili which pierce the outer membrane [164]. The transfer of an intact pilus fibre across the outer membrane is a process that needs to be carefully regulated. The diameter of the assembled pilus fiber is approximately 65 Å; and formation of channels of this size in the outer membrane could lead to the leakage of periplasmic components, including small proteins. It seems likely that pilus assembly and its transfer across the outer membrane are tightly coupled events.

PilQ shares some sequence homology within its C-terminus with the PulD secretin from *K. oxytoca*, which is involved in the transfer of pullulanase across the outer membrane [165, 166], and the pIV multimer, which plays a similar role in the secretion of filamentous bacteriophage [167]. PilQ can be purified from meningococci and, in common with other secretins, forms a large oligomeric structure. Examination of purified PilQ preparations by electron microscopy under negative stain reveals large ring-shaped particles, measuring approximately 165 Å across, with a central cavity of approximately 65 Å in diameter [168]. Other secretins have also been observed to have annular projection structures by electron microscopy [165, 167]. Furthermore, the internal diameter of the ring seems to match the approximate dimensions of the secreted protein, or pilus fiber in the case of meningococcal PilQ. Analysis of the projection structures has led to the identification of 12-fold rotational symmetry in the cases of PulD [165] and PilQ [168], 14-fold in the case of the pIV multimer [167] and 13-fold for the YscC secretin from the type III secretion system from *Yersinia* [169]. These observations suggested a structural model for PilQ which involved assembly of individual PilQ monomers into a ring, with a pore in the centre of appropriate dimensions for passage of the pilus fibre. Determination of the 3-D reconstruction of purified PilQ by two independent methods have shown, however, that this model might require some modification. The first study was conducted on samples in negative stain, using random conical tilt methodology [170]. This relatively low resolution reconstruction revealed a bowl-like structure, with a cavity measuring approximately 90 Å deep by 65 Å across

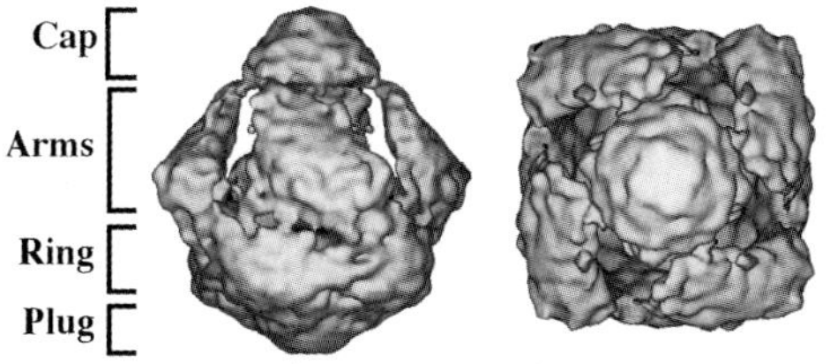

Fig. 10.7 Detailed 3-D reconstruction of purified PilQ at 12-Å resolution. The structure is anchored at the bottom by a "plug" and a "ring", which are surmounted by four arm-like features which join at the top to form a "cap". There appears to be a high degree of flexibility to the cap and arms sections.

[170]; and 12-fold rotational symmetry averaging was imposed on the complex. A second study, using data obtained with cryonegative staining methods, produced a more detailed 3-D reconstruction at 12-Å resolution [171], which is shown in Chapter 12 (Fig. 12.4). At higher resolution, four distinct features of the structure can be discerned: the structure is anchored at the bottom by a "plug" and a "ring", which are surmounted by four arm-like features which join at the top to form a "cap" (Fig. 10.7). There appears to be a higher degree of flexibility to the cap and arms sections, which may explain why the cap feature was not apparent in the reconstruction at lower resolution [170]. The higher resolution reconstruction also revealed a more complex quaternary structure: the complex apparently had C4 rotational symmetry, but with C12 quasi-symmetry. More recently, we have shown that it is possible to reconstitute a specific interaction between the PilQ oligomer and purified type IV pili [172]. Intriguingly, the PilQ oligomer appears to bind specifically to the end of the pilus fiber when the two proteins are mixed together in vitro. Analysis of the structure of the complex reveals that the cavity within the PilQ complex is filled when the pilus fiber is bound. These observations have some interesting ramifications for potential mechanisms of pilus biogenesis. It is difficult to reconcile the structure of PilQ determined by Collins et al. [171] with the more open structure required to allow passage of an assembled pilus fiber through the secretin. The width of the pilus fiber is almost as large as the diameter of the ring feature in PilQ, which seems to hold the structure together; and it is hard to imagine how this structure would dissociate and retain any structural integrity on its own. The structure of the complex of the PilQ oligomer with the fiber, in contrast, provides a different model for structural change on association with the pilus. The cap feature must presumably dissociate and the arms move laterally to allow the pilus to fill the central cavity. The question how the pilus fiber passes through the secretin, if indeed it does so in an assembled state, remains open at present.

References

1 Tsai, C.M., Frasch, C.E., Mocca, L.F. **1981**, *Journal of Bacteriology* 146, 69–78.
2 Hitchcock, P.J. **1989**, *Clin Microbiol Rev* 2[Suppl], S64–S65.
3 Blake, M.S., Gotschlich, E.C. **1987**, Functional and immunologic properties of pathogenic *Neisseria* surface proteins, in *Bacterial Outer Membranes as Model Systems*, J. Wiley, Chichester.
4 Tommassen, J., Vermeij, P., Struyve, M., Benz, R., Poolman, J.T. **1990**, *Infection and Immunity* 58, 1355–1359.
5 Frasch, C.E., Zollinger, W.D., Poolman, J.T. **1985**, *Reviews of Infectious Diseases* 7, 504–510.
6 van der Ende, A., Hopman, C.P., Zaat, S., Oude Essink, B.B., Berkhout, B., Dankert, J. **1995**, *Journal of Bacteriology* 177, 2475–2480.
7 van der Ley, P., Heckels, J.E., Virji, M., Hoogerhout, P., Poolman, J.T. **1991**, *Infection and Immunity* 59, 2963–2971.
8 McGuinness, B.T., Lambden, P.R., Heckels, J.E. **1993**, *Molecular Microbiology* 7, 505–514.
9 McGuinness, B.T., Barlow, A.K., Clarke, I.N., Farley, J.E., Anilionis, A., Poolman, J.T., Heckels, J.E. **1990**, *Journal of Experimental Medicine* 171, 1871–1882.
10 Russell, J.E., Jolley, K.A., Feavers, I., Maiden, M.C., Suker, J. **2005**, *Emerging Infectious Diseases* 10, 674–678.
11 Bash, M.C., Lesiak, K.B., Banks, S.D., Frasch, C.E. **1995**, *Infection and Immunity* 63, 1484–1490.
12 Sacchi, C.T., Lemos, A.P., Whitney, A.M., Solari, C.A., Brandt, M.E., Melles, C.E., Frasch, C.E., Mayer, L.W. **1998**, *Clin Diagn Lab Immunol* 5, 348–354.
13 Feavers, I.M., Gray, S.J., Urwin, R., Russell, J.E., Bygraves, J.A., Kaczmarski, E.B., Maiden, M.C.J. **1999**, *Journal of Clinical Microbiology* 37, 3883–3887.
14 Saukkonen, K., Abdillahi, H., Poolman, J.T., Leinonen, M. **1987**, *Microbial Pathogenesis* 3, 261–267.
15 Saukkonen, K., Leinonen, M., Abdillahi, H., Poolman, J.T. **1989**, *Vaccine* 7, 325–328.
16 Mandrell, R.E., Zollinger, W.D. **1989**, *Infection and Immunity* 57, 1590–1598.
17 Guttormsen, H.K., Wetzler, L.M., Solberg, C.O. **1994**, *Infection and Immunity* 62, 1437–1443.
18 Jones, G.R., Christodoulides, M., Brooks, J.L., Miller, A.R.O., Cartwright, K.A.V., Heckels, J.E. **1998**, *Journal of Infectious Diseases* 178, 451–459.
19 Jordens, J.Z., Williams, J.N., Jones, G.R., Christodoulides, M., Heckels, J.E. **2004**, *Infect Immun* 72, 6503–6510.
20 Bjune, G., Hoiby, E.A., Gronnesby, J.K., Arnesen, O., Holstfredriksen, J., Halstensen, A., Holten, E., Lindbak, A.K., Nokleby, H., Rosenqvist, E., Solberg, L.K., Closs, O., Eng, J., Froholm, L.O., Lystad, A., Bakketeig, L.S., Hareide, B. **1991**, *Lancet* 338, 1093–1096.
21 Boslego, J., Garcia, J., Cruz, C., Zollinger, W., Brandt, B., Ruiz, S., Martinez, M., Arthur, J., Underwood, P., Silva, W., Moran, E., Hankins, W., Gilly, J., Mays, J. **1995**, *Vaccine* 13, 821–829.
22 Milagres, L.G., Ramos, S.R., Sacchi, C.T., Melles, C.E.A., Vieira, V.S.D., Sato, H., Brito, G.S., Moraes, J.C., Frasch, C.E. **1994**, *Infection and Immunity* 62, 4419–4424.
23 Rosenqvist, E., Hoiby, E.A., Wedege, E., Bryn, K., Kolberg, J., Klem, A., Ronnild, E., Bjune, G., Nokleby, H. **1995**, *Infection and Immunity* 63, 4642–4652.
24 Wedege, E., Hoiby, E.A., Rosenqvist, E., Bjune, G. **1998**, *Infection and Immunity* 66, 3223–3231.
25 Guttormsen, H.K., Wetzler, L.M., Naess, A. **1993**, *Infection and Immunity* 61, 4734–4742.
26 Michaelsen, T.E., Aase, A., Kolberg, J., Wedge, E., Rosenqvist, E. **2001**, *Vaccine* 19, 1526–1533.
27 Wright, J.C., Williams, J.N., Christodoulides, M., Heckels, J.E. **2002**, *Infection and Immunity* 70, 4028–4034.
28 van der Ley, P., van der Biezen, J., Poolman, J.T. **1995**, *Vaccine* 13, 401–407.
29 de Kleijn, E.D., De Groot, R., Labadie, J., Lafeber, A.B., van den Dobbelsteen, G., van Alphen, L., van Dijken, H., Kuipers, B., van Omme, G.W., Wala, M., Juttmann, R., Rumke, H.C. **2000**, *Vaccine* 18, 1456–1466.

30 de Kleijn, E., Vermont, C., Kuipers, B., Vermont, C., van Dijken, H., Rumke, H., De Groot, R., van Alphen, L., van den Dobbelsteen, G. **2001**, *Vaccine* 20, 352–358.

31 Humphries, H.E., Williams, J.N., Blackstone, R., Jolley, K.A., Yuen, H.M., Christodoulides, M., Heckels, J.E. **2005**, *Vaccine* (in press).

32 O'Hallahan, J., Lennon, D., Oster, P., Lane, R., Reid, S., Mulholland, K., Stewart, J., Penney, L., Percival, T., Martin, D. **2005**, *Vaccine* 23, 2197–2201.

33 Lynch, E.C., Blake, M.S., Gotschlich, E.C., Mauro, A. **1984**, *Biophysical Journal* 45, 104–107.

34 Weel, J.F.L., van Putten, J.P.M. **1991**, *Research In Microbiology* 142, 985–993.

35 van Putten, J.P.M., Duensing, T.D., Carlson, J. **1998**, *Journal of Experimental Medicine* 188, 941–952.

36 Muller, A., Gunther, D., Dux, F., Naumann, M., Meyer, T.F., Rudel, T. **1999**, *EMBO Journal* 18, 339–352.

37 Massari, P., King, C.A., Ho, A.Y., Wetzler, L.M. **2003**, *Cellular Microbiology* 5, 99–109.

38 Fusco, P.C., Michon, F., Laude-Sharp, M., Minetti, C.A.S.A., Huang, C.H., Heron, I., Blake, M.S. **1998**, *Vaccine* 16, 1842–1849.

39 Wetzler, L.W., Ho, Y., Reiser, H. **1996**, *Journal of Experimental Medicine* 183, 1151–1159.

40 Mackinnon, F.G., Ho, Y., Blake, M.S., Michon, F., Chandraker, A., Sayegh, M.H., Wetzler, L.M. **1999**, *Journal of Infectious Diseases* 180, 755–761.

41 Al-Bader, T., Jolley, K., Humphries, H.E., Holloway, J., Heckels, J.E., Semper, A.S., Friedmann, P., Christodoulides, M. **2004**, *Cellular Microbiology* 6, 651–662.

42 Swanson, J. **1981**, *Infection and Immunity* 34, 804–816.

43 Klugman, K.P., Gotschlich, E.C., Blake, M.S. **1989**, *Infection and Immunity* 57, 2066–2071.

44 Jansen, C., Wiese, A., Reubsaet, L., Dekker, N., de Cock, H., Seydel, U., Tommassen, J. **2000**, *Biochimica et Biophysica Acta-Biomembranes* 1464, 284–298.

45 Prinz, T., Tommassen, J. **2000**, *FEMS Microbiology Letters* 183, 49–53.

46 Wolff, K., Stern, A. **1995**, *FEMS Microbiol Lett* 125, 255–263.

47 Troncoso, G., Sanchez, S., Kolberg, J., Rosenqvist, E., Veiga, M., Ferreiros, C.M., Criado, M.T. **2001**, *FEMS Microbiology Letters* 199, 171–176.

48 Rice, P.A., Vayo, H.E., Tam, M.R., Blake, M.S. **1986**, *Journal of Experimental Medicine* 164, 1735–1748.

49 Virji, M., Heckels, J.E. **1988**, *Journal of General Microbiology* 134, 2703–2711.

50 Plummer, F.A., Chubb, H., Simonsen, J.N., Bosire, M., Slaney, L., Maclean, I., Ndinyaachola, J.O., Waiyaki, P., Brunham, R.C. **1993**, *Journal of Clinical Investigation* 91, 339–343.

51 Munkley, A., Tinsley, C.R., Virji, M., Heckels, J.E. **1991**, *Microbial Pathogenesis* 11, 447–452.

52 Claassen, I., Meylis, J., van der Ley, P., Peeters, C., Brons, H., Robert, J., Borsboom, D., van der Ark, A., van Stratten, I., Roholl, P., Kuipers, B., Poolman, J. **1996**, *Vaccine* 14, 1001–1008.

53 Rosenqvist, E., Musacchio, A., Aase, A., Hoiby, E.A., Namork, E., Kolberg, J., Wedege, E., Delvig, A., Dalseg, R., Michaelsen, T.E., Tommassen, J. **1999**, *Infection and Immunity* 67, 1267–1276.

54 Carson, S.D.B., Klebba, P.E., Newton, S.M.C., Sparling, P.F. **1999**, *Journal of Bacteriology* 181, 2895–2901.

55 Perkins-Balding, D., Ratliff-Griffin, M., Stojiljkovic, I. **2004**, *Microbiology and Molecular Biology Reviews* 68, 154–171.

56 Lissolo, L., Maitrewilmotte, G., Dumas, P., Mignon, M., Danve, B., Quentin-Millet, M.J. **1995**, *Infection and Immunity* 63, 884–890.

57 West, D., Reddin, K., Matheson, M., Heath, R., Funnell, S., Hudson, M., Robinson, A., Gorringe, A. **1903**, *Infection and Immunity* 69, 1561–1567.

58 Rokbi, B., Renauld-Mongenie, G., Mignon, M., Danve, B., Poncet, D., Chabanel, C., Caugant, D.A., Quentin-Millet, M.J. **2000**, *Infection and Immunity* 68, 4938–4947.

59 Prinz, T., Meyer, M., Pettersson, A., Tommassen, J. **1999**, *Journal of Bacteriology* 181, 4417–4419.

60 Johnson, A.S., Gorringe, A.R., Mackinnon, F.G., Fox, A.J., Borrow, R., Robin-

son, A. **1999**, *FEMS Immunology and Medical Microbiology* 25, 349–354.
61 Pettersson, A., van der Biezen, J., Joosten, V., Hendriksen, J., Tommassen, J. **1999**, *Gene* 231, 105–110.
62 Urwin, R., Russell, J. E., Thompson, E. A., Holmes, E. C., Feavers, I. M., Maiden, M. C. **2004**, *Infection and Immunity* 72, 5955–5962.
63 Pettersson, A., Kuipers, B., Pelzer, M., Verhagen, E., Tiesjema, R. H., Tommassen, J., Poolman, J. T. **1990**, *Infection and Immunity* 58, 3036–3041.
64 Hardy, S. J., Christodoulides, M., Weller, R. O., Heckels, J. E. **2000**, *Mol Microbiol* 36, 817–829.
65 Virji, M., Watt, S. M., Barker, S., Makepeace, K., Doyonnas, R. **1996**, *Mol Microbiol* 22, 929–939.
66 Unkmeir, A., Latsch, K., Dietrich, G., Wintermeyer, E., Schinke, B., Schwender, S., Kim, K. S., Eigenthaler, M., Frosch, M. **2002**, *Mol Microbiol* 46, 933–946.
67 Bradley, C. J., Griffiths, N. J., Rowe, H. A., Heyderman, R. S., Virji, M. **2005**, *Cell Microbiol* 7, 1490–1503.
68 Virji, M., Makepeace, K., Peak, I. R., Ferguson, D. J., Jennings, M. P., Moxon, E. R. **1995**, *Mol Microbiol* 18, 741–754.
69 Toleman, M., Aho, E., Virji, M. **2001**, *Cell Microbiol* 3, 33–44.
70 Aho, E. L., Dempsey, J. A., Hobbs, M. M., Klapper, D. G., Cannon, J. G. **1991**, *Mol Microbiol* 5, 1429–1437.
71 Malorny, B., Morelli, G., Kusecek, B., Kolberg, J., Achtman, M. **1998**, *J Bacteriol* 180, 1323–1330.
72 Stern, A., Brown, M., Nickel, P., Meyer, T. F. **1986**, *Cell* 47, 61–71.
73 Belland, R. J., Morrison, S. G., Carlson, J. H., Hogan, D. M. **1997**, *Mol Microbiol* 23, 123–135.
74 Meyer, T. F., Gibbs, C. P., Haas, R. **1990**, *Annu Rev Microbiol* 44, 451–477.
75 Olyhoek, A. J., Sarkari, J., Bopp, M., Morelli, G., Achtman, M. **1991**, *Microb Pathog* 11, 249–257.
76 Achtman, M., Neibert, M., Crowe, B. A., Strittmatter, W., Kusecek, B., Weyse, E., Walsh, M. J., Slawig, B., Morelli, G., Moll, A., Blake, M. **1988**, *Journal of Experimental Medicine* 168, 507–525.
77 Achtman, M., Wall, R. A., Bopp, M., Kusecek, B., Morelli, G., Saken, E., Hassan-King, M. **1991**, *J Infect Dis* 164, 375–382.
78 Crowe, B. A., Wall, R. A., Kusecek, B., Neumann, B., Olyhoek, T., Abdillahi, H., Hassan-King, M., Greenwood, B. M., Poolman, J. T., Achtman, M. **1989**, *J Infect Dis* 159, 686–700.
79 Seiler, A., Reinhardt, R., Sarkari, J., Caugant, D. A., Achtman, M. **1996**, *Mol Microbiol* 19, 841–856.
80 Virji, M., Makepeace, K., Ferguson, D. J., Achtman, M., Sarkari, J., Moxon, E. R. **1992**, *Mol Microbiol* 6, 2785–2795.
81 Sarkari, J., Pandit, N., Moxon, E. R., Achtman, M. **1994**, *Mol Microbiol* 13, 207–217.
82 Zhu, P. X., Morelli, G., Achtman, M. **1999**, *Molecular Microbiology* 33, 635–650.
83 Zhu, P. X., Klutch, M. J., Derrick, J. P., Prince, S. M., Tsang, R. S. W., Tsai, C.-M. **2003**, *Gene* 307, 31–40.
84 Virji, M., Makepeace, K., Moxon, E. R. **1994**, *Molecular Microbiology* 14, 173–184.
85 Wright, S. D., Levin, S. M., Jong, M. T., Chad, Z., Kabbash, L. G. **1989**, *J Exp Med* 169, 175–183.
86 Cheresh, D. A., Pytela, R., Pierschbacher, M. D., Klier, F. G., Ruoslahti, E., Reisfeld, R. A. **1987**, *J Cell Biol* 105, 1163–1173.
87 Sokolova, O., Heppel, N., Jagerhuber, R., Kim, K. S., Frosch, M., Eigenthaler, M., Schubert-Unkmeir, A. **2004**, *Cell Microbiol* 6, 1153–1166.
88 Rostand, K. S., Esko, J. D. **1997**, *Infect Immun* 65, 1–8.
89 de Vries, F. P., Cole, R., Dankert, J., Frosch, M., van Putten, J. P. M. **1998**, *Molecular Microbiology* 27, 1203–1212.
90 Chen, T., Belland, R. J., Wilson, J., Swanson, J. **1995**, *J Exp Med* 182, 511–517.
91 van Putten, J. P., Paul, S. M. **1995**, *EMBO J* 14, 2144–2154.
92 Virji, M., Evans, D., Hadfield, A., Grunert, F., Teixeira, A. M., Watt, S. M. **1999**, *Mol Microbiol* 34, 538–551.
93 Prince, S. M., Achtman, M., Derrick, J. P. **2002**, *Proceedings of the National Academy of Sciences of the United States of America* 99, 3417–3421.
94 Hauck, C. R., Meyer, T. F. **2003**, *Curr Opin Microbiol* 6, 43–49.

95 Merz, A. J., So, M. **2000**, *Annu Rev Cell Dev Biol* 16, 423–457.

96 Duensing, T. D., Putten, J. P. **1998**, *Biochem J* 334, 133–139.

97 Grant, C. C., Bos, M. P., Belland, R. J. **1999**, *Mol Microbiol* 32, 233–242.

98 Gorby, G. L., Ehrhardt, A. F., Apicella, M. A., Elkins, C. **2001**, *J Infect Dis* 184, 460–472.

99 Blake, M. S., Blake, C. M., Apicella, M. A., Mandrell, R. E. **1995**, *Infect Immun* 63, 1434–1439.

100 Porat, N., Apicella, M. A., Blake, M. S. **1995**, *Infect Immun* 63, 2164–2172.

101 Moore, J., Bailey, S. E., Benmechernene, Z., Tzitzilonis, C., Griffiths, N. J., Virji, M., Derrick, J. P. **2005**, *J Biol Chem* 280, 31489–31497.

102 Bos, M. P., Kuroki, M., Krop-Watorek, A., Hogan, D., Belland, R. J. **1998**, *Proc Natl Acad Sci USA* 95, 9584–9589.

103 Chen, T., Gotschlich, E. C. **1996**, *Proc Natl Acad Sci USA* 93, 14851–14856.

104 de Jonge, M. I., Hamstra, H. J., van Alphen, L., Dankert, J., van der Ley, P. **2003**, *Mol Microbiol* 50, 1005–1015.

105 Gray-Owen, S. D., Dehio, C., Haude, A., Grunert, F., Meyer, T. F. **1997**, *EMBO J* 16, 3435–3445.

106 Virji, M., Makepeace, K., Ferguson, D. J., Watt, S. M. **1996**, *Mol Microbiol* 22, 941–950.

107 Hammarstrom, S. **1999**, *Semin Cancer Biol* 9, 67–81.

108 Billker, O., Popp, A., Gray-Owen, S. D., Meyer, T. F. **2000**, *Trends Microbiol* 8, 258–261.

109 Bos, M. P., Hogan, D., Belland, R. J. **1999**, *J Exp Med* 190, 331–340.

110 Hauck, C. R., Meyer, T. F., Lang, F., Gulbins, E. **1998**, *EMBO J* 17(2), 443–454.

111 Pantelic, M., Kim, Y. J., Bolland, S., Chen, I., Shively, J., Chen, T. **2005**, *Infect Immun* 73, 4171–4179.

112 Boulton, I. C., Gray-Owen, S. D. **2002**, *Nat Immunol* 3, 229–236.

113 Hammarstrom, S., Baranov, V. **2001**, *Trends Microbiol* 9, 119–125.

114 McCaw, S. E., Liao, E. H., Gray-Owen, S. D. **2004**, *Infect Immun* 72, 2742–2752.

115 Hill, D. J., Virji, M. **2003**, *Mol Microbiol* 48, 117–129.

116 Virji, M., Evans, D., Griffith, J., Hill, D., Serino, L., Hadfield, A., Watt, S. M. **2000**, *Mol Microbiol* 36, 784–795.

117 Hill, D. J., Edwards, A. M., Rowe, H. A., Virji, M. **2005**, *Mol Microbiol* 55, 1515–1527.

118 Dansky-Ullmann, C., Salgaller, M., Adams, S., Schlom, J., Greiner, J. W. **1995**, *Cytokine* 7, 118–129.

119 Fahlgren, A., Baranov, V., Frangsmyr, L., Zoubir, F., Hammarstrom, M. L., Hammarstrom, S. **2003**, *Scand J Immunol* 58, 628–641.

120 Muenzner, P., Dehio, C., Fujiwara, T., Achtman, M., Meyer, T. F., Gray-Owen, S. D. **2000**, *Infect Immun* 68, 3601–3607.

121 Tran Van Nhieu, G., Isberg, R. R. **1993**, *EMBO J* 12, 1887–1895.

122 Estabrook, M. M., Jack, D. L., Klein, N. J., Jarvis, G. A. **2004**, *J Immunol* 172, 3784–3792.

123 Milagres, L. G., Gorla, M. C., Sacchi, C. T., Rodrigues, M. M. **1998**, *Infect Immun* 66, 4755–4761.

124 de Jonge, M. I., Vidarsson, G., van Dijken, H. H., Hoogerhout, P., van Alphen, L., Dankert, J., van der Ley, P. **2003**, *Infection And Immunity* 71, 2331–2340.

125 de Jonge, M. I., Hamstra, H. J., Jiskoot, W., Roholl, P., Williams, N. A., Dankert, J., van Alphen, L., van der Ley, P. **2004**, *Vaccine* 22, 4021–4028.

126 Rosenqvist, E., Hoiby, E. A., Wedege, E., Kusecek, B., Achtman, M. **1993**, *J Infect Dis* 167, 1065–1073.

127 Wedege, E., Kuipers, B., Bolstad, K., van Dijken, H., Froholm, L. O., Vermont, C., Caugant, D. A., van den Dobbelsteen, G. **2003**, *Infect Immun* 71, 3775–3781.

128 Carmenate, T., Mesa, C., Menendez, T., Falcon, V., Musacchio, A. **2001**, *Biotechnol Appl Biochem* 34, 63–69.

129 Jolley, K. A., Appleby, L., Wright, J. C., Christodoulides, M., Heckels, J. E. **2001**, *Infect Immun* 69, 3809–3816.

130 Grifantini, R., Bartolini, E., Muzzi, A., Draghi, M., Frigimelica, E., Berger, J., Ratti, G., Petracca, R., Galli, G., Agnusdei, M., Giuliani, M.M., Santini, L., Brunelli, B., Tettelin, H., Rappuoli, R., Randazzo, F., Grandi, G. **2002**, *Nat Biotechnol* 20, 914–921.

131 Merz, A.J., So, M. **1997**, *Infect. Immun* 65, 4341–4349.

132 Pujol, C., Eugene, E., de Saint Martin, L., Nassif, X. **1997**, *Infect Immun* 65, 4836–4842.

133 Martin, D., Cadieux, N., Hamel, J., Brodeur, B.R. **1997**, *J Exp Med* 185, 1173–1183.

134 Plante, M., Cadieux, N., Rioux, C.R., Hamel, J., Brodeur, B.R., Martin, D. **1999**, *Infect Immun* 67, 2855–2861.

135 Vandeputte-Rutten, L., Bos, M.P., Tommassen, J., Gros, P. **2003**, *Journal Of Biological Chemistry* 278, 24825–24830.

136 Moe, G.R., Tan, S., Granoff, D.M. **1999**, *Infect Immun* 67, 5664–5675.

137 Moe, G.R., Zuno-Mitchell, P., Hammond, S.N., Granoff, D.M. **2002**, *Infect Immun* 70, 6021–6031.

138 Hou, V.C., Moe, G.R., Raad, Z., Wuorimaa, T., Granoff, D.M. **2003**, *Infect Immun* 71, 6844–6849.

139 O'Dwyer C, A., Reddin, K., Martin, D., Taylor, S.C., Gorringe, A.R., Hudson, M.J., Brodeur, B.R., Langford, P.R., Kroll, J.S. **2004**, *Infect Immun* 72, 6511–6518.

140 Martin, P., Makepeace, K., Hill, S.A., Hood, D.W., Moxon, E.R. **2005**, *Proc Natl Acad Sci USA* 102, 3800–3804.

141 Comanducci, M., Bambini, S., Brunelli, B., Adu-Bobie, J., Arico, B., Capecchi, B., Giuliani, M.M., Masignani, V., Santini, L., Savino, S., Granoff, D.M., Caugant, D.A., Pizza, M., Rappuoli, R., Mora, M. **2002**, *J Exp Med* 195, 1445–1454.

142 Litt, D.J., Savino, S., Beddek, A., Comanducci, M., Sandiford, C., Stevens, J., Levin, M., Ison, C., Pizza, M., Rappuoli, R., Kroll, J.S. **2004**, *J Infect Dis* 190, 1488–1497.

143 Capecchi, B., Adu-Bobie, J., Di Marcello, F., Ciucchi, L., Masignani, V., Taddei, A., Rappuoli, R., Pizza, M., Arico, B. **2005**, *Mol Microbiol* 55, 687–698.

144 Serruto, D., Adu-Bobie, J., Scarselli, M., Veggi, D., Pizza, M., Rappuoli, R., Arico, B. **2003**, *Mol Microbiol* 48, 323–334.

145 Hadi, H.A., Wooldridge, K.G., Robinson, K., Ala'Aldeen, D.A. **2001**, *Mol Microbiol* 41, 611–623.

146 Peak, I.R., Srikhanta, Y., Dieckelmann, M., Moxon, E.R., Jennings, M.P. **2000**, *FEMS Immunol Med Microbiol* 28, 329–334.

147 Wimley, W.C. **2003**, *Current Opinion In Structural Biology* 13, 404–411.

148 Prince, S.M., Feron, C., Janssens, D., Lobet, Y., Achtman, M., Kusecek, B., Bullough, P.A., Derrick, J.P. **2001**, *Acta Crystallographica* D57, 1164–1166.

149 Buchanan, S.K. **1999**, *Current Opinion in Structural Biology* 9, 455.

150 Hwang, P.M., Choy, W.Y., Lo, E.I., Chen, L., Forman-Kay, J.D., Raetz, C.R.H., Prive, G.G., Bishop, R.E., Kay, L.E. **2002**, *Proceedings Of The National Academy Of Sciences Of The United States Of America* 99, 13560–13565.

151 Dehio, C., Gray-Owen, S.D., Meyer, T.F. **1998**, *Trends in Microbiology* 6, 489–495.

152 Oomen, C.J., van Ulsen, P., Van Gelder, P., Feijen, M., Tommassen, J., Gros, P. **2004**, *EMBO Journal* 23, 1257–1266.

153 Nikaido, H. **2003**, *Microbiology And Molecular Biology Reviews* 67, 593–656.

154 Derrick, J.P., Urwin, R., Suker, J., Feavers, I.M., Maiden, M.C.J. **1999**, *Infection and Immunity* 67, 2406–2413.

155 Urwin, R., Holmes, E.C., Fox, A.J., Derrick, J.P., Maiden, M.C.J. **2002**, *Molecular Biology and Evolution* 19, 1686–1694.

156 Zeth, K., Diederichs, K., Welte, W., Engelhardt, H. **2000**, *Structure* 8, 981–992.

157 van den Elsen, J., Vandeputte-Rutten, L., Kroon, J., Gros, P. **1999**, *Journal Of Biological Chemistry* 274, 1495–1501.

158 van den Elsen, J.M.H., Herron, J.N., Hoogerhout, P., Poolman, J.T., Boel, E., Logtenberg, T., Wilting, J., Crommelin, D.J.A., Kroon, J., Gros, P. **1997**, *Proteins Structure Function And Genetics* 29, 113–125.

159 Tzitzilonis, C., Prince, S.M., Collins, R.F., Achtman, M., Feavers, I.M., Mai-

den, M. C. J., Derrick, J. P. **2005**, *Proteins* (in press).

160 Derrick, J. P., Maiden, M. C. J., Feavers, L. M. **1999**, *Journal Of Molecular Biology* 293, 81–91.

161 Ferguson, A. D., Deisenhofer, J. **2002**, *Biochimica Et Biophysica Acta Biomembranes* 1565, 318–332.

162 Perkins-Balding, D., Baer, M. T., Stojiljkovic, I. **2003**, *Microbiology* 149, 3423–3435.

163 Carbonnelle, E., Helaine, S., Prouvensier, L., Nassif, X., Pelicic, V. **2005**, *Molecular Microbiology* 55, 54–64.

164 Wolfgang, M., van Putten, J. P. M., Hayes, S. F., Dorward, D., Koomey, M. **2000**, *EMBO Journal* 19, 6408–6418.

165 Nouwen, N., Ranson, N., Saibil, H., Wolpensinger, B., Engel, A., Ghazi, A., Pugsley, A. P. **1999**, *Proceedings of the National Academy of Sciences of the United States of America* 96, 8173–8177.

166 Nouwen, N., Stahleberg, H., Pugsley, A. P., Engel, A. **2000**, *EMBO Journal* 19, 2229–2236.

167 Opalka, N., Beckmann, R., Boisset, N., Simon, M. N., Russel, M., Darst, S. A. **2003**, *Journal of Molecular Biology* 325, 461–470.

168 Collins, R. F., Davidsen, L., Derrick, J. P., Ford, R. C., Tonjum, T. **2001**, *Journal of Bacteriology* 183, 3825–3832.

169 Burghout, P., van Boxtel, R., Van Gelder, P., Ringler, P., Muller, S. A., Tommassen, J., Koster, M. **2004**, *Journal Of Bacteriology* 186, 4645–4654.

170 Collins, R. F., Ford, R. C., Kitmitto, A., Olsen, R., Tonjum, T., Derrick, J. P. **2003**, *Journal of Bacteriology* 185, 2611–2617.

171 Collins, R. F., Frye, S. A., Kitmitto, A., Ford, R. C., Tonjum, T., Derrick, J. P. **2004**, *Journal Of Biological Chemistry* 279, 39750–39756.

172 Collins, R. F., Frye, S. A., Balasingham, S., Ford, R. C., Tonjum, T., Derrick, J. P. **2005**, *Journal Of Biological Chemistry* 280, 18923–18930.

173 Salyers, A. A., Wa, D. D. **1994** *Bacterial Pathogenesis, A Molecular Approach*, ASM Press, St Paul.

174 Kraulis, P. J. **1991**, *Journal of Applied Crystallography* 24, 946–950.

175 Nicholls, A., Sharp, K. A., Honig, B. **1991**, *Proteins* 11, 281–296.

11
Iron Metabolism in *Neisseria meningitidis*

Andrew Ekins and Anthony B. Schryvers

11.1
Iron Homeostasis in Humans

Iron is an essential element for most living organisms due to its role as a cofactor for many proteins and enzymes that mediate critical functions such as energy metabolism and biosynthesis. Iron can assume a wide range of redox potentials depending on the mode of coordination by the protein and thus is a versatile redox catalyst for a variety of different biological reactions. Most living organisms have devised specialized strategies for transporting and storing iron due to its solubility characteristics in neutral aqueous solutions and its potential to generate toxic byproducts through reaction with oxygen.

In humans and other mammals, the relatively small amount of dietary iron required to maintain iron homeostasis is taken up by transporters on the apical surface of enterocytes. The transporter that has been implicated as playing a major role in host dietary iron acquisition is the ferrous ion transporter Nramp2 (DMT1) [1]. Excess iron taken up by the enterocytes is exported through the membrane on the basolateral surface of the enterocyte through the exporter ferroportin1 (MTP1) and with the assistance of ceruloplasmin and/or hephaestin, the exported iron is oxidized to the ferric form and bound by the serum glycoprotein, transferrin [1].

Transferrin (Tf) is largely responsible for transport of iron throughout the body from areas of uptake and storage to areas of need. Actively growing cells obtain iron from Tf for growth by capturing the iron-loaded form of Tf with a specific Tf receptor at the cell surface and internalizing the Tf–receptor complex into an endosome. The relatively low pH of the endosome and possibly iron chelators such as citrate or ATP are involved in the removal of iron from Tf [1]. After removal of iron, the Tf–receptor complex is returned to the cell surface where the apo form of Tf is readily released by the recycled surface receptor protein. Excess intracellular iron is stored within a large complex formed by the iron storage protein ferritin and can readily be retrieved to maintain an adequate intracellular iron concentration. The iron requirements are particularly

Handbook of Meningococcal Disease. Infection Biology, Vaccination, Clinical Management.
Edited by M. Frosch and M.C.J. Maiden

ISBN: 3-527-31260-9

large for growing reticulocytes for the production of hemoglobin, which ultimately constitutes 70% of the total iron content in the human body.

There are efficient systems for retention of iron within the body, particularly for the large reservoir of iron present in erythrocyte hemoglobin. Hemoglobin that is released by erythrocyte lysis is rapidly complexed by the circulating glycoprotein haptoglobin and the resulting hemoglobin–haptoglobin complex is taken up by the liver where the iron is retrieved and transferred to Tf [60]. Similarly, any hemin that is released from hemoglobin or other heme containing proteins is rapidly complexed by the circulating serum glycoprotein hemopexin, which is subsequently taken up by the liver for recycling into the transferrin pool. Circulating Tf is only partially saturated ($\sim$30%) with respect to its iron-binding capacity and thus is capable of rapidly binding any released ferric ion [1]. At sights of inflammation free ferric ion would readily be complexed by lactoferrin (Lf), an iron-binding protein related to Tf, which is released by neutrophils and is capable of binding iron at the lower pH levels that may be present.

11.2
Potential Sources of Iron in the Host for the Meningococcus

The meningococcus is a host-restricted pathogen whose primary ecological niche is on the mucosal surface of the human nasopharynx. This organism is not adapted for survival outside of the host and thus there is no known reservoir for this bacterium outside of the human body. While the meningococcus is primarily transmitted by respiratory droplets [57], more direct person-to-person modes of transmission may also be involved, particularly for the infrequent occasions when the meningococcus is isolated from the genital mucosa.

The nature of the association of the meningococcus with the mucosal surface during colonization of the human nasopharynx likely involves anchoring of the bacteria to the epithelial cells through interactions mediated by the type IV pilus via the PilC1 protein [33]. Although meningococci are capable of initiating much more intimate associations with epithelial cells, including endocytosis and intracellular survival, the degree to which these occur during normal carriage is uncertain. Since host-to-host transmission undoubtedly primarily involves extracellular meningococci residing on the surface of the epithelial cells, it is likely the predominant mode during carriage.

In contrast to the gastrointestinal tract where there is a reasonably steady supply of iron from environmental sources, exposure to potential iron sources from the environment would be sporadic in the nasopharynx, thus host-derived iron sources would have to be sufficient to support bacterial growth. Studies with a human gonococcal infection model provide compelling evidence that Tf serves as an important source of iron for growth on the male urethral mucosa [13]. Although there are clear differences between the urethral and nasopharyngeal mucosal environments, it is probable that Tf would also comprise an important iron source for meningococci colonizing the nasopharynx. Further support for the importance of Tf as a source of iron for growth on the nasopharyngeal mucosa comes from studies with the host-restricted pathogen, *Actinobacillus pleuropneumoniae,* which normally colonizes the nasopharynx of the pig [8]. The observation that growth was attained in a gonococcal infection model with expression of the Lf receptor in the absence of the Tf receptor indicates that Lf can also serve as an iron source on mucosal surfaces [5]. It seems reasonable to extrapolate these findings to the human nasopharynx and suggest that Lf could serve as an iron source for meningococci, particularly since the ability to use Lf is present in all strains, contrasting its variable presence in gonococci [34].

The inability of Tf and Lf receptor deficient gonococci or Tf receptor deficient *A. pleuropneumoniae* to thrive in authentic infection models in the natural host, indicates that alternative iron sources were not sufficient to support growth *in vivo.* Although this might suggest that alternative forms of iron may not be able to serve as the sole source of iron for growth in the human nasopharynx, this does not preclude them from being important supplemental sources of iron. There must be sufficient quantities of heme, or heme-containing proteins available in the nasopharynx to support the growth of *Haemophilus influenzae,* an organism that has an absolute dependence on exogenously supplied heme or protoporphyrin during aerobic growth. However, greater quantities of heme are required to fulfill the iron requirements during growth under aerobic conditions *in vitro* [14] suggesting that alternative iron sources may also be required *in vivo.*

The mixed microflora present on the nasopharyngeal mucosal surface presents a potentially competitive environment for acquiring the limited amount of available iron. Thus, in spite of the fact that the meningococcus does not synthesize and secrete iron-chelating siderophores, it might exploit siderophores secreted by neighboring organisms and acquire iron from the resulting iron-siderophore complex. However, such proposals remain speculative in the absence of information on the repertoire of siderophores produced in this environment and the ability of meningococci to specifically bind and utilize these siderophores.

Due to factors not completely understood, meningococci will on occasion invade the bloodstream and disseminate, leading to septicemia and meningitis. In order to gain access to the bloodstream the meningococcus must first traverse through the epithelial cell it has associated with, a process taking up to 18 h [33]. While it is not known to what extent, or if, meningococci require an extracellular iron source while within epithelial cells *in vivo,* studies on intracellular replication of meningococci within cultured epithelial cells have revealed that Tf, Lf and hemoglobin do not serve as iron sources [24]. At present it is known that the acquisition of iron for intracellular growth involves TonB and presumably an associated receptor. The nature or state of the acquired iron is not known, however it is believed that the iron is derived from degraded host cell ferritin [25]. During the bacteremic phase, meningococci target to the endothelial cells of the blood–brain barrier and, after traversing this cell barrier, they replicate within the normally sterile cerebrospinal fluid, inducing the typical symptoms associated with meningitis.

Meningococci are thought to reside primarily in the extracellular environment, regardless of whether they are invading the bloodstream or cerebrospinal fluid and therefore the majority of iron for continued growth during the invasive stage is likely acquired from extracellular iron sources. The majority of host iron is found in the intracellular compartment and is bound to either hemoglobin or ferritin. While some hemoglobin and heme may be released into the extracellular environment due to hemolysis or cellular damage caused by an invading pathogen, such iron sources are only transiently available. As stated earlier, hemoglobin and heme are quickly bound by haptoglobin and hemopexin or albumin, respectively, and these iron-containing complexes are cleared from circulation by the liver [35, 60]. There is little evidence for the production of hemolysins by meningococci and hemolysis is not a characteristic feature of meningococcal infection, particularly in the early phases, suggesting that these iron sources may not play a major role in establishment of infection.

Within the body, the majority of extracellular iron is bound by the iron-binding glycoprotein Tf that is present in significant concentrations in serum (approximately 30 μM or 2 mg ml^{-1}). The pool of Tf in the circulatory system is typically one-third saturated with iron, such that the predominant species is a monoferric form of Tf with the iron bound in the N-lobe of the protein [27]. The hypoferremic response to infection results in a reduction in the levels of iron in the circulating Tf pool. Although the normal concentration of Lf in serum is very low, it can reach high levels at local sites of infection and inflammation. Lf is released by neutrophils and is capable of complexing with iron that is released upon destruction and lysis of cells even when the pH of the localized environment is reduced. Thus, Tf is probably the predominant iron source during the invasive phase of infection but the ability to acquire iron from Lf might be advantageous to meningococci at site-localized inflammation.

11.3
Iron Acquisition from Transferrin and Lactoferrin

Transferrin (Tf) and lactoferrin (Lf) are related bilobed glycoproteins, with both the N- and C-lobes of the protein capable of binding a single iron ion with a cognate carbonate ion. The two lobes are virtually identical in overall structure and mode of iron coordination (Fig. 11.1 A). The lobes consist of two domains separated by an interdomain cleft connected by two antiparallel beta-strands. The iron atom is bound at the base of the interdomain cleft with amino acid side-chains from residues in both domains and the interconnecting beta-strand contributing to the octahedral iron coordination complex (Fig. 11.1 B). There is a substantial separation of the two domains in the apo form of Lf, indicating that the process of iron binding involves substantial movement of the rigid domains to complete the iron coordination complex (Fig. 11.2). The relatively high affinity of Tf and Lf for binding iron effectively lowers the level of free iron below that required to support microbial growth and precludes effective competition

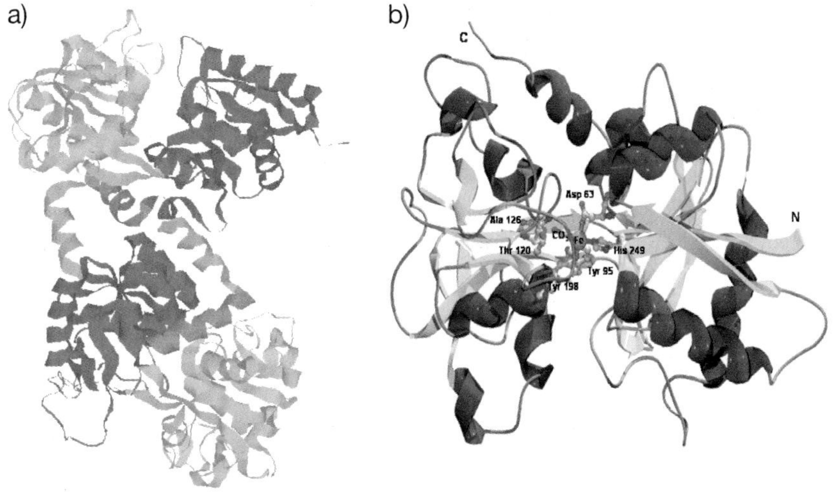

Fig. 11.1 Structure of transferrin and lactoferrin. (A) Ribbon model of human lactoferrin, illustrating the domain structure of both the N-lobe (top) and C-lobe (bottom). Domain 1 (green) is connected to domain 2 (white) by antiparallel beta-strands forming the base of an interdomain cleft. The two lobes are connected by an inter-domain bridge consisting of two alpha-helices (pink and yellow) equivalent to the C-terminal tail of the C-lobe. (B) Ribbon model of the human lactoferrin N-lobe, illustrating the amino acids from both domains and the anion that form the iron coordination complex. (This figure also appears with the color plates.)

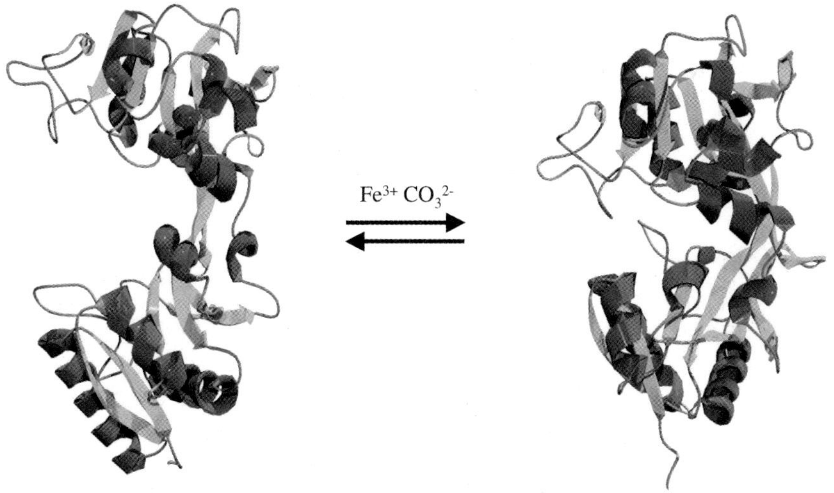

Fig. 11.2 Domain closure associated with iron binding. Ribbon model of the apo-form (left) and iron-loaded form (right) of the human lactoferrin N-lobe. (This figure also appears with the color plates.)

by weak iron chelators. Iron removal from Tf and Lf is thus limited to very high affinity iron chelators (siderophores) or to mechanisms involving direct interaction with these glycoproteins.

Meningococci do not produce siderophores, yet are able to acquire iron for growth from Tf [7] or Lf [34] in iron-limited media. They express specific receptors capable of binding these glycoproteins when grown in iron restricted conditions [51, 52] that not only discriminate between Tf and Lf but are specific for the human form of these proteins. Human but not cattle Tf was capable of promoting lethal infection in mice, indicating that alternative receptor-independent routes of acquiring iron from Tf are not available *in vivo* [50].

The Tf receptor is comprised of two iron-regulated outer membrane proteins, Tf binding protein A (TbpA) and B (TbpB), that can readily be identified and isolated by affinity capture with human Tf [51]. The Lf receptor has a similar composition but the second receptor protein, LbpB, can only be affinity captured using modified isolation conditions [10]. The genes encoding the Tf and Lf receptor proteins are arranged in operons with the *tbpB/lbpB* gene preceding the *tbpA/lbpA* gene (Fig. 11.3) [9, 26].

The TbpA and LbpA proteins are integral outer membrane proteins that are members of the TonB-dependent receptor family that includes proteins involved in the transport of siderophores, heme and vitamin B12 across the outer membrane. Since the structures of several siderophore receptors and the vitamin B12 receptor have been determined and shown to consist of a 22-strand C-terminal beta-barrel and an N-terminal plug region, it is reasonable to assume that TbpA

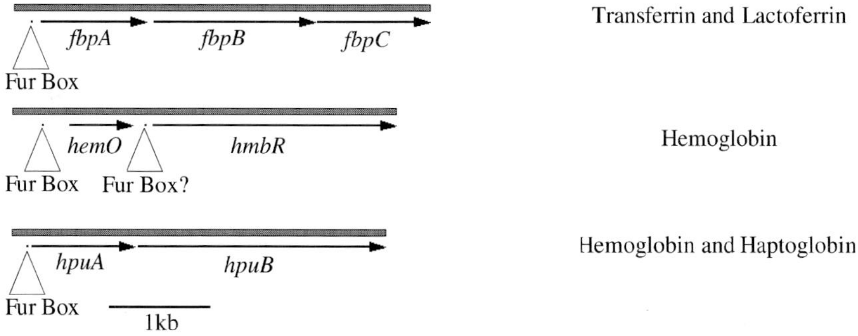

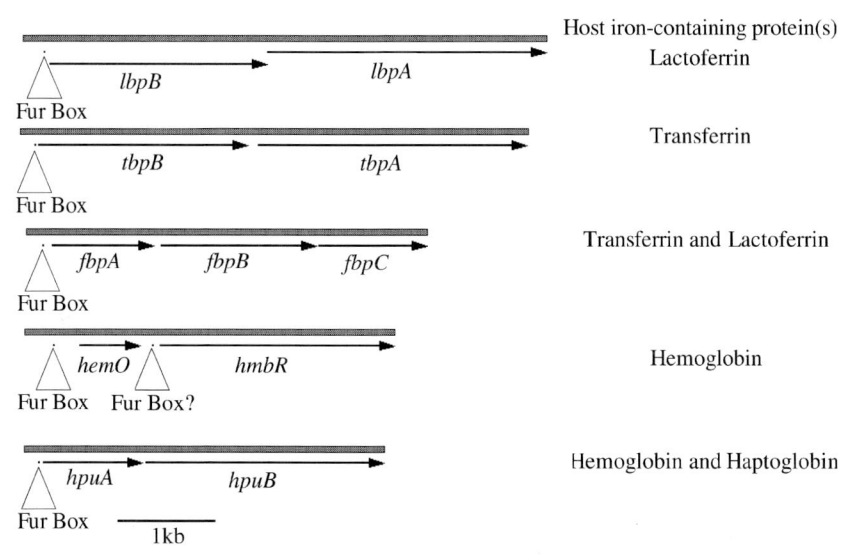

Fig. 11.3 The genetic organization of genes whose encoded products are involved in acquiring iron from the indicated host iron-containing proteins.

and LbpA share these overall structural features. Comparisons of the TbpA or LbpA sequence with that of the receptors whose structures are known have been used to develop topology models for TbpA and LbpA, and, more recently, a structural model for a meningococcal TbpA [36]. Although the validity of the topology models, and particularly the structural model, can readily be challenged, they do serve as useful guides for designing experiments probing the functional and immunological properties of these proteins.

TbpA and LbpA are proposed to form the channel that the "extracted" iron passes through to enter the periplasm of the cell (Fig. 11.4). This is consistent with the experimental observation that TbpA and LbpA are absolutely required for the acquisition of iron from Tf or Lf, respectively, based on insertional mutagenesis [9, 19]. The importance of TbpA for causing meningococcal infection is inferred from mouse infection experiments with insertional mutants [42], and perhaps even more compelling evidence is provided from a human gonococcal model of infection where TbpA and/or LbpA were shown to be required for survival in the human host [5, 13]. Clearly these results indicate that TbpA would be an ideal target for vaccine development providing that issues regarding antigenic variation and feasibility of antigen production are addressed.

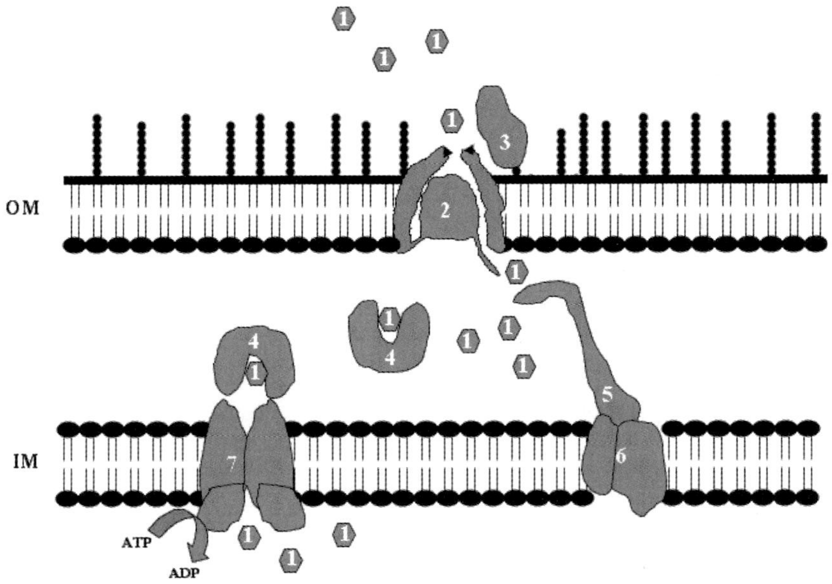

Fig. 11.4 General model of iron acquisition pathways. Ferrisiderophore, heme-bound iron, or transferrin- or lactoferrin-derived iron (1) are transported through the outer membrane by a TonB-dependent receptor (2), which may require the activities of an associated lipoprotein (3) anchored to the outer membrane. The transport process requires energy derived from the TonB (5) ExbBD (6) complex. Iron or iron complex present in the periplasm is bound by a periplasmic binding protein (4) which delivers the iron or iron-complex to the cytoplasmic membrane ATP-dependent permease complex (7).

The mature TbpB and LbpB proteins contain an N-terminal cysteine that is lipidated and serves as the primary anchor for attaching these proteins to the outer membrane surface. There is evidence of internal amino acid sequence homology in these proteins, indicating that they are bilobed proteins, analogous to the glycoproteins that they bind to. Experimental evidence suggesting that both lobes of TbpB are capable of binding to Tf, in a similar if not identical fashion [44], have not been reproduced in recent studies in which the C-lobe was incapable of binding to Tf [23]. A combination of structural and functional studies will be required to resolve this issue, but unfortunately there is no structural information currently available for TbpB, LbpB or any known homologs.

The role of TbpB and LbpB in iron acquisition is still unclear. In contrast to TbpA, TbpB has been shown to have a strong preference for binding the iron-loaded form of Tf [45], leading to the suggestion that TbpB may be involved in the initial capture of Tf or on changing the specificity of the receptor. Insertional activation of the tbpB gene from some meningococcal strains results in a loss of the ability to utilize Tf iron for growth, suggesting that TbpB plays an important role in the iron removal and uptake process [19]. However, insertional activation of the *tbpB* gene in other strains has only minor effects on growth *in vitro* with Tf as the sole iron source [42]. The minor impact of this mutation on survival and disease causation in a mouse infection model has led to questioning the importance of this protein *in vivo* and its suitability as a vaccine target [42]. However, it is unlikely that coadministration of large quantities of Tf and bacteria into the intraperitoneal cavity of a mouse reflects the natural human infection. The demonstration that TbpB was essential for infection of pigs by *A. pleuropneumoniae,* even though *in vitro* growth did not require TbpB, argues against extrapolation of the mouse model experiments to human infection. Aside from performing similar experiments in the human gonococcal model, the experiments with *A. pleuropneumoniae* are probably the best we can do to evaluate the role of TbpB *in vivo,* since this pathogen occupies a similar niche (nasopharynx) and was administered to its natural host in a physiologically relevant mode of transmission (aerosol). Although *in vitro* growth studies suggest that LbpB is not involved in iron acquisition from Lf [9], based on the results with TbpB, it is clearly premature to reach that conclusion.

Studies performed with enzymatically deglycosylated human Tf and Lf demonstrated that the N-linked oligosaccharide chains are not involved in binding to the bacterial receptors [2, 37] indicating that the specificity is determined solely by protein–protein interactions. Binding studies with proteolytically derived Tf subfragments [3] demonstrated that the regions involved in binding to TbpA and TbpB were primarily located in the C-lobe, an observation later confirmed in studies with hybrid recombinant cattle–human Tfs, that also demonstrated that the N-lobe of TbpB primarily recognizes regions in the C-lobe of Tf [43]. Studies with hybrid recombinant cattle Tf–human Lf proteins indicated that LbpA bound to the C-lobe of Lf and recognized binding determinants on both domains. Collectively, these results suggest that there may be a conserved mode of interaction in which the C-lobe of Tf or Lf docks onto the TonB-dependent receptor protein (TbpA or LbpA) as illustrated in Fig. 11.5 and it would logically follow that the anchored N-lobe of TbpB which is in close proximity would primarily interact with the C-lobe of Tf. Although this proposed orientation raises obvious questions regarding interaction with the N-lobe of Tf and iron removal from this lobe, it is consistent with the demonstrated binding interactions.

A fairly extensive interaction between TbpB and Tf has been inferred from studies in which recombinant TbpBs from different species identified an identical set of peptides from a synthetic overlapping peptide library representing human Tf [44]. The binding peptides mapped to adjacent regions on the surface of Tf, nearly encircling it. Loss of reactivity to these peptides by sequential truncation of the TbpB N-lobe from *Moraxella catarrhalis* provided additional evidence that the binding regions were authentic [53]. The truncations were designed to remove peptides from the TbpB N-lobe from *M. catarrhalis* that were shown to bind Tf when probing a synthetic peptide library representing the TbpB N-lobe. Two of these binding regions were equivalent to those identified in the *N. meningitidis* TbpB by a sequence-based predictive method and verified by site-directed mutagenesis [41]. Collectively these results indicate that the interaction between TbpB and Tf is complex and a full appreciation of the interaction may only be revealed when structures of receptor–ligand complexes are obtained.

Regions of the gonococcal TbpA that are involved in binding to Tf have been localized to subfragments of 128 amino acids (predicted surface loops 4 and 5) and 53 amino acids (loop 5) [31]. Although insertional mutagenesis experiments

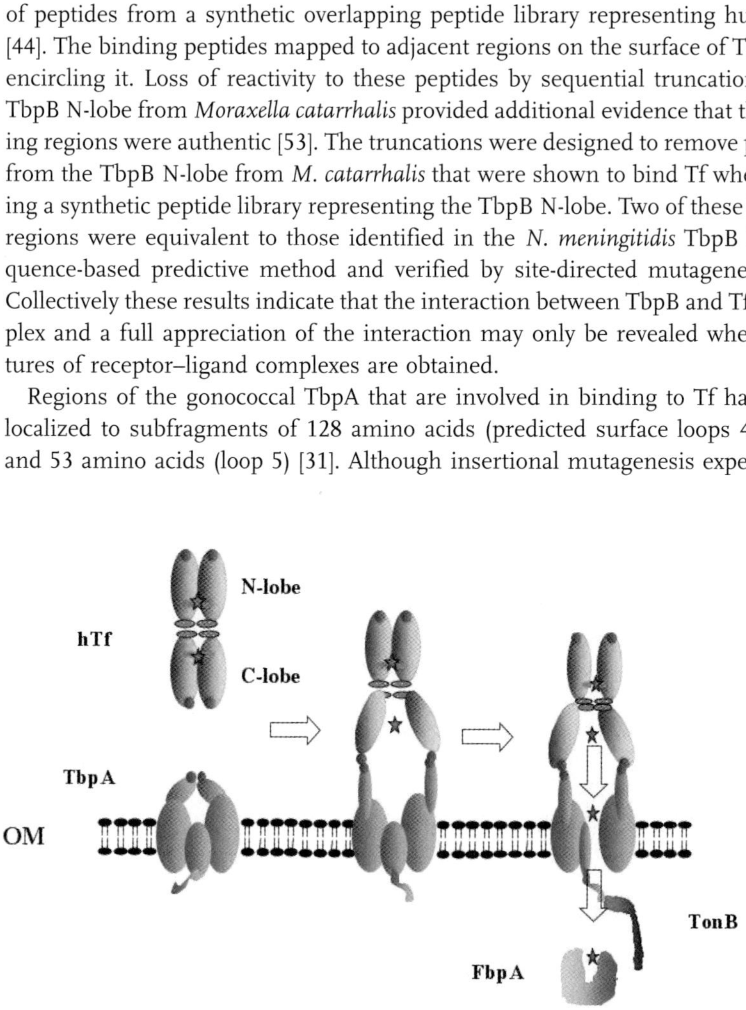

Fig. 11.5 Model of iron removal from transferrin. The binding of transferrin by the receptor is accompanied by conformational changes that result in domain separation and concomitant lowering of iron binding affinity. Once a channel is formed across the outer membrane by TonB interaction (by removal or conformational change in the cork domain), the iron atom is transported across the outer membrane partly driven by the higher affinity of FbpA for iron.

only implicated one additional Tf binding determinant in predicted surface loop 3, it failed to identify the loop 5 binding determinant, indicating that insertional mutagenesis is not a very effective means of delineating the Tf binding regions [62]. Thus, although the interaction between TbpA and Tf is likely quite extensive, we currently do not have a good appreciation of the regions of TbpA and Tf involved. The insertional mutagenesis study also yielded a series of interesting mutants that retained Tf binding ability but became dependent upon TbpB for Tf iron utilization [62] but the mechanistic implications of these observations are still unclear.

The Tf receptor is responsible for binding Tf at the cell surface, removing iron from Tf and transporting it across the outer membrane. The overall process requires energy provided by the TonB complex (Fig. 11.4) [56]. Although a number of interesting insertion mutants have been isolated that interfere with this process [62], they have not yielded significant insights into the mechanisms involved. Since it is known that there are large conformational changes involved in iron binding by Tf and Lf (Fig. 11.2), it seems logical to propose that domain separation upon receptor binding could contribute to the iron removal process (Fig. 11.5). The domain separation would effectively reduce the affinity of Tf for iron and facilitate transport of iron across the outer membrane when a path is made available through TonB interaction. The iron transported across the outer membrane is subsequently bound by a periplasmic ferric iron-binding protein A (FbpA) (Fig. 11.4) which has a similar iron coordination strategy and affinity for iron as Tf. Insertional mutatgenesis of the fbpA gene effectively demonstrated that this pathway is essential for the transport of Tf- and Lf-derived iron [22]. A prediction of the conformational model for iron transport is that the high-affinity binding of iron by the periplasmic binding protein, FbpA, is required to drive the transport of iron across the outer membrane. This prediction has been verified in studies with a series of site-directed mutants of the Haemophilus influenzae FbpA (Schryvers, unpublished data) and likely also applies to removal and transport of iron from Tf and Lf in *N. meningitidis.*

The FbpA protein subsequently delivers iron to an inner membrane transport complex comprised of the FbpB and FbpC proteins (Fig. 11.4). These proteins are predicted to serve as the cytoplasmic membrane permease protein (FbpB) and the ATPase (FbpC) that provides the energy for transport through ATP hydrolysis. Studies using the FbpABC pathway from *H. influenzae* have effectively demonstrated that this transport system is dependent upon ATP for transport [4] and while mechanisms of iron release from FbpA and transport across the inner membrane involving displacement of anion and reduction of the ferric ion to a ferrous ion have been proposed [16], the demonstration that gallium, a trivalent metal ion that cannot be reduced to the divalent form, is transported by the FbpABC pathway effectively rules out a reduction step in transport [4].

11.4
Acquisition of Heme Iron

Hemoglobin found within erythrocytes constitutes the majority of iron within the body. Native hemoglobin consists of an $\alpha_2\beta_2$ tetramer with a heme moiety bound to each of the four hydrophobic heme-binding clefts of the individual subunits. The heme is held in place not only by the hydrophobic interactions within the binding pocket, but also by a histidine residue that coordinates to iron in addition to the four nitrogens from the porphyrin ring. Hemoglobin that is released by erythrocyte lysis readily dissociates into two $\alpha_1\beta_1$ dimers which are rapidly complexed by excess circulating haptoglobin for retrieval and processing by the liver. Haptoglobin is a tetrameric ($\alpha_2\beta_2$) glycoprotein capable of binding two $\alpha_1\beta_1$ hemoglobin dimers. In individuals expressing the Hp2 allele, large polymers of the haptoglobin tetramer are present due to crosslinking via the additional cysteine residues in the alpha subunit encoded by this allele. Heme that dissociates from the heme-binding pocket of hemoglobin, or that is released by proteolysis of hemoglobin, is rapidly bound by the serum glycoprotein hemopexin for capture and recycling by the liver.

Meningococci are capable of utilizing a variety of different heme-containing preparations as a source of iron for growth, including heme, hemoglobin and hemoglobin–haptoglobin complexes [6, 17]. However, unlike *H. influenzae*, they are incapable of utilizing heme that is bound by hemopexin or albumin. The ability to utilize heme-containing preparations is mediated by two distinct TonB-dependent receptors, Hpu (hemoglobin–haptoglobin utilization) [28] and HmbR (hemoglobin receptor) [55]. Although the majority of clinical isolates of *N. meningitidis* possess the genetic loci for both of these receptors [46], phase variation occurs in both of these loci [29], perhaps suggesting that they may be useful in different microenvironments.

The Hpu receptor is comprised of two iron-regulated outer membrane proteins, HpuA and HpuB. The 85-kDa HpuB protein can be isolated by affinity capture with a hemoglobin-haptoglobin complex [28], whereas identification of HpuA was based on the location of the hpuA gene upstream of the hpuB gene [30] (Fig. 11.3). The receptor is capable of binding hemoglobin, hemoglobin–haptoglobin or apo-haptoglobin [30] and insertional mutants demonstrate that both HpuA and HpuB are required for utilization of hemoglobin or hemoglobin–haptoglobin complexes as a source of iron for growth [28, 30].

HpuB is an integral outer membrane protein related to the TonB-dependent receptors and is thus proposed to be comprised of a 22-strand C-terminal beta-barrel and an N-terminal plug region [48]. Although the HpuB protein undoubtedly serves as the channel for transport of heme across the outer membrane, it is incapable of acquiring iron from hemoglobin or haptoglobin–hemoglobin complexes independent of HpuA. Binding of hemoglobin, hemoglobin–haptoglobin or apo-haptoglobin by HpuB in the absence of HpuA was not detected by solid-phase binding assays, but was revealed by the use of a more sensitive flow cytometry-based assay [47]. The dissociation of hemoglobin or haptoglobin–

hemoglobin from the receptor was inhibited in a TonB mutant or by addition of the protonophore, CCCP, suggesting that the release may be dependent upon heme removal and uptake.

HpuA is a 35-kDa surface-accessible lipoprotein that clearly must be involved in the binding of hemoglobin or hemoglobin–haptoglobin and heme removal, since it is required for heme uptake from these proteins. However, there is no direct evidence for independent binding of either protein in the absence of HpuB, even with sensitive methods; and the binding interaction can only be inferred from indirect experiments such as protection from protease activity by ligand binding [49].

The HmbR receptor is comprised of a single integral outer membrane protein [55]. HmbR is only capable of binding and acquiring heme from hemoglobin and not hemoglobin–haptoglobin complexes. A topology model was developed for HmbR, based on homology to known TonB-dependent receptors, and was used to target mutations to the predicted outer membrane loops and the plug region using a HmbR-mediated uptake system reconstituted in *Escherichia coli* [38]. In this study, it was shown that deletion of predicted loops 2 or 3 reduced or eliminated hemoglobin binding without compromising heme uptake, whereas deletion of predicted loops 6 or 7 abrogated heme uptake without impairment of hemoglobin binding. Although these studies localized functional epitopes to individual surface loops and provided some insights into the heme-uptake process, the mechanism of heme removal and uptake is still not understood.

The transport of heme from the periplasm to the cytoplasm is likely mediated by a heme-specific ABC transport system (Fig. 11.4), similar to the HemTUV system employed by *Yersinia enterocolitica* [54], but none has been identified to date. Insertional inactivation of the FbpA protein did not influence growth on hemoglobin [22], refuting prior suggestions that it was involved in heme iron uptake. The heme molecule is transported into the cytoplasm where iron removal is mediated by a heme oxygenase enzyme encoded by hemO [63]. The activity of this enzyme is absolutely required for use of heme-containing compounds as iron sources; and interestingly enough the hemO gene is found immediately upstream of the hemoglobin receptor gene hmbR (Fig. 11.3) and is transcribed in the same orientation [63]. Although hmbR appears to have its own promoter and Fur box sequences immediately upstream, insertional mutagenesis of hemO results in essentially no HmbR expression, suggesting that the mutation has a polar effect on the transcription of hmbR and that the two genes are cotranscribed. The unlinked hpuAB genes were unaffected in the hemO mutant [63].

11.5
Acquisition of Siderophore Iron

It is clear that siderophores do not facilitate acquisition of iron for growth of meningococci during the invasive phase of infection, since they do not produce siderophores and they invade otherwise sterile body compartments. However, during colonization, there may be a diversity of different siderophores being produced by the resident microflora that could potentially serve as an iron source for meningococci. Since siderophore receptors are characteristically highly specific for a given siderophore, it is difficult to systematically evaluate the ability of meningococci to utilize siderophore iron in the absence of the knowledge of what siderophores would be available in the mucosal environment of the human nasopharynx.

The phenolate siderophore from *E. coli*, aerobactin, can provide iron for growth to gonococci [61] and meningococci, but no homolog of the aerobactin receptor, IutA, has been detected in gonococci. High levels of the catecholate siderophore from *E. coli*, enterobactin, can enhance the growth of iron-limited meningococci [11]; and insertional inactivation of the ferric enterobactin receptor, FetA, abrogated the growth enhancement. However, while this receptor can bind and transport enterobactin, it is a relatively low-affinity receptor for this ligand, suggesting it is not the natural substrate. The meningococcal genomes contain genes encoding a number of TonB-dependent receptor homologs whose function have not been determined and it is likely that most of these are receptors for siderophores that meningococci could encounter on the mucosal surface.

11.6
Regulation of Iron Import and Storage

Although iron is an essential element required by *N. meningitidis* and other bacteria, there are serious consequences associated with iron overload. In the absence of known mechanisms for the secretion of iron, regulating its entry into the cell is the obvious first step to avoid iron overload. Regulation of iron-uptake systems in most Gram-negative bacteria is accomplished by regulation at the level of transcription by the ferric uptake regulatory (Fur) protein [18]. In the presence of iron, Fur recognizes and binds to a consensus sequence, known as the Fur or iron box, either within or nearby the promoter region of iron-regulated genes and blocks transcription by RNA polymerase. Increased intracellular iron levels also induces the enhanced expression of loci involved in iron storage, a process also mediated by Fur. However, the positive regulation by Fur is not due to direct interaction with the promoter regions of these genes but by repressing the synthesis of regulatory RNA molecules that repress these loci [32]. Thus, both the negative and positive regulation by Fur is by the same mechanism of inhibition of transcription.

The structure of the *Pseudomonas aeruginosa* Fur protein demonstrates that Fur is present as a dimer through interactions of the C-terminal domains of the protein, while the N-terminal portion is involved in DNA binding [40]. The protein has two metal ion-binding sites. One site is for binding a zinc ion, which may be important for maintenance of overall structure, while the second site, which binds a ferrous ion, apparently induces a conformational change that allows the dimerized regulator to bind DNA [40].

N. meningitidis possesses a Fur homolog and many genes involved in iron acquisition are regulated by this protein, including *tbp* [15], *lbp*, *fbp* [21, 59], *hpuA* [30] and *hmbR* [55].

Little is known about the proteins that are involved in capturing and distributing iron once it enters the cytoplasm, where it will either be used for production of the various proteins that use iron or iron complexes as a cofactor, or stored for future use. However, it is apparent that a different set of proteins are required for initially handling iron obtained from heme iron, siderophore iron or ferric iron-uptake pathways.

Once the capacity of the systems for production of iron-containing proteins is exceeded, the excess iron must be stored in a form that reduces its ability to participate in the Fenton reaction [39], which generates the extremely reactive hydroxyl radical that is capable of damaging a variety of biological molecules including DNA [20]. Bacteria store excess iron in ferritin or bacterioferritin protein complexes. It appears that meningococci only have bacterioferritin, based on analysis of the meningococcal genomes. While the function and role of bacterioferritin has not been specifically studied in *N. meningitidis*, studies in the closely related species *N. gonorrhoeae* should readily be extrapolated to meningococci. Bfr is a large complex ($\sim$400 kDa), made up of subunits of BfrA (18 kDa) and BfrB (22 kDa), with an internal cavity that is believed to be capable of storing several thousand iron atoms [12]. Insertional mutagenesis of *bfrB* led to reduced growth under iron-restricted conditions and rendered the cell more sensitive to hydrogen peroxide and the superoxide anion-generating compound paraquat [12], suggesting Bfr may serve as a potential iron source during periods of transient iron-depravation and additionally helps the bacterium deal with oxidative stress. The structural genes encoding BfrA and B are arranged in an operon [58] and a potential Fur box was identified within the promoter region of the operon, however Fur- or iron-dependent regulation of *bfrAB* remains to be demonstrated.

References

1 Aisen, P., C. Enns, M. Wessling-Resnick **2001**, Chemistry and biology of eukaryotic iron metabolism, Int J Biochem Cell Biol 33, 940–959.

2 Alcantara, J., J. S. Padda, A. B. Schryvers **1992**, The N-linked oligosaccharides of human lactoferrin are not required for binding to bacterial lactoferrin receptors, Can J Microbiol 38, 1202–1205.

3 Alcantara, J., R.-H. Yu, A. B. Schryvers **1993**, The region of human transferrin involved in binding to bacterial transferrin receptors is localized in the C-lobe, Mol Microbiol 8, 1135–1143.

4 Anderson, D. S., P. Adhikari, A. J. Nowalk, C. Y. Chen, T. A. Mietzner **2004**, The hFbpABC transporter from Haemophilus influenzae functions as a binding protein-dependent ABC transporter with high specificity and affinity for ferric iron, J Bacteriol 186, 6220–6229.

5 Anderson, J. E., M. M. Hobbs, G. D. Biswas, P. F. Sparling **2003**, Opposing selective forces for expression of the gonococcal lactoferrin receptor, Mol Microbiol 48, 1325–1337.

6 Archibald, F. S., I. W. DeVoe **1980**, Iron acquisition by Neisseria meningitidis in vitro, Infect Immun 27, 322–334.

7 Archibald, F. S., I. W. DeVoe **1979**, Removal of iron from human transferrin by Neisseria meningitidis, FEMS Microbiol Lett 6, 159–162.

8 Baltes, N., I. Hennig-Pauka, G. F. Gerlach **2002**, Both transferrin binding proteins are virulence factors in Actinobacillus pleuropneumoniae serotype 7 infection, FEMS Microbiol Lett 209, 283–287.

9 Bonnah, R. A., A. B. Schryvers **1998**, Preparation and characterization of Neisseria meningitidis mutants deficient in the production of the human lactoferrin binding proteins LbpA and LbpB, J Bacteriol 180, 3080–3090.

10 Bonnah, R. A., R.-H. Yu, A. B. Schryvers **1995**, Biochemical analysis of lactoferrin receptors in the neisseriaceae: identification of a second bacterial lactoferrin receptor protein, Microb Pathog 19, 285–297.

11 Carson, S. D., P. E. Klebba, S. M. Newton, P. F. Sparling **1999**, Ferric enterobactin binding and utilization by Neisseria gonorrhoeae, J Bacteriol 181, 2895–2901.

12 Chen, C. Y., S. A. Morse **1999**, Neisseria gonorrhoeae bacterioferritin: structural heterogeneity, involvement in iron storage and protection against oxidative stress, Microbiology 145, 2967–2975.

13 Cornelissen, C. N., M. Kelley, M. M. Hobbs, J. E. Anderson, J. G. Cannon, M. S. Cohen, P. F. Sparling **1998**, The transferrin receptor expressed by gonococcal strain FA1090 is required for the experimental infection of human male volunteers, Mol Microbiol 27, 611–616.

14 Coulton, J. W., J. C. S. Pang **1983**, Transport of hemin by Haemophilus influenzae type b, Curr Microbiol 9, 93–98.

15 Delany, I., R. Ieva, C. Alaimo, R. Rappuoli, V. Scarlato **2003**, The iron-responsive regulator Fur is transcriptionally autoregulated and not essential in Neisseria meningitidis, J Bacteriol 185, 6032–6041.

16 Dhungana, S., C. H. Taboy, D. S. Anderson, K. G. Vaughan, P. Aisen, T. A. Mietzner, A. L. Crumbliss **2003**, The influence of the synergistic anion on iron chelation by ferric binding protein, a bacterial transferrin, Proc Natl Acad Sci USA 100, 3659–3664.

17 Dyer, D. W., E. P. West, P. F. Sparling **1987**, Effects of serum carrier proteins on the growth of pathogenic neisseriae with heme-bound iron, Infect Immun 55, 2171–2175.

18 Escolar, L., J. Perez-Martin, V. de Lorenzo **1999**, Opening the iron box: transcriptional metalloregulation by the Fur protein, J Bacteriol 181, 6223–6229.

19 Irwin, S. W., N. Averill, C. Y. Cheng, A. B. Schryvers **1993**, Preparation and analysis of isogenic mutants in the transferrin receptor protein genes, tbp1 and tbp2, from Neisseria meningitidis, Mol Microbiol 8, 1125–1133.

20 Keyer, K., A. S. Gort, J. A. Imlay **1995**, Superoxide and the production of oxidative DNA damage, J Bacteriol 177, 6782–6790.

21 Khun, H.H., V. Deved, H. Wong, B.C. Lee **2000**, fbpABC gene cluster in Neisseria meningitidis is transcribed as an operon, Infect Immun 68, 7166–7171.

22 Khun, H.H., S.D. Kirby, B.C. Lee **1998**, A Neisseria meningitidis fbpABC mutant is incapable of using nonheme iron for growth, Infect Immun 66, 2330–2336.

23 Krell, T., G. Renauld-Mongenie, M.C. Nicolai, S. Fraysse, M. Chevalier, Y. Berard, J. Oakhill, R.W. Evans, A. Gorringe, L. Lissolo **2003**, Insight into the structure and function of the transferrin receptor from Neisseria meningitidis using microcalorimetric techniques, J Biol Chem 278, 14712–14722.

24 Larson, J.A., D.L. Higashi, I. Stojiljkovic, M. So **2002**, Replication of Neisseria meningitidis within epithelial cells requires TonB-dependent acquisition of host cell iron, Infect Immun 70, 1461–1467.

25 Larson, J.A., H.L. Howie, M. So **2004**, Neisseria meningitidis accelerates ferritin degradation in host epithelial cells to yield an essential iron source, Mol Microbiol 53, 807–820.

26 Legrain, M., E. Jacobs, S.W. Irwin, A.B. Schryvers, M.J. Quentin-Millet **1993**, Cloning and characterization of Neisseria meningitidis genes encoding the transferrin binding proteins Tbp1 and Tbp2, Gene 130, 73–80.

27 Leibman, A., P. Aisen **1979**, Distribution of iron between the binding sites of transferrin in serum: methods and results in normal human subjects, Blood 53, 1058–1065.

28 Lewis, L.A., D.W. Dyer **1995**, Identification of an iron-regulated outer membrane protein of Neisseria meningitidis involved in the utilization of hemoglobin complexed to haptoglobin, J Bacteriol 177, 1299–1306.

29 Lewis, L.A., M. Gipson, K. Hartman, T. Ownbey, J. Vaughn, D.W. Dyer **1999**, Phase variation of HpuAB and HmbR, two distinct haemoglobin receptors of Neisseria meningitidis DNM2, Mol Microbiol 32, 977–989.

30 Lewis, L.A., E. Gray, Y.P. Wang, B.A. Roe, D.W. Dyer **1997**, Molecular characterization of hpuAB, the haemoglobin-haptoglobin-utilization operon of Neisseria meningitidis, Mol Microbiol 23, 737–749.

31 Masri, H.P., C.N. Cornelissen, **2002**, Specific ligand binding attributable to individual epitopes of gonococcal transferrin binding protein A, Infect Immun 70, 732–740.

32 Masse, E., S. Gottesman **2002**, A small RNA regulates the expression of genes involved in iron metabolism in Escherichia coli, Proc Natl Acad Sci USA 99, 4620–4625.

33 Merz, A.J., M. So **2000**, Interactions of pathogenic neisseriae with epithelial cell membranes, Annu Rev Cell Dev Biol 16, 423–457.

34 Mickelsen, P.A., E. Blackman, P.F. Sparling **1982**, Ability of Neisseria gonorrhoeae, Neisseria meningitidis, commensal Neisseria species to obtain iron from lactoferrin, Infect Immun 35, 915–920.

35 Mietzner, T.A., S.A. Morse **1994**, The role of iron-binding proteins in the survival of pathogenic bacteria, Annu Rev Nutr 14, 471–493.

36 Oakhill, J.S., B.J. Sutton, A.R. Gorringe, R.W. Evans **2005**, Homology modelling of transferrin-binding protein A from Neisseria meningitidis, Protein Eng Des Sel 18, 221–228.

37 Padda, J.S., A.B. Schryvers **1990**, N-linked oligosaccharides of human transferrin are not required for binding to bacterial transferrin receptors, Infect Immun 58, 2972–2976.

38 Perkins-Balding, D., M.T. Baer, I. Stojiljkovic **2003**, Identification of functionally important regions of a haemoglobin receptor from Neisseria meningitidis, Microbiology 149, 3423–3435.

39 Pierre, J.L., M. Fontecave **1999**, Iron and activated oxygen species in biology: the basic chemistry, Biometals 12, 195–199.

40 Pohl, E., J.C. Haller, A. Mijovilovich, W. Meyer-Klaucke, E. Garman, M.L. Vasil **2003**, Architecture of a protein central to iron homeostasis: crystal structure and spectroscopic analysis of the ferric uptake regulator, Mol Microbiol 47, 903–915.

41 Renauld-Mongenie, G., L. Lins, T. Krell, L. Laffly, M. Mignon, M. Dupuy, R.M.

Delrue, F. Guinet-Morlot, R. Brasseur, L. Lissolo **2004**, Transferrin-binding protein B of Neisseria meningitidis: sequence-based identification of the transferrin-binding site confirmed by site-directed mutagenesis, J Bacteriol 186, 850–857.

42 Renauld-Mongenie, G., D. Poncet, M. Mignon, S. Fraysse, C. Chabanel, B. Danve, T. Krell, M.-J. Quentin-Millet **2004**, Role of transferrin receptor from a Neisseria meningitidis tbpB isotype II strain in human transferrin binding and virulence, Infect Immun 72, 3461–3470.

43 Retzer, M. D., A. Kabani, L. Button, R.-H. Yu, A. B. Schryvers **1996**, Production and characterization of chimeric transferrins for the determination of the binding domains for bacterial transferrin receptors, J Biol Chem 271, 1166–1173.

44 Retzer, M. D., R.-H. Yu, A. B. Schryvers **1999**, Identification of sequences in human transferrin that bind to the bacterial receptor protein, transferrin-binding protein B, Mol Microbiol 32, 111–121.

45 Retzer, M. D., R.-H. Yu, Y. Zhang, G. C. Gonzalez, A. B. Schryvers **1998**, Discrimination between apo and iron-loaded forms of transferrin by transferrin binding protein B and its N-terminal subfragment, Microb Pathog 25, 175–180.

46 Richardson, A. R., I. Stojiljkovic **1999**, HmbR, a hemoglobin-binding outer membrane protein of Neisseria meningitidis, undergoes phase variation, J Bacteriol 181, 2067–2074.

47 Rohde, K. H., D. W. Dyer **2004**, Analysis of haptoglobin and hemoglobin-haptoglobin interactions with the Neisseria meningitidis TonB-dependent receptor HpuAB by flow cytometry, Infect Immun 72, 2494–2506.

48 Rohde, K. H., D. W. Dyer **2003**, Mechanisms of iron acquisition by the human pathogens Neisseria meningitidis and Neisseria gonorrhoeae, Front Biosci 8, D1186–D1218.

49 Rohde, K. H., A. F. Gillaspy, M. D. Hatfield, L.aA. Lewis, D. W. Dyer **2002**, Interactions of haemoglobin with the Neisseria meningitidis receptor HpuAB: the role of TonB and an intact proton motive force, Mol Microbiol 43, 335–354.

50 Schryvers, A. B., G. C. Gonzalez **1989**, Comparison of the abilities of different protein sources of iron to enhance Neisseria meningitidis infection in mice, Infect Immun 57, 2425–2429.

51 Schryvers, A. B., L. J. Morris **1988**, Identification and characterization of the human lactoferrin-binding protein from Neisseria meningitidis, Infect Immun 56, 1144–1149.

52 Schryvers, A. B., L. J. Morris **1988**, Identification and characterization of the transferrin receptor from Neisseria meningitidis, Mol Microbiol 2, 281–288.

53 Sims, K. L., A. B. Schryvers **2003**, Peptide–peptide interactions between human transferrin and transferrin binding protein B from Moraxella catarrhalis, J Bacteriol 185, 2603–2610.

54 Stojiljkovic, I., K. Hantke **1994**, Transport of haemin across the cytoplasmic membrane through a haemin-specific periplasmic binding protein-dependent transport system in Yersinia enterocolitica, Mol Microbiol 13, 719–732.

55 Stojiljkovic, I., V. Hwa, L. de Saint Martin, P. O'Garoa, X. Nassif, F. Heffron, M. So **1995**, The Neisseria meningitidis haemoglobin receptor: its role in iron utilization and virulence, Mol Microbiol 15, 531–541.

56 Stojiljkovic, I., N. Srinivasan **1997**, Neisseria meningitidis tonB, exbB, exbD genes: Ton-dependent utilization of protein-bound iron in neisseriae, J Bacteriol 179, 805–812.

57 Taha, M. K., A. E. Deghmane, A. Antignac, M. L. Zarantonelli, M. Larribe, J. M. Alonso **2002**, The duality of virulence and transmissibility in Neisseria meningitidis, Trends Microbiol 10, 376–382.

58 Tettelin, H., N. J. Saunders, J. Heidelberg, A. C. Jeffries, K. E. Nelson, J. A. Eisen, K. A. Ketchum, D. W. Hood, J. F. Peden, R. J. Dodson, W. C. Nelson, M. L. Gwinn, R. DeBoy, J. D. Peterson, E. K. Hickey, D. H. Haft, S. L. Salzberg, O. White, R. D. Fleischmann, B. A. Dougherty, T. Mason, A. Ciecko, D. S. Parksey, E. Blair **2000**, Complete genome sequence of Neisseria meningitidis serogroup B strain MC58, Science 287, 1809–1815.

59 Thomas, C. E., P. F. Sparling, **1994**, Identification and cloning of a fur homologue from Neisseria meningitidis, Mol Microbiol 11, 725–737.
60 Wandersman, C., I. Stojiljkovic **2000**, Bacterial heme sources: the role of heme, hemoprotein receptors and hemophores, Curr Opin Microbiol 3, 215–220.
61 West, S. E. H., P. F. Sparling **1987**, Aerobactin utilization by Neisseria gonorrhoeae and cloning of a genomic DNA fragment that complements Escherichia coli fhuB mutations, J Bacteriol 169, 3414–3421.
62 Yost-Daljev, M. K., C. N. Cornelissen **2004**, Determination of surface-exposed, functional domains of gonococcal transferrin-binding protein A, Infect Immun 72, 1775–1785.
63 Zhu, W. M., D. J. Hunt, A. R. Richardson, I. Stojiljkovic **2000**, Use of heme compounds as iron sources by pathogenic neisseriae requires the product of the hemO gene, J Bacteriol 182, 439–447.

12
Genetics, Structure and Function of Pili

Philippe C. Morand and Thomas Rudel

12.1
Introduction

Among the bacterial factors that contribute to the pathophysiology of meningococcal infection, the type IV pili (tfp) are of central importance. Together with other virulence factors, like Opa proteins or the capsule, they can consistently be found in clinical isolates [1]. Recent findings challenge the simple historical view of pili as colonization factors. Although there is no doubt about their importance in mediating the contact of *N. meningitidis* to the host cells surface, tfp are also involved in bacterial movement and transformation competence, induce multiple signalling events in host cells, mediate bacterial aggregation and communication. Moreover, pili of pathogenic *Neisseria* undergo spontaneous phase and antigenic variation, resulting in mixed bacterial populations expressing pili or not, or with structurally different pili. Beside its role in escaping the host immune response, pilus variation also affects functions associated with tfp.

Tfp are found in a variety of Gram negative bacteria. They are flexible filaments that are extremely thin (50–80 Å), are up to several micrometers long (Fig. 12.1) and can sustain considerable mechanical stress. The major component of the tfp is the pilin subunit, the helical assembly of which constitutes the scaffold of the fiber. Two subclasses of tfp have been identified on the basis of sequence homologies between pilin subunits (for a review, see [2]). Pilins in the type IVa group have an average length of about 150 amino acids, a signal peptide not exceeding six amino acids and have a +1 N-methylated N-terminal residue which is a phenylalanine. Neisserial tfp belong to type IVa. In contrast, the pilins in group IVb show a longer mature sequence, as well as longer signal peptides (up to 30 amino acids). Whereas group IVa tfp are expressed by a wide range of bacteria found in mammals or plants, all group IVb tfp have been described in bacteria that have a tropism for the human intestine.

Tfp also share structural similarities with other biological systems that, at least at first sight, serve different functions. For example, proteins required for the assembly of filamentous phages are structurally related to tfp. Moreover, tfp

Handbook of Meningococcal Disease. Infection Biology, Vaccination, Clinical Management.
Edited by M. Frosch and M.C.J. Maiden

ISBN: 3-527-31260-9

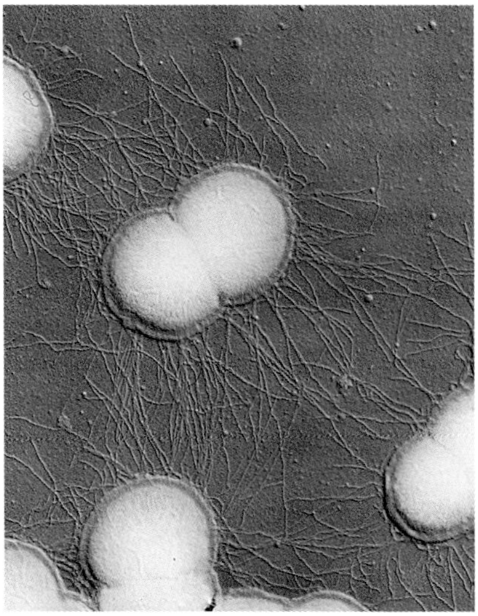

Fig. 12.1 Scanning electron micrograph of neisserial tfp (in this case *N. gonorrhoeae*; by courtesy of J. A. Tainer).

and type II secretion systems (general secretory pathway, GSP) share common architectural components. The similarity is so close that both systems, when they are concomitantly found in bacteria, can share components. This is the case for the prepilin peptidase of *P. aeruginosa*, which is at the same time part of the tfp machinery and of the type II secretion system in the same host. The similarity between the GSP and tfp is also strengthened by the finding that some components of the GSP, the pseudopilins, can form pili that extend on the bacterial surface. Thus, analogy between the two systems suggests that the tfp might be seen as a particular form of a secretion system. Similarly, the GSP may function by alternating cycles of assembly and disassembly of a "pseudopilus" in the periplasm, resulting in the propelling of substrates through the outer membrane.

12.2 Macromolecular Structure and Biogenesis

12.2.1 The tfp Machinery in *N. meningitidis*

Although sharing similar architectures, tfp systems found in different bacterial species each have their particularities, which is also reflected in the nomenclature diversity for different orthologs (for reviews, see [3, 4]). The tfp of pathogenic *Neisseria* spp. have been studied in both the closely related *N. meningitidis* and *N. gonorrhoeae* species and it is generally assumed that most observations made in one system are also valid for the other. This is however not always the case and we will try to emphasize structural or functional differences that distinguish *N. meningitidis* from *N. gonorrhoeae*.

Neisserial tfp are highly dynamic structures which undergo rapid cycles of extension and retraction. They stem from the inner membrane to the bacterial surface, passing through the outer membrane. The components involved in tfp assembly, retraction and specific functions are distributed at the vicinity of the bacterial membranes, from the inner side of the cytoplasmic membrane to the outer membrane, and at the pilus fiber (Fig. 12.2). A recent systematic screen

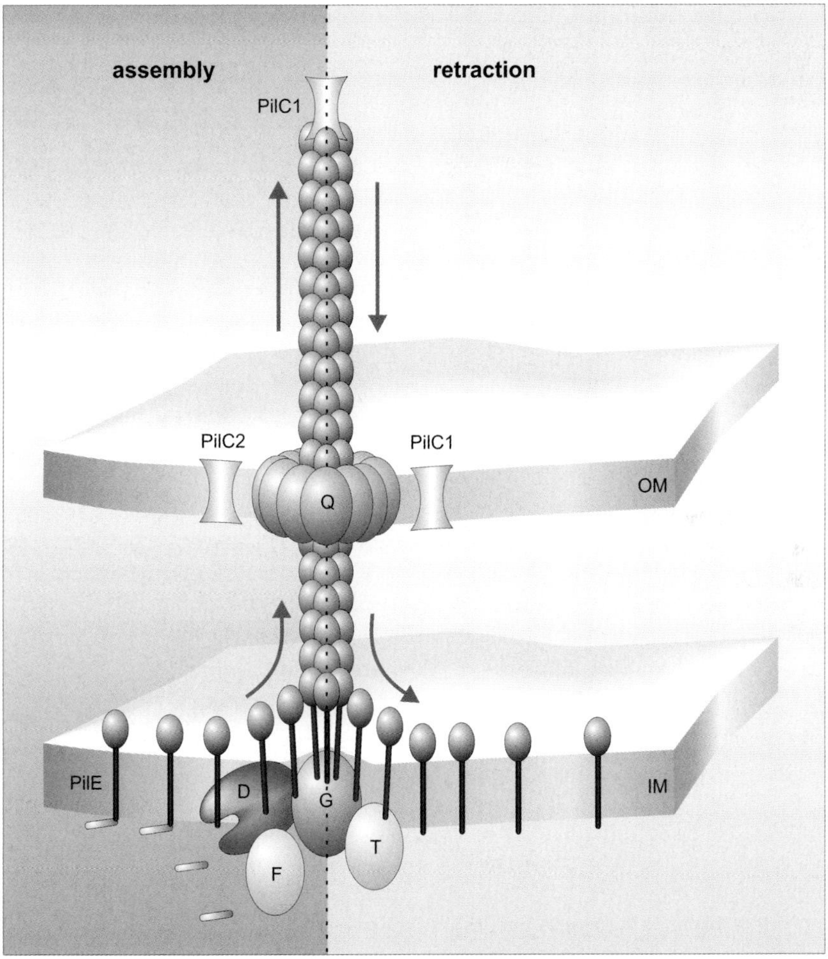

Fig. 12.2 Functional architecture of neisserial tfp. The helical assembly of pilin (PilE) into fibers relies on proteins located in or in the vicinity of the cytoplasmic membrane (PilD, PilG, PilF) and extrusion to the bacterial surface through an outer membrane macromolecular complex (PilQ, stabilized by PilP and PilW, not shown). Retraction is mediated by the ATPase PilT. See text for details.

for tfp biogenesis genes on the basis of an ordered mutation library identified 15 genes required for biogenesis [5]. Most of these genes are scattered around the genome, with some exceptions like the gene coding for *pilQ*, which is located in an operon (*pilM, pilN, pilO, pilP, pilQ*, respectively). In addition to proteins required for tfp expression, PilT, PilU, PilC and the recently discovered PilX are involved in tfp function but are dispensable for assembly (see below) [5].

12.2.1.1 The Pilin: PilE

The major neisserial pilus subunit, the pilin, is encoded by the *pilE* gene. In most cases, only one intact copy of *pilE* is present on the chromosome, but some gonococcal strains may harbor two copies of *pilE*. Along with *pilE*, up to eight loci containing truncated and silent copies of the pilin gene named *pilS* (*pil*in, *s*ilent) are found on the chromosome. *pilS* copies are not expressed but serve as a source of variant pilin gene sequences which occasionally recombine with *pilE*, leading to the expression of variant PilE (see below). In *N. meningitidis*, *pilS* loci are clustered near *pilE*, whereas they are scattered across the genome in *N. gonorrhoeae*. Pilin is first synthesized as a preprotein, the prepilin, which is targeted to the inner membrane due to its hydrophobicity. It is then cleaved at the inner membrane by the prepilin peptidase PilD. The mature pilin subunit is characterized by a conserved hydrophobic N-terminal moiety, which within the pilus is involved in the cohesion of the subunits as a fiber. The polymorphic C-terminus of pilin is partially exposed at the surface of the assembled pilus. The pilin also harbors two cysteine residues that build a disulfide bridge, involved in the formation of the surface accessible, variable and immune dominant part of the pilus (Fig. 12.3).

Two classes of pilin differing in antibody reactivity can be found in *N. meningitidis*. The class I meningococcal pilins are similar to gonococcal pilins and are recognized by a monoclonal antibody (SM1), that is specific to the epitope 49–53 found in the pilin of the strain *N. gonorrhoeae* MS11. Meningococcal class II pilins are not recognized by this antibody and are encoded from a different locus than class I pilins [6]. Class II pilins are slightly shorter than class I, and lack some domains usually found in class I pilins. Commensal *Neisseria* species like *N. lactamica* or *N. cinerea* also express class II pilins. So far, expression of either class I or II pilin could not be correlated to differences in pathogenicity.

Some pilin variants are processed at an additional cleavage site, leading to the removal of 39 amino-acids from the N-terminus. This truncated form of pilin, named S-pilin (soluble, in contrast to the mature protein that is not water-soluble), can not assemble to fibers and is released into the medium [7]. Strains expressing S-pilin are poorly piliated and poorly adhesive. Although initially described and more abundant in *N. gonorrhoeae*, S-pilin can also be observed in *N. meningitidis*, its formation being linked to pilin glycosylation [8].

Glycosylation is one of a number of different post-translational modifications of pilin, which, in addition to variations of the primary sequence, may account for the structural diversity of pilin. Glycosylation of bacterial proteins is an un-

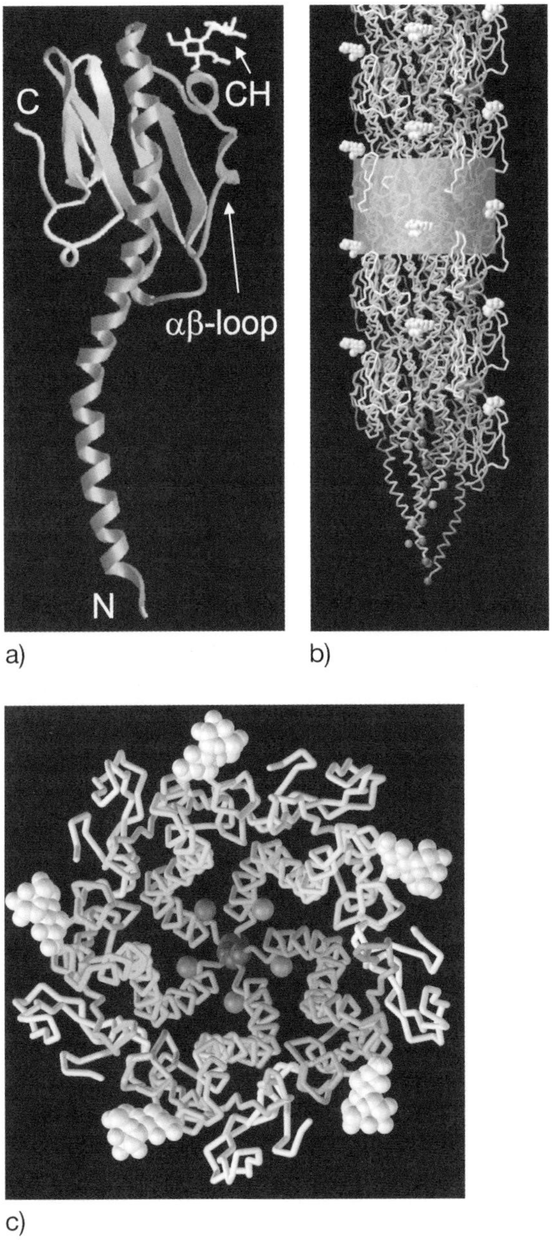

Fig. 12.3 Structural model for pilin (adapted from [11]). (a) Structure of the pilin monomer. Colors indicate different functional parts of pilin. The carbohydrate (CH), N-terminus (N) and C-terminus (C) and the *αβ*-loop is indicated. (b) The helical assembly of the monomer forms the pilus fiber. (c) Projection of a cross section of the pilus fiber. Different colors indicate individual pilin subunits (by courtesy of J. A. Tainer). (This figure also appears with the color plates.)

usual phenomenon and *Neisseria* spp. were the first pathogenic eubacteria for which pilin glycosylation could be observed (for a review, see [9, 10]). Definitive evidence for glycosylation of pilin was provided by the structural analysis of *N. gonorrhoeae* pilin crystals that identified an O-linked disaccharide Gal(alpha1,3)-GlcNAc bound to Ser63 [11]. In *N. meningitidis*, O-glycosylation of class I pilin could also be established (for a review, see [12]) and both class I and class II pilins have been found to be glycosylated [13]. Like in *N. gonorrhoeae*, the glycosylation site was located on Ser63, but instead of a disaccharide, the trisaccharide Gal(beta1,4)Gal(alpha1,3)2,4-diacetimido-2,4,6-trideoxyhexose (DATDH) was attached to pilin via the unusual sugar DATDH [14]. The nature of the sugar moiety linked to pilin was the subject of controversy since the glycosylation residue described in *N. gonorrhoeae* was also described in *N. meningitidis* [15], but a later report suggested DATDH as the only neisserial O-linked moiety in both species [16]. Apart from the observation that pilin glycosylation affects the production of S-pilin and may thereby indirectly affect tfp function [8], there is no clear evidence that pilin glycosylation significantly contributes to bacterial adhesion or other tfp functions associated with pathogenesis.

Pilin glycosylation in *N. meningitidis* is under the control of the *pgl* gene cluster [17–20], which encodes genes characterized by length polymorphisms. The meningococcal *pglA* seems to be subject to phase variation due to the presence of a poly-G stretch, which is not the case for *pgtA*, the gonococcal homolog to *pglA* [21].

Beside glycosylation, an alpha-glycerophosphate decorates Ser93 of pilin, in a serogroup B strain [22]. Although glycerophosphate is commonly found in bacterial cell surface saccharides, it is an unusual protein substituent, the function of which on pili is not known.

Crystallographic data of gonococcal pilin from strain MS11 revealed the presence of a phosphate group covalently linked to Ser68 [23]. Loss of phosphorylation alters the morphology of the pilus fiber, but has no notable effect on adhesion, piliation, twitching motility or transformation competence. However, later reports suggested that, rather than a phosphate group, Ser68 in gonococcal pilin is modified with O-linked forms of either phosphorylcholine (PC) or phosphoethanolamine (PE) [16]. Neisserial pili from both *N. meningitidis* and *N. gonorrhoeae* react with a monoclonal antibody recognizing a PC epitope [24]. Frequently attached to bacterial sugar moieties, PC also decorates the LPS of commensal *Neisseria* spp. [25] but is not bound to the pilin-linked trisaccharide [26]. The presence of this epitope correlates with the expression of the *pptA* gene (pilin phosphorylcholine transferase A), which has been shown to be subject to phase variation in *N. meningitidis*. The prepilin-like PilV, one of the proteins involved in bacterial adherence to host cells, influences the ratio of PE and PC present on Ser68 of pilin, suggesting a role for PilV in the modulation of pilus structure and antigenicity.

12.2.1.2 **Inner Membrane Proteins: PilD and PilG**

PilD is a leader peptidase localized to the inner membrane that specifically recognizes the N-terminal part of prepilin and of prepilin-like molecules. A single copy of PilD is found in the chromosome [27]. Most of our knowledge about PilD relies on studies in *P. aeruginosa*. The substrate cleavage by PilD depends on the presence of a glycine residue at position –1 of the cleavage site [28]. Moreover, PilD activity also leads to the methylation of the N-terminal phenylalanine of the mature protein product, which relies on the presence of a glutamic acid in position +5 of the substrate. However, lack of methylation seems to have little effect on tfp assembly [29].

PilG is an inner membrane protein required for tfp formation and transformation competence [30]. In *P. aeruginosa*, the accumulation of mature pilin in the inner membrane in the absence of PilG suggests that it acts downstream of PilD.

12.2.1.3 **The Secretin PilQ and Outer Membrane Components**

PilQ forms a channel in the outer membrane through which the pilus is extruded to the bacterial surface. It is a member of a family of outer membrane proteins termed secretins, which are involved in secretion of a variety of substrates. Neisserial C-terminal regions of PilQ proteins show a significant level of identity with the PulD secretin of the type II secretion system in *Klebsiella oxytoca*. In *N. gonorrhoeae*, loss of PilQ function leads to the absence of tfp expression and triggers S-pilin secretion [31]. Furthermore, concomitant deletion of *pilQ* and of the ATPase *pilT* results in the accumulation of pili in the periplasm of gonococci [32], suggesting that fiber assembly occurs independently of PilQ. Functional PilQ forms a large homododecameric complex (approx. 900 kDa). Transmission electron microscopy and cryoelectron microscopy analysis of the meningococcal PilQ complex [33, 34] revealed a donut-shaped macromolecular structure, in the center of which the pilus is thought to pass through (Fig. 12.4). The dodecameric structure has a 4-fold symmetry, which suggests that, within this complex, a PilQ monomer can have three different conformations. The complex has a gated cavity with a length of 90 Å, which suggests that the protein complex has to undergo drastic conformational changes to allow the passage of the pilus. Thus PilQ probably has an active role in tfp biogenesis, rather than just being a pore for the fiber. Stable oligomerization of PilQ requires the lipoprotein PilP [35], the presence of an outer membrane protein Omp85 [36], as well as the outer membrane lipoprotein PilW that is required for the stabilization of the pilus, but not for its formation [5].

12.2.1.4 **Nucleotide-binding Proteins**

Nucleotide (NTP)-binding proteins are basic components of all tfp machineries. They usually contain a "walker box" for the binding of ATP and belong to the family of AAA ATPases (ATPases associated with various cellular activities), which also includes chaperones and mechanoenzymes (for a review, see [37]).

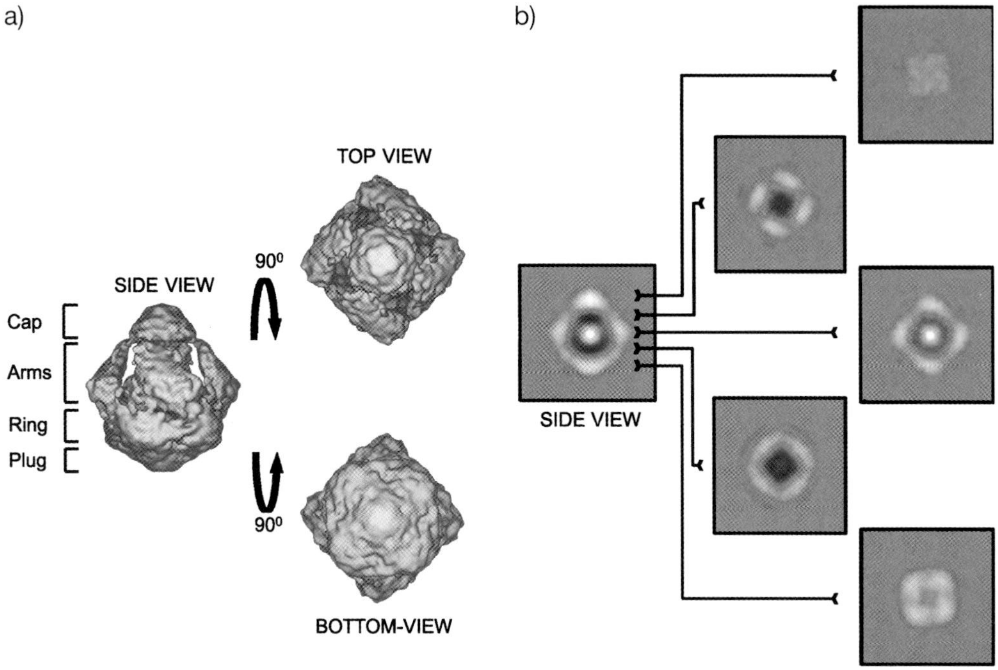

Fig. 12.4 Model for the outer membrane PilQ complex (adapted from [34]). Schematic representation of the surface (A) and two-dimensional cross sections (B) of the PilQ complex. The four-fold symmetry of the dodecameric complex and the presence of a gated channel suggest that PilQ function relies on a conformational change of the subunit (by courtesy of J. Derrick).

PilT is dispensable for assembly and expression of tfp on the cell surface, but is required for their retraction. It was initially reported as an effector for transformation competence and twitching motility [38] and plays a key role in the interaction with the host cell [39], since its absence prevents the onset of intimate adhesion. As a consequence, pili in *pilT* mutants are formed but not retracted, and the bacteria remain attached as aggregates on the cell surface, a phenotype called localized adherence.

Like other AAA ATPases, PilT has an hexameric structure [40] and, at least *in vitro*, hydrolyzes ATP [41, 42]. *In vivo*, PilT can be found both associated with the inner membrane and in the cytoplasm [42, 43].

In gonococci, pilT forms an operon with pilU. Like PilT, PilU was described as a member of the GspE/TrbB-like family of proteins, which feature centrally located domains implicated in ATP binding and hydrolysis. PilU is 33% identical to PilT but, unlike PilT is not required for transformation competence and twitching motility. The PilU mutants are also characterized by an increased adherence to human cells; and they lack the interbacterial autoagglutination that is seen in the absence of PilT. Since PilT seems to inhibit tfp-associated aggregation and PilU seems to promote it, it was proposed that PilU might be a conditional antagonist of PilT and could modulate its activity [44].

Whereas PilT is required for fiber retraction, another member of the AAA ATPases, PilF, is required for tfp expression [27]. In *N. gonorrhoeae,* PilF is encoded from the same locus as pilD. Abolition of PilF results in the absence of tfp and production of soluble pilin, a proteolytic derivative of pilin. By homology with *P. aeruginosa,* PilF is associated with the inner side of the inner membrane, and its functionality relies on the integrity of the "walker box".

12.2.1.5 **The PilC Proteins**

Among the components of the tfp machinery, the PilC proteins play a crucial but still enigmatic role [32, 45–48]. Two alleles were originally discovered in *N. gonorrhoeae* [48]. Expression of both variants is subject to phase variation as a result of frameshifting in homopolymeric "G" tracts located in the open reading frames [48]. Phase variation of PilC has also been shown in meningococcal clinical samples [49]. PilC proteins are associated with the membrane, are exposed at the bacterial surface and can also be recovered from purified pili [46, 50]. PilC-null strains show impaired pilus expression and lack the ability for transformation competence. In addition, they have been described as pilus-tip adhesins in *N. gonorrhoeae* [46].

The two *pilC* loci harbored by *N. gonorrhoeae* are functionally interchangeable. In contrast, in *N. meningitidis,* only PilC1 is equivalent to the gonococcal PilC proteins and required for adhesion. PilC2, which is expressed independently of PilC1, fails to promote adhesion despite identical functions in piliation and transformation competence [45, 51]. Abolition of *pilT* in a PilC-null background restores piliation, confirming the hypothesis that PilC acts as a conditional antagonist of PilT by preventing PilT-mediated retraction [52, 53].

PilC1 and PilC2 in *N. meningitidis* have also been shown to be differently regulated. Both loci share similar promoter regions, but the adhesion-promoting *pilC1* promoter harbors additional regions that are involved in a specific cell contact-dependent upregulation of PilC1 [54]. Upregulation of PilC1 in early stages of adhesion is necessary for full adhesion to human cells. It is however transient, and *pilC1* transcription gradually goes down to basal levels in later adhesion stages. Besides regulation, the specific role for meningococcal PilC1 in adhesion is also due to structural differences with PilC2 in the N-terminal region [51].

12.2.1.6 **The Prepilin-like Proteins**

Pilin (PilE), the major component of the tfp fiber, contains a N-terminal region which is specifically involved in the cohesion of subunits to form a fiber. Interestingly, a number of other proteins share similar N-terminal moieties. These prepilin-like proteins (or "pseudopilins"), although not directly required for tfp biogenesis, are sometimes essential in tfp-related functions.

The first prepilin-like protein identified in pathogenic *Neisseria* was ComP, which was shown to play a central role in transformation competence [55]. Like PilE, this 14-kDa protein needs processing by PilD for full function. Abolition of ComP leads to a defect in DNA uptake, but tfp expression, autoagglutination, twitching motility and adhesion to human cells are unaffected.

In addition to PilE and PilC, PilV has been shown to modulate neisserial binding to human cells [56]. The mechanism by which PilV contributes to adherence is unknown, but the fact that both PilV and PilC can be copurified with pili and that tfp in *pilV* mutants contain reduced levels of PilC suggests that PilV promotes the functional display of PilC in the pilus. Besides its role in adhesion, PilV antagonizes ComP in transformation competence [57] and modulates the levels of phosphorylcholine or phosphoethanolamine on pili [16].

pilX is present in the genomes of *N. meningitidis* as well as *N. gonorrhoeae* [58]. Like PilE, PilX is processed by the prepilin peptidase PilD and is found associated with purified pili. Lack of PilX does not impair tfp expression, transformation competence, twitching motility or pilus anchorage. However, *pilX*-null meningococci are unable to form autoaggregates, which accounts for their poor adhesion to cells. PilX is thus thought to promote inter-bacterial aggregation, but has *per se* no adhesive properties for cells.

12.2.2 Structure of *Neisseria* tfp

No three-dimensional structure is yet available for any tfp. However, atomic resolution structures of type IV pilin have been obtained for *P. aeruginosa, Vibrio cholerae* and *N. gonorrhoeae* (for a review, see [4, 59]).

The current model for the neisserial tfp fiber is largely based on the crystal structure of the gonococcal pilin [11]. The 6-nm fiber is formed by the helical assembly of five monomers of pilin per turn, with a rise of 41 Å per turn (Fig. 12.3). Like other tfp pilins, gonococcal pilin has an N-terminal alpha-helix that is about 85 Å long, the C-terminal part of which is buried in the globular domain of the protein (Fig. 12.3). The N-terminal part of the alpha-helix is involved in the cohesion of the fiber by forming a hydrophobic and flexible core at the center of the fiber, serving as a scaffold for the hydrophobic parts of the pilus. The rest of the molecule, that encompasses the C-terminal part of the alpha-helix and an antiparallel four-stranded β-sheet, forms a globular domain. Outer regions of the globular head are formed by the $\alpha\beta$-loop, that connects the N-terminal α-helix to the β-sheet, as well as by the disulfide-bridged region in the C-terminal part. The $\alpha\beta$-loop is partially exposed to the surface of the fiber and contains two unusual post-translational modifications, an O-glycosylated serine at position 63 and a phosphorylated serine at position 68. The two cysteines in pilin that form a DsbA catalyzed disulfide bridge are essential for tfp assembly and function [60]. This bridged region forms one edge on the globular head domain, opposite to the $\alpha\beta$-loop, and is immunoreactive [61].

On the macromolecular level, the fiber can be divided into three spiralling layers. The innermost part of the fiber is formed by the hydrophobic packing of the α-helixes. The central layer is built by the juxtaposition of the four strands of the antiparallel β-sheet of each subunit, as well as the corresponding sugar loops. This layer is characterized by β-sheet hydrogen bonding and is thought to provide stability of the fiber without covalent bonds between subunits. The outermost layer is composed of the regions 123–143 and 152–158, which are exposed on the surface, and comprises a hypervariable region, the C-terminal tail and the saccharide on Ser63. Although this layer is critical for the biology of the pilus, it contributes little to the cohesion of the fiber. Single meningococcal tfp fibers can associate to form bundles that correlate with increased adhesion to human cells [62].

12.2.3 Assembly, Anchorage and Retraction of tfp

The molecular processes involved in fiber biogenesis are still largely hypothetical. The fiber stems from the cytoplasmic membrane, spans the periplasm and is extruded through the outer membrane by PilQ (Fig. 12.2). Known prerequisites for fiber assembly are the maturation of prepilin by the action of the prepilin peptidase PilD, the presence of the PilG in the cytoplasmic membrane and the expression of PilF, since the lack of either of these factors is detrimental to fiber formation. The propensity of the fiber to be retracted is dependent on the amount of PilT, on ATP and on the level of expression of the PilC, which inhibits the action of PilT by a still unknown mechanism. In the absence of PilC, PilT-mediated retraction is increased and bacteria appear poorly piliated. In contrast, the accumulation of PilC prevents retraction and increases piliation [53].

This schematic view of tfp biogenesis raises numerous questions: How and where are pilin subunits assembled? How is the pilus anchored in the cell membranes and how are pulling forces generated by retraction and transmitted to the whole bacteria? How are pilin subunits redistributed towards the inner membrane during retraction?

12.3 Genetics

Neisserial pili are characterized by a high rate of polymorphism in the primary sequence of pilin referred to as antigenic variation, since pilin variants trigger different antibody responses. Antigenic variation has been extensively studied in *N. gonorrhoeae* and is believed to be similar in *N. meningitidis*. It occurs by the RecA-dependent recombination of parts of silent *pilS* copies with the expressed *pilE* gene involving reciprocal and nonreciprocal transfer. The latter event results in gene conversion, leaving the donor *pilS* sequence unchanged [63, 64]. Only the variable regions of *pilE* are susceptible to change by this mechanism; and the recombinant sequence is a mosaic of parent *pilE* and *pilS*, intercalated by regions of exact identity in both loci. Besides *pilS*, the donor sequence may also originate from exogenous DNA taken up by transformation, after release from other bacteria [65, 66].

Tfp phase variation may be the consequence of recombination events leading to loss of PilE expression or the expression of assembly deficient variant pilin [67]. On and off switching of PilC expression by frame-shift mutations is yet another cause for the gain and loss of pilus assembly [48].

An influence of pilin variation on pilus associated functions has been demonstrated for adherence [68–70] and autoagglutination. Moreover, the propensity of pili to form bundles, where fibers are organized in parallel arrays, correlates with sequence changes in the C-terminal part of pilin [62]. Although it is clear from these investigations that pilin variation has an impact on tfp function, the molecular and structural basis is not known.

12.4 Functions Associated with tfp

12.4.1 Twitching Motility

Microorganisms use different strategies to move in various environments. Tfp-mediated movement is known as twitching motility in the case of *P. aeruginosa* and *Neisseria*, or gliding motility in *Myxococcus xanthus*. In the case of pathogenic *Neisseria*, twitching motility is easy to observe among agglutinated bacteria in liquid media. In the course of infection, twitching motility is thought to be a key for the onset of intimate adhesion, which follows the early localized adherence.

Pilus retraction provides the mechanical force necessary for motility in a fishing reel-fashion: reeling the tethered pilus from its base pulls the bacterium towards the tethering point [71, 72]. The force generated by the retraction is greater than 100 pN, which, compared to its size, make tfp retraction the most powerful motor known until now [73]. The precise mechanism ruling tfp retraction is still unclear. Evidence exists that retraction involves the targeting of fiber-forming pilin to the inner membrane [53]. The dissociation of the pilus in the inner membrane vicinity would result in the "melting" of the hydrophobic moieties of pilin into this membrane. Fiber retraction relies on the availability of ATP and triggers fiber movement of about 1 $\mu m\ s^{-1}$, which corresponds to the disassembly into the cytoplasmic membrane of about 1300 subunits s^{-1}. The velocity and force of the retraction are independent of the concentration of PilT and of the length of the pilus [73]. However, the frequency of retraction events on one bacterium increases with the number of pili, as well as with the amount of PilT available. Retraction was also shown to be under the control of a force-dependent molecular switch, since external forces applied on the pilus were shown to temporarily reverse retraction into elongation [74]. Taken together, retraction appears to be an on–off system that would be independently tuned for every single pilus, depending on the availability of PilT, ATP and on mechanical forces applied to the fiber (for a review, see [75]).

12.4.2
Auto-aggregation

Auto-aggregation of capsulated *N. meningitidis* is dependent on the presence of pili. Auto-aggregates of *N. meningitidis* can be observed in liquid cultures, as well as during the adhesion process, where bacteria form localized microcolonies on the surface of the cells. Auto-aggregation mediated by tfp also provides a conformation where PilT-mediated retraction can easily be observed as non-Brownian movement of cells within a bacterial clump. However, the relationship between bacterial aggregation and adhesion is still not fully understood.

Different factors have been implicated in auto-aggregation. As described before, pili may assemble in organized arrays of fibers called bundles. The propensity to form bundles depends on the primary sequence of a polymorphic region of pilin [62]. However, bundling probably involves the association of fibers stemming from one single cell, as well as the anti-parallel bundling of fibers coming from different bacteria, which is also the case in auto-aggregation.

Besides pilin polymorphism, two other components have been shown to impair bacterial aggregation without affecting tfp expression. PilU was described in *N. gonorrhoeae* and its function is still unknown. It is closely related to and is organized in an operon with the PilT AAA ATPase [44]. PilX was described in *N. meningitidis* and is proposed to mediate interbacterial interactions; and the effect of PilX abolition can be reverted by concomitant abolition of PilT [58]. Both PilU and PilX mutants fail to form bacterial aggregates but, surprisingly, they have opposite effects on adhesion. PilU mutants displays increased adhesion, whereas a PilX mutant is poorly adhesive. Further studies are thus needed in both *N. meningitidis* and *N. gonorrhoeae* to assess the respective role of these components.

12.4.3
Transformation Competence

Natural competence for genetic transformation is a programmed physiological state which enables bacteria to take up and process exogenous DNA. It is a highly regulated process that involves sequential steps: binding and uptake of the exogenous DNA and translocation across the bacterial membranes, which subsequently allows recombination with homologous DNA counterparts in the genome. Although sequence nonspecific binding was also reported [47], pathogenic *Neisseria,* like *Haemophilus influenzae,* efficiently bind double-stranded DNA that contains specific short sequence (ten base pairs for the *Neisseria*), named DNA uptake sequence (DUS) [76]. DUS sequences are found scattered in the genomes of both *N. meningitidis* and *N. gonorrhoeae* and are thought to provide a means to discriminate DNA from unrelated species. Both PilQ and PilE are involved in sequence-specific DNA binding.

Binding and uptake of the DNA could be resolved as two separate steps. A major point is therefore whether tfp themselves are responsible for the binding and uptake of DNA. Piliation has long been closely associated with natural transformation in *N. gonorrhoeae* [77]. Competence efficiency is associated with the level of pilus expression [47, 65, 78], although low levels of pilin, leading to hardly detectable piliation, are sufficient for transformation competence, as long as PilT and PilQ are present [31, 79]. More specifically, mutants defective for PilQ [31], PilP [35], PilF, PilD [27] or PilG [30] expression lack tfp and transformation competence. Neisserial *pilE* or *pilC* mutants are unable to take up DNA [80], but complementation of a PilC-null mutant with purified PilC protein partially compensated the transformation competence defect [47].

Two proteins of the tfp machinery are dispensable for fiber expression but required for competence: PilT and ComP [38, 55]. PilT is responsible for the subsequent uptake of the DNA into the cell [81]. ComP shares structural similarities with PilE, but is expressed at very low levels compared to PilE. Abolition of ComP results in a severe defect in competence, but has no discernable effect on tfp biogenesis, adhesion to cells or twitching motility. Finally, the periplasmic ComE protein, although not part of the tfp machinery, is also necessary for DNA uptake and displays DNA-binding activities [82]. Curiously, the prepilin-like PilV, which is involved in the adhesion to cells, acts as an antagonist of ComP [57], by a mechanism that is still not understood.

12.4.4
Adhesion

Specific adhesion of capsulated meningococci to human cells has been modeled in two steps. Initial attachment, depicted as “localized adherence”, is mediated by tfp and is characterized by the formation of heavily piliated bacterial microcolonies that are localized on the cell surface. This is accompanied by transient formation of microvilli-like structures that extend from the cell surface and reach the bacteria. After 4–9 h, adhering microcolony-forming bacteria disperse on the cell surface, lose piliation and form a monolayer of bacteria that intimately interacts with the cell surface. At this stage, cells are devoid of microvilli [39]. Although not required for attachment to the cells, PilT is required for the onset of intimate attachment [39].

Tfp are the major bacterial attributes involved in the initial attachment to host cells, which is supported by studies using primary cells [83], or *post mortem* data [84]. Localized adherence is dependent on the expression of PilC1 and PilV and is modulated by sequence variation in pilin (PilE). Expression of variant pilins that have increased propensity to form tfp bundles correlates with higher adhesion levels [62]. Pilin also mediates specific binding to erythrocytes, which is distinct from pilus-mediated adhesion to other cell types [85].

The 110-kDa PilC proteins play important roles in tfp function. PilC proteins are involved in the interaction of *N. meningitidis* with human cells, highlighted by the finding that *pilC1* mutants fail to adhere to cells [45]. Interestingly, mutation of *pilC2* does not affect adhesion suggesting that PilC1 and PilC2 in *N. meningitidis* exert different functions. Gonococcal variants of PilC are in contrast functionally interchangeable since both PilC1 and PilC2 mediate binding of piliated *N. gonorrhoeae* to epithelial cells [86]. In *N. gonorrhoeae*, PilC has been localized to the tip of the pili. Moreover, purified PilC efficiently competed for the binding of piliated gonococci and meningococci to human epithelial cells, suggesting that PilC directly exerts binding properties [46]. Moreover, PilC1 of *N. meningitidis* fully complemented a piliated *N. gonorrhoeae pilC* null mutant for adherence indicating a similar function of *N. gonorrhoeae* PilC and *N. meningitidis* PilC1 [87].

Little is known about the mechanisms involved in the onset of intimate adhesion. This step involves PilT, retraction being thought to promote bacterial dispersal on the cellular surface [39]. Whereas it is upregulated in early stages, the expression of the adhesion-promoting PilC1 protein is at this stage downregulated back to basal level [54]. Downregulation of *pilC1* transcription may be under the control of CrgA, a transcriptional regulator that recognizes contact regulatory element *Neisseria* (CREN) sequences in the promoter regions of *pilC1* [88].

A proposed receptor on the human cell for tfp is CD46, a member of the superfamily of complement resistance proteins comprising at least six isoforms (for a review, see [89]). CD46 is expressed in almost all cell types, apart from erythrocytes. Pili purified from *N. meningitidis* bind to a protein of the size of CD46 and adhesion of *N. meningitidis* to cells is blocked by anti-CD46 antibodies [90]. Soluble pilin has been proposed as a binding partner for CD46 [91], and unpublished data also report an interaction between PilC and CD46 [89]. Transgenic mice expressing human CD46 were more susceptible to systemic challenge than control animals, although this was independent of the piliation status of the bacteria. In the case of intra-nasal infection, the transgenic animals developed disease when infected with piliated meningococci, whereas they remained asymptomatic after inoculation with non-piliated organisms [92]. In the case of *N. gonorrhoeae*, it could be shown that PilT was required to observe a downregulation of CD46 in the course of cellular adhesion and that infection also resulted in the shedding of CD46 in the milieu [93]. However, the finding of an inverse correlation between CD46 expression and adherence levels of piliated *N. gonorrhoeae* has challenged the perception of CD46 as a classic receptor for pathogenic *Neisseria* [94]. Moreover, *N. meningitidis* does not interact with some human cells expressing CD46 (for a review, see [89]). Also, experiments with cells which were depleted of CD46 by RNA interference or which recombinantly expressed CD46, suggested that piliated *N. gonorrhoeae* do not bind in a CD46-dependent manner [95]. Thus, the role of CD46 as receptor in neisserial infection needs to be further investigated.

12.4.5 Tfp-initiated Signaling Pathways

Tfp-mediated binding to cells is accompanied by a complex cascade of signaling events. A transient release of Ca^{2+} from the intracellular stores occurs within minutes of the onset of infection and is dependent on the presence of PilC1 and the binding of pili to CD46 [96]. This in turn triggers exocytosis, which increases the amount of LAMP1 accessible to the neisserial IgA1 protease [97]. Gonococcal infection also triggers CD46 phosphorylation at position Tyr354, in the cytoplasmic tail of the CD46 Cyt2 isoform [98]. This is mediated by c-Yes, a member of the Src tyrosine kinase family. Inhibition of Src-kinase with PP2 leads to a decrease in gonococcal adhesion to cells, which suggests that a cellular response involving Src family kinases is necessary for completion of the adhesion process. These results are supported by observations that Src inactivation leads to decreased internalization rates [99].

A second set of signaling events initiated by piliated bacteria is the induction of cortical plaques at the site of bacterial attachment [100]. These plaques are enriched in components of the cortical cytoskeleton like actin and ezrin, as well as in the integral membrane proteins CD44v3, CD44, EGFR and ICAM-1. The reorganization of the cytoskeleton is essential for the internalization of *N. meningitidis*. Tfp-induced activation of Cdc42 and Rho is required for actin recruitment at the cortical plaques, although ezrin and moesin targeting to the site of attachment is not [103]. Moreover, engulfment of *N. meningitidis* also involves the transmembrane tyrosine kinase ErbB2 [99]. Recruitment of ErbB2 at the bacterial site of attachment triggers Src activation, which in turn phosphorylates cortactin and allows cortical actin assembly.

Cortical plaque formation requires PilT, suggesting that pilus retraction is an important event of cellular signaling. Fiber retraction in *N. gonorrhoeae* also enhances the activation of the ERK, JNK and p38 MAP kinases and mediates cell cytoprotection [101]. It is however important to note that care should be taken when extrapolating data on host cell signal transduction pathways activated by *N. gonorrhoeae* to *N. meningitidis*. A comparative microarray transcriptional study of the cytokine and adhesion related genes response of the host cell showed that responses elicited by both *N. meningitidis* and *N. gonorrhoeae* are not identical [102]. Moreover, unlike *N. gonorrhoeae*, *N. meningitidis* usually expresses a capsule that is likely to affect the accessibility of bacterial ligands to host receptors, thus modifying the host–cell response.

12.4.6 Invasion of the CSF

Entry to the CSF is a prerequisite to cause meningitis. In the case of a trauma, or a meningeal breach, the bacteria can directly gain access from the nasopharynx. However, in most cases, inoculation of the CSF occurs from the bloodstream. *N. meningitidis* can be seen adhering to the endothelial cells of both the choroid plexus and the meninges. In a clinical meningococcal isolate, the adhesion level could be correlated to that of piliation, and was shown to depend on the amount of PilC expression [84]. Although no definite proof is available, evidence suggests that the crossing of the blood–brain barrier occurs via transcellular migration, rather than a paracellular route [104]. Moreover, the site where the blood–brain barrier is breached is also unclear, since two routes are possible: the meninges where the endothelial cells forming the blood–brain barrier present tight junctions, and the choroid plexus. The latter site, which is responsible for the production of the CSF, is characterized by an endothelium devoid of tight junctions, the barrier integrity being enforced by the underlying epithelial cells.

12.5 Conclusions

Recent findings on the molecular architecture and function of *N. meningitidis* tfp significantly extended our understanding of these major pathogenicity factors. There is no doubt that the initial description of *N. meningitidis* tfp as colonization factors was confirmed with the use of genetics and molecular biology. Nevertheless, after decades of intensive research, the nature of the interaction of the meningococal pilus with the host cell is still not completely elucidated at the molecular level. To this regard, the functions of most of the pseudopilins and pilus associated proteins are still unclear.

On the cellular side, the identification of CD46 as a receptor involved in tfp signaling brought important steps towards the understanding of the molecular interaction of tfp and host cell receptors. However, evidence on the presence of additional receptors accumulates; and future work should help to unravel the nature of the receptor for high affinity binding of *N. meningitidis* tfp.

Another unresolved issue is the role of twitching motility in infection. Although evidence exists for a role of twitching motility in intimate attachment of piliated *N. meningitidis*, the consequences of the pulling forces generated by tfp retraction for the cell are just starting to be unveiled. Furthermore, one may speculate that assembly and disassembly of pili may also be important in the course of invasion and transcytosis of cellular barriers. More generally, signals triggering either assembly or disassembly of tfp still need to be clarified.

Finally, although some principles on how signals can be transduced by the pili during infection have been demonstrated, the signaling elicited in the host cell by the tfp also needs to be further unravelled. Here, the basic questions have to be answered: What is the interplay between the mechanical and chemical signals transduced by the pili? What signals are required for short or long term adaptation of the bacteria to its host? Moreover, it is not clear what kind of signals are transmitted by the tfp-mediated aggregation of bacteria. Thus, we are far from understanding the complete picture on how *N. meningitidis* tfp act in infection and pathogenesis. Considering the already identified functions of these multitask organelles as anchor, grapnel and antennae for chemical and mechanical signals, one would not be surprised if future research reports unprecedented function to meningococcal tfp.

References

1 O.B. Harrison, B.D. Robertson, S.N. Faust, M.A. Jepson, R.D. Goldin, M. Levin, R.S. Heyderman **2002**, *Infect. Immun.* 70, 5193–5201.

2 M.S. Strom, S. Lory **1993**, *Annu. Rev. Microbiol.* 47, 565–596.

3 T. Tonjum, M. Koomey **1997**, *Gene* 192, 155–163.

4 L. Craig, M.E. Pique, J.A. Tainer **2004**, *Nat. Rev. Microbiol.* 2, 363–378.

5 E. Carbonnelle, S. Helaine, L. Prouvensier, X. Nassif, V. Pelicic **2005**, *Mol. Microbiol.* 55, 54–64.

6 M. Virji, J.E. Heckels, W.J. Potts, C.A. Hart, J.R. Saunders **1989**, *J. Gen. Microbiol.* 135, 3239–3251.

7 R. Haas, H. Schwarz, T.F. Meyer **1987**, *Proc. Natl Acad. Sci. USA* 84, 9079–9083.

8 M. Marceau, X. Nassif **1999**, *J. Bacteriol.* 181, 656–661.

9 I. Benz, M.A. Schmidt **2002**, *Mol. Microbiol.* 45, 267–276.

10 A. Banerjee, S.K. Ghosh **2003**, *Mol. Cell Biochem.* 253, 179–190.

11 H.E. Parge, K.T. Forest, M.J. Hickey, D.A. Christensen, E.D. Getzoff, J.A. Tainer **1995**, *Nature* 378, 32–38.

12 M. Virji **1997**, *Gene* 192, 141–147.

13 C.M. Kahler, L.E. Martin, Y.L. Tzeng, Y.K. Miller, K. Sharkey, D.S. Stephens, J.K. Davies **2001**, *Infect. Immun.* 69, 3597–3604.

14 E. Stimson, M. Virji, K. Makepeace, A. Dell, H.R. Morris, G. Payne, J.R. Saunders, M.P. Jennings, S. Barker, M. Panico **1995**, *Mol. Microbiol.* 17, 1201–1214.

15 M. Marceau, K. Forest, J.L. Beretti, J. Tainer, X. Nassif **1998**, *Mol. Microbiol.* 27, 705–715.

16 F.T. Hegge, P.G. Hitchen, F.E. Aas, H. Kristiansen, C. Lovold, W. Egge-Jacobsen, M. Panico, W.Y. Leong, V. Bull, M. Virji, H.R. Morris, A. Dell, M. Koomey **2004**, *Proc. Natl Acad. Sci. USA* 101, 10798–10803.

17 M.P. Jennings, M. Virji, D. Evans, V. Foster, Y.N. Srikhanta, L. Steeghs, L.P. van der, E.R. Moxon **1998**, *Mol. Microbiol.* 29, 975–984.

18 P.M. Power, L.F. Roddam, M. Dieckelmann, Y.N. Srikhanta, Y.C. Tan, A.W. Berrington, M.P. Jennings **2000**, *Microbiology* 146, 967–979.

19 P.M. Power, L.F. Roddam, K. Rutter, S.Z. Fitzpatrick, Y.N. Srikhanta, M.P. Jennings **2003**, *Mol. Microbiol.* 49, 833–847.

20 M.J. Warren, L.F. Roddam, P.M. Power, T.D. Terry, M.P. Jennings **2004**, *FEMS Immunol. Med. Microbiol.* 41, 43–50.

21 A. Banerjee, R. Wang, S.L. Supernavage, S.K. Ghosh, J. Parker, N.F. Ganesh, P.G. Wang, S. Gulati, P.A. Rice **2002**, *J. Exp. Med.* 196, 147–162.

22 E. Stimson, M. Virji, S. Barker, M. Panico, I. Blench, J. Saunders, G. Payne, E.R. Moxon, A. Dell, H.R. Morris **1996**, *Biochem. J.* 316, 29–33.

23 K.T. Forest, S.A. Dunham, M. Koomey, J.A. Tainer **1999**, *Mol. Microbiol.* 31, 743–752.

24 J.N. Weiser, J.B. Goldberg, N. Pan, L. Wilson, M. Virji **1998**, *Infect. Immun.* 66, 4263–4267.

25 L. Serino, M. Virji **2000**, *Mol. Microbiol.* 35, 1550–1559.

26 M.J. Warren, M.P. Jennings **2003**, *Infect. Immun.* 71, 6892–6898.

27 N.E. Freitag, H.S. Seifert, M. Koomey **1995**, *Mol. Microbiol.* 16, 575–586.

28 S. Lory, M.S. Strom **1997**, *Gene* 192, 117–121.

29 J.C. Pepe, S. Lory **1998**, *J. Biol. Chem.* 273, 19120–19129.

30 T. Tonjum, N.E. Freitag, E. Namork, M. Koomey **1995**, *Mol. Microbiol.* 16, 451–464.

31 S.L. Drake, M. Koomey **1995**, *Mol. Microbiol.* 18, 975–986.

32 M. Wolfgang, J.P. van Putten, S.F. Hayes, D. Dorward, M. Koomey **2000**, *EMBO J.* 19, 6408–6418.

33 R.F. Collins, R.C. Ford, A. Kitmitto, R.O. Olsen, T. Tonjum, J.P. Derrick **2003**, *J. Bacteriol.* 185, 2611–2617.

34 R.F. Collins, S.A. Frye, A. Kitmitto, R.C. Ford, T. Tonjum, J.P. Derrick **2004**, *J. Biol. Chem.* 279, 39750–39756.

35 S.L. Drake, S.A. Sandstedt, M. Koomey **1997**, *Mol. Microbiol.* 23, 657–668.

36 R. Voulhoux, J. Tommassen **2004**, *Res. Microbiol.* 155, 129–135.

37 R.D. Vale **2000**, *J. Cell Biol.* 150, F13–F19.

38 M. Wolfgang, P. Lauer, H.S. Park, L. Brossay, J. Hebert, M. Koomey **1998**, *Mol. Microbiol.* 29, 321–330.

39 C. Pujol, E. Eugene, M. Marceau, X. Nassif **1999**, *Proc. Natl Acad. Sci. USA* 96, 4017–4022.

40 K.T. Forest, K.A. Satyshur, G.A. Worzalla, J.K. Hansen, T.J. Herdendorf **2004**, *Acta Crystallogr. D. Biol. Crystallogr.* 60, 978–982.

41 T.J. Herdendorf, D.R. McCaslin, K.T. Forest **2002**, *J. Bacteriol.* 184, 6465–6471.

42 S. Okamoto, M. Ohmori **2002**, *Plant Cell Physiol* 43, 1127–1136.

43 L. Brossay, G. Paradis, R. Fox, M. Koomey, J. Hebert **1994**, *Infect. Immun.* 62, 2302–2308.

44 H.S. Park, M. Wolfgang, M. Koomey **2002**, *Infect. Immun.* 70, 3891–3903.

45 X. Nassif, J.L. Beretti, J. Lowy, P. Stenberg, P. O'Gaora, J. Pfeifer, S. Normark, M. So **1994**, *Proc. Natl Acad. Sci. USA* 91, 3769–3773.

46 T. Rudel, I. Scheurerpflug, T.F. Meyer **1995**, *Nature* 373, 357–359.

47 T. Rudel, D. Facius, R. Barten, I. Scheuerpflug, E. Nonnenmacher, T.F. Meyer **1995**, *Proc. Natl Acad. Sci. USA* 92, 7986–7990.

48 A.B. Jonsson, G. Nyberg, S. Normark **1991**, *EMBO J.* 10, 477–488.

49 A. Rytkonen, B. Albiger, P. Hansson-Palo, H. Kallstrom, P. Olcen, H. Fredlund, A.B. Jonsson **2004**, *J. Infect. Dis.* 189, 402–409.

50 M. Rahman, H. Kallstrom, S. Normark, A.B. Jonsson **1997**, *Mol. Microbiol.* 25, 11–25.

51 P.C. Morand, P. Tattevin, E. Eugene, J.L. Beretti, X. Nassif **2001**, *Mol. Microbiol.* 40, 846–856.

52 M. Wolfgang, H.S. Park, S.F. Hayes, J.P. van Putten, M. Koomey **1998**, *Proc. Natl. Acad. Sci. USA* 95, 14973–14978.

53 P.C. Morand, E. Bille, S. Morelle, E. Eugene, J.L. Beretti, M. Wolfgang, T.F. Meyer, M. Koomey, X. Nassif **2004**, *EMBO J.* 23, 2009–2017.

54 M.K. Taha, P.C. Morand, Y. Pereira, E. Eugene, D. Giorgini, M. Larribe, X. Nassif **1998**, *Mol. Microbiol.* 28, 1153–1163.

55 M. Wolfgang, J.P. van Putten, S.F. Hayes, M. Koomey **1999**, *Mol. Microbiol.* 31, 1345–1357.

56 H.C. Winther-Larsen, F.T. Hegge, M. Wolfgang, S.F. Hayes, J.P. van Putten, M. Koomey **2001**, *Proc. Natl Acad. Sci. USA* 98, 15276–15281.

57 F.E. Aas, C. Lovold, M. Koomey **2002**, *Mol. Microbiol.* 46, 1441–1450.

58 S. Helaine, E. Carbonnelle, L. Prouvensier, J.L. Beretti, X. Nassif, V. Pelicic **2005**, *Mol. Microbiol.* 55, 65–77.

59 K.T. Forest, J.A. Tainer **1997**, *Gene* 192, 165–169.

60 C.R. Tinsley, R. Voulhoux, J.L. Beretti, J. Tommassen, X. Nassif **2004**, *J. Biol. Chem.* 279, 27078–27087.

61 K.T. Forest, S.L. Bernstein, E.D. Getzoff, M. So, G. Tribbick, H.M. Geysen, C.D. Deal, J.A. Tainer **1996**, *Infect. Immun.* 64, 644–652.

62 M. Marceau, J.L. Beretti, X. Nassif **1995**, *Mol. Microbiol.* 17, 855–863.

63 R. Haas, T.F. Meyer **1986**, *Cell* 44, 107–115.

64 E. Segal, P. Hagblom, H.S. Seifert, M. So **1986**, *Proc. Natl Acad. Sci. USA* 83, 2177–2181.

65 C.P. Gibbs, B.Y. Reimann, E. Schultz, A. Kaufmann, R. Haas, T.F. Meyer **1989**, *Nature* 338, 651–652.

66 H.S. Seifert, R.S. Ajioka, C. Marchal, P.F. Sparling, M. So **1988**, *Nature* 336, 392–395.

67 T.F. Meyer, C.P. Gibbs, R. Haas **1990**, *Annu. Rev. Microbiol.* 44, 451–477.

68 T. Rudel, J.P. van Putten, C.P. Gibbs, R. Haas, T.F. Meyer **1992**, *Mol. Microbiol.* 6, 3439–3450.

69 M. Virji, C. Alexandrescu, D. J. Ferguson, J. R. Saunders, E. R. Moxon **1992**, *Mol. Microbiol.* 6, 1271–1279.
70 X. Nassif, J. Lowy, P. Stenberg, P. O'Gaora, A. Ganji, M. So **1993**, *Mol. Microbiol.* 8, 719–725.
71 D. E. Bradley **1980**, *Can. J. Microbiol.* 26, 146–154.
72 A. J. Merz, M. So, M. P. Sheetz **2000**, *Nature* 407, 98–102.
73 B. Maier, L. Potter, M. So, C. D. Long, H. S. Seifert, M. P. Sheetz **2002**, *Proc. Natl Acad. Sci. USA* 99, 16012–16017.
74 B. Maier, M. Koomey, M. P. Sheetz **2004**, *Proc. Natl Acad. Sci. USA* 101, 10961–10966.
75 D. Kaiser **2000**, *Curr. Biol.* 10, R777–R780.
76 C. Elkins, C. E. Thomas, H. S. Seifert, P. F. Sparling **1991**, *J. Bacteriol.* 173, 3911–3913.
77 P. F. Sparling **1966**, *J. Bacteriol.* 92, 1364–1371.
78 C. D. Long, R. N. Madraswala, H. S. Seifert **1998**, *Infect. Immun.* 66, 1918–1927.
79 C. D. Long, D. M. Tobiason, M. P. Lazio, K. A. Kline, H. S. Seifert **2003**, *Infect. Immun.* 71, 6279–6291.
80 D. Facius, M. Fussenegger, T. F. Meyer **1996**, *FEMS Microbiol. Lett.* 137, 159–164.
81 F. E. Aas, M. Wolfgang, S. Frye, S. Dunham, C. Lovold, M. Koomey **2002**, *Mol. Microbiol.* 46, 749–760.
82 I. Chen, E. C. Gotschlich **2001**, *J. Bacteriol.* 183, 3160–3168.
83 S. J. Hardy, M. Christodoulides, R. O. Weller, J. E. Heckels **2000**, *Mol. Microbiol.* 36, 817–829.
84 B. Pron, M. K. Taha, C. Rambaud, J. C. Fournet, N. Pattey, J. P. Monnet, M. Musilek, J. L. Beretti, X. Nassif **1997**, *J. Infect. Dis.* 176, 1285–1292.
85 I. Scheuerpflug, T. Rudel, R. Ryll, J. Pandit, T. F. Meyer **1999**, *Infect. Immun.* 67, 834–843.
86 T. Rudel, H. J. Boxberger, T. F. Meyer **1995**, *Mol. Microbiol.* 17, 1057–1071.
87 R. R. Ryll, T. Rudel, I. Scheuerpflug, R. Barten, T. F. Meyer **1997**, *Mol. Microbiol.* 23, 879–892.
88 A. E. Deghmane, S. Petit, A. Topilko, Y. Pereira, D. Giorgini, M. Larribe, M. K. Taha **2000**, *EMBO J.* 19, 1068–1078.
89 D. B. Gill, J. P. Atkinson **2004**, *Trends Mol. Med.* 10, 459–465.
90 H. Kallstrom, M. K. Liszewski, J. P. Atkinson, A. B. Jonsson **1997**, *Mol. Microbiol.* 25, 639–647.
91 A. Rytkonen, L. Johansson, V. Asp, B. Albiger, A. B. Jonsson **2001**, *Infect. Immun.* 69, 6419–6426.
92 L. Johansson, A. Rytkonen, P. Bergman, B. Albiger, H. Kallstrom, T. Hokfelt, B. Agerberth, R. Cattaneo, A. B. Jonsson **2003**, *Science* 301, 373–375.
93 D. B. Gill, M. Koomey, J. G. Cannon, J. P. Atkinson **2003**, *J. Exp. Med.* 198, 1313–1322.
94 D. M. Tobiason, H. S. Seifert **2001**, *Microbiology* 147, 2333–2340.
95 M. Kirchner, D. Heuer, T. F. Meyer **2005**, *Infect. Immun.* 73, 3072–3082.
96 H. Kallstrom, M. S. Islam, P. O. Berggren, A. B. Jonsson **1998**, *J. Biol. Chem.* 273, 21777–21782.
97 B. P. Ayala, B. Vasquez, S. Clary, J. A. Tainer, K. Rodland, M. So **2001**, *Cell Microbiol.* 3, 265–275.
98 S. W. Lee, R. A. Bonnah, D. L. Higashi, J. P. Atkinson, S. L. Milgram, M. So **2002**, *J. Cell Biol.* 156, 951–957.
99 I. Hoffmann, E. Eugene, X. Nassif, P. O. Couraud, S. Bourdoulous **2001**, *J. Cell Biol.* 155, 133–143.
100 A. J. Merz, C. A. Enns, M. So **1999**, *Mol. Microbiol.* 32, 1316–1332.
101 H. L. Howie, M. Glogauer, M. So **2005**, *PLoS Biol.* 3, e100.
102 L. Plant, V. Asp, L. Lovkvist, J. Sundqvist, A. B. Jonsson **2004**, *Cell Microbiol.* 6, 663–670.
103 E. Eugene, I. Hoffmann, C. Pujol, P. O. Couraud, S. Bourdoulous, X. Nassif **2002**, *J. Cell Sci.* 115, 1231–1241.
104 X. Nassif, S. Bourdoulous, E. Eugene, P. O. Couraud **2002**, *Trends Microbiol.* 10, 227–232.

Part III
Infection Biology

Handbook of Meningococcal Disease. Infection Biology, Vaccination, Clinical Management.
Edited by M. Frosch and M.C.J. Maiden

ISBN: 3-527-31260-9

13
Mechanisms of Attachment and Invasion

Sandrine Bourdoulous and Xavier Nassif

13.1
Introduction

Neisseria meningitidis is a gram-negative bacterium that is an obligate commensal of the human nasopharyngeal mucosa, the only known reservoir of infection. Colonization is necessary for both the propagation and survival of the bacterium, and is the first step in the disease process.

The strict tropism of *N. meningitidis* for humans has prevented the development of any suitable animal model for studying the mechanisms by which this bacterium colonizes and traverses host barriers. Most of the knowledge of the pathway of infection by *N. meningitidis* has been derived from studies of its interactions with organ cultures, primary cell cultures, and immortalized cell lines. Specific models have been used to reflect individual stages in the progression of infection: the interactions between the bacterium and isolated, immortalized epithelial cells have been studied to understand the process of colonization, while rodent models have been adapted to investigate the dissemination of the bacterium in the systemic circulation. Experiments with endothelial and meningeal cells have been used to represent the subsequent stages of attachment to vascular cells and entry into the cerebrospinal fluid (CSF), leading to meningitis. While none of these models is ideal, they have revealed that *N. meningitidis* is able to adhere to, enter, and traffic through human epithelial and endothelial cells and that *N. meningitidis* can also replicate in cultured cell lines. These *in vitro* models have provided valuable insights into the bacterial factors required for pathogenesis and their cellular targets.

The purpose of this chapter is to review our current knowledge on the interaction between the bacterium and host cells, particularly epithelial and endothelial cells which are critical to colonization and represent the probable route of spread to the CSF.

Handbook of Meningococcal Disease. Infection Biology, Vaccination, Clinical Management.
Edited by M. Frosch and M. C. J. Maiden

ISBN: 3-527-31260-9

13.2 Mechanisms of Attachment

N. meningitidis interacts with many different cell types effectively to colonize the nasopharynx, enter the systemic circulation, and cause disease. To mediate association with a range of host cells, this bacterium expresses a number of adhesins. However, virulent strains of *N. meningitidis* express a polysaccharide capsule, which can affect the accessibility of some bacterial ligands to host receptors. This is especially relevant for serogroups of *N. meningitidis* (B, C) that express a capsule consisting of polymers of negatively charged sialic acid, which is also present on human cells. The major adhesin in initial attachment to many host cells is therefore their type IV pilus. This adhesin confers the capacity for the primary attachment of *N. meningitidis* to host cells, which can be further facilitated by lipooligosaccharide (LOS), opacity (Opa) proteins, and glycolipid adhesins.

13.2.1 Type IV Pili

Type IV pili are polymeric filaments found on many Gram-negative bacteria. These structures, formed from multiprotein complexes with the pilus filament being composed of a multimer of a pilin sub-unit protein encoded by the gene *pilE,* play a crucial role in the pathogenesis of *N. meningitidis* infections in humans. Nonpiliated mutants (PilE defective mutants) of encapsulated strains of *N. meningitidis* do not efficiently interact with host cells [1, 2], indicating that virulent encapsulated meningococci mainly adhere by means of type IV pili [3].

The pilin protein can be modified by glycosylation [4]. This modification is subject to phase variation but does not have a major effect on the function of the type IV pili: nonglycosylated mutants have slightly enhanced binding to epithelial cells compared with glycosylated bacteria [5]. However, the pilin subunit undergoes extensive antigenic variation that regulates adhesion of *N. meningitidis* to human cells [2, 6]. The high adhesiveness of some pilin variants has been correlated with their ability to form bundles of pili that bind bacteria together and allow them to grow as colonies on infected cell monolayers [7]. Recently a pilin-like protein PilX has been identified that copurifies with type IV pili and that is essential for bacterial aggregation and adhesiveness [8]. Indeed, *pilX* mutants (even though piliated) are not only unable to form clumps of bacteria but also unable to adhere to host cells, thus stressing the importance of bacterium–bacterium connections in pilus-mediated adhesion.

Among the components of the neisserial type IV pili machinery, the PilC proteins play a crucial role [2]. The PilC proteins, PilC1 and PilC2, are key elements in the formation of pili, as the production of at least one PilC protein is required for pilus assembly. In addition, PilC1 but not PilC2 modulates adhesiveness. Mutation in the *pilC2* gene does not affect adhesion, but *pilC1* mutants do not associate with host cells, even though piliated [2]. Early work suggested that the PilC proteins may be the adhesin. These proteins are associated with the outer membrane but can also be recovered from purified pili [9, 10]. Each of these genes presents a different promoter, indicating that they may be under independent transcriptional control. Expression of PilC1, but not PilC2, is transiently induced by contact between bacteria and host cells [11]. The loss of cell contact-dependent upregulation of *pilC1* leads to a dramatic decrease in bacterial adhesiveness. Moreover, upregulation of *pilC1* expression is detected in the cerebrospinal fluid and choroid plexus, supporting a role for the upregulation of this protein during the development of meningitis [12].

Another pilus component, PilT, is required for association with host cells after initial attachment. PilT promotes pilus retraction, which is required for twitching motility, and also plays a central role in the interactions of pathogenic *Neisseriae* with human cells [13, 14]. PilT protein is a member of the AAA superfamily of proteins, which act as multimeric mechanoenzymes able to disassemble stable protein–protein complexes [14]. PilT is an active motor molecule generating force in excess of 100 pN, making PilT the strongest molecular motor reported so far [15]. The force generated by pili retraction is thought to be the motive force that brings the pathogen into close association with the host cell. Moreover, such force is strong enough to cause membrane protrusions and possibly membrane puncture [15, 16].

The proposed host cell receptor for the type IV pili of *N. meningitidis* and the closely related pathogen *N. gonorrhoeae* is CD46, or membrane cofactor protein (MCP) [17]. This receptor is a member of a superfamily of complement resistance proteins, of which at least six isoforms have been described, that are found expressed in nearly all human cell types, except erythrocytes. CD46 is a well characterized receptor protein for a number of viruses such as measles [18] and human herpes virus-6 [19]. Using Chinese hamster ovary (CHO) cells transfected with CD46 isoforms, Kallström and colleagues showed that piliated neisseriae bind to BC1 and BC2 isoforms but not to C1 or C2 isoforms, and that this binding was blocked by recombinant CD46 or by anti-CD46 antibodies [17]. Mice expressing human CD46 were more susceptible to systemic challenge by *N. meningitidis* than were control animals, although this was independent of the piliation status of the infecting bacterium [20]. Following infection by the intranasal route, which is the site of the proposed interaction between *N. meningitidis* and CD46, a low proportion of transgenic animals developed disease if they received piliated meningococci, whereas all mice remained well if given nonpiliated organisms [20].

However, most of the recent published data support the notion that pilus-mediated infection of host cells occurs in a CD46-independent manner:

1. Adhesion of *N. meningitidis* to CD46 expressed in otherwise nonpermissive cells was weak compared with the adhesion supported by human epithelial cells [17]; and it was not reproduced by other groups [21]. Inhibition of pilus-mediated adhesion of *Neisseriae* to epithelial cells by incubation with anti-CD46 antibodies was not reproduced by several other groups [21–24].
2. In primary epithelial cells, CD46 is expressed on the basolateral surface and is not transcytosed to the apical surface, therefore rendering most unlikely its

availability to serve as initial, predominant pilus receptor on the mucosal surface of epithelial cells [24].

3. No correlation has been observed between the level of CD46 expression by cell lines and the degree of adhesion with piliated *Neisseriae* [21, 25]. Moreover, a specific downregulation of CD46 expression in human epithelial cell lines by RNA interference did not alter the binding efficiency of piliated gonococci [21]. These data therefore call into question the function of CD46 as an essential pilus receptor for pathogenic *Neisseriae.*

New studies to identify pilus receptors have highlighted a potential interaction with the I-domain of some integrin alpha chains (α_M, α_1, α_2), since adhesion of gonococci on primary urethral cells may be blocked by recombinant, soluble I domain or anti-alpha chain antibodies [22, 24]. However, only 20–40% adherence inhibition was observed on some epithelial cell lines (Chang, ME180), while no inhibition was observed on others (T84), suggesting that another, yet undefined, pilus receptor exists.

13.2.2
Opacity Proteins: Opa and Opc

For unencapsulated meningococci, several mechanisms of bacterial internalization have been described involving the interaction of cellular receptors with bacterial surface components, such as the Opa and Opc outer membrane proteins [26–28].

Opa proteins consist of eight transmembrane β-strands and four surface-exposed loops. The transmembrane and periplasmic sections are highly conserved, while the first three surface exposed loops display antigenic variation. There are 4–5 loci encoding Opa proteins in *N. meningitidis,* and expression varies between strains. Thus, a single bacterium may express any number of Opa proteins at any one time, and variation is enhanced by horizontal transfer of *opa* alleles promoting the formation of hybrid recombinant *opa* loci [26]. This has important functional consequences, as expression of different Opa proteins confers tropism to different cell lines [29, 30].

Several groups have shown that many different Opas bind to members of the large CD66/CEACAM family of proteins [26]. CD66-related proteins can mediate cell–cell adhesion, are encoded by different genes, and are often produced as multiple splice variants [31]. Different CD66 family members are variably expressed on different cell types. Most family members encode transmembrane proteins, whereas a few encode peripheral membrane proteins with glycosylphosphatidylinositol (GPI) membrane anchors. Opa proteins have been observed to bind to a number of variants of CD66; and Opa structure can be altered to determine CD66 specificity [32]. Depending on the particular CD66 variant(s) and Opa protein(s) expressed, different host cell responses occur, including binding, uptake, and the activation of different signal transduction pathways.

In the gonococcus, one class of Opas established binding with heparan sulfate proteoglycans (HSPG) present on certain epithelial cells [33]. Two pathways then mediate bacterial entry into the cell, either through localized recruitment of lipid hydrolysis [34], or through a vitronectin-dependent mechanism [35]. Interaction between Opa proteins (via vitronectin) and thence integrins can be sufficient to facilitate bacterial uptake in certain cell lines. However, no interaction between HSPG and meningococcal Opa proteins has yet been described.

Opc proteins share physiochemical properties and a weak homology with the Opa group, but differ in their structure and genetic control. The *opc* gene is present in many but not all *N. meningitidis* strains and is associated with virulence [36, 37]. The expression of Opc proteins is governed by alterations in the length of a homopolymeric tract in the promoter region [38]. Expression of *opc* in nonencapsulated *N. meningitidis* confers on the bacteria the ability to adhere to and invade endothelial cells independently of Opa and pili [29, 39–41]. The action of Opc follows interaction with the serum glycoprotein, vitronectin, which acts as a molecular bridge to $\alpha v\beta 3$ integrins on the surface of umbilical vein endothelial cells, facilitating entry of the bacterium into these cells [40]. Opc also affects internalization of bacteria into human brain microvascular endothelial cells. This, however, is mediated through the interaction of Opc with fibronectin in serum and then with $\alpha v\beta 3$ integrins [42].

13.2.3
Other Adhesins

Other molecules expressed at the bacterial cell surface have also been implicated in adhesion. Recently, a novel antigen of *N. meningitidis*, NadA, contributing to meningococcal adhesion to and invasion into epithelial cells, has been described [43]. NadA is present in three of the four known hypervirulent lineages [44] and is a bacterial invasin which, when expressed on the surface of *Escherichia coli*, promotes adhesion to and invasion of Chang epithelial cells [43]. Deletion of the N-terminal globular domain of recombinant NadA or pronase treatment of human cells abrogates the adhesive phenotype. Moreover, a hypervirulent strain of *N. meningitidis* where the NadA gene was inactivated had a reduced ability to adhere and to invade epithelial cells *in vitro*.

The structure of the lipooligosaccharide (LOS) of the meningococcus is similar to the lipopolysaccharide (LPS) of the Enterobacteriaceae, but lacks a repeating O-antigen. Differences in side-chain composition underlie the individual immunotypes of different strains [45]. Some immunotypes express the lacto-N-neotetraose epitope that mimics human asialocarbohydrates; and the contribution of LOS to *N. gonorrhoeae* binding to the host cell may be through interaction with asialocarbohydrate receptors [46]. In *N. meningitidis*, LOS can be further modified by the addition of terminal sialic acid moieties. LOS sialylation is a phenotypic variable, increasing the bacterium's negative surface charge density, which may produce an antiadhesive effect [28].

The effects of the capsule composition on meningococcal adhesion have been mostly studied in strains expressing the polysialic acid, serogroup B polysaccharide. The capsule is antiphagocytic and antibactericidal due to surface-exposed polysaccharides [47, 48]. Thus, the capsule is commonly seen in strains isolated from the blood and CSF. The capsule and sialylated LOS inhibit Opa- and Opc-mediated adhesion to host cells, possibly due to negatively charged molecules that repel host cells, but do not strongly inhibit type IV pilus-mediated adhesion [41, 49], presumably because pili extend far enough from the bacterial cell surface that electrostatic repulsion between bacterial sialic acids and the negatively charged host cell surface is negligible [50].

13.3 Mechanisms of Cellular Invasion

The invasion of host cells by *N. meningitidis* appears to be essential for meningococcal pathogenesis, since *in vitro* and *in vivo* evidence indicates that *N. meningitidis* uses a transcytosis pathway to cross cell monolayers [51]. *N. meningitidis* appears to replicate within host cells and is capable of traversing polarized epithelial or endothelial monolayers without disrupting barrier function [52–54]. It is unknown to what extent the intracellular bacteria egress through basolateral versus apical cellular membranes. Moreover, the mechanisms by which intracellular bacteria obtain nutrients are just beginning to be addressed.

13.3.1 Initial Attachment to Host Cells

Initial attachment of wild-type virulent capsulated bacteria to the host cell, a process mediated by the type IV pili, is characterized by a transient release of Ca^{2+} from intracellular stores. Semipurified pili also trigger a cytosolic Ca^{2+} flux in human epithelial cells [55]. This Ca^{2+} signal has a long latency, occurring $\sim$10 min after the addition of bacteria or pili, can be blocked by anti-CD46 antibodies, and depends on the presence of PilC1 which, as mentioned above, is required for strong pilus-mediated adherence. These data suggest that pili are necessary for the Ca^{2+} signal but do not exclude the possibility that a copurifying component is also required. Depletion of intracellular Ca^{2+} stores or treatment with protein kinase inhibitors results in diminished bacterial adherence [55]. *N. meningitidis* pili may therefore elicit a host cell response that reinforces an initial, weak attachment.

13.3.2 Cortical Plaque Formation and Invasion

After their initial attachment to host cells, encapsulated meningococci proliferate, locally forming a colony at their site of attachment on the cell surface. When adhering to the apical membrane of epithelial cells, *N. meningitidis* induces the local elongation of microvilli towards the bacteria, leading to their engulfment and internalization [52, 53]. Adhesion of *N. meningitidis* to endothelial cells promotes the local formation of membrane protrusions reminiscent of epithelial microvilli structures that surround bacteria and initiate their internalization within intracellular vacuoles [54]. Interestingly, the formation of such protrusions was also observed *ex vivo*, by transmission electron microscopic analysis of brain sections from a child who died from fulminant meningitis [51]. These observations strongly suggest that such morphological modifications of the host cell membrane may be essential for *N. meningitidis* to cross human vascular endothelium via a transcytosis pathway.

The formation of membrane protrusions by encapsulated *N. meningitidis* stems from the organization of specific molecular complexes, referred to as cortical plaques, beneath bacterial colonies (Fig. 13.1). Cortical plaques result from the recruitment of the molecular linkers ezrin and moesin, that cluster several membrane integral proteins such as CD44 or ICAM-1, and from the localized polymerization of cortical actin [54, 56, 57]. Ezrin and moesin are members of the ezrin/radixin/moesin (ERM) family that act as a linker between the plasma membrane and the actin cytoskeleton and play a critical role in the cortical morphogenesis required for the formation of microvilli [58]. Moreover, pilus-mediated adhesion of encapsulated *N. meningitidis* on human endothelial cells induces the clustering and tyrosine phosphorylation of the host cell tyrosine kinase receptor ErbB2 [59]. Activation of ErbB2 is required to elicit an efficient bacterial uptake by promoting the phosphorylation of the actin-binding protein cortactin, an essential step in the control of cortical actin assembly [59, 60]. Cor-

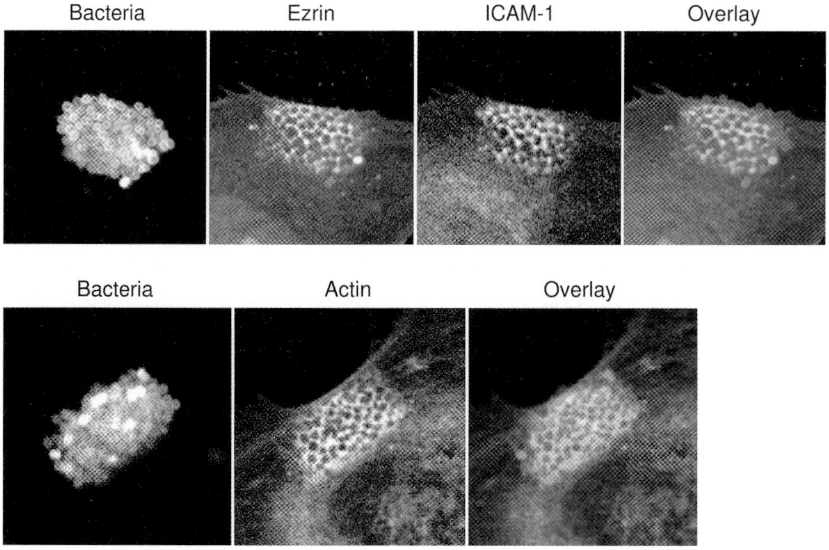

Fig. 13.1 Infection of human endothelial cells by *Neisseria meningitidis* induces the formation of cortical plaques beneath bacterial colonies. Human endothelial cells infected for 3 h with the 2C43 strain of *N. meningitidis* were stained for bacteria (blue), ezrin (green), and ICAM-1 (red), or double-stained for bacteria (red) and actin (green), and were analysed by confocal microscopy. (This figure also appears with the color plates.)

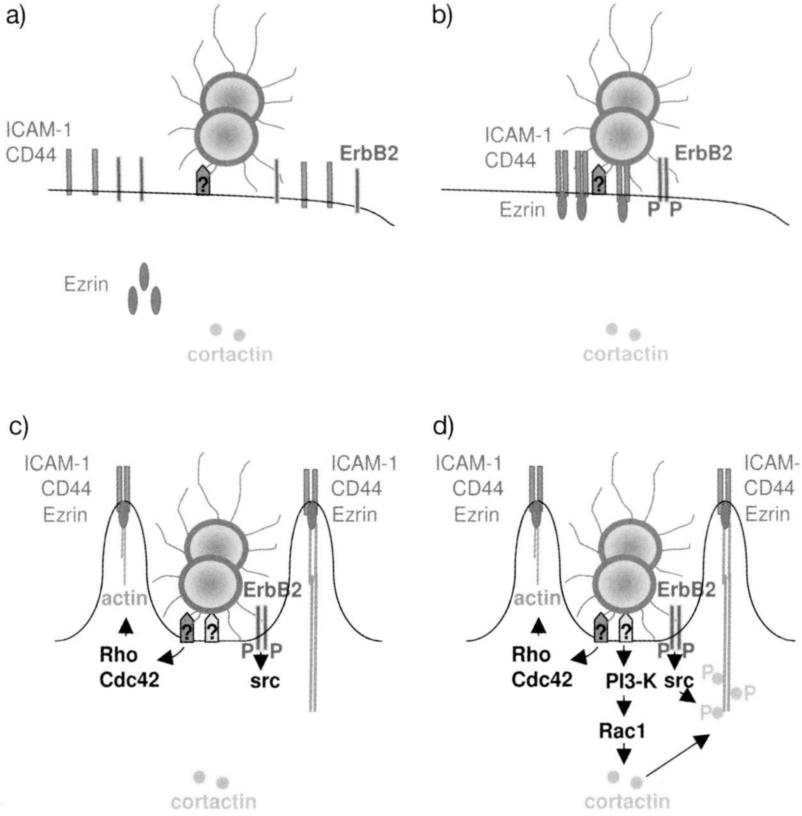

Fig. 13.2 Schematic representation of the signaling pathways activated by *N. meningitidis*, leading to their internalization into human endothelial cells. (A) Type IV pili initiate the interaction of virulent, encapsulated *N. meningitidis* with human endothelial cells by interacting with a cellular receptor, possibly CD46 [17]. (B) This pili-dependent adhesion induces the recruitment of ezrin and the clustering of several transmembrane proteins: the ErbB2 tyrosine kinase receptor and the ezrin-binding proteins CD44 and ICAM-1. (C) The activation of both Rho and Cdc42 GTPases induces a local polymerization of cortical actin. ErbB2 clustering leads to the activation of src tyrosine kinase. (D) In parallel, LOS of *N. meningitidis*, by a mechanism which remains to be identified, provides a costimulatory signal leading to PI3-K and Rac1 activation and the subsequent translocation of cortactin to the site of cortical actin rearrangements. When localized at the cell plasma membrane, cortactin is tyrosine-phosphorylated by src kinase and contributes to the formation of dynamic actin structures, leading to the formation of membrane projections which surround bacteria and induce their internalization within endothelial intracellular vacuoles. (This figure also appears with the color plates.)

tical actin polymerization induced by *N. meningitidis* relies on the activation of both Rho and Cdc42 Rho GTPases, along with the activation of a PI3-K/Rac1GTPase signaling pathway involved in cortactin recruitment at the bacterial entry site [54, 60]. The signaling pathways triggered by *N. meningitidis* interaction with human endothelial cells are summarized in Fig. 13.2.

The rearrangements require pili and PilT, which is involved in pilus retraction and is greatly enhanced when mechanical force is exerted on the host cell membrane. The force exerted by pilus retraction is thought to be the motive force that induces elongation of microvilli [28]. Moreover, recent data indicate that LOS integrity is required for efficient bacterial uptake. Bacteria expressing a truncated LOS structure elicit the formation of altered cortical plaques [60, 61]. Indeed, LOS provides a costimulatory signal, leading to the activation of the PI3-K/Rac1 GTPase signaling pathway, which is required for cortactin recruitment to the bacterial adhesion sites and its subsequent phosphorylation downstream of the ErbB2/src pathway. By controlling cortactin localization, LOS contributes to the formation of actin structures and membrane protrusions associated with the internalization of *N. meningitidis* [60].

13.3.3
Intimate Adhesion

After 8–16 h of *N. meningitidis* interaction with host cells, diffuse adherence occurs, during which process bacteria disperse at the cell surface, lose their pili, and adhere tightly to the host cell plasma membrane [13, 53]. During this step, the loss of the host cell membrane protrusions seen during localized adhesion is observed. Two main processes are responsible for diffuse adherence. The first is bacterial dispersal over the cell surface, which is mediated by PilT, and a reduction in pilus expression [13]. The second is the intimate attachment of the bacteria, characterized by PilC1 downregulation and capsule downregulation [11, 62–64].

13.4
N. meningitidis Survival and Replication Within Host Cells

Adhesion is usually followed by internalization of the bacterium, occurring predominantly during the stage of localized adhesion [54]. Intracellular bacteria apparently reside within a membranous vacuole, since the presence of a phagosomal membrane surrounding bacteria is visible by electron microscopy. However, the immediate environment of intracellular neisseriae is unclear at present. After internalization, the bacterium is able to survive within the membranous vacuole and to progress completely through the epithelial or endothelial layer by 18–40 h post-infection [28].

13.4.1
Intracellular Survival

Like a number of other mucosal pathogens, *N. meningitidis* secretes one of two closely related types of IgA1 proteases which cleave at different sites within the hinge of the human IgA1 (hIgA1) subclass of immunoglobulins. Type 1 protease cleaves at a specific proline–serine (P-S) bond, while type 2 protease cleaves at a proline–threonine (P-T) bond in the hIgA1 hinge. Indirect evidence suggests that the protease cleaves hIgA1 *in vivo*. hIgA1 activity, anti-hIgA1 antibodies, and hIgA1 fragments of the sizes predicted to result from IgA1 protease cleavage have been found in the nasal mucus of infected individuals [28]. The IgA1 protease may therefore promote bacterial colonization through cleavage of protective secretory antibodies.

A second biological function has been identified for the neisseria type 2 IgA1 protease: that of altering the levels of a major lysosomal protein, thereby promoting intracellular survival of the bacteria [65]. Lysosomes are terminal degradative compartments in the endocytic route [66]. They perform key functions within a eukaryotic cell, among them the digestion of foreign compounds and macromolecules that have been endocytosed. Numerous hydrolases sequestered in the lysosome lumen degrade a wide range of biological materials, including proteins, carbohydrates, lipids, and nucleic acids. Associated with the lysosomal membrane are enzymes that participate in the acidification of the lumen, selective transport of metabolites from the lumen to the cytoplasm, and fusion of the lysosome with other compartments and organelles. A unique class of glycoproteins known as lysosome-associated membrane proteins (LAMPs), of which LAMP1 and LAMP2 are members, is located in the lysosomal membrane [67]. LAMP1 and LAMP2 contain a proline-rich hinge with striking similarities to the hIgA1 hinge. The function of LAMPs is unknown, although they have been hypothesized to play a role in protecting the lysosome from its associated hydrolases.

The *Neisseria* type 2 IgA1 protease cleaves Lamp1 [65, 68]. Protease cleavage of Lamp1 accelerates its degradation and reduces its steady-state levels in infected epithelial cells [65]. Such cleavage apparently occurs at the cell plasma membrane. The flux in cytosolic free Ca^{2+} levels induced by the *Neisseria* pilus triggers lysosome exocytosis and an increase in cell surface Lamp1 levels [69]. Surface Lamp1 is then quickly cleaved by IgA1 protease secreted by bacteria adhered to the cell surface [69]. By cleaving Lamp1, the protease also indirectly reduces the levels of several other lysosomal constituents, such as Lamp2, CD63, and lysosomal acid phosphatase, thereby altering the lysosomes of *Neisseria*-infected cells [70]. A mutant with a defined deletion in the IgA1 protease gene (*iga*) is negatively affected during intracellular growth [65] and in the early stages of passage through polarized epithelial cells [71], therefore confirming that IgA1 protease-mediated alterations in lysosomes play a role in *Neisseria* intracellular survival and trafficking.

13.4.2
Intracellular Replication

Once having entered the host cells, *N. meningitidis* is able to replicate within cultured epithelial cell lines [65]. Transmission electron micrographs of infected nasopharyngeal organ cultures reveal *N. meningitidis* in large numbers, apparently within phagosomes, suggesting that intracellular replication also occurs in this *ex vivo* setting [72]. The significance of intracellular *N. meningitidis* replication is unclear, although it is likely to play a role in promoting disease. A mutant identified in the closely related species, *N. gonorhoeae*, traffics through polarized epithelial cells at an enhanced rate [73]. This mutant, named *fitA*, for fast intracellular trafficker A, also had an accelerated intracellular replication phenotype, suggesting that replication may be part of the transcytotic process for pathogenic *Neisseriae*. Alternatively, such a strategy may promote bacterial persistence, thereby facilitating the transmission of infection.

Replication of *N. meningitidis* within host cells requires the acquisition of iron, an essential nutrient for *N. meningitidis*. Chelation of iron from infected tissue culture cells strongly inhibited intracellular replication of *N. meningitidis*, suggesting that iron must be acquired from the host cell [74]. Interestingly, while multiple iron uptake systems – hemoglobin, transferrin, and lactoferrin – have been shown to perform essential functions for *N. meningitidis* replication at extracellular sites within the human host [75], these systems are not involved in iron uptake by intracellular bacteria [76]. A HmbR mutant (unable to use hemoglobin iron) or a fbpA mutant (unable to utilize human transferrin iron or lactoferrin iron) replicate normally within cells. In contrast, *N. meningitidis* lacking TonB are unable to replicate intracellularly unless infected cultures are supplemented with ferric nitrate [76]. The TonB complex is a highly conserved macromolecule located in the inner membrane and periplasm. Proteins in this complex, TonB, ExbB, and ExbD, cooperate in translating the proton motive force across the inner membrane into conformational changes in TonB-dependent outer membrane receptors [77]. A yet undefined TonB-dependent receptor is therefore implicated in the acquisition of intracellular iron.

The vast majority of nonhemoglobin iron in humans is localized intracellularly within the storage molecule ferritin. A recent study indicates that *N. meningitidis* accelerates ferritin degradation in host epithelial cells to yield an essential iron source [74]. Cytosolic ferritin is then aggregated and recruited to intracellular meningococci. Inhibition of such ferritin redistribution and degradation prevents intracellular *N. meningitidis* from replicating. Since *N. meningitidis* can interfere with transferrin uptake by infected cells [78], it has been proposed that accelerated ferritin degradation occurs as a response to an iron starvation state induced by *N. meningitidis* infection. Ferritin degradation therefore provides intracellular bacteria with a critical source of iron.

13.5
Interactions with Extracellular Matrix Proteins

Between endothelial and epithelial layers, the invading meningococcus encounters the extracellular matrix (ECM). Traversal of this macromolecular complex is imperative for progression of the infection, but our current knowledge of this process is extremely limited. Observational studies have described a degradation of the ECM as the pathogen interacts with it. Adhesion assays were carried out using different strains tested with ECM preparations; and these isolated matrix protein components [79]. Results showed that all the strains adhered to the ECM, especially to fibronectin and collagen types I, III, and V. Further work involved blocking specific parts of the interacting proteins, leading to the identification of the cell-binding domain on the bacterial cell surface and the discovery that the binding seen in the meningococcus is unlike the binding by other bacteria in that it does not involve the C- or N-terminal of the host fibronectin molecules [79]. It was also discovered that binding occurred regardless of the expression of Opa and Opc proteins. Further work is required to elucidate the mechanisms by which the bacterium invades and traverses this important layer around the vascular system, and also around the brain and spinal cord.

13.6
Conclusions

Recent progress has opened the way to a molecular understanding of neisserial attachment and invasion in the pathogenesis of neisserial infection. A number of adhesive factors have been characterized and their cognate receptors defined. Recent exciting findings have considerably expanded our understanding of the cellular events involved in *N. meningitidis* invasion processes, underlining the complex sequence of signaling events induced by *N. meningitidis* to elicit its uptake in nonphagocytic cells. However, in spite of recent advances in our understanding of these molecular mechanisms, much remains to be discovered about the complex molecular networks involved. Among major issues is the identification of the receptor for meningococcal pili, which would constitute a significant breakthrough in the field and pave the way to the future development of novel vaccinal strategies. Future research should also focus on the identification of key proteins that may functionally link cortical actin cytoskeletal reorganization to the endocytic machinery responsible for the formation of intracellular vacuoles containing bacteria and their subsequent transcytosis through cellular barriers. In addition to the importance of the elucidation of this pathway for our current knowledge of *N. meningitidis* pathogenesis, these results would also certainly bring new insights in the understanding of fundamental cellular mechanisms of infection.

References

1 Virji, M., et al. **1991**, The role of pili in the interactions of pathogenic Neisseria with cultured human endothelial cells, *Mol Microbiol* 5, 1831–1841.

2 Nassif, X., et al. **1994**, Roles of pilin and PilC in adhesion of Neisseria meningitidis to human epithelial and endothelial cells, *Proc Natl Acad Sci USA* 91, 3769–3773.

3 Nassif, X., et al. **1997**, Type-4 pili and meningococcal adhesiveness, *Gene* 192, 149–153.

4 Virji, M., et al. **1996**, Posttranslational modifications of meningococcal pili,

Identification of a common trisaccharide substitution on variant pilins of strain C311, *Ann NY Acad Sci* 797, 53–64.
5 Marceau, M., et al. **1998**, Consequences of the loss of O-linked glycosylation of meningococcal type IV pilin on piliation and pilus-mediated adhesion, *Mol Microbiol* 27, 705–715.
6 Nassif, X., et al. **1993**, Antigenic variation of pilin regulates adhesion of Neisseria meningitidis to human epithelial cells, *Mol Microbiol* 8, 719–725.
7 Marceau, M., J. L. Beretti, X. Nassif **1995**, High adhesiveness of encapsulated Neisseria meningitidis to epithelial cells is associated with the formation of bundles of pili, *Mol Microbiol* 17, 855–863.
8 Helaine, S., et al. **2005**, PilX, a pilus-associated protein essential for bacterial aggregation, is a key to pilus-facilitated attachment of Neisseria meningitidis to human cells, *Mol Microbiol* 55, 65–77.
9 Rahman, M., et al. **1997**, PilC of pathogenic Neisseria is associated with the bacterial cell surface, *Mol Microbiol* 25, 11–25.
10 Rudel, T., I. Scheurerpflug, T. F. Meyer **1995**, Neisseria PilC protein identified as type-4 pilus tip-located adhesin, *Nature* 373, 357–359.
11 Taha, M. K., et al. **1998**, Pilus-mediated adhesion of Neisseria meningitidis: the essential role of cell contact-dependent transcriptional upregulation of the PilC1 protein, *Mol Microbiol* 28, 1153–1163.
12 Pron, B., et al. **1997**, Interaction of Neisseria meningitidis with the components of the blood–brain barrier correlates with an increased expression of PilC, *J Infect Dis* 176, 1285–1292.
13 Pujol, C., et al. **1999**, The meningococcal PilT protein is required for induction of intimate attachment to epithelial cells following pilus-mediated adhesion, *Proc Natl Acad Sci USA* 96, 4017–4022.
14 Merz, A. J., M. So, M.P. Sheetz **2000**, Pilus retraction powers bacterial twitching motility, *Nature* 407, 98–102.
15 Maier, B. **2005**, Using laser tweezers to measure twitching motility in Neisseria, *Curr Opin Microbiol* 8, 344–349.
16 Maier, B., M. Koomey, M.P. Sheetz **2004**, A force-dependent switch reverses type IV pilus retraction, *Proc Natl Acad Sci USA* 101, 10961–10966.
17 Kallstrom, H., et al. **1997**, Membrane cofactor protein (MCP or CD46) is a cellular pilus receptor for pathogenic Neisseria, *Mol Microbiol* 25, 639–647.
18 Dorig, R. E., et al. **1993**, The human CD46 molecule is a receptor for measles virus (Edmonston strain), *Cell* 75, 295–305.
19 Santoro, F., et al. **1999**, CD46 is a cellular receptor for human herpes virus 6, *Cell* 99, 817–827.
20 Johansson, L., et al. **2003**, CD46 in meningococcal disease, *Science* 301, 373–375.
21 Kirchner, M., D. Heuer, T. F. Meyer **2005**, CD46-independent binding of neisserial type IV pili and the major pilus adhesin, PilC, to human epithelial cells, *Infect Immun* 73, 3072–3082.
22 Edwards, J. L., et al. **2002**, A co-operative interaction between Neisseria gonorrhoeae and complement receptor 3 mediates infection of primary cervical epithelial cells, *Cell Microbiol* 4, 571–584.
23 Gill, D. B., et al. **2003**, Down-regulation of CD46 by piliated Neisseria gonorrhoeae, *J Exp Med* 198, 1313–1322.
24 Edwards, J. L., M. A. Apicella **2005**, I-domain-containing integrins serve as pilus receptors for Neisseria gonorrhoeae adherence to human epithelial cells, *Cell Microbiol* 7, 1197–1211.
25 Tobiason, D. M., H. S. Seifert **2001**, Inverse relationship between pilus-mediated gonococcal adherence and surface expression of the pilus receptor, CD46, *Microbiology* 147, 2333–2340.
26 Dehio, C., S. D. Gray-Owen, T. F. Meyer **1998**, The role of neisserial Opa proteins in interactions with host cells, *Trends Microbiol* 6, 489–495.
27 Nassif, X. **1999**, Interaction mechanisms of encapsulated meningococci with eucaryotic cells: what does this tell us about the crossing of the blood-brain barrier by Neisseria meningitidis? *Curr Opin Microbiol* 2, 71–77.
28 Merz, A. J., M. So **2000**, Interactions of pathogenic neisseriae with epithelial cell membranes, *Annu Rev Cell Dev Biol* 16, 423–457.

29 Virji, M., et al. **1993**, Meningococcal Opa and Opc proteins: their role in colonization and invasion of human epithelial and endothelial cells, *Mol Microbiol* 10, 499–510.
30 Makino, S., J. P. van Putten, T. F. Meyer **1991**, Phase variation of the opacity outer membrane protein controls invasion by Neisseria gonorrhoeae into human epithelial cells, *EMBO J* 10, 1307–1315.
31 Hammarstrom, S. **1999**, The carcinoembryonic antigen (CEA) family: structures, suggested functions and expression in normal and malignant tissues, *Semin Cancer Biol* 9, 67–81.
32 Virji, M., et al. **1999**, Critical determinants of host receptor targeting by Neisseria meningitidis and Neisseria gonorrhoeae: identification of Opa adhesiotopes on the N-domain of CD66 molecules, *Mol Microbiol* 34, 538–551.
33 van Putten, J. P., S. M. Paul **1995**, Binding of syndecan-like cell surface proteoglycan receptors is required for Neisseria gonorrhoeae entry into human mucosal cells, *EMBO J* 14, 2144–2154.
34 Grassme, H., et al. **1997**, Acidic sphingomyelinase mediates entry of N. gonorrhoeae into nonphagocytic cells, *Cell* 91, 605–615.
35 Gomez-Duarte, O. G., et al. **1997**, Binding of vitronectin to opa-expressing Neisseria gonorrhoeae mediates invasion of HeLa cells, *Infect Immun* 65, 3857–3866.
36 Olyhoek, A. J., et al. **1991**, Cloning and expression in Escherichia coli of opc, the gene for an unusual class 5 outer membrane protein from Neisseria meningitidis (meningococci/surface antigen), *Microb Pathog* 11, 249–257.
37 Seiler, A., et al. **1996**, Allelic polymorphism and site-specific recombination in the opc locus of Neisseria meningitidis, *Mol Microbiol* 19, 841–856.
38 Sarkari, J., et al. **1994**, Variable expression of the Opc outer membrane protein in Neisseria meningitidis is caused by size variation of a promoter containing poly-cytidine, *Mol Microbiol* 13, 207–217.
39 Virji, M., et al. **1992**, Expression of the Opc protein correlates with invasion of epithelial and endothelial cells by Neisseria meningitidis, *Mol Microbiol* 6, 2785–2795.
40 Virji, M., K. Makepeace, E. R. Moxon **1994**, Distinct mechanisms of interactions of Opc-expressing meningococci at apical and basolateral surfaces of human endothelial cells; the role of integrins in apical interactions, *Mol Microbiol* 14, 173–184.
41 Virji, M., et al. **1995**, Opc- and pilus-dependent interactions of meningococci with human endothelial cells: molecular mechanisms and modulation by surface polysaccharides, *Mol Microbiol* 18, 741–754.
42 Unkmeir, A., et al. **2002**, Fibronectin mediates Opc-dependent internalization of Neisseria meningitidis in human brain microvascular endothelial cells, *Mol Microbiol* 46, 933–946.
43 Capecchi, B., et al. **2005**, Neisseria meningitidis NadA is a new invasin which promotes bacterial adhesion to and penetration into human epithelial cells, *Mol Microbiol* 55, 687–698.
44 Comanducci, M., et al. **2002**, NadA, a novel vaccine candidate of Neisseria meningitidis, *J Exp Med* 195, 1445–1454.
45 Kahler, C. M., D. S. Stephens **1998**, Genetic basis for biosynthesis, structure, and function of meningococcal lipooligosaccharide (endotoxin), *Crit Rev Microbiol* 24, 281–334.
46 Porat, N., M. A. Apicella, M. S. Blake **1995**, A lipooligosaccharide-binding site on HepG2 cells similar to the gonococcal opacity-associated surface protein Opa, *Infect Immun* 63, 2164–2172.
47 Estabrook, M. M., D. Zhou, M. A. Apicella **1998**, Nonopsonic phagocytosis of group C Neisseria meningitidis by human neutrophils, *Infect Immun* 66, 1028–1036.
48 Unkmeir, A., et al. **2002**, Lipooligosaccharide and polysaccharide capsule: virulence factors of Neisseria meningitidis that determine meningococcal interaction with human dendritic cells, *Infect Immun* 70, 2454–2462.
49 van Putten, J. P. **1993**, Phase variation of lipopolysaccharide directs interconversion of invasive and immuno-resistant

phenotypes of Neisseria gonorrhoeae, *EMBO J* 12, 4043–4051.
50 Tzeng, Y. L., D. S. Stephens **2000**, Epidemiology and pathogenesis of Neisseria meningitidis, *Microbes Infect* 2, 687–700.
51 Nassif, X., et al. **2002**, How do extracellular pathogens cross the blood–brain barrier? *Trends Microbiol* 10, 227–232.
52 Merz, A. J., et al. **1996**, Traversal of a polarized epithelium by pathogenic Neisseriae: facilitation by type IV pili and maintenance of epithelial barrier function, *Mol Med* 2, 745–754.
53 Pujol, C., et al. **1997**, Interaction of Neisseria meningitidis with a polarized monolayer of epithelial cells, *Infect Immun* 65, 4836–4842.
54 Eugene, E., et al. **2002**, Microvilli-like structures are associated with the internalization of virulent capsulated Neisseria meningitidis into vascular endothelial cells, *J Cell Sci* 115, 1231–1241.
55 Kallstrom, H., et al. **1998**, Cell signaling by the type IV pili of pathogenic Neisseria, *J Biol Chem* 273, 21777–21782.
56 Merz, A. J., M. So **1997**, Attachment of piliated, Opa- and Opc-gonococci and meningococci to epithelial cells elicits cortical actin rearrangements and clustering of tyrosine-phosphorylated proteins, *Infect Immun* 65, 4341–4349.
57 Merz, A. J., C. A. Enns, M. So **1999**, Type IV pili of pathogenic Neisseriae elicit cortical plaque formation in epithelial cells, *Mol Microbiol* 32, 1316–1332.
58 Bretscher, A., K. Edwards, R. G. Fehon **2002**, ERM proteins and merlin: integrators at the cell cortex, *Nat Rev Mol Cell Biol* 3, 586–599.
59 Hoffmann, I., et al. **2001**, Activation of ErbB2 receptor tyrosine kinase supports invasion of endothelial cells by Neisseria meningitidis, *J Cell Biol* 155, 133–143.
60 Lambotin, M., et al. **2005**, Invasion of endothelial cells by Neisseria meningitidis requires cortactin recruitment by a PI3-Kinase/Rac1 signalling pathway triggered by the lipo-oligosaccharide, *J Cell Sci* (in press).
61 Bonnah, R. A., et al. **2005**, Lipooligosaccharide-independent alteration of cellular homeostasis in Neisseria meningitidis-infected epithelial cells, *Cell Microbiol* 7, 869–885.
62 Deghmane, A. E., et al. **2000**, Intimate adhesion of Neisseria meningitidis to human epithelial cells is under the control of the crgA gene, a novel LysR-type transcriptional regulator, *EMBO J* 19, 1068–1078.
63 Deghmane, A. E., et al. **2002**, Down-regulation of pili and capsule of Neisseria meningitidis upon contact with epithelial cells is mediated by CrgA regulatory protein, *Mol Microbiol* 43, 1555–1564.
64 Morelle, S., E. Carbonnelle, X. Nassif **2003**, The REP2 repeats of the genome of Neisseria meningitidis are associated with genes coordinately regulated during bacterial cell interaction, *J Bacteriol* 185, 2618–2627.
65 Lin, L., et al. **1997**, The Neisseria type 2 IgA1 protease cleaves LAMP1 and promotes survival of bacteria within epithelial cells, *Mol Microbiol* 24, 1083–1094.
66 Winchester, B. **2005**, Lysosomal metabolism of glycoproteins, *Glycobiology* 15, 1R–15R.
67 Winchester, B. G. **2001**, Lysosomal membrane proteins, *Eur J Paediatr Neurol* 5[Suppl A], 11–19.
68 Hauck, C. R., T. F. Meyer **1997**, The lysosomal/phagosomal membrane protein h-lamp-1 is a target of the IgA1 protease of Neisseria gonorrhoeae, *FEBS Lett* 405, 86–90.
69 Ayala, B. P., et al. **2001**, The pilus-induced Ca^{2+} flux triggers lysosome exocytosis and increases the amount of Lamp1 accessible to Neisseria IgA1 protease, *Cell Microbiol* 3, 265–275.
70 Ayala, P., et al. **1998**, Infection of epithelial cells by pathogenic neisseriae reduces the levels of multiple lysosomal constituents, *Infect Immun* 66, 5001–5007.
71 Hopper, S., et al. **2000**, Effects of the immunoglobulin A1 protease on Neisseria gonorrhoeae trafficking across polarized T84 epithelial monolayers, *Infect Immun* 68, 906–911.
72 Stephens, D. S., L. H. Hoffman, Z. A. McGee **1983**, Interaction of Neisseria meningitidis with human nasopharyngeal mucosa: attachment and entry into

columnar epithelial cells, *J Infect Dis* 148, 369–376.

73 Hopper, S., et al. **2000**, Isolation of Neisseria gonorrhoeae mutants that show enhanced trafficking across polarized T84 epithelial monolayers, *Infect Immun* 68, 896–905.

74 Larson, J. A., H. L. Howie, M. So **2004**, Neisseria meningitidis accelerates ferritin degradation in host epithelial cells to yield an essential iron source, *Mol Microbiol* 53, 807–820.

75 Schryvers, A. B., I. Stojiljkovic **1999**, Iron acquisition systems in the pathogenic Neisseria, *Mol Microbiol* 32, 1117–1123.

76 Larson, J. A., et al. **2002**, Replication of Neisseria meningitidis within epithelial cells requires TonB-dependent acquisition of host cell iron, *Infect Immun* 70, 1461–1467.

77 Moeck, G. S., J. W. Coulton **1998**, TonB-dependent iron acquisition: mechanisms of siderophore-mediated active transport, *Mol Microbiol* 28, 675–681.

78 Bonnah, R. A., et al. **2000**, Alteration of epithelial cell transferrin–iron homeostasis by Neisseria meningitidis and Neisseria gonorrhoeae, *Cell Microbiol* 2, 207–218.

79 Eberhard, T., et al. **1998**, Binding to human extracellular matrix by Neisseria meningitidis, *Infect Immun* 66, 1791–1794.

14
Role of Complement in Defense Against Meningococcal Infection

Sanjay Ram and Ulrich Vogel

14.1
Introduction

The importance of complement in the innate immune defenses against neisserial infections is well established. The interaction of the complement system with *Neisseria meningitidis* is of pivotal importance for our understanding of differences in virulence among strains and their propensities to cause deadly invasive disease, as opposed to coexisting in the nasopharynx as an asymptomatic carrier strain. The dynamic nature of the complement system and the several functions it subserves accounts for its complexity. The discussion of the interaction of the bacteria with this system is therefore preceded by a brief introduction into the biology of this arm of the innate immune system.

14.2
The Complement Cascade

The complement system comprises about 30 different fluid-phase proteins circulating in plasma and several membrane-associated complement receptor proteins. There are three pathways by which complement can be activated, called the classical, alternative, and lectin pathways. For a detailed review of the complement cascade, the reader is referred to textbooks of immunology or a recent review by Walport [1, 2]. A schematic of complement activation and its regulation in the fluid phase is shown in Fig. 14.1.

14.2.1
The Classical Pathway

The classical pathway was the first to be described and is triggered by the binding of an antibody molecule to an antigen. This results in the binding of the activated C1 complex (composed of a C1q molecule and two molecules each of

Handbook of Meningococcal Disease. Infection Biology, Vaccination, Clinical Management.
Edited by M. Frosch and M. C. J. Maiden

ISBN: 3-527-31260-9

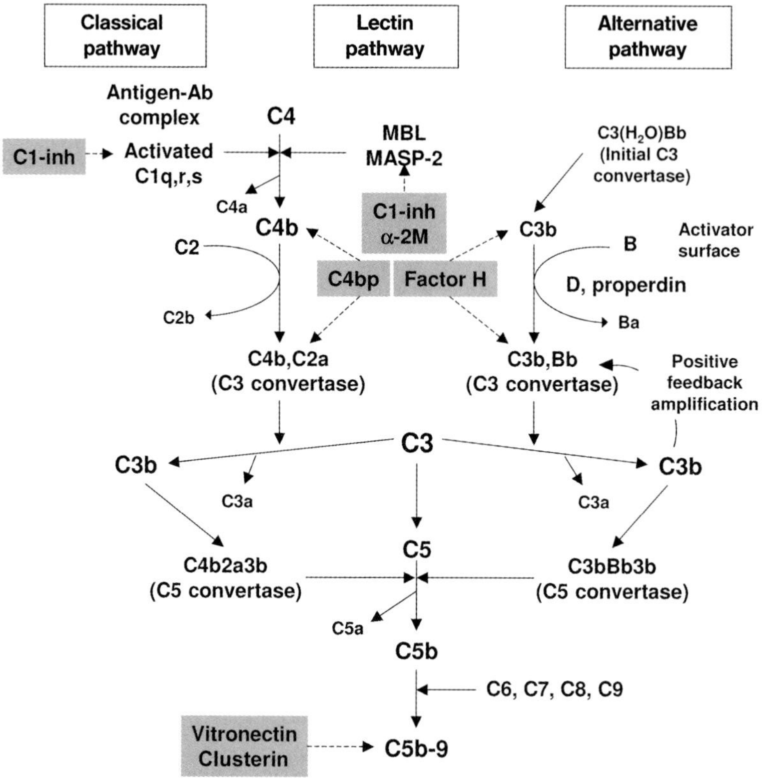

Fig. 14.1 Schematic of the complement cascade. The key soluble phase negative regulatory molecules are indicated by gray shaded boxes.

C1r and C1s). Activated C1s in the complex first cleaves C4, which results in the separation of 77 amino acids (C4a) from the N-terminal end of the C4 α-chain and the subsequent formation of the metastable C4b molecule. This results in the activation of the internal thioester bond of C4b, so that the carbonyl group linked to sulfur (the native thioester) becomes more electrophilic (i.e. an electron acceptor) and reacts readily with nucleophilic groups (i.e., electron-donating groups) such as –OH to form an ester linkage, or with $-NH_2$ to form an amide linkage. Alternatively, the carbonyl group can react with water and become hydrolyzed. C1s also cleaves C2; and the C2a fragment binds to C4b to form C4b2a, which is the C3 convertase of the classical pathway. Binding of a C3 molecule at or close to the classical pathway C3 convertase imparts C5 convertase activity to the enzyme complex.

14.2.2
The Alternative Pathway

Akin to C4, C3 also possesses a highly reactive internal thioester bond. Initiation of the alternative pathway occurs by spontaneous low-rate hydrolysis of the thioester in C3 and the resultant continuous supply of C3(H_2O) in solution. Binding of Factor B to C3(H_2O) in the presence of Factor D leads to the formation of the alternative pathway initiation C3 convertase [C3(H_2O)Bb]. This initiation fluid-phase C3 convertase can cleave C3 to release C3a and C3b. The C3b fragment covalently binds to cellular and microbial surfaces. If the cell or microbe surface is an activator, alternative pathway activation will proceed. If the C3b fragment covalently binds to a cell or microbe surface that is not an activator, alternative pathway activation will stop. The binding of Factor B to a C3b fragment covalently bound to an activator, in the presence of Factor D, will lead to the formation of an alternative pathway C3 convertase (C3bBb) on the activator surface, which can cleave more C3 molecules. This positive C3 amplification loop is a key feature of the alternative pathway. The binding of an additional C3b to the C3 convertase leads to the formation of the C5 convertase (C3bBb3b). Factor P (properdin) stabilizes both the C3 and C5 alternative pathway convertases from decay dissociation. The importance of properdin and the alternative pathway positive feedback loop is illustrated by the observation that properdin-deficient individuals are predisposed to meningococcal infections and suffer a higher mortality than persons with a normal complement system [3–5].

14.2.3
The Lectin Pathway

Although most recently described, the lectin pathway is phylogenetically older than the classical pathway. The lectin pathway is activated when mannose-binding lectin (MBL) binds to membrane carbohydrates or other ligands on microorganisms. Mannan-binding lectin (MBL) is a member of the collectin family of proteins. MBL is associated with three novel MBL-associated serine proteases (MASPs): MASP-1, MASP-2, and MASP-3. Most of the protease activity is mediated by MASP-2, which cleaves C4. MASP-1 has only marginal C3 and C2 cleaving activity; and its role in complement activation is uncertain. Although the function of MASP-3 is not resolved, recombinant MASP-3 can inhibit C4-cleaving activity of recombinant as well as naturally occurring MBL/MASP-2 complexes. Upon activation, the MBL–MASP-2 complex is able to cleave C4 and C2 to form C4b2a, the C3 convertase that is able to enzymatically split hundreds of molecules of C3 into C3a and C3b.

MBL binds to a wide array of carbohydrate structures on microbial surfaces and is believed to mediate direct killing via complement activation or by enhancing phagocytosis by acting as an opsonin. Complement receptor 1 (CR1/CD35) has been defined as the cellular receptor for MBL [6], a finding consistent with the structural relatedness of MBL to C1q, which also binds to CR1.

14.2.4
Assembly of the Terminal Complement Components (Membrane Attack Complex)

In all three activation pathways, the cleavage of C5 leads to the assembly of the C5b-9 membrane attack complex (MAC, or C5b-9). The C5 convertases cleave the C5 component to generate C5a and C5b fragments. C5a serves as an inflammatory mediator that can activate a variety of cells through G protein-linked receptors. The MAC is composed of one molecule each of C5b, C6, C7, and C8 and as many as 10–12 molecules of C9. When C5 is cleaved by C5 convertase, nascent C5b binds to C6 and forms a stable bimolecular complex that binds C7. The C5b67 complex has amphiphilic properties and commits MAC assembly to a membrane site. The binding of one C8 molecule to each C5b67 complex gives rise to small transmembrane channels that perturb the target membrane. Each membrane-bound C5b678 complex acts as a receptor for multiple C9 molecules. The binding of the first C9 initiates a process of C9 oligomerization at the site of membrane attack. The MAC, once assembled in the cell membrane (for example, the membrane of a gram-negative bacterium), creates transmembrane channels, leading to osmotic lysis of the cell. The transmembrane channels formed vary in size, depending on the number of C9 molecules incorporated into the complex.

14.2.5
Regulation of the Complement Cascade in the Fluid Phase

Uncontrolled activation of the complement cascade can be detrimental to the host and therefore must be tightly regulated. Activation is confined to sites of tissue damage and on foreign surfaces, while kept to a minimum under physiological conditions. Regulation is mediated by several soluble as well as membrane-bound proteins at various stages of the cascade. A soluble phase regulator of the early part of the classical pathway is C1-inhibitor, a serpin (*ser*ine *p*rotease *in*hibitor) that binds to and inactivates C1r, C1s, and the MASPs. The MBL pathway is also regulated by α2-macroglobulin.

Another important regulator of the classical pathway at the level of C4 is C4b-binding protein (C4bp). C4bp acts as a cofactor in the factor I-mediated cleavage of C4b to C4d (hemolytically inactive). In addition, C4bp can cause irreversible dissociation of the classical pathway C3 convertase (C4b2a) into its component molecules, which is termed decay-accelerating activity.

The analogous regulator of the alternative pathway of complement is factor H, which acts as a cofactor in the factor I-mediated cleavage and inactivation of C3b to iC3b. It also possesses decay-accelerating activity by virtue of its ability to cleave C3bBb to C3b and factor Bb. Several bacteria, including the pathogenic *Neisseriae*, can bind to human factor H and C4bp and regulate complement activation on their surface; and the role of these regulatory molecules in neisserial pathogenesis is discussed in more detail below.

The formation of the C5b-9 (MAC) is controlled by the S-protein (vitronectin) in serum, which prevents C9 polymerization and blocks the attachment of

C5b67 to the cell surface. This protects cells proximate to sites of complement activation from accidental attack.

14.2.6 Membrane-associated Complement Receptors and Regulators

Several host cell surface-associated molecules act as ligands for complement molecules, including the C1q receptor (C1qR), the complement receptors (CRs) 1, 2, 3, and 4, and receptors for complement activation products, such as the C5a receptor. These molecules subserve important biological functions – e.g., the CR3 receptor binds iC3b and plays a key role in the opsonophagocytic clearance of bacteria.

The function of preventing host cells from complement-mediated lysis during periods of complement activation, as may occur during meningococcemia, is performed by several membrane-bound regulators of complement, which include complement receptor 1 (CR1), membrane cofactor protein (MCP, or CD46), decay-accelerating factor (DAF, or CD55), and homologous restriction factor (protectin, or CD59). A detailed description of these receptors is beyond the scope of this chapter.

14.3 Complement Deficiencies and Meningococcal Infections

The complement system forms a key arm of the innate immune defenses against the pathogenic neisseriae (*N. meningitidis, N. gonorrhoeae*). Evidence for the importance of complement in combating neisserial infections is provided by the strong association between persons with deficiencies of the terminal complement components (C5–C9) with recurrent meningococcal infections. Hereditary deficiencies of complement components are very rare; and their incidence varies with ethnic groups. For example, C9 deficiency is most commonly encountered in the Japanese population ($\sim$1 in 1000 persons) [7], while C6 deficiency is more frequent among African-Americans ($\sim$1 in 1600) than Caucasians, in a survey conducted in the south-eastern United States [8]. C6 deficiency has also been reported in several families in the western Cape region of South Africa [9]. Disease caused by serogroups W-135, Y, and other rarer serogroups [10–13] are more frequently seen in persons with terminal complement deficiencies [10–13]. Despite the higher frequency of unusual serogroups isolated from complement-deficient persons, the more common serogroups (such as B and C) are still the most frequently isolated strains in persons with complement defects [14]. Diseases caused by serogroups B and C strains do not seem to be associated with complement defects. Siblings of individuals with complement deficiency, who share the same defect, often lead a healthy life and do not get meningococcal disease.

Defects of the alternative pathway have also been associated with meningococcal infections. These include deficiencies of factor D and properdin. While persons with terminal complement defects suffer recurrent disease, they have substantially milder episodes and enjoy a lower mortality per episode than their complement-sufficient counterparts. In contrast, a higher mortality than normal individuals has been reported in persons with properdin deficiency [4]. Deficiencies of regulatory proteins of the alternative pathway, factor H [15] and factor I [16], are also associated with meningococcal infections. Lack of regulators leads to uninhibited C3 activation and complement consumption in vivo, resulting in the lack of functional C3.

MBL deficiency may also be associated with meningococcal infections. Bax et al. [17] reported a case of an 18-year-old male with meningococcal meningitis who had low MBL levels. His mother and grandfather also had low MBL levels and suffered meningitis in early childhood [17].

Most persons with meningococcal disease do not have complement deficiencies. This is probably because naturally occurring antibodies against subcapsular antigens (probably induced by colonization with nonpathogenic neisseriae such as *N. lactamica*) [18, 19] are the more important line of defense against meningococcal disease, lack of which contributes to the development of meningococcal disease after acquisition of a pathogenic isolate. Colonization with *N. meningitidis* is common (prevalence of ∼5–10%) and is an "immunizing process" [20]. The importance of protective antibodies in preventing meningococcal disease is reflected by the observation that infants under the age of 3 months do not usually get the disease because of protective maternal antibodies. Waning of maternal antibodies is associated with a higher incidence of disease among infants between 3 months and 12 months of age. A second peak of high incidence is seen among teenagers, in whom outbreaks are associated with residence in dormitories, barracks, and other crowded conditions.

14.3.1
Correlation of Disease Severity with Complement Activation

The severity of meningococcal disease directly correlates with plasma levels of meningococcal endotoxin (or lipooligosaccharide): a high circulating endotoxin level portends a poor prognosis [21] (also, see chapter 21). The concentrations of endotoxin detected in the blood of persons with fulminant meningococcemia are substantially (10- to 10 000-fold) higher than those found in the blood of individuals with sepsis due to other gram-negative bacteria. Tesh and his colleagues [22] demonstrated that *E. coli* J5 released LPS when incubated with normal human serum. Release of endotoxin from intact *E. coli* (strain J5) appears to require complement activation to completion (i.e., through the final step of C9 activation) [23]. The extent of complement activation *in vivo*, as measured by terminal complement complex (C5b-9) generation, correlates positively with meningococcal disease severity [21]. Persons with complement deficiencies have a less severe disease and lower circulating endotoxin levels. This was exemplified in the case report of a C6-deficient person, who received a fresh-frozen plasma (FFP) infusion [24]. The initial endotoxin levels were low, but rose sharply following FFP infusion. These *in vivo* findings were simulated *in vitro* with *E. coli* J5, where endotoxin release by the individual's serum was augmented by FFP. Taken together, these observations suggest that at least one possible mechanism of disease severity in meningococcemia is the release of LOS from bacteria mediated by complement activation on the bacterial surface. The relatively innocuous disease course in persons with terminal complement deficiencies may be related to lower circulating endotoxin levels, which in turn may be due to lack of C5b-9 insertion in the bacterial membrane. In contrast, individuals with properdin deficiency tend to have a more fulminant disease course with higher mortality. The molecular basis for this phenomenon is not fully understood, but points to an important role for the alternative pathway in fighting meningococcal infections, especially if the levels of bactericidal antibodies are low.

14.3.2
Complement Activation on Meningococci

The classical pathway is required to initiate efficient complement-dependent killing of *Neisseriae*. Ingwer et al. [25] showed that Mg-EGTA-treated serum (inactive classical pathway) was unable to support the killing of gonococci. The absorption of bacteria-specific antibodies also abrogates the complement-dependent killing of *Neisseriae* [26, 27]. Collectively, these observations suggest that the antibody-dependent classical pathway is important for initiating complement activation on meningococci. Efficient killing of meningococci may also require a fully functional alternative pathway. Söderström et al. [28] showed a synergy between properdin levels and the amount of "presensitizing" IgG needed for the killing of certain serogroup A, B, and E strains. Jarvis and Griffiss [29] demonstrated that bactericidal killing of certain serogroup C strains was initiated by monomeric IgA1 directed against somatic antigens. The MBL pathway has been shown to activate complement on meningococci when the bacteria are "preincubated" with purified MBL, followed by the addition of serum [30, 31].

Classical pathway activation is initiated by binding of the activated C1 complex to appropriately spaced Fc domains of surface-bound IgG molecules (or adjacent Fc domains of a single IgM molecule). C1s cleaves the a-chain of C4 to release the C4a fragment, which results in activation of the labile internal thioester bond of C4 that can bind covalently to electron donors on the bacterial surface. There are two isoforms of C4 in human serum, called C4A and C4B, each with distinct properties. C4A forms amide linkages with its targets, while C4B preferentially forms ester linkages. C4A is believed to engage the CR1 more efficiently than C4B, while C4B may be hemolytically more active than C4A. The role of these isoforms of C4 in protection against *N. meningitidis* infection remains controversial. Two studies suggested an increased risk of meningitis associated with homozygous C4B deficiency [32, 33], while a larger study by Cates et al. did not confirm these findings [34].

LOS was recently found to be a target for C4b. The inner core phosphoethanolamine (PEA) residues were important in determining C4b binding to LOS

[35]. The C4A isoform formed amide linkages with PEA residues on the second heptose (HepII) of LOS. PEA at the 6-position of HepII preferentially bound C4b over PEA at the 3-position. Strains that expressed 6-PEA were found to be more serum-sensitive than those that possessed a 3-PEA. These findings may provide an explanation for the observation that 6-PEA-bearing strains comprise less than 30% of all clinical meningococcal isolates [36].

Ongoing work in our laboratory suggests that opacity-associated protein (Opa) is also an acceptor for C4b. McGee and Stevens have shown that most *N. meningitidis* isolated from patients with meningitis and septicemia formed in predominantly transparent colonies, whereas meningococci isolated from asymptomatic carriers generally formed opaque or a mixture of opaque and transparent colonies [37]. It is possible that non-opaque meningococci can resist higher levels of complement and can cause invasive disease.

C3 binding to the bacterial surface is another key event in complement activation. C3b is an integral component of the C5 convertases of the classical and alternative pathways, which is essential for C5b-9 formation and direct complement-dependent killing. In addition, C3b and its degradation product iC3b can promote opsonophagocytosis via engagement of CR1 and CR3, respectively. Jarvis demonstrated that all major serogroups of *N. meningitidis* bound C3b via ester linkages and that most of the deposited C3b was converted to iC3b [38]. The total amount of C3 deposited appeared to be independent of the cell surface sialic acid content and the resistance of the organism to killing by serum. C3 deposition and degradation was subsequently examined using isogenic mutant strains derived from the serogroup B strain B1940 that either lacked capsular polysaccharide but had sialylated LOS (*siaD*), had a truncated LOS molecule (Glc → HepI) that lacked the ability to sialylate (*galE*), or had a "double" mutation (unencapsulated, with truncated LOS; designated Δ*cps*). Despite similar amounts and "patterns" of C3b (indicative of the C3b targets on the bacterium) binding to the wild-type strain and the *siaD* mutant, only the former was serum-resistant. Truncation of LOS resulted in high levels of IgM binding, enhanced C3b binding and a serum-sensitive phenotype. Again, the pattern of C3b binding did not differ among these mutants [39]. This study pointed to important roles of capsular polysaccharide as well as LOS structure in mediating serum resistance. The *galE* mutant was used to evaluate the effects of LOS sialic acid because the LOS sialyltransferase gene had not been published at that time, but it is possible that the loss of three additional hexoses of the lacto-N-neotetraose LOS may have contributed to the dramatic effects on serum resistance and C3b binding seen with the *galE* and Δ*cps* mutants. Kahler et al. [40] subsequently demonstrated that, in the meningococcal strain NMB, a *galE* mutation did not alter the serum resistant phenotype, pointing to the central role of the capsule in mediating serum resistance [40]. It is noteworthy that the NMB *galE* mutant (in contrast to the truncated B1940 *galE* LOS) possessed a higher molecular weight LOS, containing multiple Glc residues off the HepI residue (Glc_n → HepI). We speculate that the differences in serum resistance between strains B1940 and NMB may relate to structural differences in the LOS or to other differences in the bacterial surface.

14.4
Capsular Polysaccharide and Serum Resistance

Almost all meningococci recovered from the blood or cerebrospinal fluid of persons with invasive disease possess a polysaccharide capsule. The chemical composition of capsular polysaccharide forms the basis of serogrouping of meningococci. Serogroup A polysaccharide is a homopolymer of N-acetylmannosamine phosphate; serogroup B and C capsules are homopolymers of $\alpha(2,8)$- and $\alpha(2,9)$-linked sialic acids, respectively; and serogroup W-135 and Y capsules comprise disaccharide repeating units of 6-D-Gal $\alpha(1,4)$-NANA $\alpha(2,6)$- and 6-D-Glc $\alpha(1,4)$-NANA $\alpha(2,6)$-, respectively. The polysaccharides of serogroups A, C, W-135, and Y are also variably O-acetylated.

Encapsulated meningococci are more serum-resistant than their unencapsulated counterparts [26, 39, 40]. Interruption of the polysialyltransferase (*siaD*) gene results in loss of the ability to synthesize the capsular polysaccharide of serogroup B and C strains; and the resultant mutants are serum-sensitive [39, 40]. The mechanism by which capsular polysaccharide mediates serum resistance has not been fully determined, but appears to occur at or before the level of C3 binding. Using chemical mutagenesis, Jarvis and Vedros [26] showed that a capsule-deficient mutant of a serogroup B mutant was unable to regulate the alternative pathway and was killed by serum lacking bacteria-specific immunoglobulins. They also showed that enzymatic desialylation of the wild-type strain augmented C3 deposition. This study was undertaken before neisserial LOS sialylation was described and therefore did not discriminate between LOS and capsular sialic acid. It was speculated that the presence of sialic acid may have resulted in enhanced interaction of factor H with C3b, favoring C3b inactivation. A subsequent *in vitro* study showed that colominic acid [also a homopolymer of $\alpha(2,8)$-linked sialic acid that is derived from *E. coli* K1 capsule] did not enhance the interaction between C3b and factor H [41, 42]. Therefore, the role of capsular polysaccharide in regulating the alternative pathway by this mechanism is questionable and merits further study.

Unpublished data in our laboratory has shown that unencapsulated isogenic mutant strains derived from all five major meningococcal serogroups (A, B, C, W-135, Y) bound more C3 and C4 than their wild-type parent progenitors. It is possible that capsular polysaccharide regulates the classical pathway, which could in turn lead to less alternative pathway activation. Serogroup A capsule lacks sialic acid, which indicates that the mechanism of complement regulation mediated by the meningococcal capsule is not necessarily related to the sialic acid moiety. We speculate that capsular polysaccharide may decrease the binding of naturally occurring antibodies to subcapsular antigens.

De-O-acetylated polysaccharide conjugated to proteins has been shown to be slightly more immunogenic than acetylated polysaccharide [43]. However, no difference in serum resistance was detected when mutants defective in O-acetyltransferase were compared to the wild-type strains (Claus and Vogel, unpublished data).

Lipooligosaccharide Sialylation and Serum Resistance

In 1970, Ward made the observation that *N. gonorrhoeae* recovered directly from human urethral exudates were resistant to killing by normal human serum [44]. This property was lost upon culture on standard gonococcal media and was termed "unstable" serum resistance. The seminal work of Harry Smith and his colleagues [45–47] led to the discovery that gonococci were able to use 5′-cytidinemonophospho-*N*-acetylneuraminic acid (CMP-NANA) from the host to sialylate their LOS, which led to the serum-resistant phenotype [45–47]. LOS sialylation was shown to unequivocally enhance serum resistance in *N. gonorrhoeae*. Sialylation of gonococci has been shown to increase binding of the alternative complement pathway regulatory molecule, factor H, which forms at least one mechanism of sialic acid-enhanced serum resistance [48].

Shortly after the discovery of gonococcal LOS sialylation, it was observed that *N. meningitidis* could sialylate their LOS even without the addition of CMP-NANA to growth media [49]. Strains belonging to serogroups B, C, W-135, and Y, but not serogroup A, have the ability to synthesize CMP-NANA, which acts as the donor molecule for sialic aid for biosynthesis of capsular polysaccharide and for LOS sialylation.

The role of LOS sialylation in conferring serum resistance in meningococci is not as well defined as it is for gonococci. An earlier report by Fox et al. suggested that LOS sialylation did not enhance serum resistance [50]. Another report using epidemiologically related serogroup C strains suggested that LOS sialylation did impact serum resistance [51]. The amount of killing of the strains examined correlated directly with the amount of unsialylated lacto-*N*-neotetraose expressed by the strains. The protection conferred by LOS sialylation is probably strain-specific, as evidenced by the observation that isogenic mutants lacking the ability to sialylate LOS (LOS sialyltransferase, or *lst* mutants) were slightly more serum sensitive than the wild-type strain at higher ($\geq 25\%$) serum concentrations in two strains (serogroup B strain B1940, serogroup C strain 2120), but did not impact survival in a third strain (serogroup B strain MC58) [52].

There is an important difference in the mechanism of complement regulation by LOS sialic acid on the two pathogenic neisserial species. Our preliminary observations have shown that meningococcal lacto-*N*-neotetraose LOS sialylation, in contrast to gonococcal LOS sialylation, does not enhance factor H binding. A cooperative interaction between LOS sialic acid and the gonococcal porin (Por) molecule appears to be necessary for factor H binding to *N. gonorrhoeae* [53]. Replacement of meningococcal Por with the Por molecule from *N. gonorrhoeae* results in enhanced factor H binding and a serum-resistant phenotype. LOS has been identified as a target for C3b on *Neisseriae* [54] and the low level of serum resistance that is seen with sialylation of the LOS of certain meningococcal strains may be because of obscuring of C3b targets.

The contribution of meningococcal LOS sialic acid in causing experimental infection in the infant rat model was studied using a wild-type strain and its *lst* mutant that lacked the ability to sialylate LOS. The *lst* mutant was able to cause disseminated disease to the same extent as the wild-type strain [52]. It may be concluded that meningococcal LOS sialylation plays only a minor role in enhancing serum resistance and probably is not critical for pathogenesis, at least in experimental animal models. The recovery of meningococcal isolates from blood and CSF of patients that express LOS species that lack the ability to sialylate [such as the L8 immunotype (Gal → Glc → HepI)] suggests that LOS sialylation is not essential for meningococcal pathogenesis or serum resistance. One might speculate that LOS sialylation improves the survival of unencapsulated meningococci, which are frequently observed during healthy carriage [55] and which might encounter low concentrations of complement in the oral cavity [56]. However, a systematic analysis of this question has not yet been conducted.

14.6
Complement Evasion by Meningococci

14.6.1
Binding of Host Complement Regulatory Molecules

Microbes use several mechanisms to limit complement activation on their surfaces [57]. Restriction of complement activation decreases the opsonophagocytosis of bacteria and prevents direct complement-mediated killing of gram-negative pathogens. One mechanism utilized by microbes to regulate complement activation is to bind host complement regulatory proteins, such as factor H and C4b-binding protein (C4bp). Factor H and C4bp act as cofactors for the factor I-mediated cleavage of C3b and C4b to their hemolytically inactive fragments iC3b and C4d, respectively. In addition, factor H and C4bp both possess decay-accelerating activity, which results in irreversible dissociation of the C3-convertases of the alternative (C3bBb) and classical (C4b2a) pathway, respectively. Decay-acceleration limits the total amount of C3b deposited on the organism.

Factor H binds to group A [58] and group B streptococci [59], *Borrelia burgdorferi* [60], *Streptococcus pneumoniae* [61–64], *Yersinia enterocolitica* [65], *Candida albicans* [66], human immunodeficiency virus-1 [67, 68], microfilariae of *Onchocerca volvulus* [69], and *N. gonorrhoeae* [48, 70]. C4bp has been demonstrated binding to group A streptococci [71–73], *Moraxella catarrhalis* [74], *Bordetella pertussis* [75] and *N. gonorrhoeae* [76, 77]. The ligand for both C4bp and factor H on *N. gonorrhoeae* is the porin (Por) protein.

C4bp binding to the PorA protein of serogroup B *N. meningitidis* strain H44/76 has recently been demonstrated [78]. There are salient differences in the binding of C4bp to *N. gonorrhoeae* and *N. meningitidis*. While the binding of C4bp to *N. gonorrhoeae* occurs under normotonic conditions, binding to *N. meningitidis* is best observed in hypotonic conditions, with ~90% decrease in binding seen at physiological buffers. Capsular polysialic acid was shown to impede to C4bp binding to PorA [78].

Our unpublished data has shown that factor H binds to *N. meningitidis*. The ligand for factor H is the lipoprotein GNA1870, which currently is being intensely investigated as a meningococcal vaccine candidate [79–81]. Based on amino acid sequences derived from a diverse collection of strains, GNA1870 has been classified into three variants. Our preliminary data suggests that factor H can bind to strains that represent all three variants. Deleting GNA1870 abrogates factor H binding and results in enhanced killing of bacteria by normal human serum, suggesting that this lipoprotein plays an important role in protecting *N. meningitidis* against complement-dependent killing.

14.6.2
Modulation of Sialic Acid Biosynthesis

Recent work by Exley et al. [82] has shown that interruption of the lactate permease gene (*lctP*) gene decreased the ability of *N. meningitidis* to grow in cerebrospinal fluid (CSF). The *lctP* mutant was also attenuated during bloodstream infection and decreased virulence was attributed to increased sensitivity to complement-mediated killing. The role of complement was confirmed by restoration of virulence of the *lctP* mutant in a C3-deficient mouse. The mutant strain had a defect in the sialic acid biosynthetic pathway, underscoring the importance of sialic acid of both the capsule and the LOS in complement resistance and highlights the intimate relationship between bacterial physiology and the ability to evade the innate immune system.

14.7
The MBL Pathway

Since its discovery, considerable interest has focused on the role of the MBL pathway in defending against infections. Although MBL deficiency is common and is believed to be associated with predisposition to a myriad of infections [83], the role of this pathway in defense against infection is still debated [84]. MBL preferentially recognizes glucans, lipophosphoglycans, and glycoinositol phospholipids that contain mannose, glucose, fucose, or *N*-acetylglucosamine (GlcNAc) as their terminal hexose (Hex) [85]. Thus, MBL is efficient in recognizing microbial surfaces with a high content of repetitive (and terminal) mannose and/or GlcNAc residues, such as those presented by *Saccharomyces cerevisae* [86], *Candida albicans* [87], *Escherichia coli* strain K12 [88], *Salmonella Typhimurium* and *S. Montevideo* [88–92], gp120 of HIV-1, gp110 of HIV-2 [93, 94], and *N. gonorrhoeae* [92]. Such carbohydrate micropatterns are found in limited amounts in glycoproteins of higher animals and these are not arranged in a repetitive pattern in the membrane that would be suitable for binding to MBL. Furthermore, mammalian carbohydrates (and some bacterial carbohydrates, such as neisserial lipooligosaccharide) often terminate in sialic acid residues, which shield the relevant neutral sugars and thus are not recognized by MBL.

Van Emmerik et al. [88] examined binding of MBL to various pathogens causing bacterial meningitis. They found high binding to unencapsulated variants of *N. meningitidis, Listeria monocytogenes, Haemophilus influenzae,* intermediate binding to serogroup A *N. meningitidis, E. coli* K1, and *Streptococcus pneumoninae,* and weak binding to *N. meningitidis* belonging to serogroups other than A and *H. influenzae* type B [88].

The role of capsular polysaccharide and LOS structure and sialylation in modulating MBL binding was examined by Jack et al. [31], using isogenic mutants of strain B1940 that either lacked a capsule but expressed the sialylated lacto-*N*-neotetraose LOS (*siaD* mutant), or an encapsulated mutant that expressed a truncated (Glc → HepI) LOS molecule (*galE*), or its unencapsulated derivative [31]. MBL bound to mutants with truncated LOS (*galE*), and only weakly to the unencapsulated *siaD* mutant, but not to the wild type strain, suggesting that the LOS structure modulated MBL binding. MBL-MASP complexes bound to the bacterial surface were able to activate both isoforms of C4 (C4A, C4B). In a subsequent study using strains that expressed the lacto-*N*-neotetraose LOS species but varied in the amount of sialylation, it was shown that MBL bound best to the strain that was minimally sialylated; and addition of exogenous CMP-NANA (the donor molecule for sialic acid) to the growth media to enhance sialylation of this strain resulted in decreased MBL binding and decreased killing of organisms preopsonized with MBL followed by addition of complement [30]. Similarly, decreased MBL binding upon sialylation of gonococcal LOS was also demonstrated [92]. A recent study showed direct binding of MBL to PorB3 and opacity-associated protein (Opa). Binding occurred in the absence of calcium and was not inhibited by mannose or *N*-acetylglucosamine, which are the natural carbohydrate MBL ligands [95]. MBL did not bind directly to purified LOS. Taken together, these data suggest that the binding of MBL may bind to PorB3 and Opa; and binding to these ligands may be modulated by LOS structure and sialylation.

Studies examining the function of MBL in mediating direct bactericidal killing of meningococci have used bacteria preincubated with MBL, followed by the addition of a complement source. An examination of the ability of MBL to activate complement on the surface of *N. gonorrhoeae* showed that only bacteria that were preincubated with MBL followed by addition of complement were killed [96]. The addition of MBL and complement simultaneously to bacteria did not result in killing. C1-inhibitor and α2-macroglobulin were the factors in serum that could regulate MBL function on the gonococcal surface. While MBL may not serve an important function in direct bactericidal killing in normal serum, it may play a role in enhancing opsonophagocytosis by virtue of its ability to bind to CR1 (CD35) [6], or by enhancing complement activation in individuals who lack adequate levels of protective antibody.

14.8 Blocking Antibodies

Antibodies directed against certain epitopes of the reduction-modifiable protein (Rmp or PIII protein; the homologue of class 4 protein in *N. meningitidis*) of *N. gonorrhoeae* have been shown to block killing by otherwise bactericidal antibodies directed against other outer membrane molecules such as LOS or Por [97]. Blocking antibodies could activate complement on the bacterial surface, evidenced by increased C3 and C9 binding to bacteria. $F(ab')_2$ fragments derived from intact blocking IgG also demonstrated blocking activity. The mechanism of blocking antibodies has not been fully elucidated, but one proposed mechanism is diversion of C3 away from bactericidal targets on to alternative targets [98]. The resultant complement activation at these alternative site(s) could result in the insertion of "non-bactericidal" C5b-9 [99]. Rosenqvist et al. [100] examined antibodies induced by a meningococcal outer membrane vesicle vaccine preparation which included Class 4 protein for possible blocking properties. The anti-Class 4 antibodies that were elicited reacted strongly against the antigen in immunoblot assays, but failed to bind to whole bacteria, suggesting that these antibodies were directed against regions in the Class 4 molecule that were not normally surface exposed. Among the 27 vaccinees, only one individual that had anti-Class 4 antibodies could block the bactericidal effects of an anti-PorA (Class 1) mAb. This blocking effect was presumed not to be vaccine-induced because the "blocking" effect was also seen in preimmune serum.

IgA antibodies purified from sera of individuals recovering from infection with serogroups B, C, and Y disease were shown to block the bactericidal activity of IgG and IgM isolated from the same sera. Inhibition of killing by IgA was dependent on the ratio of lytic to blocking antibody, was strain-specific, and was greater for IgG than IgM [101–103]. The specificity of IgA binding may determine whether it acts as a blocking or bactericidal antibody. IgA1 directed against outer membrane proteins can initiate complement-dependent killing, which is dependent on the Fc portion of the antibody [29]. Killing was not associated with an increase in C3 binding to bacteria. In contrast, IgA1 directed against serogroup C capsular polysaccharide can block the lytic activity of capsule-specific IgG. Both, the F(ab')2 and Fab derivatives of IgA1 blocked lysis in a manner that was quantitatively similar to intact IgA1. IgA1 and its Fab and F(ab')2 fragments blocked IgG-initiated lysis via either the classical pathway (as seen in factor B-depleted and properdin-deficient serum), the alternative pathway (using Mg-EGTA-chelated serum), or both pathways combined (intact normal serum). The mechanism of IgA1-mediated blockade was not because of competition for IgG binding. The blocking effect is not restricted to anticapsular IgA, but has also been described in an individual who received the quadrivalent meningococcal vaccine, where IgG directed against serogroup W-135 capsule blocked killing of the strain by C2-deficient serum [104].

14.9 Summary

Complement is a critical arm of the innate immune defenses against meningococcal infections. Persons deficient in terminal and alternative complement components are highly predisposed to recurrent and disseminated neisserial infections. Evasion of complement-mediated killing is necessary for survival of meningococci in the bloodstream and for dissemination of infection. *N. meningitidis* has evolved several strategies to evade complement. The presence of capsular polysaccharide is the most important factor for imparting high-level serum resistance and for causing disseminated disease in humans and in animal models. LOS sialylation and structure may also contribute to serum resistance, although its role is not as well defined as for *N. gonorrhoeae*. A summary of the role of meningococcal surface components that are known to interact with the complement system is provided in Table 14.1.

Table 14.1 Summary of interactions of the complement system with *N. meningitidis* surface molecules.

Meningococcal molecule	Interaction(s) with the complement system [reference]
Capsular polysaccharide	Required for high level serum resistance [39, 40] and for virulence in animal model [52]. Regulates the alternative pathway [26] as well as the classical pathway. In some instances, a target for "blocking" IgA [102, 103] and IgG [104] Ab
Lipooligosaccharide (LOS)	Sialylation of lacto-*N*-neotetraose LOS regulates the alternative and classical pathway [51], and may also decrease MBL binding [30]. Meningococcal LOS sialylation does not enhance factor H binding (in contrast to *N. gonorrhoeae* LOS sialylation [53]). LOS is a target for C3b and C4b [35]
Opa (class 5 protein)	Binds MBL [95] and is probably a target for C3b and C4b (our unpublished observations), both of which may enhance complement-dependent killing
PorB3 (class 3 protein)	Ligand for MBL [95]
PorA (class 1 protein)	PorA binds C4b-binding protein (C4bp) under hypotonic conditions, and may regulate the classical pathway [78]
GNA1870/LP2086	Lipoprotein that may be the target for the alternative pathway regulatory protein, factor H (our unpublished observations)

References

1 Walport, M. J. **2001**, Complement, Second of two parts, *N Engl J Med* 344, 1140–1144.

2 Walport, M. J. **2001**, Complement, First of two parts, *N Engl J Med* 344, 1058–1066.

3 Söderström, C., J. H. Braconier, H. Käyhty, A. G. Sjöholm, B. Thuresson **1989**, Immune response to tetravalent meningococcal vaccine: opsonic and bactericidal functions of normal and properdin deficient sera, *Eur J Clin Microbiol Infect Dis* 8, 220–224.

4 Sjöholm, A. G., J. H. Braconier, C. Söderström **1982**, Properdin deficiency in a family with fulminant meningococcal infections, *Clin Exp Immunol* 50, 291–297.

5 Braconier, J. H., A. G. Sjöholm, C. Söderström **1983**, Fulminant meningococcal infections in a family with inherited deficiency of properdin, *Scand J Infect Dis* 15, 339–345.

6 Ghiran, I., S. F. Barbashov, L. B. Klickstein, S. W. Tas, J. C. Jensenius, A. Nicholson-Weller **2000**, Complement receptor 1/CD35 is a receptor for mannan-binding lectin, *J Exp Med* 192, 1797–1808.

7 Hayama, K., N. Sugai, S. Tanaka, S. Lee, H. Kikuchi, J. Ito, J. Suzuki, Y. Nagata, H. Kondo, O. Harayama, et al. **1989**, High-incidence of C9 deficiency throughout Japan: there are no significant differences in incidence among eight areas of Japan, *Int Arch Allergy Appl Immunol* 90, 400–404.

8 Zhu, Z. B., K. Totemchokchyakarn, T. P. Atkinson, J. E. Volanakis **1998**, Molecular defects leading to human complement component C6 deficiency in an African-American family, *Clin Exp Immunol* 111, 91–96.

9 Hobart, M. J., B. A. Fernie, K. A. Fijen, A. Orren **1998**, The molecular basis of C6 deficiency in the western Cape, South Africa, *Hum Genet* 103, 506–512.

10 Fijen, C. A., E. J. Kuijper, M. T. te Bulte, M. R. Daha, J. Dankert **1999**, Assessment of complement deficiency in patients with meningococcal disease in The Netherlands, *Clin Infect Dis* 28, 98–105.

11 Fijen, C. A., E. J. Kuijper, A. J. Hannema, A. G. Sjöholm, J. P. van Putten **1989**, Complement deficiencies in patients over ten years old with meningococcal disease due to uncommon serogroups [see comments], *Lancet* 2, 585–588.

12 Ross, S. C., P. Densen **1984**, Complement deficiency states and infection: epidemiology, pathogenesis and consequences of neisserial and other infections in an immune deficiency, *Medicine* 63, 243–273.

13 Mayatepek, E., M. Grauer, G. M. Hansch, H. G. Sonntag **1993**, Deafness, complement deficiencies and immunoglobulin status in patients with meningococcal diseases due to uncommon serogroups, *Pediatr Infect Dis J* 12, 808–811.

14 Orren, A., D. A. Caugant, C. A. Fijen, J. Dankert, E. J. van Schalkwyk, J. T. Poolman, G. J. Coetzee **1994**, Characterization of strains of *Neisseria meningitidis* recovered from complement-sufficient and complement-deficient patients in the Western Cape Province, South Africa, *J Clin Microbiol* 32, 2185–2191.

15 Zipfel, P. F., J. Hellwage, M. A. Friese, G. Hegasy, S. T. Jokiranta, S. Meri **1999**, Factor H and disease: a complement regulator affects vital body functions, *Mol Immunol* 36, 241–248.

16 Vyse, T. J., P. J. Spath, K. A. Davies, B. J. Morley, P. Philippe, P. Athanassiou, C. M. Giles, M. J. Walport **1994**, Hereditary complement factor I deficiency, *Q J Med* 87, 385–401.

17 Bax, W. A., O. J. Cluysenaer, A. K. Bartelink, P. C. Aerts, R. A. Ezekowitz, H. van Dijk **1999**, Association of familial deficiency of mannose-binding lectin and meningococcal disease, *Lancet* 354, 1094–1095.

18 Zorgani, A. A., V. S. James, J. Stewart, C. C. Blackwell, R. A. Elton, D. M. Weir **1996**, Serum bactericidal activity in a secondary school population following an outbreak of meningococcal disease: effects of carriage and secretor status, *FEMS Immunol Med Microbiol* 14, 73–81.

19 Gold, R., I. Goldschneider, M. L. Lepow, T. F. Draper, M. Randolph **1978**, Carriage

of *Neisseria meningitidis* and *Neisseria lactamica* in infants and children, *J Infect Dis* 137, 112–121.

20 Goldschneider, I., E.C. Gotschlich, M.S. Artenstein **1969**, Human immunity to the meningococcus, I. The role of humoral antibodies, *J Exp Med* 129, 1307–1326.

21 Brandtzaeg, P., T.E. Mollnes, P. Kierulf **1989**, Complement activation and endotoxin levels in systemic meningococcal disease, *J Infect Dis* 160, 58–65.

22 Tesh, V.L., R.L. Duncan, Jr., D.C. Morrison **1986**, The interaction of *Escherichia coli* with normal human serum: the kinetics of serum-mediated lipopolysaccharide release and its dissociation from bacterial killing, *J Immunol* 137, 1329–1335.

23 O'Hara, A.M., A.P. Moran, R. Würzner, A. Orren **2001**, Complement-mediated lipopolysaccharide release and outer membrane damage in *Escherichia coli* J5: requirement for C9, *Immunology* 102, 365–372.

24 Lehner, P.J., K.A. Davies, M.J. Walport, A.P. Cope, R. Würzner, A. Orren, B.P. Morgan, J. Cohen **1992**, Meningococcal septicaemia in a C6-deficient patient and effects of plasma transfusion on lipopolysaccharide release, *Lancet* 340, 1379–1381.

25 Ingwer, I., B.H. Petersen, G. Brooks **1978**, Serum bactericidal action and activation of the classic and alternate complement pathways by *Neisseria gonorrhoeae*, *J Lab Clin Med* 92, 211–220.

26 Jarvis, G.A., N.A.Vedros **1987**, Sialic acid of group B *Neisseria meningitidis* regulates alternative complement pathway activation, *Infect Immun* 55, 174–180.

27 McQuillen, D.P., S. Gulati, P.A. Rice **1994**, Complement-mediated bacterial killing assays, *Methods Enzymol* 236, 137–147.

28 Söderström, C., J.H. Braconier, D. Danielsson, A.G. Sjöholm **1987**, Bactericidal activity for *Neisseria meningitidis* in properdin-deficient sera, *J Infect Dis* 156, 107–112.

29 Jarvis, G.A., J.M. Griffiss **1989**, Human IgA1 initiates complement-mediated killing of *Neisseria meningitidis*, *J Immunol* 143, 1703–1709.

30 Jack, D.L., G.A. Jarvis, C.L. Booth, M.W. Turner, N.J. Klein **2001**, Mannose-binding lectin accelerates complement activation and increases serum killing of *Neisseria meningitidis* serogroup C, *J Infect Dis* 184, 836–845.

31 Jack, D.L., A.W. Dodds, N. Anwar, C.A. Ison, A. Law, M. Frosch, M.W. Turner, N.J. Klein **1998**, Activation of complement by mannose-binding lectin on isogenic mutants of *Neisseria meningitidis* serogroup B, *J Immunol* 160, 1346–1353.

32 Bishof, N.A., T.R. Welch, L.S. Beischel **1990**, C4B deficiency: a risk factor for bacteremia with encapsulated organisms, *J Infect Dis* 162, 248–250.

33 Rowe, P.C., R.H. McLean, R.A. Wood, R.J. Leggiadro, J.A. Winkelstein **1989**, Association of homozygous C4B deficiency with bacterial meningitis, *J Infect Dis* 160, 448–451.

34 Cates, K.L., P. Densen, J.C. Lockman, R.P. Levine **1992**, C4B deficiency is not associated with meningitis or bacteremia with encapsulated bacteria, *J Infect Dis* 165, 942–944.

35 Ram, S., A.D. Cox, J.C. Wright, U. Vogel, S. Getzlaff, R. Boden, J. Li, J.S. Plested, S. Meri, S. Gulati, D.C. Stein, J.C. Richards, E.R. Moxon, P.A. Rice **2003**, Neisserial lipooligosaccharide is a target for complement component C4b: inner core phosphoethanolamine residues define C4b linkage specificity, *J Biol Chem* 278, 50853–50862.

36 Plested, J.S., K. Makepeace, M.P. Jennings, M.A. Gidney, S. Lacelle, J. Brisson, A.D. Cox, A. Martin, A.G. Bird, C.M. Tang, F.M. Mackinnon, J.C. Richards, E.R. Moxon **1999** Conservation and accessibility of an inner core lipopolysaccharide epitope of Neisseria meningitidis, *Infect Immun* 67, 5417–5426.

37 McGee, Z., C. Clemens, J. Klein, L. Barley, G. Gorby **1990**, Role of tumor necrosis factor in gonococcal damage to human fallopian tube mucosa, in *Seventh International Pathogenic Neisseria Conference*, eds. M. Achtmann, et al., Neisseria Conf., Berlin.

38 Jarvis, G.A. **1994**, Analysis of C3 deposition and degradation on *Neisseria meningitidis* and *Neisseria gonorrhoeae*, *Infect Immun* 62, 1755–1760.

39 Vogel, U., A. Weinberger, R. Frank, M.A., J. Köhl, J.P. Atkinson, M. Frosch **1997**, Complement factor C3 deposition and serum resistance in isogenic capsule and lipooligosaccharide sialic acid mutants of serogroup B *Neisseria meningitidis*, *Infect Immun* 65, 4022–4029.

40 Kahler, C.M., L.E. Martin, G.C. Shih, M.M. Rahman, R.W. Carlson, D.S. Stephens **1998**, The (alpha → 28)-linked polysialic acid capsule and lipooligosaccharide structure both contribute to the ability of serogroup B *Neisseria meningitidis* to resist the bactericidal activity of normal human serum, *Infect Immun* 66, 5939–5947.

41 Meri, S., M.K. Pangburn **1994**, Regulation of alternative pathway complement activation by glycosaminoglycans: specificity of the polyanion binding site on factor H, *Biochem Biophys Res Commun* 198, 52–59.

42 Meri, S., M.K. Pangburn **1990**, Discrimination between activators and nonactivators of the alternative pathway of complement: regulation via a sialic acid/polyanion binding site on factor H, *Proc Natl Acad Sci USA* 87, 3982–3986.

43 Richmond, P., R. Borrow, D. Goldblatt, J. Findlow, S. Martin, R. Morris, K. Cartwright, E. Miller **2001**, Ability of 3 different meningococcal C conjugate vaccines to induce immunologic memory after a single dose in UK toddlers, *J Infect Dis* 183, 160–163.

44 Ward, M.E., P.J. Watt, A.A. Glynn **1970**, Gonococci in urethral exudates possess a virulence factor lost on subculture, *Nature* 227, 382–384.

45 Parsons, N.J., P.V. Patel, E.L. Tan, J.R.C. Andrade, C.A. Nairn, M. Goldner, J.A. Cole, H. Smith **1988**, Cytidine 5′-monophospho-N-acetyl neuraminic acid and a low molecular weight factor from human red blood cells induce lipopolysaccharide alteration in gonococci when conferring resistance to killing by human serum, *Microb Pathog* 5, 303–309.

46 Nairn, C.A., J.A. Cole, P.V. Patel, N.J. Parsons, J.E. Fox, H. Smith **1988**, Cytidine 5′-monophospho-N-acetylneuraminic acid or a related compound is the low Mr factor from human red blood cells which induces gonococcal resistance to killing by human serum, *J Gen Microbiol* 134, 3295–3306.

47 Tan, E.L., P.V. Patel, N.J. Parsons, P.M. Martin, H. Smith **1986**, Lipopolysaccharide alteration is associated with induced resistance of *Neisseria gonorrhoeae* to killing by human serum, *J Gen Microbiol* 132, 1407–1413.

48 Ram, S., A.K. Sharma, S.D. Simpson, S. Gulati, D.P. McQuillen, M.K. Pangburn, P.A. Rice **1998**, A novel sialic acid binding site on factor H mediates serum resistance of sialylated *Neisseria gonorrhoeae*, *J Exp Med* 187, 743–752.

49 Mandrell, R.E., J.J. Kim, C.M. John, B.W. Gibson, J.V. Sugai, M.A. Apicella, J.M. Griffiss, R. Yamasaki **1991**, Endogenous sialylation of the lipooligosaccharides of *Neisseria meningitidis*, *J Bacteriol* 173, 2823–2832.

50 Fox, A.J., D.M. Jones, S.M. Scotland, B. Rowe, A. Smith, M.R. Brown, R.G. Fitzgeorge, A. Baskerville, N.J. Parsons, J.A. Cole, et al. **1989**, Serum killing of meningococci and several other gram-negative bacterial species is not decreased by incubating them with cytidine 5′-monophospho-N-acetyl neuraminic acid [letter], *Microb Pathog* 7, 317–318.

51 Estabrook, M.M., J.M. Griffiss, G.A. Jarvis **1997**, Sialylation of *Neisseria meningitidis* lipooligosaccharide inhibits serum bactericidal activity by masking lacto-N-neotetraose, *Infect Immun* 65, 4436–4444.

52 Vogel, U., H. Claus, G. Heinze, M. Frosch **1999**, Role of lipopolysaccharide sialylation in serum resistance of serogroup B and C meningococcal disease isolates, *Infect Immun* 67, 954–957.

53 Madico, G., S. Ram, S. Getzlaff, A. Prasad, S. Gulati, J. Ngampasutadol, U. Vogel, P.A. Rice **2004**, Sialylation of lacto-N-tetraose lipooligosaccharide in gonococci, but not meningococci, results in enhanced factor H binding: the modula-

tory role of gonococcal porin, *Int Pathogen Neisseria Conf* 14, 230.

54 Edwards, J. L., M. A. Apicella **2002**, The role of lipooligosaccharide in *Neisseria gonorrhoeae* pathogenesis of cervical epithelia: lipid A serves as a C3 acceptor molecule, *Cell Microbiol* 4, 585–598.

55 Claus, H., M. C. Maiden, D. J. Wilson, N. D. McCarthy, K. A. Jolley, R. Urwin, F. Hessler, M. Frosch, U. Vogel **2005**, Genetic analysis of meningococci carried by children and young adults, *J Infect Dis* 191, 1263–1271.

56 Andoh, A., Y. Fujiyama, T. Kimura, H. Uchihara, H. Sakumoto, H. Okabe, T. Bamba **1997**, Molecular characterization of complement components (C3, C4, and factor B) in human saliva, *J Clin Immunol* 17, 404–407.

57 Würzner, R. **1999**, Evasion of pathogens by avoiding recognition or eradication by complement, in part via molecular mimicry, *Mol Immunol* 36, 249–260.

58 Horstmann, R. D., H. J. Sievertsen, J. Knobloch, V. A. Fischetti **1988**, Antiphagocytic activity of streptococcal M protein: selective binding of complement control protein factor H, *Proc Natl Acad Sci USA* 85, 1657–1661.

59 Areschoug, T., M. Stalhammar-Carlemalm, I. Karlsson, G. Lindahl **2002**, Streptococcal beta protein has separate binding sites for human factor H and IgA-Fc, *J Biol Chem* 277, 12642–12648.

60 Kraiczy, P., C. Skerka, M. Kirschfink, V. Brade, P. F. Zipfel **2001**, Immune evasion of *Borrelia burgdorferi* by acquisition of human complement regulators FHL-1/reconectin and Factor H, *Eur J Immunol* 31, 1674–1684.

61 Dave, S., A. Brooks-Walter, M. K. Pangburn, L. S. McDaniel **2001**, PspC, a pneumococcal surface protein, binds human factor H, *Infect Immun* 69, 3435–3437.

62 Jarva, H., R. Janulczyk, J. Hellwage, P. F. Zipfel, L. Björck, S. Meri **2002**, *Streptococcus pneumoniae* evades complement attack and opsonophagocytosis by expressing the pspC locus-encoded Hic protein that binds to short consensus repeats 8–11 of factor H, *J Immunol* 168, 1886–1894.

63 Neeleman, C., S. P. Geelen, P. C. Aerts, M. R. Daha, T. E. Mollnes, J. J. Roord, G. Posthuma, H. van Dijk, A. Fleer **1999**, Resistance to both complement activation and phagocytosis in type 3 pneumococci is mediated by the binding of complement regulatory protein factor H, *Infect Immun* 67, 4517–4524.

64 Duthy, T. G., R. J. Ormsby, E. Giannakis, A. D. Ogunniyi, U. H. Stroeher, J. C. Paton, D. L. Gordon **2002**, The human complement regulator factor H binds pneumococcal surface protein PspC via short consensus repeats 13 to 15, *Infect Immun* 70, 5604–5611.

65 China, B., M. P. Sory, B. T. N'Guyen, M. De Bruyere, G. R. Cornelis **1993**, Role of the YadA protein in prevention of opsonization of *Yersinia enterocolitica* by C3b molecules, *Infect Immun* 61, 3129–3136.

66 Meri, T., A. Hartmann, D. Lenk, R. Eck, R. Würzner, J. Hellwage, S. Meri, P. F. Zipfel **2002**, The yeast *Candida albicans* binds complement regulators factor H and FHL-1, *Infect Immun* 70, 5185–5192.

67 Stoiber, H., C. Ebenbichler, R. Schneider, J. Janatova, M. P. Dierich **1995**, Interaction of several complement proteins with gp120 and gp41, the two envelope glycoproteins of HIV-1, *Aids* 9, 19–26.

68 Stoiber, H., C. Pinter, A. G. Siccardi, A. Clivio, M. P. Dierich **1996**, Efficient destruction of human immunodeficiency virus in human serum by inhibiting the protective action of complement factor H and decay accelerating factor (DAF, CD55), *J Exp Med* 183, 307–310.

69 Meri, T., T. S. Jokiranta, J. Hellwage, A. Bialonski, P. F. Zipfel, S. Meri **2002**, *Onchocerca volvulus* microfilariae avoid complement attack by direct binding of factor H, *J Infect Dis* 185, 1786–1793.

70 Ram, S., D. P. McQuillen, S. Gulati, C. Elkins, M. K. Pangburn, P. A. Rice **1998**, Binding of complement factor H to loop 5 of porin protein 1A: a molecular mechanism of serum resistance of nonsialylated *Neisseria gonorrhoeae, J Exp Med* 188, 671–680.

71 Thern, A., L. Stenberg, B. Dahlback, G. Lindahl **1995**, Ig-binding surface proteins of *Streptococcus pyogenes* also bind human C4b-binding protein (C4BP), a

regulatory component of the complement system, *J Immunol* 154, 375–386.
72 Johnsson, E., A. Thern, B. Dahlbäck, L. O. Hedén, M. Wikström, G. Lindahl **1997**, Human C4BP binds to the hypervariable N-terminal region of many members in the streptococcal M protein family, *Adv Exp Med Biol* 418, 505–510.
73 Johnsson, E., A. Thern, B. Dahlbäck, L. O. Hedén, M. Wikström, G. Lindahl **1996**, A highly variable region in members of the streptococcal M protein family binds the human complement regulator C4BP, *J Immunol* 157, 3021–3029.
74 Nordström, T., A. M. Blom, A. Forsgren, K. Riesbeck **2004**, The emerging pathogen *Moraxella catarrhalis* interacts with complement inhibitor C4b binding protein through ubiquitous surface proteins A1 and A2, *J Immunol* 173, 4598–4606.
75 Berggard, K., E. Johnsson, F. R. Mooi, G. Lindahl **1997**, *Bordetella pertussis* binds the human complement regulator C4BP: role of filamentous hemagglutinin, *Infect Immun* 65, 3638–3643.
76 Blom, A. M., A. Rytkonen, P. Vasquez, G. Lindahl, B. Dahlback, A. B. Jonsson **2001**, A novel interaction between type IV pili of *Neisseria gonorrhoeae* and the human complement regulator C4B-binding protein, *J Immunol* 166, 6764–6770.
77 Ram, S., M. Cullinane, A. Blom, S. Gulati, D. McQuillen, B. Monks, C. O'Connell, R. Boden, C. Elkins, M. Pangburn, B. Dahlback, P. Rice **2001**, Binding of C4b-binding Protein to Porin: A molecular mechanism of serum resistance of neisseria gonorrhoeae, *J Exp Med* 193, 281–296.
78 Jarva, H., S. Ram, U. Vogel, A. M. Blom, S. Meri **2005**, Binding of the complement inhibitor C4bp to serogroup B *Neisseria meningitidis, J Immunol* 174, 6299–6307.
79 Masignani, V., M. Comanducci, M. M. Giuliani, S. Bambini, J. Adu-Bobie, B. Arico, B. Brunelli, A. Pieri, L. Santini, S. Savino, D. Serruto, D. Litt, S. Kroll, J. A. Welsch, D. M. Granoff, R. Rappuoli, M. Pizza **2003**, Vaccination against *Neisseria meningitidis* using three variants of the lipoprotein GNA1870, *J Exp Med* 197, 789–799.
80 Pillai, S., A. Howell, K. Alexander, B. E. Bentley, H. Q. Jiang, K. Ambrose, D. Zhu, G. Zlotnick **2005**, Outer membrane protein (OMP) based vaccine for *Neisseria meningitidis* serogroup B, *Vaccine* 23, 2206–2209.
81 Welsch, J. A., R. Rossi, M. Comanducci, D. M. Granoff **2004**, Protective activity of monoclonal antibodies to genome-derived neisserial antigen 1870, a *Neisseria meningitidis* candidate vaccine, *J Immunol* 172, 5606–5615.
82 Exley, R. M., J. Shaw, E. Mowe, Y. H. Sun, N. P. West, M. Williamson, M. Botto, H. Smith, C. M. Tang **2005**, Available carbon source influences the resistance of *Neisseria meningitidis* against complement, *J Exp Med* 201, 1637–1645.
83 Eisen, D. P., R. M. Minchinton **2003**, Impact of mannose-binding lectin on susceptibility to infectious diseases, *Clin Infect Dis* 37, 1496–1505.
84 Cartwright, K. A., J. M. Stuart, D. M. Jones, N. D. Noah **1987**, The Stonehouse survey: nasopharyngeal carriage of meningococci and *Neisseria lactamica, Epidemiol Infect* 99, 591–601.
85 Weis, W. I., K. Drickamer, W. A. Hendrickson **1992**, Structure of a C-type mannose-binding protein complexed with an oligosaccharide, *Nature* 360, 127–134.
86 Turner, M. W. **1998**, Mannose-binding lectin (MBL) in health and disease, *Immunobiology* 199, 327–339.
87 Hoppe, H. C., B. J. de Wet, C. Cywes, M. Daffe, M. R. Ehlers **1997**, Identification of phosphatidylinositol mannoside as a mycobacterial adhesin mediating both direct and opsonic binding to nonphagocytic mammalian cells, *Infect Immun* 65, 3896–3905.
88 van Emmerik, L. C., E. J. Kuijper, C. A. Fijen, J. Dankert, S. Thiel **1994**, Binding of mannan-binding protein to various bacterial pathogens of meningitis, *Clin Exp Immunol* 97, 411–416.
89 Schweinle, J. E., M. Nishiyasu, T. Q. Ding, K. Sastry, S. D. Gillies, R. A. Ezekowitz **1993**, Truncated forms of mannose-binding protein multimerize and bind to mannose-rich Salmonella montevideo

but fail to activate complement in vitro, *J Biol Chem* 268, 364–370.

90 Schweinle, J. E., R. A. Ezekowitz, A. J. Tenner, M. Kuhlman, K. A. Joiner **1989**, Human mannose-binding protein activates the alternative complement pathway and enhances serum bactericidal activity on a mannose-rich isolate of Salmonella, *J Clin Invest* 84, 1821–1829.

91 Kuhlman, M., K. Joiner, R. A. Ezekowitz **1989**, The human mannose-binding protein functions as an opsonin, *J Exp Med* 169, 1733–1745.

92 Devyatyarova-Johnson, M., I. H. Rees, B. D. Robertson, M. W. Turner, N. J. Klein, D. L. Jack **2000**, The lipopolysaccharide structures of *Salmonella enterica* serovar Typhimurium and *Neisseria gonorrhoeae* determine the attachment of human mannose-binding lectin to intact organisms, *Infect Immun* 68, 3894–3899.

93 Ezekowitz, R. A., M. Kuhlman, J. E. Groopman, R. A. Byrn **1989**, A human serum mannose-binding protein inhibits in vitro infection by the human immunodeficiency virus, *J Exp Med* 169, 185–196.

94 Haurum, J. S., S. Thiel, I. M. Jones, P. B. Fischer, S. B. Laursen, J. C. Jensenius **1993**, Complement activation upon binding of mannan-binding protein to HIV envelope glycoproteins, *Aids* 7, 1307–1313.

95 Estabrook, M. M., D. L. Jack, N. J. Klein, G. A. Jarvis **2004**, Mannose-binding lectin binds to two major outer membrane proteins, opacity protein and porin, of *Neisseria meningitidis, J Immunol* 172, 3784–3792.

96 Gulati, S., K. Sastry, J. C. Jensenius, P. A. Rice, S. Ram **2002**, Regulation of the mannan-binding lectin pathway of complement on *Neisseria gonorrhoeae* by C1-inhibitor and alpha(2)-macroglobulin, *J Immunol* 168, 4078–4086.

97 Rice, P. A., H. Vayo, M. Tam, M. S. Blake **1986**, Immunoglobulin G antibodies directed against protein III block killing of serum-resistant *Neisseria gonorrhoeae* by immune serum, *J Exp Med* 164, 1735–1748.

98 Joiner, K. A., R. Scales, K. A. Warren, M. M. Frank, P. A. Rice **1985**, Mechanism of action of blocking immunoglobulin G for *Neisseria gonorrhoeae, J Clin Invest* 76, 1765–1772.

99 Joiner, K. A., K. A. Warren, C. Hammer, M. M. Frank **1985**, Bactericidal but not nonbactericidal C5b-9 is associated with distinctive outer membrane proteins in *Neisseria gonorrhoeae, J Immunol* 134, 1920–1925.

100 Rosenqvist, E., A. Musacchio, A. Aase, E. A. Hoiby, E. Namork, J. Kolberg, E. Wedege, A. Delvig, R. Dalseg, T. E. Michaelsen, J. Tommassen **1999**, Functional activities and epitope specificity of human and murine antibodies against the class 4 outer membrane protein (Rmp) of *Neisseria meningitidis, Infect Immun* 67, 1267–1276.

101 Griffiss, J. M., D. K. Goroff **1983**, IgA blocks IgM and IgG-initiated immune lysis by separate molecular mechanisms, *J Immunol* 130, 2882–2885.

102 Griffiss, J. M. **1975**, Bactericidal activity of meningococcal antisera, Blocking by IgA of lytic antibody in human convalescent sera, *J Immunol* 114, 1779–1784.

103 Jarvis, G. A., J. M. Griffiss **1991**, Human IgA1 blockade of IgG-initiated lysis of *Neisseria meningitidis* is a function of antigen-binding fragment binding to the polysaccharide capsule, *J Immunol* 147, 1962–1967.

104 Selander, B., H. Kayhty, E. Wedege, E. Holmstrom, L. Truedsson, C. Soderstrom, A. G. Sjoholm **2000**, Vaccination responses to capsular polysaccharides of *Neisseria meningitidis* and *Haemophilus influenzae* type b in two C2-deficient sisters: alternative pathway-mediated bacterial killing and evidence for a novel type of blocking IgG, *J Clin Immunol* 20, 138–149.

15
Cellular Immune Responses in Meningococcal Disease

Oliver Kurzai and Matthias Frosch

15.1
Introduction

One of the hallmarks in our understanding of meningococcal epidemiology and the development of invasive disease is the observation that *N. meningitidis* is exclusively encountered in humans (Rosenstein et al. 2001). Currently, there is no other recognized ecological niche for this species. This immediately implies that a considerable percentage of healthy humans (in fact 10–15% and, in some cohorts, up to 40%) are colonized with meningococci in their nasopharynx, a fact that had been recognized very early (Bennett et al. 2005; Bogaert et al. 2005; Rage 1934; Yazdankhah and Caugant 2004). Although the vast majority of these colonizations will never proceed to invasive disease, it is already at this early stage of interaction that intricate mechanisms controlling immunological homeostasis at the epithelial borderlines of the human body are activated (Jordens et al. 2004; Robinson et al. 2002; Yazdankhah and Caugant 2004). Whereas the essential function of specific antibodies in protection against invasive meningococcal disease has been evident since the studies of Goldschneider, ancient mechanisms of innate immunity are likely to predominate during the first encounter of the human host with *N. meningitidis* (Goldschneider et al. 1969a, b; Zhang and Finn 2004). Although not in the focus of this summary, epithelial cells exert major immune functions essential for controlling the response to harmless commensals as well as invading pathogens (Plant et al. 2004; Rescigno and Chieppa 2005). However, the epithelial barrier already contains several specialized cell types of the human immune system (Kelsall and Rescigno 2004; Pollard and Frasch 2001; Rescigno and Chieppa 2005; Fig. 15.1). Among those are dendritic cells, linking innate and adaptive immunity and shuttling relevant antigens from the epithelium to regional lymph nodes, as well as resident macrophages (Mowat 2003; Sasmono and Hume 2004). In addition, cells of the adaptive immune system, especially T-lymphocytes, can home to the epithelium after activation and B-cell-derived IgA-producing plasma cells reside in the *lamina propria* of all human epithelial barriers (Cheroutre 2004;

Handbook of Meningococcal Disease. Infection Biology, Vaccination, Clinical Management.
Edited by M. Frosch and M. C. J. Maiden

ISBN: 3-527-31260-9

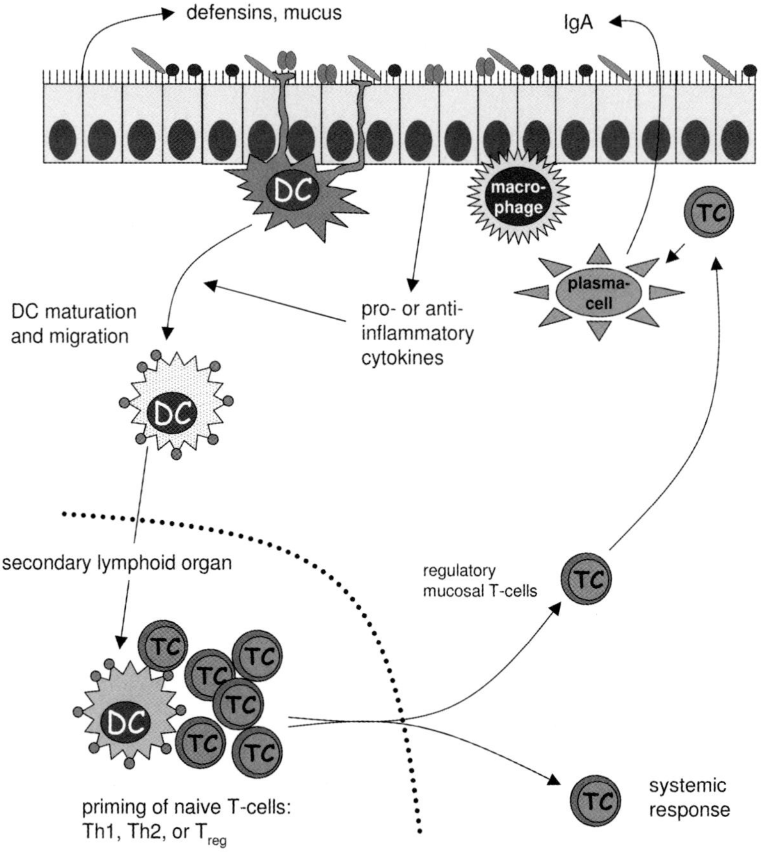

Fig. 15.1 Cells contributing to mucosal immunity. The nasopharyngeal mucosa is the port of entry for invasive *N. meningitidis*. Several mechanisms control immunity at this barrier. Resident macrophages and dendritic cells (DC) can sample antigen from apical and invading bacteria. DC can shuttle ingested antigen to regional secondary lymphoid organs during phenotypic maturation and induce an appropriate T-cell response. T-cells can disseminate further in the case of a systemic response or home to the epithelium (mostly regulatory T-cells contributing to immune homeostasis). The majority of human plasma cells is associated with epithelial barriers and secretes IgA, which is shuttled aross the epithelium and represents a major humoral constituent of mucosal immunity. Epithelial cells also contribute to immune homeostasis. They produce mucus and several antimicrobial peptides or proteins (defensins, lysozyme) regulating the composition of the apical flora. In addition, they can secrete antiinflammatory as well as proinflammatory mediators in response to environmental stimuli that regulate DC and macrophage activity. (This figure also appears with the color plates.)

Fig. 15.1). In this chapter we will summarize our current understanding of the interaction between *N. meningitidis* and specialized immune cells. We will start with cells residing in the nasopharyngeal epithelium, likely to mediate early immune effects and trigger the induction of protective immunity. Afterwards, neutrophil granulocytes, the major type of cells present in the cerebrospinal fluid of patients suffering from meningococcal meningitis will be discussed, before the last part of the chapter will focus on cells of the adaptive immune system.

15.2 Cellular Immunity Against *N. meningitidis* at the Mucosal Barrier

Mucosal surfaces represent the point of entry – not only for *N. meningitidis* but for most human pathogenic bacteria (Zhang and Finn 2004). Mucosal immunity is a subtly regulated system programmed to induce tolerance against the majority of encountered antigens, including food antigens in the intestine and inhaled antigens in the respiratory tract (Kiyono and Fukuyama 2004; Mowat 2003). However, in the case of invading pathogens, mucosal immunity must be capable of rapidly switching from the generation of tolerance to the induction of protective immunity (Rescigno and Chieppa 2005). This complex function is maintained by a variety of immune cells and their interplay with epithelial cells (Fig. 15.1). Among the immune cells, dendritic cells have been shown to exert central regulatory functions.

15.2.1 Dendritic Cells – an Early Encounter Linking Innate and Adaptive Immunity

After the first description of dendritic cells it took more than 100 years until immunologists realized that this cell type was likely to play a central role in activating, governing and regulating the human immune system (Banchereau and Steinman 1998; Granucci et al. 2004; Palucka and Banchereau 1999). Although it is currently well accepted that dendritic cell precursors arise constantly from the hematopoietic stem cell system and are dispersed in all human tissues, although at low numbers, the definition of dendritic cell types and subtypes is still complex and largely provisional (Banchereau et al. 2000; Maldonado-Lopez and Moser 2001; Shortman and Liu 2002). In their immature form, dendritic cells carry out a sentinel function, sensing and phagocytosing potential pathogens. Upon contact with invading microorganisms, so-called "danger signals" induce a maturation process, leading to the downregulation of pathogen recognition receptors and the upregulation of costimulatory signals and antigen presentation receptors (Banchereau and Steinman 1998). During the maturation process, dendritic cells migrate to secondary lymphoid tissues, where they induce and direct T-cell activation. Thus, dendritic cells are not only potent initiators of an immune response but also display the unique ability to direct the T-cell response towards Th1 or Th2. It has been a fundamental step towards a better understanding of the initial contact between the human immune system and invading pathogens that Rescigno et al. were able to show how dendritic cells can take up bacteria, even in the presence of an intact epithelial layer in the gastrointestinal system (Kelsall and Rescigno 2004; Rescigno et al. 2001 a, b;

Rescigno and Chieppa 2005). The basis of this trans-epithelial sentinel function of immature dendritic cells is a subtle interaction with certain barrier functions of the epithelial layer, for example by a maturity-dependent up- and downregulation of proteins like occludin involved in the organization of tight junctions (Kelsall and Rescigno 2004; Rimoldi et al. 2005).

15.2.2
How do Dendritic Cells Recognize *N. meningitidis*?

Two fundamentally diverse mechanisms for pathogen recognition have evolved in the human immune system. Subtly organized DNA recombination events enable recognition of an incredible diversity of putative epitopes by the acquired immune system. Antibody diversity and the variety of T-cell receptors are generated this way. In contrast, the innate immune system is focussed on sensing the evolutionary conserved attributes of pathogens, so-called pathogen associated molecular patterns (PAMPs) – a concept known as pattern recognition. The targets of pattern recognition are products of unique aspects in microbial metabolism or structure (Barton et al. 2004; Janeway and Medzhitov 2002; Medzhitov and Janeway 1997). The receptors involved in the recognition of these patterns are ancient and some of them are conserved throughout the metazoan organisms.

15.2.3
Toll-like Receptors

Since their first description in humans, Toll-like receptors (TLR) have become one of the best studied classes of pattern recognition receptors (Barton et al. 2004; Medzhitov et al. 1997; Takeda and Akira 2004). All of the so far characterized ten members of the human TLR family recognize microbial products. Among those are a lipopolysaccharide (TLR4), lipoproteins and lipoteichoic acid (TLR2), flagellin (TLR5), unmethylated CpG DNA motives (TLR9) and several forms of viral RNA (TLR3, TLR7; Barton et al. 2004). TLRs are type 1 transmembrane proteins with a leucine repeat rich extracellular domain and a cytoplasmic moiety homologous to the IL-1 receptor (Netea et al. 2004; Pasare and Medzhitov 2005; Takeda and Akira 2005). Toll itself is a *Drosophila* receptor that was primarily characterized as a regulator of dorsal–ventral polarity (Anderson et al. 1985 a, b). Years later it was established that Toll is an essential mediator of antifungal immunity in *Drosophila* (Lemaitre et al. 1996; Lemaitre 2004). Interestingly, *Drosophila* Toll does not directly recognize fungal pathogens. Rather, it detects an endogenous ligand called spaetzle, which is proteolytically released after the activation of a serine protease cascade in the presence of fungal pathogens (Fitzgerald et al. 2004; Weber et al. 2003). In contrast, human TLRs most likely directly recognize pathogen associated molecular patterns – although formal experimental proof for this is in most cases still not available (Medzhitov and Janeway 1997, 2000 a, b). Several TLR-associated adaptor molecules, characterized by the presence of a Toll-interleukin 1-receptor domain (TIR) have been found in human cells (O'Neill et al. 2003). These include MyD88, which has long been known to be an adaptor protein for the IL-1 receptor and also has a homologue in the *Drosophila* Toll signaling cascade, TIRAP/Mal, TRIF/TICAM-1, TRAM/TIRP/TICAM-2 and SARM (Charatsi et al. 2003; O'Neill et al. 2003). Specificity for single TLRs for a subset of these adaptors might confer signaling specificity (Beutler 2004). Mainly two TLRs have been shown to contribute to the recognition of *N. meningitidis*: TLR4 and TLR2.

15.2.4
TLR4 – a Receptor for Recognition of Lipopolysaccharide

TLR4 is the central receptor for recognition of the predominant gram-negative surface molecule lipopolysaccharide in the innate immune system (Miller et al. 2005). It functions in a complex with the co-receptor MD-2, which is bound to TLR4 in the Golgi (Fitzgerald et al. 2004). MD-2 binds LPS in its monomeric form (Fitzgerald et al. 2004). Beside MD-2, other proteins act synergistically to TLR4 in LPS recognition. LPS-binding protein (LBP) is an acute phase serum protein synthesized in the liver and the lung (Fitzgerald et al. 2004; Schumann et al. 1990, 1996; Wurfel et al. 1997). It accelerates binding of LPS to another LPS recognition protein, CD14, thereby enhancing the sensitivity to LPS (Jack et al. 1997). CD14 is present in two forms in the human body, a soluble serum form and a membrane-bound form which is attached to the cell surface via a GPI anchor and is probably the most important cofactor for LPS recognition by TLR4/MD-2 (Fitzgerald et al. 2004). However, recent results point towards the possibility that beta-2 integrins can at least partially substitute for CD14, especially in recognizing bacterium-associated LPS (Ingalls and Golenbock 1995; Moore et al. 2000). Activation of immune cells by meningococcal LPS has been shown to be mediated by TLR4 and depends on the lipid A moiety of meningococcal LPS (Zughaier et al. 2004, 2005; Fig. 15.2). The LPS-devoid Δ*lpxA N. meningitidis* mutant induces significantly lower levels of proinflammatory cytokines and fails to signal via TLR4, although it can activate immune cells through TLR4-independent mechanisms, which will be discussed below (Pridmore et al. 2001; Steeghs et al. 2004; Unkmeir et al. 2002). However, the covalent linkage of a keto-deoxy-D-manno-octulosonic acid to lipid A is necessary for efficient activation of the TLR4 and full biologic activity (Zughaier et al. 2004). Secretion of the proinflammatory cytokine TNF-alpha and release of nitric oxide and reactive oxygen species are severely diminished in KDO-deficient meningococcal LPS. Recognition of meningococcal LPS, which displays an extraordinary capacity of TLR4 activation, by TLR4 induces both MyD88-dependent and -independent signaling (Zughaier et al. 2005; Fig. 15.2). MyD88 is required for induction of proinflammatory cytokines like TNF-alpha, whereas MyD88-independent signaling leads to induction of IFN-beta and nitric oxide (Zughaier et al. 2005). Meningococcal LPS has long been known to be one of the key players in the activation of the human immune response. Levels of LPS in the plasma of patients

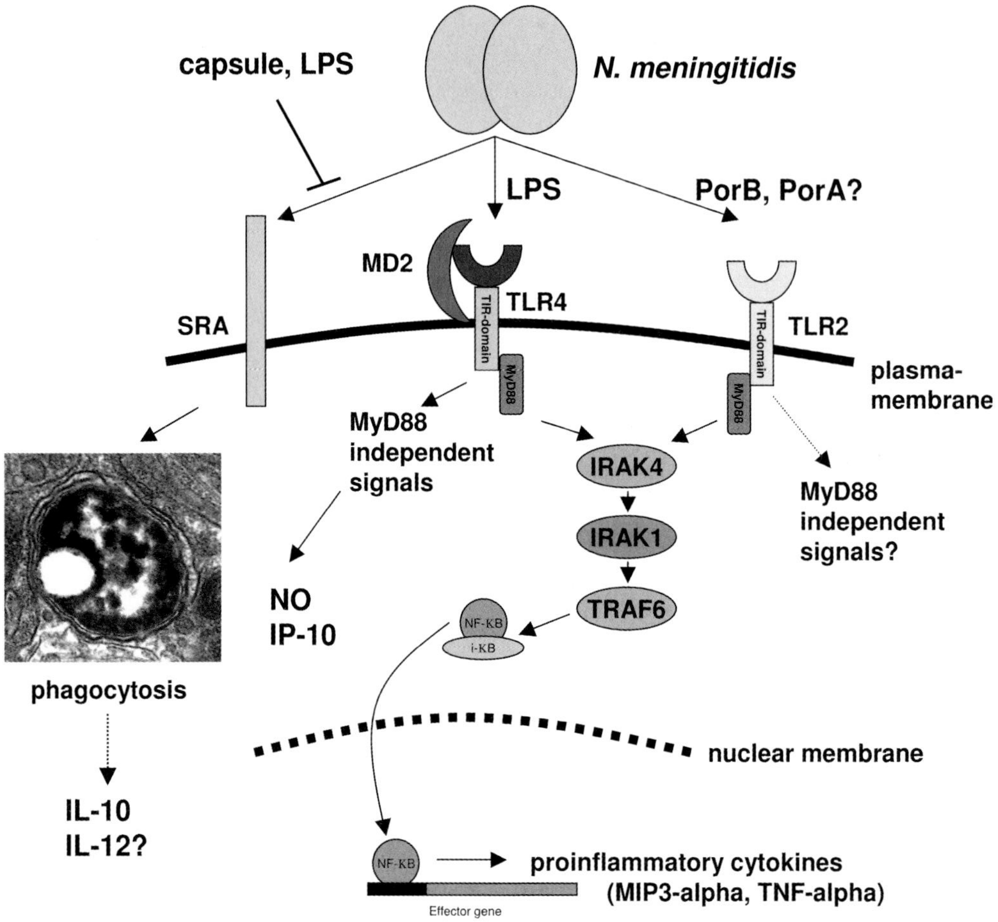

Fig. 15.2 Receptors and signaling events induced by *N. meningitidis* in dendritic cells. Several receptors on the DC surface are involved in recognition of meningococci. LPS interaction with TLR4 requires the TLR4 associated LPS recognition proteins MD2 and CD14 as well as some structural components of the meningococcal LPS (see text). This interaction is probably responsible for rapid activation of the immature DC and the induction of cytokine secretion. Beside LPS, other outer membrane components might also stimulate DC activation. This has been shown for PorB which interacts with TLR2, thereby inducing DC maturation and cytokine secretion. The graphic depicts only the common MyD88 dependent signaling pathway. This cascade can potentially branch to activate MAPK-pathways. In addition, MyD88 independent signaling pathways have been described for TLRs. For phagocytosis of *N. meningitidis*, the Scavenger Receptor A seems to be the predominant receptor on macrophages and dendritic cells. Although the internalization of *N. meningitidis* by DC can potentially lead to signaling, as contact to several TLRs might occur after phagosomal fusion, a direct role of SRA in signaling has yet to be determined. (This figure also appears with the color plates.)

correlate with the outcome of disease and *in vitro* studies clearly indicate that LPS is likely to be one of the major stimuli for cytokine release during the course of infection (Moller et al. 2005). Given this central function of meningococcal LPS as a mediator of inflammation, together with the observation that the majority of its immunostimulatory effects is likely to be mediated via the TLR4 receptor, it was intriguing to study whether polymorphisms in the TLR4 gene might be the background of a genetic predisposition for increased susceptibility to meningococcal disease. TLR4 diversity has been found both in the extracellular domain of this receptor, responsible for LPS recognition, and in the cytoplasmic domain, modulating the majority of signaling events in response to the detection of LPS (Miller et al. 2005). Examples for TLR4 polymorphisms are the Asp299Gly and Thr399Ile substitutions, which are present in among 10% of the white population and have been linked to several infectious diseases (Schröder and Schumann 2005). Both affect amino acids in the extracellular domain of TLR4 and result in decreased responsiveness to *Escherichia coli* LPS (Lorenz et al. 2002; Miller et al. 2005; Schröder and Schumann 2005). There is clear evidence that these substitutions might be relevant for the individual risk of infection caused by gram-negatives; and it has been demonstrated that patients with less responsive alleles have an increased risk of septic shock in an ICU setting (Lorenz et al. 2002). However, no association has been observed between these substitutions and meningococcal disease in two studies (Allen et al. 2003; Read et al. 2001). In contrast, some rare amino acid exchanges in TLR4 have been implicated in the individual susceptibility to meningococcal septicemia (Emonts et al. 2003; Schröder and Schumann 2005; Smirnova et al. 2000, 2001, 2003). Within a collective of patients suffering from meningococcal disease, 14 out of 220 individuals were found to display nonsynonymous single-nucleotide exchanges, in contrast to two out of 283 healthy individuals. In the same study, no association of the frequent Asp229Gly and Thr399Ile TLR4 SNPs with meningococcal disease could be detected (Schröder and Schumann 2005; Smirnova et al. 2001). It has been speculated that mutations associated with an increased risk for highly fatal infections like meningococcal disease should be rare rather than common, due to negative selective pressure. However, as TLR4 SNPs have also been implicated in the pathogenesis of atherosclerosis, they might also be evolutionary favorable (Schröder and Schumann 2005). Given the fact that polymorphisms not only occur in the TLR4 receptor, but also in multiple genes encoding components of the downstream pathways, our understanding of the role of LPS-induced signaling for individual susceptibility to meningococcal disease is only at its beginning.

15.2.5
TLR2 Mediates LPS Independent Ways to Recognize *N. meningitidis*

Although LPS certainly holds a central position in the events leading to immune activation by *N. meningitidis*, it is not the only player in the game. When Steeghs et al. were able to construct a *N. meningitidis* mutant completely devoid of LPS by inactivation of the *lpxA* gene, this opened up a unique possibility to examine the role of other factors on the bacterial surface (Steeghs et al. 1998; van der Ley and Steeghs 2003). Although researchers have to be aware of the fact that the outer membrane composition of the $\Delta lpxA$ mutant is altered in comparison to the wild type, important lessons have been learned from this strain (Steeghs et al. 2001; van der Ley and Steeghs 2003). The LPS-deficient mutant is still a capable inducer of a proinflammatory response in immune cells like monocytes; and the proinflammatory activity of the LPS-deficient mutant is retained in the outer membrane (Ingalls et al. 2001; Pridmore et al. 2001). Although less potent than the wild-type parental strain, it elicits a TNF-alpha release from peripheral blood mononuclear cells comparable to that induced by gram-positive pathogens like *Staphylococcus aureus*. This activation is completely independent of TLR4. It has however been shown that TLR2 and the CD14 molecule, which is an important receptor for several microbial products beside LPS, are necessary for at least part of the LPS-independent immune activation, although there is evidence also for CD14 independent effects (Ingalls et al. 2001; Sprong et al. 2001, 2002). Whereas it is generally accepted that LPS is the most important exogenous ligand of TLR4, the specificity of TLR2 is less clear. This may at least partially be due to the fact that TLR2 recognizes its ligands in heterodimers with TLR1 and TLR6, whereas homodimers do not seem to possess signaling activity (Kirschning and Schumann 2002; Wetzler 2003). TLR2 signaling has been shown to depend on at least two adaptor proteins, MyD88 and TIRAP, both of which also collaborate with TLR4 (Beutler 2004; Kirschning and Schumann 2002). Among the TLR2 ligands characterized so far are peptidoglycan and lipoteichoic acids. For *N. meningitidis*, PorB has been shown to induce maturation of mouse dendritic cells via TLR2, leading to increased expression of surface CD86 and class I and II MHC molecules (Massari et al. 2003; Singleton et al. 2005; Fig. 15.2). This process of maturation augmented the T-cell costimulatory capacity of dendritic cells in such a way that PorB-matured dendritic cells displayed enhanced allostimulatory activity and increased ability to stimulate naive, Ag-specific T cells (Singleton et al. 2005). The ability of PorB to upregulate expression of CD86, CD40, and MHC molecules on dendritic cells is dependent on MyD88-mediated TLR2 signaling, exactly as in mouse B-lymphocytes (see below). Meningococcal PorA also induces secretion of IL-6, IL-8, RANTES, MIP1-alpha, and MIP1-beta in human dendritic cells, leads to upregulation of CD80 and CD86 and augments the capacity of dendritic cells to activate T-cells (Al Bader et al. 2003, 2004). The receptor responsible for PorA-induced dendritic cell activation has however yet to be determined. Although the role of TLR2 contribution to the recognition of *N. meningitidis* is not fully understood at the moment, it has to be noted that LPS-free outer membrane preparations require higher concentrations and achieve less effect in the activation of human dendritic cells than LPS replete preparations (Al Bader et al. 2003).

15.2.6
Phagocytosis of *N. meningitidis* by Dendritic Cells: LPS and Capsule Versus Scavenger Receptor

The TLR-mediated aspects of dendritic cell–*N. meningitidis* interaction as described so far lead to the activation of dendritic cells and the secretion of mainly proinflammatory cytokines. However, to initiate a systemic response, uptake of *N. meningitidis* by dendritic cells and presentation of antigens to T-cells is crucial. Although surface structures of *N. meningitidis* that are required for phagocytosis have so far not been unequivocally defined, several meningococcal features preventing phagocytosis by dendritic cell have been well characterized. The polysaccharide capsule, which has been implicated in serum resistance and modulates *N. meningitidis* interaction with epithelial cells, is also a key player in the dendritic cell–*N. meningitidis* interaction. While capsule-deficient meningococci are found to be highly adherent to dendritic cells, encapsulated wild-type bacteria adhere to a much lesser extent (Kolb-Mäurer et al. 2001; Unkmeir et al. 2002). In line with these results, the capsule prevents phagocytosis of the bacteria by dendritic cells. Up to now, no serogroup-specific features in capsule interaction with dendritic cells have been described. However, the role of more subtle alterations of capsule composition, as for example the acetylation of serogroup A, C, W-135, and Y capsules, which has been suggested to modulate capsule immunogenicity, has not yet been addressed. In contrast to many other gram-negatives, the carbohydrate moiety of meningococcal LPS consists of only a few sugar residues. In addition, meningococcal LPS is a highly diverse and variable molecule with regard to the composition of the carbohydrate moiety (Hood and Moxon 1999; Jennings et al. 1999; Verheul et al. 1993). Two different factors contribute to this diversity. First, different strains of *N. meningitidis* are equipped with diverse sets of genes encoding the enzymes involved in biosynthesis of the LPS carbohydrate. Second, several of these genes are subject to phase variation and the composition of the LPS sugar chain can change depending on whether or not these genes are transcribed. A detailed summary of these mechanisms and the role of LPS diversity in meningococcal disease can be found in Chapter 9 of this book. Sialylation of L3 meningococcal LPS impairs recognition of unencapsulated meningococci at least during the phase of initial contact (Kurzai et al. 2005; Unkmeir et al. 2002). For this effect, complete LPS sialylation does not seem to be necessary, as partial sialylation is already effective in reducing the recognition of *N. meningitidis* by human dendritic cells. Further truncation of the LPS alpha-chain leads to an increase in the number of cell-associated bacteria, directly related to the length of the remaining alpha-chain (Kurzai et al. 2005). Phagocytosis is also increased for these mutants and they are more rapidly inactivated by dendritic cells, once internalized. In contrast to the alpha-chain, central parts of the *N. meningitidis* LPS oligosaccharide, including the beta- and gamma-chains, seem to play only a minor role in the interaction with human dendritic cells (Kurzai et al. 2005). The presence of the meningococcal capsule prevents recognition of meningococci by dendritic cells, even in the presence of a strong LPS oligosaccharide chain truncation. However, as a significant percentage of apathogenic carriage isolates has been shown to completely lack the genes necessary for capsule biosynthesis, these effects might contribute to the development of natural immunity during colonization with apathogenic *N. meningitidis* (Claus et al. 2002, 2005). Phagocytosis of *N. meningitidis* by human dendritic cells leads to efficient killing of the bacteria and only a low proportion of the intracellular bacteria that were observed microscopically were found to be alive in assays determining the numbers of viable intracellular bacteria (ca. 0.1% for encapsulated and 0.01% for unencapsulated meningococci; Kolb-Mäurer et al. 2001). These data show that human dendritic cells are capable of efficiently eliminating *N. meningitidis* by phagocytosis and suggest that they may play an important role in controlling neisserial infections by their bactericidal activity and efficiently present neisserial antigens to T-cells. The influence of human plasma on the adherence and phagocytosis of the bacteria was negligible (Unkmeir et al. 2002). This clearly indicates that, in contrast to other pathogenic bacteria, antibody opsonization is not a necessary prerequisite for uptake of meningococci by dendritic cells (Kolb-Mäurer et al. 2003). Engineering *N. meningitidis* mutants with a truncated LPS in an adhesion assay with human dendritic cells, it could be shown that the scavenger receptor A (SRA) is the major receptor on the dendritic cells surface responsible for phagocytosis of meningococci (Fig. 15.2). The poly-anionic inhibitor poly-G severely diminishes phagocytosis of *N. meningitidis* by human dendritic cells, indicating that SRA might be the single most important uptake receptor for meningococci on dendritic cells (Kurzai et al. 2005). Peiser et al. (2002) had already shown that SRA is almost the exclusive uptake receptor for *N. meningitidis* on macrophages, starting from a very elegant model using macrophages from wild-type and SRA knockout mice. SRA is a receptor synthesized in three isoforms (I–III), of which isoform III is nonfunctional, resulting from alternative splicing of a single gene. SRA I and II are structurally related to another scavenger receptor called MARCO (macrophage collagenous receptor), which also plays a role in innate immunity (Gordon 2004; Mukhopadhyay and Gordon 2004). Beside *N. meningitidis*, other human pathogens like *Staphylococcus aureus* or *Escherichia coli* have been shown to undergo opsonization-independent phagocytosis by SRA (Mukhopadhyay and Gordon 2004). Interestingly, lipid A has long been considered a ligand of SRA and this receptor family is probably implicated in the elimination of LPS from the circulation. However, whereas LPS has been suggested to be a mediator for the uptake of inactivated meningococci by human dendritic cells, no correlation was found between the presence or absence of LPS expression in viable meningococci and their SRA-dependent uptake by mouse macrophages (Mukhopadhyay and Gordon 2004; Mukhopadhyay et al. 2004; Peiser et al. 2002; Uronen-Hansson et al. 2004b). Thus, the meningococcal ligand for SRA has yet to be identified. There is some evidence that the secretion of regulatory cytokines like IL-10 and IL-12 might depend on phagocytosis of *N. meningitidis* by human dendritic cells (Kurzai et al. 2005; Uronen-Hansson et al. 2004b). A significant difference was found between the encapsulated wild-type strain MC58 and an unencapsulated strain in terms of IL-10 secretion. MC58 induces significantly lower levels of this regulatory cytokine 24 h post-infection than its unencapsulated mutant, an effect which is due to the antiphagocytotic properties of the meningococcal capsule. However, levels of IL-10 are not directly related to the number of phagocytosed bacteria, as truncation of the LPS-alpha chain, which clearly increases the number of intracellular bacteria, does not lead to a further increase in the levels of this cytokine. Uronen-Hansson et al. (2004a,b) have shown that the induction of IL-12 in human dendritic cells by inactivated meningococci is also dependent on phagocytosis; and they linked this observation to the presence of intracellular TLR in dendritic cells (Uronen-Hansson et al. 2004a,b). The molecular mechanisms leading to the secretion of IL-10 and IL-12, two cytokines which are key regulators in balancing an immune reaction, will have to be addressed in further studies (Fig. 15.2).

15.2.7
Macrophages

Macrophages are one of the earliest cell types that have been recognized as part of an organism's immune response (Sasmono and Hume 2004). They form part of the innate immune system in humans, recognizing and phagocytosing a wide variety of pathogenic microorganisms and making them accessible for recognition by the adaptive immune system by MHC-mediated presentation. Although generally considered to be less potent antigen presenting cells than dendritic cells, they nevertheless play a central role in linking innate and adaptive immunity. As macrophages and dendritic cells share many features in common, it has been suggested that they should rather be considered as different forms in a continuum of mononuclear phagocyte cell-types (Sasmono and Hume 2004). Macrophages are derived from bone marrow stem cells and finally develop from blood monocytes, a process involving the action of several cytokines, including the central regulator M-CSF. Resident macrophages are encountered nearly anywhere throughout the human body. Similar to dendritic cells, they are also closely associated with the borderlines of the human body, including the gastrointestinal mucosa as well as the respiratory tract epithelial lining (Fig. 15.1). Resident macrophages are one of the predominant cell types in the nasopharyngeal epithelium and have also been described to be present at the blood–brain barrier (Peiser et al. 2002; Pipkorn et al. 1988; Williams et al. 2001). Furthermore, macrophages can be found in the CSF of patients suffering from meningococcal meningitis. Meningococci can be found within macrophages during invasive infection and, indeed, this setting is described in early publications of meningococcal infection. Like other cells of the innate immune system, macrophages express a variety of pattern recognition receptors. As described previously for dendritic cells, the meningococcal polysaccharide capsule has been found to inhibit recognition of *N. meningitidis* by human macrophages (Read et al. 1996). Similar to dendritic cells, uptake of *N. meningitidis* by macrophages is independent of antibody opsonization and, once internalized by macrophages, meningococci are rapidly inactivated in phagolysosomal compartments whether or not they are encapsulated. However, presence of the polysaccharide capsule seems to delay phagolysosomal fusion for some time (Read et al. 1996) – altogether a situation very similar to that found with dendritic cells. Indeed, the mechanisms for recognition of *N. meningitidis* seem to be similar for macrophages and dendritic cells; and it was in macrophages that the role of SRA as a pattern recognition receptor for *N. meningitidis* was initially revealed (Mukhopadhyay et al. 2004a; Peiser et al. 2002). Interestingly, identification of SRA was achieved in mouse macrophages, using a SRA knockout mouse model (Peiser et al. 2002). Macrophage activation and cytokine release, in contrast, occurred independent from the SRA-mediated interaction and was dependent on the presence of LPS and TLR4 (Peiser et al. 2002). With regard to TLR-dependent activation, many of the mechanisms described above for dendritic cells are likely to be equally efficient in macrophages and some of the studies on LPS activity have been primarily performed in macrophages or macrophage cell lines (Zughaier et al. 2004). Until now, no macrophage or dendritic cell specific effect of *N. meningitidis* has been unequivocally ascertained.

15.3
Neutrophils and Invasive Meningococcal Disease

Neutrophil granulocytes are not only the major leukocyte cell type in peripheral blood (about 50–70% of total leukocytes in a healthy adult individual), they are also the predominant type of cells found in the cerebrospinal fluid of patients suffering from meningococcal meningitis during the acute phase of infection. Grossly elevated neutrophil counts in the CSF are a diagnostic hallmark of severe bacterial meningitis (Fig. 15.3). Neutrophils differentiate from myelopoietic stem cells in the bone marrow and circulate with the bloodstream. Upon the release of chemotactic factors such as C5a, several lipid mediators (PAF, leukotriene B4) and certain chemokines (IL-8 and many other CXC-type cytokines), neutrophils are recruited to the site of infection, crossing the endothelial barrier in a process called diapedesis, a complex interaction between endothelial cells of postcapillary venules and activated neutrophils (Kuijpers and Roos 2004; Mayer-Scholl et al. 2004). At the site of infection, neutrophils represent an essential component of first-line immunity, rapidly internalizing invading bacteria and inactivating them in the phagolysosomal compartment. However, neutrophils have also been shown to build up extracellular networks called neutrophil extracellular traps (NETs), composed of DNA, histones, and neutrophil elastase, that are capable of inactivating bacteria and degrading virulence-associated proteins of several pathogenic bacteria (Brinkmann et al. 2004; Mayer-Scholl et al. 2004; Weinrauch et al. 2002). As in other cell types of the innate immune system, pattern recognition receptors on the surface of these cells play a major role in the identification and uptake of pathogens. Some important pattern recogni-

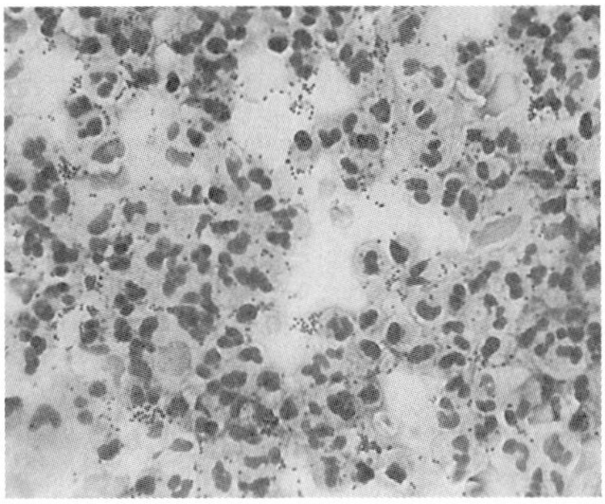

Fig. 15.3 Neutrophil granulocytes are the predominant cell type in the cerebrospinal fluid of patients suffering from meningococcal meningitis (Gram-stain, 1000×, oil immersion).

tion receptors are expressed by neutrophils at lower levels than by other cell types, like monocytes, macrophages and dendritic cells. These include TLR2, TLR4 and CD14 (Kuijpers and Roos 2004; Kurt-Jones et al. 2002). This may well account for the observation that purified neutrophils are less sensitive to activation by LPS than monocytes. In a rat model, depletion of neutrophils leads to a 100% mortality after challenging with *N. meningitidis* even after vaccination, further emphasizing the important function of these cells in meningococcal disease (Perez et al. 2001). The activation of neutrophils, resulting in upregulation of CD11b, is possibly one of the early events in *N. meningitidis* septicemia, already detectable within a few hours after the onset of symptoms and starting to decrease again after 24 h. Interestingly, this activation has also been linked to coagulation and the activity of platelets (Peters et al. 1999, 2003). Human neutrophils are responsible for efficient elimination of opsonized *N. meningitidis*, a function that is considered crucial for limiting meningococcal disease (Delvig et al. 1997). Antibodies targeted against the PorB protein might play an important role in the opsonization of *N. meningitidis*. In a study by Delvig et al. (1995, 1997), antibodies directed against the N-terminal linear epitope of the PorB VR1 loop region were shown to significantly contribute to opsonization of *N. meningitidis* in the serum of vaccines immunized with the Norwegian serogroup B outer membrane vesicle vaccine. Roughly half of the bulk serum opsonic activity could be assigned to IgG targeted against this region (Delvig et al. 1995, 1997). Although these antibodies were only marginally bactericidal, they contributed to efficient elimination of *N. meningitidis* by neutrophils (Delvig et al. 1997). In addition to this, neisserial porins have been shown to significantly influence neutrophil activation. Purified porins inhibit the responsiveness of neutrophils towards chemoattractants and degranulation. Furthermore, these neisserial surface proteins might impair expressional regulation of Fc-receptors and complement receptors and thereby inhibit uptake of *N. meningitidis* by neutrophils (Bjerknes et al. 1995). Opa proteins have also been described to be involved in *N. meningitidis*–neutrophil interaction, at least in an unencapsulated background (McNeil and Virji 1997). Indeed, Opa proteins might contribute to nonopsonic phagocytosis of *N. meningitidis* by neutrophils, which has been described for some isolates (Estabrook et al. 1998). Some intriguing insights into the interaction between pathogenic *Neisseriae* and neutrophils have been gained from studies concerning the role of gonococcal Opa proteins; and the interaction of *N. gonorrhoeae* with human neutrophils is an immunological hallmark of gonococcal infections. Members of the carcinoembryonic antigen-related cell adhesion molecule family (CEACAM, CD66) have been characterized as host cell receptors for gonococci expressing specific Opa proteins (called Opa_{CEA}), like Opa52 (Bos et al. 2002; de Jonge et al. 2003). Opa_{CEA} proteins from gonococci and meningococci can be recognized by at least four members of the human CEACAM family, namely CEACAM1, CEACAM3, CEA, and CEACAM6 (Hauck 2002; Hauck et al. 1998; Schmitter et al. 2004). CEACAM3 is a granulocyte-specific receptor in this family. CD66-mediated phagocytosis of Opa52-expressing *N. gonorrhoeae* into human cells results in a rapid activation of acid sphingomyelinase. This in turn has been shown to activate signaling cascades via Src-like protein tyrosine kinases, Rac1 and PAK, to Jun-N-terminal kinase, finally leading to tyrosine phosphorylation of CEACAM and actin-dependent nonopsonic uptake of *N. gonorrhoeae* (Hauck 2002; Hauck et al. 1998). In addition, the activity of the host cell tyrosine phosphatase SHP-1 is downregulated after Opa–CEACAM interaction, resulting in an increase in the level of tyrosine phosphorylation of several cellular proteins (McCaw et al. 2003, 2004). *N. meningitidis* has also been shown to express Opa proteins, which can be ligands for members of the CEACAM family (de Jonge et al. 2003). Taking into account the observation that a set of other human-specific pathogens can also be internalized by neutrophils in a CEACAM-dependent manner, it has been speculated that CEACAM3 has evolved as a human-specific pathogen uptake receptor (Schmitter et al. 2004). Interestingly, pathogenic *Neisseriae* have evolved variants of their CEACAM-binding adhesins that retain association with CEACAM family members expressed on epithelial cells (such as CEA or CEACAM1), but are no longer recognized by CEACAM3 (Schmitter et al. 2004).

15.4 Cells of the Adaptive Immune System

In contrast to the innate immune system, which engineers the differentiation between self and nonself by focusing on conserved, pathogen-associated patterns as outlined previously, the adaptive immune response relies on complex mechanisms of gene rearrangement to allow identification of a broad spectrum of nonself epitopes. B- and T-lymphocytes, named after their different priming locations, are the cellular armament of adaptive immunity. Like all hematopoietic cells, lymphocytes are derived from precursor cells in the bone marrow; however, whereas B-lymphocytes undergo most of their development in this organ, T-cell precursors migrate to the thymus, where they undergo a complex process of maturation. The antigenic specificity of a lymphocyte is determined early in its developmental programming by rearrangement of the variable immunoglobulin segment coding genetic regions in B-cells and genetic rearrangement of the T-cell receptor gene segments in T-cells. Once the antigen-recognizing receptor is expressed on the surface of a lymphocyte, the cell is able to bind ligands and will undergo a process of positive and negative selection, ensuring that only lymphocytes capable of correctly interacting with other immune cells and not recognizing self structures will survive. Whereas B-cells are produced throughout lifetime, the production of T-cells decreases in adolescence.

15.4.1
The Role of T-cells in Protection Against *N. meningitidis*

The first clues to the importance of a cellular participation in the immune response against meningococci came from studies on cytokine levels. In children suffering from meningitis, IL-12 and IFN-gamma levels were found to be elevated both in the serum and in the CSF (Kornelisse et al. 1997). Both cytokines are major stimuli for a Th1 directed immune response. In contrast, levels of IL-6, IL-8 and IL-10 were largely unaffected in this study. In another study, peripheral blood mononuclear cells from convalescent older children displayed a significantly higher IL-10/IFN-gamma rate than those from younger children that are more susceptible to the infection. This could point towards a necessity of Th2 induction or subtle downregulation of the immune response and the authors of this study concluded that IL-10 induction might be an important feature for a potential vaccine. In this background, the data described earlier on the dependence of IL-10 secretion by human dendritic cells on phagocytosis are especially interesting. The interaction of neisserial Opa proteins with receptors of the CEACAM family has already been described for neutrophils. Interestingly, Opa mediated binding to T-cells via CEACAM1 has been found to have a profound influence on T-cell activation in the case of gonococci (Boulton and Gray-Owen 2002). Whether meningococci can exhibit a similar activitity has yet to be determined. Meningococcal carriage has long been implicated in immune events leading to individual protection (Jordens et al. 2004; Maiden 2004; Pollard and Frasch 2001; Robinson et al. 2002; Yazdankhah and Caugant 2004). It has been shown that colonization with meningococci leads to both humoral and cellular immune reactions and it has been known for quite a time that carriage of a meningococcal strain results in the induction of bactericidal antibodies specifically directed against this particular strain but also cross-reactive against other meningococcal isolates. Similarly, the carriage of apathogenic *N. lactamica* strains has been associated with the induction of cross-reactive bactericidal antibodies, a mechanism which might be especially important in childhood, as the carriage rate of *N. meningitidis* seems to be particularly high in this age group (Bennett et al. 2005; Yazdankhah and Caugant 2004). Davenport et al. (2003) reported a proliferative response of T-cells isolated from the palatine tonsils of healthy humans, who were undergoing tonsillectomy, to *N. meningitidis* serogroup B outer membrane vesicles. This response was entirely B-cell independent and induced by protein components of the vesicles rather than LPS, as shown by the fact that proliferative responses induced by OMVs derived from the *ΔlpxA* mutant were in fact stronger than those found for the parental strain. Both CD45RA+ and CD45RO+ T-cells were capable of responding to OMV. A clear positive correlation between age and OMV response could be demonstrated in this study. In contrast, no correlation between peak responses in T-cell activation and serum bactericidal activity could be demonstrated. Despite these first glimpses of the role of T-cells in meningococcal disease, their exact function is still largely not understood. This is not only the case for T-cell specific function, but perhaps even more so for their function in B-cell activation, leading to the induction of protective antibodies.

15.4.2
B-cells: the Cellular Base for Specific Humoral Immunity

B-lymphocytes are generated in the bone marrow from precursor cells characterized by the B-cell line specific markers CD19 and CD22. During their development to antibody secreting plasma-cells, they acquire the capacity to form membrane-bound and soluble immunoglobulins and as such can be considered to be the production site for the adaptive immune system's humoral response. However, B-cells are also the cell type responsible for recognition of the meningococcal capsule polysaccharides during the course of infection or in the case of vaccination with a polysaccharide preparation. Studies have assigned the functional deficit in early childhood to B-cells rather than to T-cells (Rijkers et al. 1998). Meningococcal capsule polysaccharides are T-cell independent antigens (Mond et al. 1995; Vos et al. 2000b). T-independent antigens can be subgrouped in type 1, capable of initiating an antigen-independent polyclonal proliferative response in naïve and mature B-lymphocytes, and type 2, having no intrinsic capability to stimulate B-lymphocytes (Weintraub 2003). The latter are typically repetitive, high molecular weight polysaccharides and include the meningococcal capsule antigens. The antibody response to type 2 T-independent (TI-2) antigens is restricted both in idiotype and isotype and does not lead to immunological memory (Weintraub 2003). Although these antigens are named T-independent, experiments in T-cell depleted mice suggest that T-lymphocytes play a role in the regulation of B-cell activation by TI-2 antigens (Vos et al. 2000b). The T-cells that back up an anti-TI-2 antibody response are neither MHC-restricted nor antigen-specific in their action (Rijkers et al. 1998). They have been termed amplifier cells to differentiate them from the classic CD4+ T-helper cells that stimulate B-cell activation in response to T-dependent antigens in an MHC-restricted manner. The amplifier activity has in some studies mainly been assigned to CD4+ α,β-TCR T-cells, although the molecular interactions responsible for their regulatory function are poorly understood (Rijkers et al. 1998). Current hypotheses include the possibility that a T-cell surface molecule other than TCR could recognize epitopes on TI-2 antigens and thereby induce release of cytokines as well as a possible role for subgroups of T-cells recognizing antigens presented via MHC class 1-related molecules like CD1. The most common assumption for the process leading to B-cell activation by capsule polysaccharides is that binding of these macromolecules to specific membrane bound immunoglobulin molecules on mature B-lymphocytes leads to crosslinking and subsequent induction of antibody production by the specific cell (Vos et al. 2000 b; Weintraub 2003; Fig. 15.4). The formation of a small number of membrane-bound Ig clusters containing 10–20 receptors induce membrane association of activated Bruton's tyrosine kinase (btk) and subsequently persistent calcium flux (Vos et al. 2000 b). It has however been shown *in vitro* that ligation of membrane-bound immunoglobulins in the absence of a proper costimulatory signal may lead to anergy rather than activation of the B-cell (Vos et al. 2000 a).

Since the characterization of Toll-like receptors, their role in B-cell activation has become a focus of interest. B-lymphocytes express specific antigen-recognizing receptors (the B-cell receptor) in parallel with pattern recognition receptors like TLR (Iwasaki and Medzhitov 2004). TLR1 and TLR6–TLR10 are clearly expressed in B-cells and might be upregulated during maturation (Bernasconi et al. 2003; Bourke et al. 2003). In addition, mRNA-based studies indicate that the other TLRs might also be expressed by B-cells (Peng 2005). TLR2 has been shown to mediate PorB-induced activation of B-cells (Massari et al. 2002). The activity of neisserial porins, the major outer membrane protein of the pathogenic *Neisseria*, to stimulate B cells and upregulate the surface expression of the costimulatory receptor B7 has long been known and neisserial porins have been used as adjuvants in a variety of vaccines (Donnelly et al. 1990; Giebink et al. 1993; Lowell et al. 1988). Massari et al. (2002) have shown that the capacity of meningococcal porins to activate B-cells is due to TLR2-induced signaling via MyD88 in mouse B-cells. Costimulation of B-cells via crosslinking of membrane-bound Ig and parallel activation of a TLR cascade can lead to efficient B-cell activation (Leadbetter et al. 2002). Therefore, meningococcal porins might constitute a secondary signal via TLR2 for B-cell activation by capsule polysaccharide (Snapper et al. 1997; Wetzler et al. 1996). Other meningococcal products, including CpG DNA motives signaling via TLR9, might also be capable of providing a second signal for T-cell independent B-cell activation (Vos et al. 2000 a). A possible clue to explain the early childhood functional deficit comes from studies on the role of the complement system in the targeting of polysaccharide antigens to B-cells (Rijkers et al. 1998). Polysaccharide macromolecules can activate the complement cascade via the alternative pathway, leading to the formation of C3 fragments, which can be deposited on the polysaccharide (Dempsey et al. 1996; Fearon 1998; Fearon and Carroll 2000). C3d, a cleavage product of C3b, has been shown to be deposited on bacterial capsule polysaccharide antigens (Fig. 15.4). These complexes (C3d–polysaccharide) are ligands for CD21, a complement receptor (CR2), which is mainly expressed on mature B-lymphocytes and to a lesser degree on follicular dendritic cells and some T-cells. CD21 is part of a molecular complex together with CD19, a glycoprotein of the immunoglobulin superfamily expressed on cells of the B-lymphocyte lineage (Fearon and Carroll 2000). Via crosslinking of membrane-bound antigen-specific immunoglobulin and CD21, the latter molecule might provide a syner-

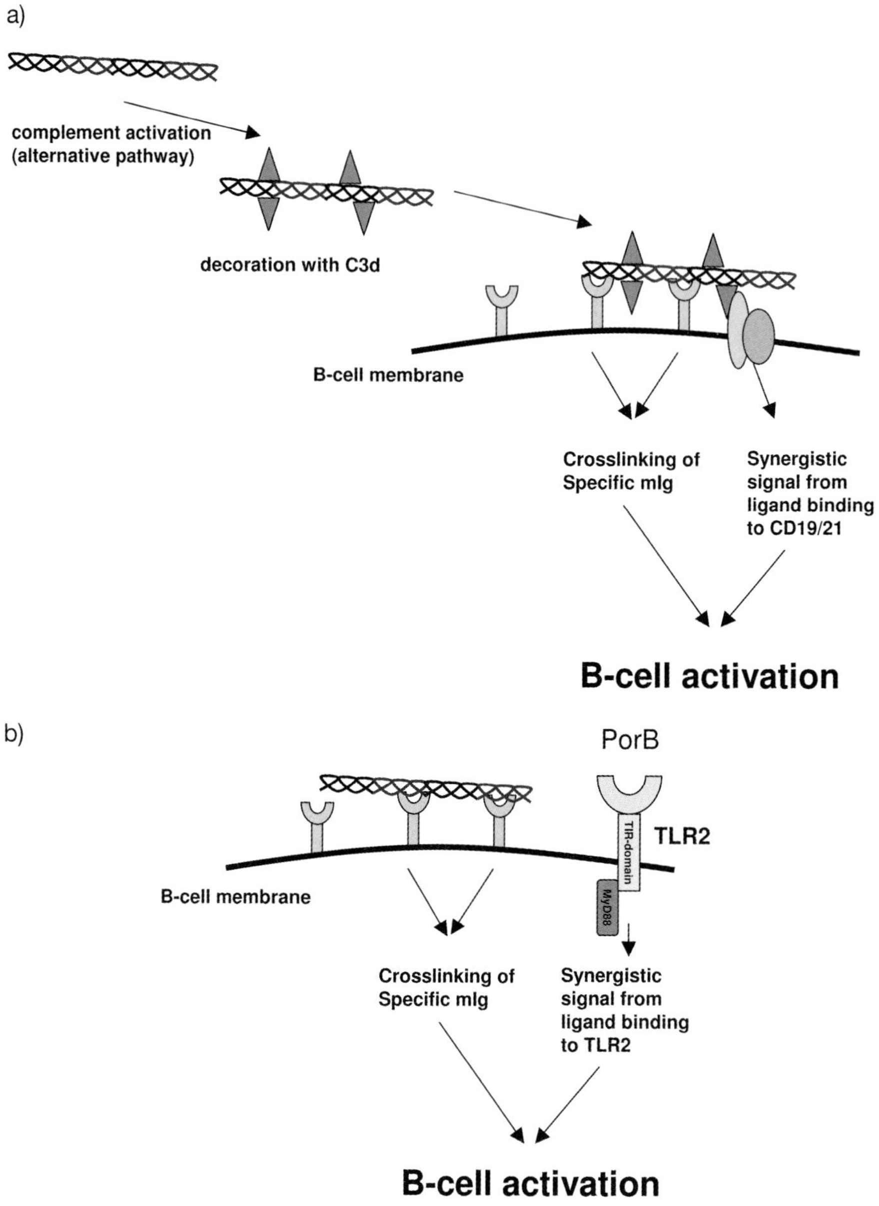

Fig. 15.4 Mechanisms leading to B-cell activation by meningococcal capsular polysaccharide. Crosslinking of B-cell membrane bound immunoglobulin receptors provides the first signal for B-cell activation. Second signals might be provided by the activation of the CD19/CD21 complement receptor complex by proteolytically released C3d, which is attached to capsule polysaccharide after activation of the complement cascade (a). Alternatively, Toll-like receptors might provide a second signal, due to the unique situation, that B-cells simultaneously express antigen-specific and pattern recognition receptors. Meningococcal PorB has been shown to activate B-cells via TLR2 (b). (This figure also appears with the color plates.)

gistic stimulus for B-cell activation via CD19, as activation of CD19 by specific antibodies has been shown to provide a costimulatory signal for B-cell activation via the B-cell receptor (Fig. 15.4). Intriguingly, B-lymphocytes of newborns and children up to 2 years of age have been found to express reduced levels of CD21 (Griffioen et al. 1992; Timens et al. 1989a, b). Some data even suggest that, in contrast to the situation in adult B-lymphocytes, cocrosslinking of membrane-bound IgG and CD21 in neonatal B-lymphocytes does not lead to synergistic activation effects (Griffioen et al. 1993). Although these models have considerably advanced our understanding of the processes leading to antibody formation against T-independent antigens, the immunological background is certainly far from being understood. Research targeted towards the elucidation of this fascinating aspect of immunology and the question why young children are unable to respond properly will certainly have to continue.

15.5 Conclusions and Perspectives

A wide variety of different cell types in the human immune system contributes to the defense against meningococcal disease. The underlying mechanisms span from pattern recognition by sentinel cells of innate immunity to highly sophisticated regulatory networks governing the activation of adaptive immunity and the induction of protective antibodies. Although our understanding of these issues has advanced considerably over the past year, there is still much to learn. In this process, the role of the innate immune system in meningococcal infection but also in the establishment of natural or vaccine induced immunity and advancements in our understanding of B-cell activation will probably be central. It is certainly a stimulating idea for everyone working in the field that one day this understanding may contribute to a possibility for protecting everyone against meningococcal disease.

References

Al Bader, T., Christodoulides, M., Heckels, J. E., Holloway, J., Semper, A. E., Friedmann, P. S. **2003**, Activation of human dendritic cells is modulated by components of the outer membranes of Neisseria meningitidis, *Infect Immun* 71, 5590–5597.

Al Bader, T., Jolley, K. A., Humphries, H. E., Holloway, J., Heckels, J. E., Semper, A. E., Friedmann, P. S., Christodoulides, M. **2004**, Activation of human dendritic cells by the PorA protein of Neisseria meningitidis, *Cell Microbiol* 6, 651–662.

Allen, A., Obaro, S., Bojang, K., Awomoyi, A. A., Greenwood, B. M., Whittle, H., Sirugo, G., Newport, M. J. **2003**, Variation in Toll-like receptor 4 and susceptibility to group A meningococcal meningitis in Gambian children, *Pediatr Infect Dis J* 22, 1018–1019.

Anderson, K.V., Bokla, L., Nusslein-Volhard, C. **1985a**, Establishment of dorsal-ventral polarity in the Drosophila embryo: the induction of polarity by the Toll gene product, *Cell* 42, 791–798.

Anderson, K.V., Jurgens, G., Nusslein-Volhard, C. **1985b**, Establishment of dorsal–ventral polarity in the Drosophila embryo: genetic studies on the role of the Toll gene product, *Cell* 42, 779–789.

Banchereau, J., Briere, F., Caux, C., Davoust, J., Lebecque, S., Liu, Y.J., Pulendran, B., Palucka, K. **2000**, Immunobiology of dendritic cells, *Annu Rev Immunol* 18, 767–811.

Banchereau, J., Steinman, R.M. **1998**, Dendritic cells and the control of immunity, *Nature* 392, 245–252.

Barton, G.M., Chandrashekhar, P., Medzhitov, R. **2004**, Toll-like receptors and control of innate immunity, in *The Innate Immune Response to Infection*, eds. Kaufmann, S.H.E., Medzhitov, R., Gordon, S. ASM, Washington, D.C., pp. 271–286.

Bennett, J.S., Griffiths, D.T., McCarthy, N.D., Sleeman, K.L., Jolley, K.A., Crook, D.W., Maiden, M.C. **2005**, Genetic diversity and carriage dynamics of Neisseria lactamica in infants, *Infect Immun* 73, 2424–2432.

Bernasconi, N.L., Onai, N., Lanzavecchia, A. **2003**, A role for Toll-like receptors in acquired immunity: up-regulation of TLR9 by BCR triggering in naive B cells and constitutive expression in memory B cells, *Blood* 101, 4500–4504.

Beutler, B. **2004**, Inferences, questions and possibilities in Toll-like receptor signalling, *Nature* 430, 257–263.

Bjerknes, R., Guttormsen, H.K., Solberg, C.O., Wetzler, L.M. **1995**, Neisserial porins inhibit human neutrophil actin polymerization, degranulation, opsonin receptor expression, and phagocytosis but prime the neutrophils to increase their oxidative burst, *Infect Immun* 63, 160–167.

Bogaert, D., Hermans, P.W., Boelens, H., Sluijter, M., Luijendijk, A., Rumke, H.C., Koppen, S., van Belkum, A., de Groot, R., Verbrugh, H.A. **2005**, Epidemiology of nasopharyngeal carriage of Neisseria meningitidis in healthy Dutch children, *Clin Infect Dis* 40, 899–902.

Bos, M.P., Kao, D., Hogan, D.M., Grant, C.C., Belland, R.J. **2002**, Carcinoembryonic antigen family receptor recognition by gonococcal Opa proteins requires distinct combinations of hypervariable Opa protein domains, *Infect Immun* 70, 1715–1723.

Boulton, I.C., Gray-Owen, S.D. **2002**, Neisserial binding to CEACAM1 arrests the activation and proliferation of CD4+ T lymphocytes, *Nat Immunol* 3, 229–236.

Bourke, E., Bosisio, D., Golay, J., Polentarutti, N., Mantovani, A. **2003**, The toll-like receptor repertoire of human B lymphocytes: inducible and selective expression of TLR9 and TLR10 in normal and transformed cells, *Blood* 102, 956–963.

Brinkmann, V., Reichard, U., Goosmann, C., Fauler, B., Uhlemann, Y., Weiss, D.S., Weinrauch, Y., Zychlinsky, A. **2004**, Neutrophil extracellular traps kill bacteria, *Science* 303, 1532–1535.

Charatsi, I., Luschnig, S., Bartoszewski, S., Nusslein-Volhard, C., Moussian, B. **2003**, Krapfen/dMyd88 is required for the establishment of dorsoventral pattern in the Drosophila embryo, *Mech Dev* 120, 219–226.

Cheroutre, H. **2004**, Starting at the beginning: new perspectives on the biology of mucosal T cells, *Annu Rev Immunol* 22, 217–246.

Claus, H., Maiden, M.C., Maag, R., Frosch, M., Vogel, U. **2002**, Many carried meningococci lack the genes required for capsule synthesis and transport, *Microbiology* 148, 1813–1819.

Claus, H., Maiden, M.C., Wilson, D.J., McCarthy, N.D., Jolley, K.A., Urwin, R., Hessler, F., Frosch, M., Vogel, U. **2005**, Genetic analysis of meningococci carried by children and young adults, *J Infect Dis* 191, 1263–1271.

Davenport, V., Guthrie, T., Findlow, J., Borrow, R., Williams, N.A., Heyderman, R.S. **2003**, Evidence for naturally acquired T cell-mediated mucosal immunity to Neisseria meningitidis, *J Immunol* 171, 4263–4270.

de Jonge, M.I., Hamstra, H.J., van Alphen, L., Dankert, J., van der Ley, P. **2003**, Mapping the binding domains on meningococcal Opa proteins for CEACAM1 and CEA receptors, *Mol Microbiol* 50, 1005–1015.

Delvig, A.A., Michaelsen, T.E., Aase, A., Hoiby, E.A., Rosenqvist, E. **1997**, Vaccine-induced IgG antibodies to the linear epitope on the PorB outer membrane protein promote opsonophagocytosis of Neisseria meningitidis by human neutrophils, *Clin Immunol Immunopathol* 84, 27–35.
Delvig, A.A., Wedege, E., Caugant, D.A., Dalseg, R., Kolberg, J., Achtman, M., Rosenqvist, E. **1995**, A linear B-cell epitope on the class 3 outer-membrane protein of Neisseria meningitidis recognized after vaccination with the Norwegian group B outer-membrane vesicle vaccine, *Microbiology* 141, 1593–1600.
Dempsey, P.W., Allison, M.E., Akkaraju, S., Goodnow, C.C., Fearon, D.T. **1996**, C3d of complement as a molecular adjuvant: bridging innate and acquired immunity, *Science* 271, 348–350.
Donnelly, J.J., Deck, R.R., Liu, M.A. **1990**, Immunogenicity of a Haemophilus influenzae polysaccharide–Neisseria meningitidis outer membrane protein complex conjugate vaccine, *J Immunol* 145, 3071–3079.
Emonts, M., Hazelzet, J.A., de Groot, R., Hermans, P.W. **2003**, Host genetic determinants of Neisseria meningitidis infections, *Lancet Infect Dis* 3, 565–577.
Estabrook, M.M., Zhou, D., Apicella, M.A. **1998**, Nonopsonic phagocytosis of group C Neisseria meningitidis by human neutrophils, *Infect Immun* 66, 1028–1036.
Fearon, D.T. **1998**, The complement system and adaptive immunity, *Semin Immunol* 10, 355–361.
Fearon, D.T., Carroll, M.C. **2000**, Regulation of B lymphocyte responses to foreign and self-antigens by the CD19/CD21 complex, *Annu Rev Immunol* 18, 393–422.
Fitzgerald, K.A., Rowe, D.C., Golenbock, D.T. **2004**, Endotoxin recognition and signal transduction by the TLR4/MD2 complex, *Microbes Infect* 6, 1361–1367.
Giebink, G.S., Koskela, M., Vella, P.P., Harris, M., Le, C.T. **1993**, Pneumococcal capsular polysaccharide-meningococcal outer membrane protein complex conjugate vaccines: immunogenicity and efficacy in experimental pneumococcal otitis media, *J Infect Dis* 167, 347–355.
Goldschneider, I., Gotschlich, E.C., Artenstein, M.S. **1969a**, Human immunity to the meningococcus, I. The role of humoral antibodies, *J Exp Med* 129, 1307–1326.
Goldschneider, I., Gotschlich, E.C., Artenstein, M.S. **1969b**, Human immunity to the meningococcus, II. Development of natural immunity, *J Exp Med* 129, 1327–1348.
Gordon, S. **2004**, Antigen-presenting cell receptors and innate immunity: diversity, recognition and responses, in *The Innate Immune Response to Infection*, eds. Kaufmann, S.H.E., Medzhitov, R., Gordon, S., ASM Press, Washington, D.C., pp. 287–300.
Granucci, F., Feau, S., Zanoni, I., Raimondi, G., Pavelka, N., Vizzardelli, C., et al. **2004**, The regulatory role of dendritic cells in the innate immune response, in *The Innate Immune Repsonse to Infection*, eds. Kaufmann, S.H.E., Medzhitov, R., Gordon, S., ASM Press, Washington D.C., pp. 95–110.
Griffioen, A.W., Franklin, S.W., Zegers, B.J., Rijkers, G.T. **1993**, Expression and functional characteristics of the complement receptor type 2 on adult and neonatal B lymphocytes, *Clin Immunol Immunopathol* 69, 1–8.
Griffioen, A.W., Toebes, E.A., Zegers, B.J., Rijkers, G.T. **1992**, Role of CR2 in the human adult and neonatal in vitro antibody response to type 4 pneumococcal polysaccharide, *Cell Immunol* 143, 11–22.
Hauck, C.R. **2002**, Cell adhesion receptors – signaling capacity and exploitation by bacterial pathogens, *Med Microbiol Immunol* 191, 55–62.
Hauck, C.R., Meyer, T.F., Lang, F., Gulbins, E. **1998** CD66-mediated phagocytosis of Opa52 Neisseria gonorrhoeae requires a Src-like tyrosine kinase- and Rac1-dependent signalling pathway, *EMBO J* 17, 443–454.
Hood, D.W., Moxon, E.R. **1999**, Lipopolysaccharide phase variation in Haemophilus and Neisseriae, in *Endotoxin in Health and Disease*, eds. Brade, H., Opal, S.M., Vogel, S.N., Morrison, D.C., Marcel Dekker, New York, pp. 39–54.
Ingalls, R.R., Golenbock, D.T. **1995**, CD11c/CD18, a transmembrane signaling receptor for lipopolysaccharide, *J Exp Med* 181, 1473–1479.

Ingalls, R.R., Lien, E., Golenbock, D.T. **2001**, Membrane-associated proteins of a lipopolysaccharide-deficient mutant of Neisseria meningitidis activate the inflammatory response through toll-like receptor 2, *Infect Immun* 69, 2230–2236.

Iwasaki, A., Medzhitov, R. **2004**, Toll-like receptor control of the adaptive immune responses, *Nat Immunol* 5, 987–995.

Jack, R.S., Fan, X., Bernheiden, M., Rune, G., Ehlers, M., Weber, A., Kirsch, G., Mentel, R., Furll, B., Freudenberg, M., Schmitz, G., Stelter, F., Schutt, C. **1997**, Lipopolysaccharide-binding protein is required to combat a murine gram-negative bacterial infection, *Nature* 389, 742–745.

Janeway, C.A., Jr., Medzhitov, R. **2002**, Innate immune recognition, *Annu Rev Immunol* 20, 197–216.

Jennings, M.P., Srikhanta, Y.N., Moxon, E.R., Kramer, M., Poolman, J.T., Kuipers, B., van der Ley, P. **1999**, The genetic basis of the phase variation repertoire of lipopolysaccharide immunotypes in Neisseria meningitidis, *Microbiology* 145, 3013–3021.

Jordens, J.Z., Williams, J.N., Jones, G.R., Christodoulides, M., Heckels, J.E. **2004**, Development of immunity to serogroup B meningococci during carriage of Neisseria meningitidis in a cohort of university students, *Infect Immun* 72, 6503–6510.

Kelsall, B.L., Rescigno, M. **2004**, Mucosal dendritic cells in immunity and inflammation, *Nat Immunol* 5, 1091–1095.

Kirschning, C.J., Schumann, R.R. **2002**, TLR2: cellular sensor for microbial and endogenous molecular patterns, *Curr Topics Microbiol Immunol* 270, 121–144.

Kiyono, H., Fukuyama, S. **2004**, NALT – versus Peyer's patch-mediated mucosal immunity, *Nat Rev Immunol* 4, 699–710.

Kolb-Mäurer, A., Kurzai, O., Goebel, W., Frosch, M. **2003**, The role of human dendritic cells in meningococcal and listerial meningitis, *Int J Med Microbiol* 293, 241–249.

Kolb-Mäurer, A., Unkmeir, A., Kammerer, U., Hubner, C., Leimbach, T., Stade, A., Kampgen, E., Frosch, M., Dietrich, G. **2001**, Interaction of Neisseria meningitidis with human dendritic cells, *Infect Immun* 69, 6912–6922.

Kornelisse, R.F., Hack, C.E., Savelkoul, H.F., van der Pouw Kraan, T.C., Hop, W.C., van Mierlo, G., Suur, M.H., Neijens, H.J., de Groot, R. **1997**, Intrathecal production of interleukin-12 and gamma interferon in patients with bacterial meningitis, *Infect Immun* 65, 877–881.

Kuijpers, T.W., Roos, D. **2004**, Neutrophils: the power within, in *The Innate Immune Response to Infection*, eds. Kaufmann, S.H.E., Medzhitov, R., Gordon, S., ASM Press, Washington D.C., pp. 47–70.

Kurt-Jones, E.A., Mandell, L., Whitney, C., Padgett, A., Gosselin, K., Newburger, P.E., Finberg, R.W. **2002**, Role of toll-like receptor 2 (TLR2) in neutrophil activation: GM-CSF enhances TLR2 expression and TLR2-mediated interleukin 8 responses in neutrophils, *Blood* 100, 1860–1868.

Kurzai, O., Schmitt, C., Claus, H., Vogel, U., Frosch, M., Kolb-Mäurer, A. **2005**, Carbohydrate composition of meningococcal lipopolysaccharide modulates the interaction of *Neisseria meningitidis* with human dendritic cells, *Cell Microbiol* 7, 1319–1334.

Leadbetter, E.A., Rifkin, I.R., Hohlbaum, A.M., Beaudette, B.C., Shlomchik, M.J., Marshak-Rothstein, A. **2002**, Chromatin-IgG complexes activate B cells by dual engagement of IgM and Toll-like receptors, *Nature* 416, 603–607.

Lemaitre, B. **2004**, The road to Toll, *Nat Rev Immunol* 4, 521–527.

Lemaitre, B., Nicolas, E., Michaut, L., Reichhart, J.M., Hoffmann, J.A. **1996**, The dorsoventral regulatory gene cassette spatzle/Toll/cactus controls the potent antifungal response in Drosophila adults, *Cell* 86, 973–983.

Lorenz, E., Mira, J.P., Frees, K.L., Schwartz, D.A. **2002**, Relevance of mutations in the TLR4 receptor in patients with gram-negative septic shock, *Arch Intern Med* 162, 1028–1032.

Lowell, G.H., Ballou, W.R., Smith, L.F., Wirtz, R.A., Zollinger, W.D., Hockmeyer, W.T. **1988**, Proteosome-lipopeptide vaccines: enhancement of immunogenicity for malaria CS peptides, *Science* 240, 800–802.

Maiden, M.C. **2004**, Dynamics of bacterial carriage and disease: lessons from the me-

ningococcus, *Adv Exp Med Biol* 549, 23–29.
Maldonado-Lopez, R,Moser, M. **2001**, Dendritic cell subsets and the regulation of Th1/Th2 responses, *Semin Immunol* 13, 275–282.
Massari, P., Henneke, P., Ho, Y., Latz, E., Golenbock, D.T., Wetzler, L.M. **2002**, Cutting edge: immune stimulation by neisserial porins is toll-like receptor 2 and MyD88 dependent, *J Immunol* 168, 1533–1537.
Massari, P., Ram, S., Macleod, H., Wetzler, L.M. **2003**, The role of porins in neisserial pathogenesis and immunity, *Trends Microbiol* 11, 87–93.
Mayer-Scholl, A., Averhoff, P., Zychlinsky, A. **2004**, How do neutrophils and pathogens interact? *Curr Opin Microbiol* 7, 62–66.
McCaw, S.E., Liao, E.H., Gray-Owen, S.D. **2004**, Engulfment of Neisseria gonorrhoeae: revealing distinct processes of bacterial entry by individual carcinoembryonic antigen-related cellular adhesion molecule family receptors, *Infect Immun* 72, 2742–2752.
McCaw, S.E., Schneider, J., Liao, E.H., Zimmermann, W., Gray-Owen, S.D. **2003**, Immunoreceptor tyrosine-based activation motif phosphorylation during engulfment of Neisseria gonorrhoeae by the neutrophil-restricted CEACAM3 (CD66d) receptor, *Mol Microbiol* 49, 623–637.
McNeil, G., Virji, M. **1997**, Phenotypic variants of meningococci and their potential in phagocytic interactions: the influence of opacity proteins, pili, PilC and surface sialic acids, *Microb Pathog* 22, 295–304.
Medzhitov, R., Janeway, C., Jr. **2000a**, Innate immunity, *N Engl J Med* 343, 338–344.
Medzhitov, R., Janeway, C., Jr. **2000b**, The Toll receptor family and microbial recognition, *Trends Microbiol* 8, 452–456.
Medzhitov, R., Janeway, C.A., Jr. **1997**, Innate immunity: the virtues of a nonclonal system of recognition, *Cell* 91, 295–298.
Medzhitov, R., Preston-Hurlburt, P., Janeway, C.A., Jr. **1997**, A human homologue of the Drosophila Toll protein signals activation of adaptive immunity, *Nature* 388, 394–397.
Miller, S.I., Ernst, R.K., Bader, M.W. **2005**, LPS, TLR4 and infectious disease diversity, *Nat Rev Microbiol* 3, 36–46.
Moller, A.S., Bjerre, A., Brusletto, B., Joo, G.B., Brandtzaeg, P., Kierulf, P. **2005**, Chemokine patterns in meningococcal disease, *J Infect Dis* 191, 768–775.
Mond, J.J., Vos, Q., Lees, A., Snapper, C.M. **1995**, T cell independent antigens, *Curr Opin Immunol* 7, 349–354.
Moore, K.J., Andersson, L.P., Ingalls, R.R., Monks, B.G., Li, R., Arnaout, M.A., Golenbock, D.T., Freeman, M.W. **2000**, Divergent response to LPS and bacteria in CD14-deficient murine macrophages, *J Immunol* 165, 4272–4280.
Mowat, A.M. **2003**, Anatomical basis of tolerance and immunity to intestinal antigens, *Nat Rev Immunol* 3, 331–341.
Mukhopadhyay, S., Gordon, S. **2004**, The role of scavenger receptors in pathogen recognition and innate immunity, *Immunobiology* 209, 39–49.
Mukhopadhyay, S., Peiser, L., Gordon, S. **2004a**, Activation of murine macrophages by Neisseria meningitidis and IFN-gamma in vitro: distinct roles of class A scavenger and Toll-like pattern recognition receptors in selective modulation of surface phenotype, *J Leukoc Biol* 76, 577–584.
Netea, M.G., van der Graaf, C., van der Meer, J.W., Kullberg, B.J. **2004**, Toll-like receptors and the host defense against microbial pathogens: bringing specificity to the innate-immune system, *J Leukoc Biol* 75, 749–755.
O'Neill, L.A., Fitzgerald, K.A., Bowie, A.G. **2003**, The Toll-IL-1 receptor adaptor family grows to five members, *Trends Immunol* 24, 286–290.
Palucka, K., Banchereau, J. **1999**, Linking innate and adaptive immunity, *Nat Med* 5, 868–870.
Pasare, C., Medzhitov, R. **2005**, Toll-like receptors: linking innate and adaptive immunity, *Adv Exp Med Biol* 560, 11–18.
Peiser, L., De Winther, M.P., Makepeace, K., Hollinshead, M., Coull, P., Plested, J., Kodama, T., Moxon, E.R., Gordon, S. **2002**, The class A macrophage scavenger receptor is a major pattern recognition receptor for Neisseria meningitidis which is independent of lipopolysaccharide and not re-

quired for secretory responses, *Infect Immun* 70, 5346–5354.

Peng, S. L. **2005**, Signaling in B cells via Toll-like receptors, *Curr Opin Immunol* 17, 230–236.

Perez, O., Lastre, M., Lapinet, J., Bracho, G., Diaz, M., Zayas, C., Taboada, C., Sierra, G. **2001**, Immune response induction and new effector mechanisms possibly involved in protection conferred by the Cuban anti-meningococcal BC vaccine, *Infect Immun* 69, 4502–4508.

Peters, M. J., Dixon, G., Kotowicz, K. T., Hatch, D. J., Heyderman, R. S., Klein, N. J. **1999**, Circulating platelet–neutrophil complexes represent a subpopulation of activated neutrophils primed for adhesion, phagocytosis and intracellular killing, *Br J Haematol* 106, 391–399.

Peters, M. J., Heyderman, R. S., Faust, S., Dixon, G. L., Inwald, D. P., Klein, N. J. **2003**, Severe meningococcal disease is characterized by early neutrophil but not platelet activation and increased formation and consumption of platelet-neutrophil complexes, *J Leukoc Biol* 73, 722–730.

Pipkorn, U., Karlsson, G., Enerback, L. **1988**, A brush method to harvest cells from the nasal mucosa for microscopic and biochemical analysis, *J Immunol Methods* 112, 37–42.

Plant, L., Asp, V., Lovkvist, L., Sundqvist, J., Jonsson, A. B. **2004**, Epithelial cell responses induced upon adherence of pathogenic Neisseria, *Cell Microbiol* 6, 663–670.

Pollard, A. J., Frasch, C. **2001**, Development of natural immunity to Neisseria meningitidis *Vaccine* 19, 1327–1346.

Pridmore, A. C., Wyllie, D. H., Abdillahi, F., Steeghs, L. van der Ley, P., Dower, S. K., Read, R. C. **2001**, A lipopolysaccharide-deficient mutant of Neisseria meningitidis elicits attenuated cytokine release by human macrophages and signals via toll-like receptor (TLR) 2 but not via TLR4/MD2, *J Infect Dis* 183, 89–96.

Rage, G. **1934**, Studies on meningococcus infection, VI. The carrier problem, *J Exp Med* 59, 553.

Read, R. C., Pullin, J., Gregory, S., Borrow, R., Kaczmarski, E. B., di Giovine, F. S., Dower, S. K., Cannings, C., Wilson, A. G. **2001**, A functional polymorphism of toll-like receptor 4 is not associated with likelihood or severity of meningococcal disease, *J Infect Dis* 184, 640–642.

Read, R. C., Zimmerli, S., Broaddus, C., Sanan, D. A., Stephens, D. S., Ernst, J. D. **1996**, The (alpha → 28)-linked polysialic acid capsule of group B Neisseria meningitidis modifies multiple steps during interaction with human macrophages, *Infect Immun* 64, 3210–3217.

Rescigno, M., Chieppa, M. **2005**, Gut-level decisions in peace and war, *Nat Med* 11, 254–255.

Rescigno, M., Rotta, G., Valzasina, B., Ricciardi-Castagnoli, P. **2001 a**, Dendritic cells shuttle microbes across gut epithelial monolayers, *Immunobiology* 204, 572–581.

Rescigno, M., Urbano, M., Valzasina, B., Francolini, M., Rotta, G., Bonasio, R., Granucci, F., Kraehenbuhl, J. P., Ricciardi-Castagnoli, P. **2001 b**, Dendritic cells express tight junction proteins and penetrate gut epithelial monolayers to sample bacteria, *Nat Immunol* 2, 361–367.

Rijkers, G. T., Sanders, E. A., Breukels, M. A., Zegers, B. J. **1998**, Infant B cell responses to polysaccharide determinants, *Vaccine* 16, 1396–1400.

Rimoldi, M., Chieppa, M., Salucci, V., Avogadri, F., Sonzogni, A., Sampietro, G. M., Nespoli, A., Viale, G., Allavena, P., Rescigno, M. **2005**, Intestinal immune homeostasis is regulated by the crosstalk between epithelial cells and dendritic cells, *Nat Immunol* 6, 507–514.

Robinson, K., Neal, K. R., Howard, C., Stockton, J., Atkinson, K., Scarth, E., Moran, J., Robins, A., Todd, I., Kaczmarski, E., Gray, S., Muscat, I., Slack, R., Ala'Aldeen, D. A. **2002**, Characterization of humoral and cellular immune responses elicited by meningococcal carriage, *Infect Immun* 70, 1301–1309.

Rosenstein, N. E., Perkins, B. A., Stephens, D. S., Popovic, T., Hughes, J. M. **2001**, Meningococcal disease, *N Engl J Med* 344, 1378–1388.

Sasmono, R. T., Hume, D. A. **2004**, The biology of macrophages, in *The Innate Immune Response To Infection*, eds. Kaufmann, S. H. E., Medhzitov, R., Gordon, S., ASM Press, Washington D. C., pp. 71–94.

Schmitter, T., Agerer, F., Peterson, L., Munzner, P., Hauck, C.R. **2004**, Granulocyte CEACAM3 is a phagocytic receptor of the innate immune system that mediates recognition and elimination of human-specific pathogens, *J Exp Med* 199, 35–46.

Schröder, N.W., Schumann, R.R. **2005**, Single nucleotide polymorphisms of Toll-like receptors and susceptibility to infectious disease, *Lancet Infect Dis* 5, 156–164.

Schumann, R.R., Kirschning, C.J., Unbehaun, A., Aberle, H.P., Knope, H.P., Lamping, N., Ulevitch, R.J., Herrmann, F. **1996**, The lipopolysaccharide-binding protein is a secretory class 1 acute-phase protein whose gene is transcriptionally activated by APRF/STAT/3 and other cytokine-inducible nuclear proteins, *Mol Cell Biol* 16, 3490–3503.

Schumann, R.R., Leong, S.R., Flaggs, G.W., Gray, P.W., Wright, S.D., Mathison, J.C., Tobias, P.S., Ulevitch, R.J. **1990**, Structure and function of lipopolysaccharide binding protein, *Science* 249, 1429–1431.

Shortman, K., Liu, Y.J. **2002**, Mouse and human dendritic cell subtypes, *Nat Rev Immunol* 2, 151–161.

Singleton, T.E., Massari, P., Wetzler, L.M. **2005**, Neisserial porin-induced dendritic cell activation is MyD88 and TLR2 dependent, *J Immunol* 174, 3545–3550.

Smirnova, I., Hamblin, M.T., McBride, C., Beutler, B., Di Rienzo, A. **2001**, Excess of rare amino acid polymorphisms in the Toll-like receptor 4 in humans, *Genetics* 158, 1657–1664.

Smirnova, I., Mann, N., Dols, A., Derkx, H.H., Hibberd, M.L., Levin, M., Beutler, B. **2003**, Assay of locus-specific genetic load implicates rare Toll-like receptor 4 mutations in meningococcal susceptibility, *Proc Natl Acad Sci USA* 100, 6075–6080.

Smirnova, I., Poltorak, A., Chan, E.K., McBride, C., Beutler, B. **2000**, Phylogenetic variation and polymorphism at the toll-like receptor 4 locus (TLR4), *Genome Biol* 1, research002.

Snapper, C.M., Rosas, F.R., Kehry, M.R., Mond, J.J., Wetzler, L.M. **1997**, Neisserial porins may provide critical second signals to polysaccharide-activated murine B cells for induction of immunoglobulin secretion, *Infect Immun* 65, 3203–3208.

Sprong, T., Stikkelbroeck, N., van der Ley, P., Steeghs, L., van Alphen, L., Klein, N., Netea, M.G., van der Meer, J.W., van Deuren, M. **2001**, Contributions of Neisseria meningitidis LPS and non-LPS to proinflammatory cytokine response, *J Leukoc Biol* 70, 283–288.

Sprong, T., van der Ley, P., Steeghs, L., Taw, W.J., Verver-Janssen, T.J., Netea, M.G., van der Meer, J.W., van Deuren, M. **2002**, Neisseria meningitidis can induce pro-inflammatory cytokine production via pathways independent from CD14 and toll-like receptor 4, *Eur Cytokine Netw* 13, 411–417.

Steeghs, L., de Cock, H., Evers, E., Zomer, B., Tommassen, J., van der Ley, P. **2001**, Outer membrane composition of a lipopolysaccharide-deficient Neisseria meningitidis mutant. *EMBO J* 20, 6937–6945.

Steeghs, L., den Hartog, R., den Boer, A., Zomer, B., Roholl, P., van der Ley, P. **1998**, Meningitis bacterium is viable without endotoxin, *Nature* 392, 449–450.

Steeghs, L., Tommassen, J., Leusen, J.H., van de Winkel, J.G., van der Ley, P. **2004**, Teasing apart structural determinants of 'toxicity' and 'adjuvanticity': implications for meningococcal vaccine development, *J Endotoxin Res* 10, 113–119.

Takeda, K., Akira, S. **2004**, Toll-like receptors: ligands and signaling, in *The Innate Immune Response To Infection*, eds. Kaufmann, S.H.E., Medhzitov, R., Gordon, S. ASM Press, Washington D.C., pp. 257–270.

Takeda, K., Akira, S. **2005**, Toll-like receptors in innate immunity, *Int Immunol* 17, 1–14.

Timens, W., Boes, A., Poppema, S. **1989a**, Human marginal zone B cells are not an activated B cell subset: strong expression of CD21 as a putative mediator for rapid B cell activation, *Eur J Immunol* 19, 2163–2166.

Timens, W., Boes, A., Rozeboom-Uiterwijk, T., Poppema, S. **1989b**, Immaturity of the human splenic marginal zone in infancy, Possible contribution to the deficient infant immune response, *J Immunol* 143, 3200–3206.

Unkmeir, A., Kammerer, U., Stade, A., Hubner, C., Haller, S., Kolb-Mäurer, A., Frosch, M., Dietrich, G. **2002**, Lipooligosaccharide and polysaccharide capsule: virulence factors of Neisseria meningitidis that determine meningococcal interaction with human dendritic cells, *Infect Immun* 70, 2454–2462.

Uronen-Hansson, H., Allen, J., Osman, M., Squires, G., Klein, N., Callard, R. E. **2004a**, Toll-like receptor 2 (TLR2) and TLR4 are present inside human dendritic cells, associated with microtubules and the Golgi apparatus but are not detectable on the cell surface: integrity of microtubules is required for interleukin-12 production in response to internalized bacteria, *Immunology* 111, 173–178.

Uronen-Hansson, H., Steeghs, L., Allen, J., Dixon, G. L., Osman, M., van der Ley, P., Wong, S. Y., Callard, R., Klein, N. **2004b**, Human dendritic cell activation by Neisseria meningitidis: phagocytosis depends on expression of lipooligosaccharide (LOS) by the bacteria and is required for optimal cytokine production, *Cell Microbiol* 6, 625–637.

van der Ley, P., Steeghs, L. **2003**, Lessons from an LPS-deficient Neisseria meningitidis mutant, *J Endotoxin Res* 9, 124–128.

Verheul, A. F., Snippe, H., Poolman, J. T. **1993**, Meningococcal lipopolysaccharides: virulence factor and potential vaccine component, *Microbiol Rev* 57, 34–49.

Vos, Q., Lees, A., Wu, Z. Q., Snapper, C. M., Mond, J. J. **2000a**, B-cell activation by T-cell-independent type 2 antigens as an integral part of the humoral immune response to pathogenic microorganisms, *Immunol Rev* 176, 154–170.

Vos, Q., Lees, A., Wu, Z. Q., Snapper, C. M., Mond, J. J. **2000b**, B-cell activation by T-cell-independent type 2 antigens as an integral part of the humoral immune response to pathogenic microorganisms, *Immunol Rev* 176, 154–170.

Weber, A. N., Tauszig-Delamasure, S., Hoffmann, J. A., Lelievre, E., Gascan, H., Ray, K. P., Morse, M. A., Imler, J. L., Gay, N. J. **2003**, Binding of the Drosophila cytokine Spatzle to Toll is direct and establishes signaling, *Nat Immunol* 4, 794–800.

Weinrauch, Y., Drujan, D., Shapiro, S. D., Weiss, J., Zychlinsky, A. **2002**, Neutrophil elastase targets virulence factors of enterobacteria, *Nature* 417, 91–94.

Weintraub, A. **2003**, Immunology of bacterial polysaccharide antigens, *Carbohydr Res* 338, 2539–2547.

Wetzler, L. M. **2003**, The role of Toll-like receptor 2 in microbial disease and immunity, *Vaccine* 21[Suppl 2], S55–S60.

Wetzler, L. M., Ho, Y., Reiser, H. **1996**, Neisserial porins induce B lymphocytes to express costimulatory B7-2 molecules and to proliferate, *J Exp Med* 183, 1151–1159.

Williams, K., Alvarez, X., Lackner, A. A. **2001**, Central nervous system perivascular cells are immunoregulatory cells that connect the CNS with the peripheral immune system, *Glia* 36, 156–164.

Wurfel, M. M., Monks, B. G., Ingalls, R. R., Dedrick, R. L., Delude, R., Zhou, D., Lamping, N., Schumann, R. R., Thieringer, R., Fenton, M. J., Wright, S. D., Golenbock, D. **1997**, Targeted deletion of the lipopolysaccharide (LPS)-binding protein gene leads to profound suppression of LPS responses ex vivo, whereas in vivo responses remain intact, *J Exp Med* 186, 2051–2056.

Yazdankhah, S. P., Caugant, D. A. **2004**, Neisseria meningitidis: an overview of the carriage state, *J Med Microbiol* 53, 821–832.

Zhang, Q., Finn, A. **2004**, Mucosal immunology of vaccines against pathogenic nasopharyngeal bacteria, *J Clin Pathol* 57, 1015–1021.

Zughaier, S. M., Tzeng, Y. L., Zimmer, S. M., Datta, A., Carlson, R. W., Stephens, D. S. **2004**, Neisseria meningitidis lipooligosaccharide structure-dependent activation of the macrophage CD14/Toll-like receptor 4 pathway, *Infect Immun* 72, 371–380.

Zughaier, S. M., Zimmer, S. M., Datta, A., Carlson, R. W., Stephens, D. S. **2005**, Differential Induction of the toll-like receptor 4-MyD88-dependent and -independent signaling pathways by endotoxins, *Infect Immun* 73, 2940–2950.

Part IV
Development of Vaccines

Handbook of Meningococcal Disease. Infection Biology, Vaccination, Clinical Management.
Edited by M. Frosch and M. C. J. Maiden

ISBN: 3-527-31260-9

16
Surrogates of Protection

Ray Borrow and Elizabeth Miller

16.1
Definitions: Surrogate Versus Correlate of Protection

The clinical efficacy of vaccines depends on the humoral and/or cellular immune responses that they invoke in the individual. In order to allow licensure of vaccines without the need for conducting expensive, laborious efficacy trials, it is important to have laboratory markers of immunity that can reliably predict clinical protection in the field. Such markers, termed *surrogates of protection*, are derived from evidence that the presence of the immune marker consistently predicts clinical protection in the individual and that the specific antibody or cellular response that is being measured is actually mediating the protection observed. A surrogate of protection may be obtained from studies of natural immunity, from phase III efficacy trials, or by showing that protection can be transferred passively to another individual by transferring the specific antibody class or cells that putatively confer protection. An example of the latter is the protection conferred against bacterial toxins, such as tetanus, by the transfer of antibodies with antitoxin activity either transplacentally or via administration of a specific immunoglobulin preparation [1].

Such a surrogate of protection for group C meningococcal infection was established in the classic studies by Goldschneider et al. [2, 3] in military recruits. These studies showed that the presence or absence of naturally occurring serum antibody that was bactericidal to group C organisms in the presence of human complement predicted the risk of subsequent group C disease in that individual [2]. Further studies showing that removal of serum antibody to the group C capsular polysaccharide abolished the serum bactericidal antibody (SBA) activity [3] and that vaccines composed purely of group C polysaccharide generated SBA activity to the group C organism and were protective [4, 5] established the SBA as a true surrogate marker of protection against the group C meningococcus.

In this chapter, the term *correlate of protection* is used to denote a laboratory measure that is correlated with protection and therefore with the surrogate, but may not be a direct measure of the antibody or cellular activity that is mediating

Handbook of Meningococcal Disease. Infection Biology, Vaccination, Clinical Management.
Edited by M. Frosch and M.C.J. Maiden

ISBN: 3-527-31260-9

protection. Correlates of protection are often measured by nonfunctional assays such as ELISA and may be derived from observing a relationship between the percentage of a vaccinated population achieving a threshold level in the ELISA and the percentage protection measured in that vaccinated population, as with the recent efficacy trial with a seven-valent pneumococcal conjugate vaccine [6]. This showed that the overall efficacy in the vaccinated cohort against the seven vaccine serotypes in the vaccine was best predicted by the overall proportion of vaccines achieving a threshold IgG concentration of $\geq 0.2\ \mu g\ ml^{-1}$ when summed across all seven serotypes. However, direct evidence that the children who were infected were those with serum antibody levels below this threshold and vice versa, and that inhibition of the IgG antibodies measured in the ELISA removed protection was not obtained. The presumption of efficacy for other pneumococcal conjugate vaccines producing a similar ELISA response for the same seven serotypes would therefore be based on a population correlate of protection, rather than a surrogate marker of protection in an individual, the latter being more likely mediated by the presence of a functional antibody, such as that measured by opsonophagocytosis with which the ELISA antibodies induced by vaccination are correlated [6]. A comparable example for meningococcal vaccines is the $2\ \mu g\ ml^{-1}$ concentration of anticapsular IgG antibody to group A that was shown to broadly correlate at the population level with short term protection obtained with the group A polysaccharide vaccine in a Phase III trial [7].

When using a population correlate derived with a nonfunctional assay such as ELISA, rather than a true individual surrogate of protection using a functional assay such as SBA, caution should be exercised about its universal applicability. For example, while the correlation between IgG antibody to capsular polysaccharide and the SBA activity induced by group C conjugate vaccines in young children may be high, this relationship may not hold for naturally acquired immunity nor antibody induced by a plain serogroup C polysaccharide vaccine, especially in young children [8]. The correlation between specific IgG concentration and SBA activity may be improved by trying to measure only those IgG antibodies with functional activity, for example by the use of a high avidity ELISA [1, 8, 9] but this approach has not so far lead to an agreed ELISA-based correlate of protection that is equally applicable to conjugate and polysaccharide vaccine recipients and those with natural immunity.

Finally, a distinction is sometimes made between an immunological marker that predicts short term and one that predicts long term protection. For example, for conjugate vaccines, it has been proposed that long-term protection after the initial post-vaccination antibody levels have declined can be predicted by demonstrating the persistence of immune memory, as evidenced by avidity maturation and a typical booster response on challenge with the priming antigen [10, 11]. Such immune memory markers constitute a correlate of protection, since protection against disease still requires the presence of protective antibody which, it is postulated, would be produced rapidly on exposure to the relevant organism by invoking a booster response. In the case of group C meningococcus, it would require the rapid production of serum antibody that is bactericidal to group C organisms in response to the acquisition of a group C carriage strain. Recent evidence showing that, despite immune memory, both *H. influenzae* type b (Hib) and meningococcal group C conjugate (MCC) vaccines fail to protect long term calls into question the validity of this as a correlate of long term protection [12]. With the growing understanding of the importance of reducing carriage in achieving long term disease control, it will become equally important to seek correlates or surrogates of protection that can predict the ability of a vaccine to protect against nasal carriage as well as invasive disease in the individual.

16.2 Group C Vaccines

16.2.1 Natural Protection Against Disease

The surrogate of natural protection for meningococcal group C disease was established by Goldschneider and colleagues [2] as an SBA titer with human complement (hSBA) of ≥4. This study involved bleeding army recruits at the initiation of their basic training and relating the SBA level to the risk of acquiring a meningococcal infection during the next eight weeks. It was found that three out of the 54 prospective meningococcal cases had circulating hSBA titers ≥4 prior to commencement of training as compared with 444 of 540 controls (those who did not acquire meningococcal infection) who had an hSBA titer of ≥4. The SBA antibody in these individuals was presumably acquired as a result of prior meningococcal carriage.

Additional indirect evidence to support an hSBA titer of ≥4 as a surrogate of protection was obtained by examining the relationship between the age-related incidence of disease and the presence of hSBA above the proposed cut-off [2]. Sera from children and military recruits were used to give a population sample covering the age range from 0–26 years. The percentage of individuals with an hSBA titer ≥4 in defined age groups was observed to have an inverse relationship to the incidence of group C disease, consistent with this cut-off being a marker of protection against disease. These studies have been comprehensively reviewed [13–15].

Goldschneider and colleagues then investigated whether antibody against the capsular polysaccharide was responsible for the serum bactericidal antibody response, by adsorbing sera with group C polysaccharide. This inhibited SBA activity to group C strains but not to groups A and B [3], consistent with anticapsular antibody being responsible for the SBA activity. However, little is known about the purity of the group C polysaccharide used in the inhibition studies and whether protein contaminants were present that may have adsorbed subcapsular antigens. A role for subcapsular antigens in generating a SBA response was suggested by the observation that sera from the army recruits demonstrated SBA activity against groups A and B in addition to C and that SBA activity to groups A and B also predicted protection against group C disease [2]. By using data on SBA activity of sera (hSBA ≥4) against a group A and B strain in sera obtained from recruits in their first week of basic training and relating this to whether the individuals subsequently developed group C disease [3], it can be shown that an hSBA titer of ≥4 generated against the groups A and B strains is highly predictive of protection against group C (Table 16.1). This is strongly suggestive of a role for cross-reacting subcapsular antigens in mediating protection. Hence, it is likely that the surrogate of protection against group C disease, established as a SBA titer ≥4, included both capsular polysaccharide and subcapsular antigen-specific SBA activity. As there was very little group A disease in the United States when the Goldschneider et al. studies were conducted, if the hSBA activity measured against group A was mediated by anticapsular antibody, then this would have to have been induced by exposure to other organisms with capsular polysaccharides that are cross-reactive with meningococcal group A polysaccharide. However, if this were the case, it is unlikely that such cross-reactive polysaccharides would induce SBA activity. Studies of naturally acquired hSBA activity to group A in sera from adults in Sudan, a country within the meningitis belt where group A is endemic, and Uganda and North America, countries where group A disease is rare, showed that hSBA titers were detected in 66% of Sudanese sera but in only 27% and 23%, respectively, of North American and Ugandan sera [16]. Moreover, SBA activity was inhibited by group A polysaccharide in 58% of the Sudanese bactericidal sera but only 17% and 6% of North American and Ugandan bactericidal sera. This indicates that exposure to group A via carriage generates hSBA activity that is mediated by antibodies to both capsular and subcapsular antigens, and that the hSBA to group A observed in the absence of carriage is primarily mediated by antibody to subcapsular antigens.

Table 16.1 Additional SBA-based protection data from [3]

	Case of serogroup C disease		Odds ratio[a)]	Predicted protection[a)]
	Yes	No		
hSBA to C11 strain (group C) ≥4				
Yes	2	154		
No	21	76	0.05	95%
hSBA to B11 strain (group B) ≥4				
Yes	3	179		
No	20	51	0.04	96%
hSBA to A1 strain (group A) ≥4				
Yes	4	166		
No	19	64	0.08	92%

a) Calculated as follows: Odds ratio (OR) for group C=(2×76)/(21×154); Predicted protection=(1–OR)×100.

The above data argues for a group-specific hSBA titer ≥4 serving as a generic surrogate of protection against meningococcal disease, for all groups and irrespective of whether the protection is induced by carriage or vaccination with capsular or subcapsular antigens.

16.2.2 Vaccine-induced Protection Against Disease

The classic studies performed by Goldschneider and colleagues [2, 3] established SBA as the surrogate of protection for meningococcal disease. However, this was achieved using human sera as the source of exogenous complement in the SBA assay. This is difficult to obtain and standardize, preventing significant interlaboratory comparisons of data. Thus it is now recommended that commercially available baby rabbit complement is used in a standardized bactericidal assay (rSBA) when evaluating meningococcal polysaccharide vaccines [17]. The criteria for the control of new vaccine lots requires that at least 90% of serum samples from healthy adults should show a ≥4-fold rise in rSBA titer from before to 2–4 weeks after immunization [17]. The rSBA criterion of a ≥4-fold rise (a commonly accepted marker of a response to a vaccine) is therefore being used as a correlate of protection, at least in adult recipients of a polysaccharide vaccine, whether group A, C, Y, or W135. Two large-scale field trials of group C polysaccharide vaccine among US military recruits at high risk of developing disease proved the effectiveness of this vaccine [18, 19] in older age groups, whereas a field trial conducted in 1974 in young children aged 6–36 months showed poor efficacy of 31% (95% CI from 11% to 58%) [20]. The immune response to group C polysaccharide is age-related, with poor functional responses in children less than 24 months and SBA levels then increase with age [21]. Therefore a broad correlation between immunogenicity and effectiveness of the group C polysaccharide vaccine with age has been shown.

More recently, an attempt has been made to define a threshold cutoff, using an rSBA criterion that would serve as a correlate of protection for conjugate vaccines in young children. This was necessary as meningococcal group C conjugate (MCC) vaccines were licensed in the U.K. and elsewhere without large-scale Phase III efficacy trials. Extensive pre-licensure studies funded by both the Department of Health and vaccine manufacturers demonstrated the safety and immunogenicity of the candidate MCC vaccines in the targeted age groups, including induction of immune memory in infants [22–24] and young children [25], as demonstrated either by challenge with a low dose of polysaccharide antigen following the primary series of MCC or by an increase in avidity indices post-primary to pre-challenge [25]. Immune memory after infant immunization was shown to persist to at least 4 years of age [11]. In these trials, the majority of the SBA data were generated using baby rabbit complement (for reviews, see [26, 27]). Comparison of hSBA with rSBA titers in sera from infants and toddlers vaccinated in these trials showed that sera with rSBA titers <8 or ≥128 were highly predictive of susceptibility and protection, as defined by an hSBA titer of <4 or ≥4, respectively [28]. However, there was an equivocal group of sera with a rSBA titer at 8–64, for which only a proportion were ≥4 by hSBA. It was proposed that, in the absence of an hSBA titer ≥4, a ≥4-fold rise in rSBA titer from pre- to post-vaccination, evidence of antibody avidity maturation or a typical booster response to a polysaccharide challenge should be taken as a correlate of protection in this equivocal group [28, 29]. This proposal was based on the established rSBA criterion for polysaccharide vaccines in adults and the reasonable assumption that this could be extrapolated to younger age groups. As stated by Goldschneider et al. [2], while an hSBA ≥4 predicted protection, a titer <4 did not necessarily indicate susceptibility [28]. Using the additional criteria of a ≥4-fold rise in rSBA or evidence of immune memory >98% of young children in the UK trials with an rSBA in the range 8–64 could be considered protected.

Indirect evidence supporting this postulated that rSBA ≥8 correlate for meningococcal group C conjugate (MCC) vaccines was obtained by demonstrating an inverse relationship between disease incidence and rSBA titer at the population level [30]. A total of 1689 sera from age-stratified individuals, collected prior to the introduction of the MCC vaccine were tested and rSBA titers plotted against disease incidence by age group. Using a rSBA titer ≥8, an inverse relationship between disease incidence and SBA was seen, similar to that observed by Goldschneider et al. [2]. The greater magnitude of responses seen in Goldschneider studies [2], especially in the older age groups, may be accounted for by differences in epidemiology and in selection of the study populations. The magnitude of the group C responses in the older age groups in the UK were, however, similar to that seen in a recent study in North America [31].

MCC vaccine was introduced into the UK routine immunization schedule at 2, 3 and 4 months of age in November 1999 and, in addition, the vaccine was offered as a single dose to all children aged 1–18 years, with two doses for infants aged 5–11 months in a catch-up campaign that was rolled out over 1 year. The number of cases of group C quickly fell in the targeted age groups; and early analyses showed high vaccine effectiveness in all age groups [26, 32] and significant herd immunity [33]. Estimates of age-specific vaccine effectiveness derived from post-marketing surveillance data (see Chapter 20) were used to validate the putative rSBA correlate of protection of ≥8 [34]. Effectiveness during the first year after immunization in toddlers (a group in whom about a quarter were in the range 8–64 by rSBA after a single dose) was closely predicted by the proportion achieving a rSBA titer of ≥8 at 1 month post-vaccination. Had the more conservative cut-off of rSBA ≥128 been the appropriate correlate, then efficacy during the first year should have been much lower than that observed in the toddler age group.

However, when effectiveness was measured again more than 1 year after vaccination, there was a significant decline in all age groups, most marked in infants vaccinated in the routine infant immunization program, for whom there was no demonstrable efficacy after only 1 year, and then in toddlers for whom efficacy declined to 61% (327 to 94) from 88% (65 to 96) in the first year [12]. A similar decline has now been shown in Spain where, following their routine 2-,

4-, 6-month schedule, vaccine effectiveness in infants fell from 98.4 (95% CI 95.7–99.4) within 1 year from vaccination to 78.0 (95% CI 3.1–95.0) at 1 year out from vaccination [35]. However, good disease control was maintained in Spain and the UK, with only low numbers of vaccine failures.

The original premise behind the introduction of the MCC vaccines was that: (a) they would protect infants, (b) there would be long lasting protection through immune memory even when circulating antibody had declined, (c) booster doses would therefore not be necessary and (d) the vaccine would reduce carriage thus potentially giving a beneficial effect via herd immunity. Thus, while (a) and (d) have been confirmed, the assumption that immune memory was predictive of long-term protection in the absence of a booster was shown to be wrong, at least after vaccination in infancy. The magnitude of the SBA responses of the infants in the UK studies was similar to that of young adults given a dose of meningococcal polysaccharide vaccine, an age group known to be highly protected by group C polysaccharide vaccination. Indeed, even when using the overly stringent rSBA titer of $\geq$128, greater than 96% of infants reached protective levels [22, 28].

It is well established that, following the UK 2-, 3- and 4-month schedule of MCC vaccine, specific antibody levels and rSBA titers wane rapidly [11, 22, 24]. In the toddler cohort 2 years after a single dose of MCC vaccine, only 37% still had SBA titers $\geq$8 [36]. However, in 13–16 year olds who received a single dose of MCC as part of the catch-up campaign, SBA geometric mean titers (GMT) remain elevated for the first 1.8 years, with a SBA GMT of 983 (95% CI 61–15 852) up to 1 year post-MCC and a GMT of 667 (95% CI 21–21 543) from 1.0 years to 1.8 years post-MCC (H. P. A., unpublished data). Waning of antibody therefore appears to be age-dependent, with poorer persistence in the younger age groups, in whom efficacy declines most rapidly. This raises the question of whether long-term protection requires the persistence of SBA, rather than relying on its rapid production as a result of immune memory after exposure to the meningococcus.

Concerns had been raised with the possibility that, due to meningococcal disease occurring very rapidly after acquisition of the pathogen [2, 37], immune memory may not protect. In infants vaccinated in either a 2-, 3-, 4-month or a 2-, 4-, 6-month schedule protection wanes with the decline of SBA and, although immune memory as evidenced by the ability to mount a booster response is present [11], it does not appear to provide protection from disease [12]. This failure is not specific to MCC vaccines, since a similar failure to protect against invasive Hib disease despite the presence of immune memory has been shown when Hib vaccine is given under the UK 2-, 3-, 4-month schedule [38–41]. Studies in mouse models assessing neonatal responses to human infant vaccines have shown that the neonatal bone marrow has a limited capacity to support the establishment of long-lived antibody secreting plasmocytes [42] which are important for the maintenance of circulating antibody. Whether the induction of long-lived plasma cells is similarly limited in human infants is unknown, but short-lived antibody responses are a hallmark of early-life immunization with polysaccharide-conjugate vaccines. Thus, infant immunization schedules may be effective when exposure to the pathogen occurs shortly after vaccination where antibody levels are elevated but immune memory, in the absence of circulating antibody, is not sufficient to confer full protection against encapsulated bacteria, such as meningococci and Hib, that require functional antibodies rapidly after exposure [1].

16.2.3 Protection Against Carriage

Although meningococcal polysaccharide vaccines only produce a short-term, transient effect on carriage [43], MCC vaccines have been shown to significantly reduce the prevalence of group C carriage [44] which was corroborated by a similar reduction in the attack rate in unvaccinated individuals [33]. Meningococcal carriage is low in childhood, though it starts to increase from 5 years of age and peaks in 15–19 year olds [45–47]. Therefore the catch-up campaign had a dramatic impact on the carriage of group C meningococci. Elevated serum antibody levels have now been shown to predict protection against carriage for both *S. pneumoniae* and Hib. For pneumococcal serotype 14, it was demonstrated that natural acquisition of concentrations of serum serotype-specific IgG >5 μg ml^{-1} protected against carriage [48]. While the absolute level may vary between pneumococcal serotypes, an identical level of 5.0 μg ml^{-1} correlated with protection from carriage for Hib [49]. For protection against pneumococcal carriage, the serum level is much higher than the correlate for protection against invasive disease, estimated by the WHO working group to be in the range 0.2–0.4 μg ml^{-1} [6].

A serum anticapsular antibody level has not been investigated for protection against group C meningococcal carriage, though studies have investigated salivary antibody responses following vaccination. Following conjugate vaccination in both infants and adolescents, significant increases in group C-specific IgG in saliva have been reported [50–53]. The salivary group C-specific IgG is largely derived from a serum leak into the crevicular fluid and salivary IgG correlates well with serum IgG. Studies need to be performed to investigate the serum IgG antibody concentration required to prevent colonization. Significant rises in salivary group C-specific IgA, especially secretory IgA which is more likely to represent true mucosally produced immunity, have been reported following conjugate vaccination in some studies [50, 52] but not in others [51, 53]. As meningococci possess IgA proteases and invasive isolates possess enhanced immunoglobulin A1 protease activity compared to colonizing strains [54] IgA must have some role in protection.

In retrospect, it is now clear that the success of the UK MCC immunization program was largely attributable to the catch-up campaign and generation of herd immunity. Although, in the short-term infants are protected through SBA activity, longer-term disease control in the population is dependent on the herd immunity generated by the catch-up campaign as a result of reduction in carriage [55]. Correlates of protection for encapsulated bacteria should therefore to include the effect of conjugate vaccines on carriage. While the role of immune memory following MCC vaccines requires clarification, it is already clear that a booster dose after the first year of life will be required in order to ensure more long-term protection after infant immunization with MCC vaccines, and probably other polysaccharide conjugate vaccines.

16.3 Group A Vaccines

To date, the only correlate of protection for group A disease we have is from the Finnish efficacy trials of meningococcal group A polysaccharide vaccine [7, 56] and was determined by radioimmunoassay to be 2 $\mu g\ ml^{-1}$. This value was the mean level in unimmunized adults who were assumed to be protected and corresponded to the level achieved by the majority of individuals in the age groups in whom the vaccine was shown to be effective [7]. Goldschneider et al. [2] demonstrated an inverse relationship across different age groups between SBA activity against groups A, B and C meningococci and meningococcal disease. As cases occurring in 1965 and 1966 were mainly due to groups B and C disease [57], the group A-specific SBA activity may be through either prior exposure to the group A polysaccharide, cross-reactive capsular polysaccharides [58–60] or subcapsular antigens. Adsorption studies of pooled gamma globulin fractions suggested that these cross-reacting anticapsular antibodies play only a minor role in naturally acquired SBA to group A strains [2], consistent with the observations by Amir et al. [16], described earlier.

A project to introduce a group A conjugate vaccine into Africa has been initiat-ed by World Health Organization/Program for Appropriate Technology for Health (WHO/PATH) [61]. The aim of the project is to alleviate the large epidemics of group A disease that occur in the subSaharan meningitis belt in Africa. It is hoped that the vaccine will be produced, evaluated and ready for introduction within the next 5–10 years. Although Phase II immunogenicity trials followed by surveillance after the introduction of this vaccine in Africa will assist in the establishment of correlates of protection for group A, lessons have been learnt from the UK MCC vaccine campaign in that a booster dose may be required to ensure long-term protection for the individual. However, since the vaccine can be expected to protect against carriage, a major and lasting impact on disease in the population can be expected if the group A conjugate vaccine is introduced with a catch-up that covers the age groups in whom carriage rates are highest.

16.4
Tetravalent Conjugate Vaccines

Recently a tetravalent A/C/Y/W135 conjugate vaccine was licensed in the USA [62]. Vaccine efficacy was inferred from the demonstration of immunological equivalence to a licensed tetravalent polysaccharide vaccine. The primary measure of immune response was induction of group-specific anticapsular antibody that possessed SBA activity. The antibody response to vaccination was evaluated by determining the proportion of subjects with ≥4-fold rises in rSBA to each group, based on the WHO-defined correlate of protection for polysaccharide vaccines.

16.5
Subcapsular Vaccines

For group B SBA assays, it is not currently possible to utilize baby rabbit complement, due to anticapsular group B antibodies being of low avidity, usually IgM isotype, that are not bactericidal in the presence of human complement but are strongly bactericidal in the rSBA [63]. Although attempts are being made to remove these low-avidity anticapsular antibodies from test sera by the use of colominic acid [64], to date the only acceptable complement source is of human origin for group B SBA assays.

The poor immunogenicity of the group B capsular polysaccharide [65] means that conjugating the polysaccharide as for groups A, C, Y and W135 may not be appropriate and thus alternative approaches have been investigated. A number of outer membrane vesicle (OMV) based vaccines have been trialled and utilized in an attempt to contain epidemics in Norway [66], Brazil [67], Cuba [68], Chile [69] and most recently New Zealand [70].

Using the existing data from efficacy and immunogenicity studies from the various countries, it is apparent that the efficacy of OMV vaccines against the homologous strain with the same PorA OMP increases with age and that efficacy correlates with the percentage of subjects with hSBA titers ≥4 and/or the percentages of subjects with ≥4-fold rises from pre- to post-vaccination [71]. The Norwegian OMV trial showed that vaccine efficacy wanes and was only highly protective for about 9 months after the second dose during the period when the hSBA GMT for the vaccinated population was estimated to be about 4 [72]. OMV vaccines when used against outbreaks of the homologous phenotype are likely to be effective in controlling disease, as suggested by the experience in Cuba [68] and hopefully to be confirmed by the experience in New Zealand. When used in this context an hSBA ≥4 or a ≥4-fold rise against the homologous strain should be considered as the putative protective threshold. When the vaccine strain is not the predominant outbreak phenotype, especially in relationship to the PorA OMP, the degree of heterologous protection remains unclear but may increase with the number of doses and age [73].

The new generation of meningococcal vaccines against group B disease are based on individual and/or pools of individual antigens that are broadly cross-reactive and induce functional antibodies against the meningococcus. Although a number of candidate antigens are now subject to intense research and development [74–76], it is not known whether mechanisms of protection will be the same as for the OMV vaccines. OMV vaccines, particularly in the young, rely heavily on the immunodominant PorA for the formation of SBA activity. Non-PorA-based vaccines may show other mechanisms of killing as well as or instead of SBA activity.

The whole-blood killing assay is a method that can assess the bactericidal activity of blood incorporating antibody-mediated complement lysis and phagocytosis [77–79]. The whole-blood assay is more sensitive than the SBA [78], with bactericidal activity detected in some individuals by the whole-blood assay but not by the SBA assay. However, the whole-blood assay is unlikely to be suitable for the evaluation of candidate group B vaccines due to the requirement for large volumes of fresh blood for the assay and the difficulty in standardization of the assay.

Opsonophagocytosis is one mechanism that has been demonstrated to be bactericidal against meningococci [80–82]. The opsonophagocytic assay (OPA) can also use inactivated bacteria as the target [83], but concerns have been raised that in the treatment of the meningococci, new or hidden epitopes may be exposed that have no functional relevance [84, 85]. Furthermore, there are issues of standardization between laboratories, particularly regarding the use of cultured cell lines or freshly obtained polymorphonuclear neutrophil (PMN) cells. Further validation of the OPA is required to determine if it is a suitable correlate of protection. The OPA may be a useful additional assay for the evaluation of group B vaccine candidates, where the protective epitopes are subcapsular and may involve a greater role for cell-mediated immunity, unlike groups A, C, W135 and Y where the capsular polysaccharide is the focus of the protective mechanisms. OPAs to analyze the immune responses against group B isolates have been developed [83, 85, 86]. A surface-labeling technique which detects the initial stage of antibody binding to killed meningococci has also been developed and shows potential as an additional assay for the evaluation of group B vaccines [83].

Animal models can also provide information on the impact of the host–pathogen relationship on whole tissues and the interaction between both humoral and cellular immune responses. However, there are disadvantages of the animal models, including the fact that the only natural host for *N. meningitidis* is humans and that there are no good models available that mimic the course of human disease. The mouse model has been most extensively used for assessing active protection and passive protection for evaluation of vaccine candidates [87–89], including *N. lactamica* immunization [90]. It is interesting to note that, although protection was observed against a lethal challenge, no SBA activity was observed in mouse sera. An infant rat protection assay (IRPA) has also been developed that has the advantage of not requiring an additional iron source and lower inocula are required to produce disease than in the mouse model. However, the IRPA does not allow active protection to be assessed, not all strains are virulent and the duration of bacteremia is short and mortality low. It has been used to demonstrate passive protection with antibodies against a number of meningococcal components [91, 92] and has been used in evaluating responses to group B meningococci [92–94]. A recent evaluation of a subset of sera collected before vaccination and 6 weeks after the second vaccination with either the Norwegian or the Cuban OMV vaccines or control bivalent polysaccharide vaccine using the IRPA and comparing IRPA responses with hSBA titers and antiOMV IgG demonstrated a low correlation [95]. Following the second dose of Norwegian OMV vaccine, 22% showed IRPA responses as compared to 65% in the hSBA assay, whilst the corresponding numbers for the Cuban OMV vaccine were 14% and 29%, respectively. This indicates the sensitivity of the IRPA may not be sufficient to evaluate OMV vaccine responses from clinical samples.

Further data are required to establish both the OPA and animal models as credible correlates of protection. It may be that, as stated, they are more appropriate for use in the evaluation of group B vaccines that are likely to be noncapsular polysaccharide vaccines and induce a wider range of immunological mechanisms, unlike the MCC vaccines that induce mainly SBA antibody. Mucosal antibody, whether local produced or serum-derived, may be of importance. However, to date, the limited data illustrate that there is no effect of OMV vaccination on carriage [96, 97]. Studies on natural immunity have shown that at the mucosal level *in vitro* cellular responses to OMVs are strongly associated with age and are largely T cell-mediated [98]. The influence of carriage of group B strains on salivary IgA has also been studied, with higher levels of specific IgA associated with carriage and specific IgA increased successively with age [99].

16.6 Conclusions

The classic studies by Goldschneider et al. [2] clearly established an hSBA titer of ≥4 as a correlate of protection against group C infection and, together with the subsequent experience with capsular polysaccharide and OMV vaccines, should be considered as a generic surrogate of protection against meningococcal disease irrespective of serogroup. The rSBA threshold is now an established correlate for protection against group C disease and has shown that the sensitivity of the hSBA assay may be too low such that individuals may still be protected, despite having an hSBA titer <4. Hence, the search for supporting correlates of protection for group B vaccines based on other functional assays or animal models, as was done with the rSBA correlate for group C vaccines for sera with titers below the hSBA cut-off. Immune memory can no longer be considered a correlate of long-term protection for meningococcal conjugate vaccines and the persistence of rSBA antibodies at a level of ≥8 may be the appropriate correlate, at least for group C vaccines. Prime/boost schedules that optimize antibody persistence need investigation, together with studies that promote understanding of the correlate of protection against carriage, which it is now understood is a major factor in achieving long-term control of meningococcal disease by vaccination despite waning protection against invasive disease in the individual.

References

1 P.-H. Lambert, M. Liu, C.-A. Siegrist **2005**, Can successful vaccines teach us how to induce efficient protective immune responses? *Nat. Med. Suppl.* 11, 554–559.

2 I. Goldschneider, E. C. Gotschlich, M. S. Artenstein **1969**, Human immunity to the meningococcus: I. The role of humoral antibodies, *J. Exp. Med.* 129, 1307–1326.

3 I. Goldschneider, E. C. Gotschlich, M. S. Artenstein **1969**, Human immunity to the meningococcus: II. Development of natural immunity, *J. Exp. Med.* 129, 1327–1348.

4 M. S. Artenstein, R. Gold, J. G. Zimmerly, F. A. Wyle, H. Schneider, C. Harkins **1970**, Prevention of meningococcal disease by group C polysaccharide vaccine, *N. Engl. J. Med.* 282, 417–420.

5 R. Gold, M. S. Artenstein **1971**, Meningococcal infections, 2. Field trial of group C meningococcal polysaccharide vaccine in 1969–70, *Bull. World Health Organ.* 45, 279–282.

6 L. Jodar, J. Butler, G. Carlone, R. Dagan, D. Goldblatt, H. Käyhty, K. Klugman, B. Plikaytis, G. Siber, R. Kohberger, I. Chang, T. Cherian **2003**, Serological criteria for evaluation and licensure of new pneumococcal conjugate vaccine formulations for use in infants, *Vaccine* 21, 3265–3272.

7 H. Peltola, H. Mäkelä, H. Käyhty, H. Jousimies, E. Herva, K. Hallstrom, A. Sivonen, O. V. Renkonen, O. Pettay, V. Karanko, P. Ahvonen, S. Sarna **1977**, Clinical efficacy of meningococcus group A capsular polysaccharide vaccine in children three months to five years of age, *N. Engl. J. Med.* 297, 686–691.

8 R. Borrow, P. Richmond, E. B. Kaczmarski, A. Iverson, S. L. Martin, J. Findlow, M. Acuna, E. Longworth, R. O'Connor, J. Paul, E. Miller **2000**, Meningococcal serogroup C-specific IgG antibody responses and serum bactericidal titers in children following vaccination with a meningococcal A/C polysaccharide vaccine, *FEMS Immunol. Med. Microbiol.* 28, 79–85.

9 D. M. Granoff, S. E. Maslanka, G. M. Carlone, B. D. Plikaytis, G. F. Santos, A. Mokatrin, H. V. Raff **1998**, A modified enzyme-linked immunosorbent assay for measurement of antibody responses to meningococcal C polysaccharide that correlate with bactericidal responses, *Clin. Diagn. Lab. Immunol.* 5, 479–485.

10 D. Goldblatt, E. Miller, N. McCloskey, K. Cartwright **1998**, Immunological response to conjugate vaccines in infants: follow up study, *Br. Med. J.* 316, 1570–1571.

11 R. Borrow, D. Goldblatt, N. Andrews, J. Southern, L. Ashton, S. Deane, R. Morris, K. Cartwright, E. Miller **2002**, Antibody persistence and immunological memory at age 4 years after meningococcal C conjugate vaccination in UK children, *J. Infect. Dis.* 186, 1353–1357.

12 C. L. Trotter, N. J. Andrews, E. B. Kaczmarski, E. Miller, M. E. Ramsay **2004**, Effectiveness of meningococcal serogroup C conjugate vaccine 4 years after introduction, *Lancet* 364, 365–367.

13 P. Balmer, R. Borrow **2004**, Serologic correlates of protection for evaluating the response to meningococcal vaccines, *Expert Rev. Vaccines* 3, 89–99.

14 R. Borrow, P. Balmer, E. Miller **2005**, Meningococcal surrogates of protection – serum bactericidal antibody activity, *Vaccine* 23, 2222–2227.

15 A. J. Pollard, C. Frasch **2001**, Development of natural immunity to *Neisseria meningitidis*, *Vaccine* 19, 1327–1346.

16 J. Amir, L. Louie, D. M. Granoff **2005**, Naturally-acquired immunity to *Neisseria meningitidis* group A, *Vaccine* 23, 977–983.

17 World Health Organization **1976**, Requirements for meningococcal polysaccharide vaccine, *World Health Organization Technical Report Series, no. 594*, World Health Organization, Geneva.

18 M. S. Artenstein, R. Gold, J. G. Zimmerly, F. A. Wyle, H. Schneider, C. Harkins **1970**, Prevention of meningococcal disease by group C polysaccharide vaccine, *N. Engl. J. Med.* 282, 417–420.

19 R. Gold, M. S. Artenstein **1971**, Meningococcal infections, 2. Field trial of group C meningococcal polysaccharide vaccine in 1969–70, *Bull. World Health Organ.* 45, 279–282.

20 A. E. Taunay, H. A. Feldman, C. Bastos, et al. **1978**, Avaliacao do efeito protector de vacina polissacaridica antimeningococica dos groupo C em crianzas de 6 a 36 meses, *Rev. Inst. Adolfo Lutz* 39, 77–82.

21 S. E. Maslanka, J. W. Tappero, B. D. Plikaytis, R. S. Brumberg, J. K. Dykes, L. L. Gheesling, K. B. Donaldson, A. Schuchat, J. Pullman, M. Jones, J. Bushmaker, G. M. Carlone **1998**, Age-dependent *Neisseria meningitidis* serogroup C class-specific antibody concentrations and bactericidal titers in sera from young children from Montana immunized with a licensed polysaccharide vaccine, *Infect. Immun.* 66, 2453–2459.

22 P. Richmond, R. Borrow, E. Miller, S. Clark, F. Sadler, A. J. Fox, N. T. Begg, R. Morris, K. A. V. Cartwright **1999**, Meningococcal serogroup C conjugate vaccine is immunogenic in infancy and primes for memory, *J. Infect. Dis.* 179, 1569–1572.

23 P. Richmond, R. Borrow, J. Findlow, S. Martin, C. Thornton, K. Cartwright, E. Miller **2001**, Evaluation of de-O-acetylated meningococcal C polysaccharide-tetanus toxoid conjugate vaccine in infancy: reactogenicity, immunogenicity, immunologic priming and bactericidal activity against O-acetylated and de-O-acetylated serogroup C strains, *Infect. Immun.* 69, 2378–2382.

24 J. M. MacLennan, F. Shackley, P. T. Heath, et al. **2000**, Safety, immunogenicity, and induction of immunologic memory by a serogroup C meningococcal conjugate vaccine in infants: a randomized controlled trial, *J. Am. Med. Assoc.* 283, 2795–2801.

25 P. Richmond, R. Borrow, D. Goldblatt, J. Findlow, S. Martin, R. Morris, K. Cartwright, E. Miller **2001**, Ability of 3 different meningococcal C conjugate vaccines to induce immunologic memory after a single dose in UK toddlers, *J. Infect. Dis.* 183, 160–163.

26 E. Miller, D. Salisbury, M. Ramsay **2001**, Planning, registration, and implementation of an immunisation campaign against meningococcal serogroup C disease in the UK: a success story, *Vaccine* 20, S58–S67.

27 P. Balmer, R. Borrow, E. Miller **2002**, Impact of meningococcal C conjugate vaccine in the UK, *J. Med. Microbiol.* 51, 717–722.

28 R. Borrow, N. Andrews, D. Goldblatt, E. Miller **2001**, Serological basis for use of meningococcal serogroup C conjugate vaccines in the United Kingdom: a re-evaluation of correlates of protection, *Infect. Immun.* 69, 1568–1573.

29 L. Jodar, E. Griffiths, I. Feavers **2004**, Scientific challenges for the quality control and production of group C meningococcal conjugate vaccines, *Vaccine* 22, 1047–1053.

30 C. Trotter, R. Borrow, N. Andrews, E. Miller **2003**, Seroprevalence of meningococcal serogroup C bactericidal antibody in England and Wales in the pre-vaccination era, *Vaccine* 21, 1094–1098.

31 A. J. Pollard, J. Ochnio, M. Ho, M. Callaghan, M. Bigham, S. Dobsong **2004**, Disease susceptibility to ST11 complex meningococci bearing serogroup C or W135 polysaccharide capsules, North America, *Emerg. Infect. Dis.* 10, 1812–1815.

32 M. E. Ramsay, N. Andrews, E. B. Kaczmarski, E. Miller **2001**, Efficacy of meningococcal serogroup C conjugate vaccine in teenagers and toddlers in England, *Lancet* 357, 195–196.

33 M.E. Ramsay, N.J. Andrews, C.L. Trotter, E.B. Kaczmarski, E. Miller **2003**, Herd immunity from meningococcal serogroup C conjugate vaccination in England: database analysis, *Br. Med. J.* 326, 365–366.

34 N. Andrews, R. Borrow, E. Miller **2003**, Validation of serological correlate of protection for meningococcal C conjugate vaccine using efficacy estimates from post-licensure surveillance in England, *Clin. Diag. Lab. Immunol.* 10, 780–786.

35 A. Larrauri, R. Cano, M. Garcia, S. De Mateo **2005**, Impact and effectiveness of meningococcal C conjugate vaccine following its introduction in Spain, *Vaccine* 23, 4097–4100.

36 M.D. Snape, D.F. Kelly, B. Green, E.R. Moxon, R. Borrow, A.J. Pollard **2005**, Lack of serum bactericidal activity in preschool children 2 years after a single dose of serogroup C meningococcal polysaccharide–protein conjugate vaccine, *Pediat. Infect. Dis. J.* 24, 128–131.

37 E.A. Edwards, L.F. Devine, G.H. Sengbusch, H.W. Ward **1977**, Immunological investigations of meningococcal disease. III. Brevity of group C acquisition prior to disease occurrence, *Scand. J. Infect. Dis.* 9, 105–110.

38 M.E. Ramsay, J. McVernon, N.J. Andrews, P.T. Heath, M.P. Slack **2003**, Estimating *Haemophilus influenzae* type b vaccine effectiveness in England and Wales by use of the screening method, *J. Infect. Dis.* 188, 481–485.

39 M. Ramsay, E. Miller, N. Andrews, M. Slack, P. Heath **2004**, Epidemiological data are essential (rapid response to H. Peltola, E. Salo and H. Saxen: Incidence of *Haemophilus influenzae* type b meningitis during 18 years of vaccine use: observational study using routine hospital data, *BMJ* 330, 18–19), *Br. Med. J.* online 16 December 2004.

40 D. Goldblatt, A.R. Vas, E. Miller **1998**, Antibody avidity as a surrogate marker of successful priming by *Haemophilus influenzae* type b conjugate vaccines following infant immunization, *J. Infect. Dis.* 177, 1112–1115.

41 D. Goldblatt, P. Richmond, E. Millard, C. Thornton, E. Miller **1999**, The induction of immunologic memory after vaccination with *Haemophilus influenzae* type b conjugate and acellular pertussis containing diphtheria, tetanus, and pertussis vaccine combination, *J. Infect. Dis.* 180, 538–541.

42 M. Pihlgren, N. Schallert, C. Tougne, P. Bozzotti, J. Kovarik, A. Fulurija, M. Kosco-Vilbois, P.H. Lambert, C.A. Siegrist **2001**, Delayed and deficient establishment of the long-term bone marrow plasma cell pool during early life, *Eur. J. Immunol.* 31, 939–946.

43 M.K. Hassan-King, R.A. Wall, B.M. Greenwood **1988**, Meningococcal carriage, meningococcal disease and vaccination, *J. Infect.* 16, 55–59.

44 M. Maiden, J. Stuart, UK Meningococcal Carriage Group **2002**, Reduced carriage of serogroup C meningococci in teenagers one year after the introduction of meningococcal C conjugate polysaccharide vaccine in the United Kingdom, *Lancet* 359, 1829–1851.

45 R. Gold, I. Goldschneider, M.L. Lepow, T.F. Draper, M. Randolph **1978**, Carriage of *Neisseria meningitidis* and *Neisseria lactamica* in infants and children, *J. Infect. Dis.* 137, 112–121.

46 S.F. Olsen, B. Djurhuus, K. Rasmussen, H.D. Joensen, S.O. Larsen, H. Zoffman, I. Lind **1991**, Pharyngeal carriage of *Neisseria meningitidis* and *Neisseria lactamica* in households with infants within areas with high and low incidences of meningococcal disease, *Epidemiol. Infect.* 106, 445–457.

47 K.A.V. Cartwright, J.M. Stuart, D.M. Jones, N.D. Noah **1987**, The Stonehouse survey: nasopharyngeal carriage of meningococci and *Neisseria lactamica, Epidemiol. Infect.* 99, 591–601.

48 D. Goldblatt, M. Hussain, N. Andrews, L. Ashton, C. Virta, A. Melegaro, R. Pebody, R. George, A. Soininen, J. Edmunds, N. Gay, H. Kayhty, E. Miller **2005**, Antibody responses to nasopharyngeal carriage of *Streptococcus pneumoniae* in adults: a longitudinal study, *J. Infect. Dis.* (in press).

49 J. Fernandez, O.S. Levine, J. Sanchez, et al. **2000**, Prevention of *Haemophilus influenzae* type b colonization by vaccination: correlation with serum anti-capsu-

lar IgG concentration, *J. Infect. Dis.* 182, 1553–1556.
50 R. Borrow, A. J. Fox, K. Cartwright, N. T. Begg, D. M. Jones **1999**, Salivary antibodies following parenteral immunization of infants with a meningococcal serogroup A and C conjugated vaccine, *Epidemiol. Infect.* 123, 201–208.
51 Q. Zhang, E. Pettitt, R. Burkinshaw, G. Race, L. Shaw, A. Finn **2002**, Mucosal immune responses to meningococcal conjugate polysaccharide vaccines in infants, *Pediatr. Infect. Dis. J.* 21, 209–213.
52 Q. Zhang, S. Choo, J. Everard, R. Jennings, A. Finn **2000**, Mucosal immune responses to meningococcal group C conjugate and group A and C polysaccharide vaccines in adolescents, *Infect. Immun.* 68, 2692–2697.
53 Q. Zhang, R. Lakshman, R. Burkinshaw, S. Choo, J. Everard, S. Akhtar, A. Finn **2001**, Primary and booster mucosal immune responses to meningococcal group A and C conjugate and polysaccharide vaccines administered to university students in the United Kingdom, *Infect. Immun.* 69, 4337–4341.
54 S. Vitovski, R. C. Read, J. R. Sayers **1999**, Invasive isolates of *Neisseria meningitidis* possess enhanced immunoglobulin A1 protease activity compared to colonizing strains, *FASEB J.* 13, 331–337.
55 C. L. Trotter, N. J. Gay, W. J. Edmunds **2005**, Dynamic models of meningococcal carriage, disease, and the impact of serogroup C conjugate vaccination, *Am. J. Epidemiol.* 162, 89–100.
56 P. H. Mäkelä, H. Käyhty, P. Weckström, E. Sivonen, O.-V. Renkonen **1975**, Effect of group A meningococcal vaccine in army recruits in Finland, *Lancet* 2, 883–886.
57 U. S. Department of Health **1967**, *Morbid. Mortal. Wkly Rep.* 16, 11.
58 J. B. Robbins, L. Myerowitz, J. K. Whisnant, M. Argaman, R. Schneerson, Z. T. Handzel, E. C. Gotschlich **1972**, Enteric bacteria cross-reactive with *Neisseria meningitidis* groups A and C and *Diplococcus pneumoniae* types 1 and 3, *Infect. Immun.* 6, 651–656.
59 W. F. Vann, T. Y. Liu, J. B. Robbins **1976**, *Bacillus pumilus* polysaccharide cross-reactive with meningococcal group A polysaccharide, *Infect. Immun.* 13, 1654–1662.
60 N. Guirguis, R. Schneerson, A. Bax, W. Egan, J. B. Robbins, J. Shiloach, I. Orskov, F. Orskov, A. el Kholy **1985**, *Escherichia coli* K51 and K93 capsular polysaccharides are crossreactive with the group A capsular polysaccharide of *Neisseria meningitidis*. Immunochemical, biological, and epidemiological studies, *J. Exp. Med.* 162, 1837–1851.
61 L. Jodar, F. M. LaForce, C. Ceccarini, T. Aguado, D. M. Granoff **2003**, Meningococcal conjugate vaccine for Africa: a model for development of new vaccines for the poorest countries, *Lancet* 361, 1902–1904.
62 O. O. Bilukha, N. Rosenstein, National Center for Infectious Diseases, Center for Disease Control and Prevention **2005**, Prevention and control of meningococcal disease (Recommendations of the Advisory Committee on Immunization Practices), *Morbid. Mortal. Wkly Rep. Recomm.* 54(RR-7), 1–21.
63 W. D. Zollinger, R. E. Mandrell **1983**, Importance of complement source in bactericidal activity of human antibody and murine monoclonal antibody to meningococcal group B polysachharide, *Infect. Immun.* 40, 257–264.
64 S. H. Hodge, B. T. Hu, B. M. Hovanec, R. Borrow, S. W. Hildreth **2002**, The use of nonhuman complement sources in the serogroup B *Neisseria meningitidis* serum bactericidal assay facilitated by a colonic acid absorbent, *Abstr. Int. Pathog. Neisseria Conf.* 13, 260.
65 F. A. Wyle, M. S. Artenstein, B. L. Brandt, E. C. Tramont, D. L. Kasper, P. L. Altieri, S. L. Berman, J. P. Lowenthal **1972**, Immunologic response of man to group B meningococcal polysaccharide antigens, *J. Infect. Dis.* 126, 514–522.
66 G. Bjune, E. A. Høiby, J. K. Grønnesby, O. Arnesen, J. H. Fredriksen, A. Halstensen, E. Holten, A. K. Lindbak, H. Nokleby, E. Rosenqvist, L. K. Solberg, O. Closs, J. Eng, L. O. Froholm, A. Lystad, L. S. Bakketeig, B. Hareide **1991**, Effect of outer membrane vesicle vaccine against group B meningococcal disease in Norway, *Lancet* 338, 1093–1096.

67 J.C. de Moraes, B.A. Perkins, M.C. Camargo, N.T. Hidalgo, H.A. Barbosa, C.T. Sacchi, I.M. Landgraf, V.L. Gattas, H. de G. Vasconcelos, B.D. Plikaytis, J.D. Wenger, C.V. Broome **1992**, Protective efficacy of a serogroup B meningococcal vaccine in Sao Paulo, Brazil, *Lancet* 340, 1074–1078.

68 G.V. Sierra, H.C. Campa, N.W. Varcacel, I.L. Garcia, P.L. Izquierdo, P.F. Sotolongo, G.V. Casanueva, C.O. Rico, C.R. Rodriguez, M.H. Terry **1991**, Vaccine against group B *Neisseria meningitidis*: protection trial and mass vaccination results in Cuba, *Nat. Inst. Public Health Ann.* 14, 195–207.

69 C. Cruz, G. Pavez, E. Aguilar, et al. **1990**, Serotype-specific outbreak of group B meningococcal disease in Iquique, Chile, *Epidemiol. Infect.* 105, 119–126.

70 J. Holst, I.S. Aaberge, P. Oster, D. Lennon, D. Martin, J. O'Hallahan, K. Nord, H. Nokleby, L. Meyer,Naess, K. Moyner, P. Kristiansen, A. Grethe, K. Skryten, A.Bryn, R. Aase, E. Rappuoli, A. Rosenqvist **2003**, A 'tailor made' vaccine trialled as part of public health response to group B meningococcal epidemic in New Zealand, *Eurosurv. Wkly* 7, 030724.

71 J. Boslego, J. Garcia, C. Cruz, W. Zollinger, B. Brandt, S. Ruiz, M. Martinez, J. Arthur, P. Underwood, W. Silva, E. Moran, W. Hankins, J. Gilly, J. Mays, Chilean National Committee for Meningococcal Disease **1995**, Efficacy, safety, and immunogenicity of a meningococcal group B (15:P1.3) outer membrane protein vaccine in Iquique, Chile, *Vaccine* 13, 821–829.

72 J. Holst, B. Feiring, J.E. Fuglesang, E.A. Hoiby, H. Nokleby, I.S. Aaberge, E. Rosenqvist **2003**, Serum bactericidal activity correlates with the vaccine efficacy of outer membrane vesicle vaccines against *Neisseria meningitidis* serogroup B disease, *Vaccine* 21, 734–737.

73 J.W. Tappero, R. Lagos, A.M. Ballesteros, B. Plikaytis, D. Williams, J. Dykes, L.L. Gheesling, G.M. Carlone, E.A. Hoiby, J. Holst, H. Nokelby, E. Rosenqvist, G. Sierra, C. Campa, F. Sotolongo, J. Vega, J. Garcia, P. Herrera, J.T. Poolman, B.A. Perkins **1999**, Immunogenicity of 2 serogroup B outer-membrane protein meningococcal vaccines: a randomized controlled trial in Chile, *J. Am. Med. Assoc.* 281, 1520–1527.

74 V. Masignani, M. Comanducci, M.M. Giuliani, S. Bambini, J. Adu-Bobie, B. Arico, B. Brunelli, A. Pieri, L. Santini, S. Savino, D. Serruto, D. Litt, S. Kroll, J.A. Welsch, D.M. Granoff, R. Rappuoli, M. Pizza **2003**, Vaccination against *Neisseria meningitidis* using three variants of the lipoprotein GNA1870, *J. Exp. Med.* 197, 789–799.

75 M. Comanducci, S. Bambini, B. Brunelli, J. Adu-Bobie, B. Arico, B. Capecchi, M.M. Giuliani, V. Masignani, L. Santini, S. Savino, D.M. Granoff, D.A. Caugant, M. Pizza, R. Rappuoli, M. Mora **2002**, NadA, a novel vaccine candidate of *Neisseria meningitidis*, *J. Exp. Med.* 195, 1445–1454.

76 S. Pillai, A. Howell, K. Alexander, B.E. Bentley, H.-Q. Jiang, K. Ambrose, D. Zhu, G. Zlotnick **2005**, Outer membrane protein (OMP) based vaccine for *Neisseria meningitidis* serogroup B, *Vaccine* 23, 2206–2209.

77 C.A. Ison, R.S. Heyderman, N.J. Klein, M. Peakman, M. Levin **1995**, Whole blood model for exploring host–bacterial interactions, *Microb. Pathog.* 18, 97–107.

78 C.A. Ison, N. Anwar, M.J. Cole, R. Galassini, R.S. Heyderman, N.J. Klein, J. West, A.J. Pollard, S. Morley, M. Levin, Meningococcal Research Group **1999**, Assessment of immune response to meningococcal disease: comparison of a whole-blood assay and the serum bactericidal assay, *Microb. Pathog.* 27, 207–214.

79 C.A. Ison, N. Anwar, M.J. Cole, A.J. Pollard, S.L. Morley, K. Fidler, C. Sandiford, J. Banks, S.J. Kroll, M. Levin **2003**, Age dependence of in vitro survival of meningococci in whole blood during childhood, *Pediatr. Infect. Dis. J.* 22, 868–873.

80 R.G. Bredius, B.H. Derkx, C.A. Fijen, T.P. de Wit, M. de Haas, R.S. Weening, J.G. van de Winkel, T.A. Out **1994**, Fc gamma receptor IIa (CD32) polymorphism in fulminent meningococcal shock in children, *J. Infect. Dis.* 170, 848–853.

81 M.M. Estabrook, N.C. Christopher, J.M. Griffiss, C.J. Baker, R.E. Mandrell **1994**,

Sialylation and human neutrophil killing of group C *Neisseria meningitidis*, *J. Infect. Dis.* 166, 1079–1088.
82 M. Schlesinger, R. Greenberg, J. Levy, H. Käythy, R. Levy **1994**, Killing of meningococci by neutrophils: effect of vaccination on patients with complement deficiency, *J. Infect. Dis.* 170, 449–453.
83 A. Aase, E.A. Hoiby, T.E. Michaelsen **1998**, Opsonophagocytic and bactericidal activity mediated by purified IgG subclass antibodies after vaccination with the Norwegian group B meningococcal vaccine, *Scand. J. Immunol.* 47, 388–396.
84 T.E. Michaelsen, A. Aase, J. Kolberg, E. Wedge, E. Rosenqvist **2001**, PorB3 outer membrane protein on Neisseria meningitidis is poorly accessible for antibody binding on live bacteria, *Vaccine* 19, 1526–1533.
85 A. Aase, L.M. Naess, R.H. Sandin, T.K. Herstad, F. Oftung, J. Holst, I.L. Haugen, E.A. Hoiby, T.E. Michaelsen **2003**, Comparison of functional immune responses in humans after intranasal and intramuscular immunizations with outer membrane vesicle vaccines against group B meningococcal disease, *Vaccine* 21, 2042–2051.
86 S.G.P. Funnell, S. Taylor, H. Pryer, K. Reddin, M.J. Hudson, A.R. Gorringe **2002**, Developing of meningococcal whole cell antibody surface labeling and opsonophagocytic assays for assessment of vaccines containing proteins, *Int. Pathog. Neisseria Conf.* 13, 251.
87 M. Huet, A. Suire **1981**, An animal model for testing the activity of meningococcal polysaccharide vaccine, *J. Biol. Stand.* 9, 67–74.
88 D. Martin, N. Cadieux, J. Hamel, B.R. Brodeur **1997**, Highly conserved *Neisseria meningitidis* surface protein confers protection against experimental infection, *J. Exp. Med.* 185, 1173–1183.
89 B.R. Brodeur, Y. Larose, P. Tsang, J. Hamel, A. Ryan **1985**, Protection against infection with *Neisseria meningitidis* group B serotype 2b by passive immunization with serotype-specific monoclonal antibody, *Infect. Immun.* 50, 510–516.
90 K.J. Oliver, K.M. Reddin, P. Bracegirdle, M.J. Hudson, R. Borrow, I.M. Feavers, A. Robinson, K. Cartwright, A.R. Gorringe **2002**, *Neisseria lactamica* protects against experimental meningococcal infection, *Infect. Immun.* 70, 3621–3626.
91 K. Saukkonen, M. Leinonen, H. Abdillahi, J.T. Poolman **1989**, Comparative evaluation of potential components for group B meningococcal vaccine by passive protection in the infant rat and in vitro bactericidal assay, *Vaccine* 7, 325–328.
92 M. Toropainen, H. Käyhty, L. Saarinen, E. Rosenqvist, E.A. Hoiby, E. Wedege, T. Michaelsen, P.H. Makela **1999**, The infant rat model adapted to evaluate human sera for protective immunity to group B meningococci, *Vaccine* 7, 2677–2689.
93 M. Toropainen, L. Saarinen, P. van der Ley, B. Kuipers, H. Käyhty **2001**, Murine monoclonal antibodies to PorA of *Neisseria meningitidis* show reduced protective activity in vivo against B:15:P1.7,16 subtype variants in an infant rat infection model, *Microb. Pathog.* 30, 139–148.
94 J.A. Welsch, G.R. Moe, R. Rossi, J. Adu-Bobie, R. Rappuoli, D. Granoff **2003**, Antibody to genome-derived Neisserial antigen 2132, a *Neisseria meningitidis* candidate vaccine, confers protection against bacteremia in the absence of complement-mediated bactericidal activity, *J. Infect. Dis.* 188, 1730–1740.
95 M. Toropainen, L. Saarinen, E. Wedege, K. Bolstad, H. Makela, H. Käyhty **2005**, Passive protection in the infant rat protection assay by sera taken before and after vaccination of teenagers with serogroup B meningococcal outer membrane vesicle vaccines, *Vaccine* (in press).
96 B.A. Perkins, K. Jonsdottir, H. Briem, E. Griffiths, B.D. Plikaytis, E.A. Hoiby, E. Rosenqvist, J. Holst, H. Nokelby, F. Sotolongo, G. Sierra, H.C. Campa, G.M. Carlone, D. Williams. J. Dykes, D. Kapczynski, E. Tikhomirov, J.D. Wenger, C.V. Broome **1998**, Immunogenicity of two efficacious outer membrane protein-based serogroup B meningococcal vaccines among young adults in Iceland, *J. Infect. Dis.* 177, 683–691.
97 E. Wedege, B. Kuipers, K. Bolstad, H. van Dijken, L.O. Froholm, C. Vermont, D.A. Caugant, G. van den Dobbelsteen

2003, Antibody specificities and effect of meningococcal carriage in Icelandic teenagers receiving the Norwegian serogroup B outer membrane vesicle vaccine, *Infect. Immun.* 71, 3775–3781.

98 V. Davenport, T. Guthrie, J. Findlow, R. Borrow, N. A. Williams, R. S. Heyderman **2003**, Evidence for naturally acquired T cell-mediated mucosal immunity to *Neisseria meningitidis, J. Immunol.* 171, 4263–4270.

99 R. E. Horton, J. Stuart, H. Christensen, R. Borrow, T. Guthrie, V. Davenport, A. Finn, N. A. Williams, R. S. Heyderman, ALSPAC Study Team **2005**, Influence of age and carriage status on salivary IgA to *Neisseria meningitidis, Epidemiol. Infect.* 2005, 1–7.

17
Conjugate Vaccines

Neil Ravenscoft and Ian M. Feavers

17.1
Introduction

For all practical purposes, *Neisseria meningitidis*, the meningococcus, is a commensal of the upper respiratory tract that comparatively rarely causes invasive disease [1, 2]. However, the highest attack rates for meningococcal disease are in the very young and its rapid development and progression, together with the ability of the organism to cause epidemics, make this one of the most dreaded bacterial infections [3]. Meningococcal disease is also notoriously difficult to distinguish from other febrile illnesses, often confounding rapid and accurate diagnosis [4, 5]. Despite the availability of effective antibiotics and sophisticated intensive care management, case fatality rates remain high and morbidity amongst survivors continues to be a significant problem [6]. Thus it is perhaps not surprising that immunoprophylaxis with effective vaccines against the pathogenic serogroups is at the forefront of strategies towards the elimination of the disease.

The prevention of meningococcal disease through vaccination has been a continuing challenge for the scientific community during the past century [3, 7, 8]. Attempts to produce killed whole cell vaccines early in the 20th century met with limited success, largely because such vaccines proved too reactogenic. The clinical trials that were conducted with whole-cell formulations were poorly controlled and were insufficiently powered to confirm the efficacy of this approach [9]. During the 1930s, efforts to develop an exotoxin vaccine similarly met with limited success [10, 11] and, even today with the benefit of genome science, it remains unclear whether meningococci produce functional exotoxins. The first demonstrably efficacious meningococcal vaccines were developed during the 1960s by Gotschlich and coworkers, whose serological studies revealed the importance of bactericidal anticapsular antibodies in protection against meningococcal disease [12, 13]. Based on these observations, they developed a method for the purification of high molecular weight capsular polysaccharide and demonstrated that it was immunogenic in adult volunteers [14, 15]. Subsequent clin-

Handbook of Meningococcal Disease. Infection Biology, Vaccination, Clinical Management.
Edited by M. Frosch and M.C.J. Maiden

ISBN: 3-527-31260-9

ical studies in military recruits showed that meningococcal polysaccharide vaccine was highly effective at preventing disease in adults [16–18].

The serogroup of the meningococcus is defined by the immunochemistry of its capsular polysaccharide. Of the 12 immunologically distinct serogroups, only five (A, B, C, W-135, Y) are responsible for almost all of the disease and are therefore the principal targets for vaccine development [19]. Bivalent (A, C) and tetravalent (A, C, W-135, Y) formulations of purified, high molecular weight polysaccharides have been available since the 1970s [20]. They are effective and over the past three decades have been widely used to disrupt outbreaks of meningococcal disease and to protect individuals with an elevated risk of contracting meningococcal disease. More recently, a trivalent (A, C, W-135) formulation has been licensed specifically to address the threat of outbreaks of W-135 disease in sub-Saharan Africa [21].

Polysaccharide vaccines have a number of critical drawbacks that limit their utility in immunization programs [3]. In general, the immunogenicity and efficacy of capsular polysaccharide vaccines are age-related, with the vaccines being poorly immunogenic in the very young, who are most at risk of meningococcal disease [20]. This is a consequence of age-related differences in both the quantity and the quality of antibody responses to polysaccharide vaccines, which elicit a higher proportion of high-avidity, bactericidal antibodies in older children and adults than in infants. With bactericidal antibody levels declining more rapidly in young children than adults, the duration of protective immunity induced by polysaccharide antigens is also age-related and tends not to be readily boosted by subsequent exposure to the antigen. In the case of the serogroup C polysaccharide, the administration of repeated doses of vaccine has been shown to lead to immunological hyporesponsiveness, although the clinical significance of such hyporesponsiveness remains unclear. Finally, current evidence shows that vaccination with polysaccharide vaccines induces only transient and incomplete protection against nasopharyngeal carriage of the meningococcus, which suggests that, at best, polysaccharide vaccines are only likely to provide limited herd immunity.

The immunobiological shortcomings of capsular polysaccharides are largely attributable to the fact that they are T cell-independent antigens and induce serum antibody responses in the absence of T cell help [22–24]. Capsular polysaccharides exhibit repetitive epitopes and induce antibody production after cross-linking B cell receptors, which explains the requirement that purified polysaccharides exceed a minimum molecular size to be immunogenic [25]. Evidence suggests that the ability to respond to purified polysaccharide is restricted to a limited set of B lymphocytes; and the failure of infants to respond to specific polysaccharides is taken as evidence that the antipolysaccharide antibodies are produced by a subset of B cells that develops late in ontogeny [26].

The problems associated with the use of T cell-independent polysaccharide vaccines are largely solved by conversion of the polysaccharide into a T cell-dependent antigen [24, 27, 28]. Protein antigens are usually T cell-dependent and the conversion is achieved by chemical conjugation of the antigen to a carrier protein, a technique that had long been known to make nonantigenic small molecules immunogenic. After uptake and processing by antigen-presenting cells (APCs), peptides derived from them are presented on the surface of the APCs by MHC class II molecules, where they are recognized by CD4 T cells [29]. These T-helper cells secrete cytokines which activate B cell proliferation and differentiation, affecting the antibody response in a number of ways, including: (a) the development of memory, resulting in the induction of a more rapid and higher titer secondary response, (b) isotype-switching from IgM to IgG and (c) the affinity maturation of antibodies. If polysaccharide is linked to a protein that is processed by APCs, B cells that recognize the saccharide epitopes are similarly stimulated by T-helper cells, resulting in improved antipolysaccharide antibody and memory responses. Significantly, this T cell-dependence makes the vaccine more immunogenic in infants.

The successful introduction of the *Haemophilus influenzae* type b glycoconjugate vaccine in the late 1980s highlighted the advantages of the conjugation approach [30] and paved the way for the development of conjugates prepared from pneumococcal and meningococcal polysaccharides [27]. In 1999, conjugated group C meningococcal vaccines were first licensed in the UK [31] and, more recently, a tetravalent A, C, W135 and Y combination has been licensed in the USA [32]. Table 17.1 lists the currently licensed meningococcal conjugate vaccines.

17.2 Preparation of Conjugate Vaccines

17.2.1 Background

The essential requirement of glycoconjugate vaccines is that the saccharide antigen is covalently linked to an appropriate carrier protein. Approaches to the preparation of meningococcal conjugate vaccines are largely based on the successful strategies employed for the production of Hib conjugate vaccines (Fig. 17.1).

The saccharide component is either a long-chain polysaccharide or an oligosaccharide comprising the repeating unit of the capsular polysaccharide, which is activated and attached to the protein carrier. The polysaccharide starting material may be high molecular weight or partly size-reduced prior to random activation (Fig. 17.1, i) and attachment, whereas the saccharide component of oligosaccharide-based vaccines is generated by degradation of the polysaccharide to form active functional groups at both terminals (ii), or at only one terminal (iii), which may be used directly or modified prior to conjugation. The third and most recent approach involves the synthesis of a short saccharide chain (iv) from readily available chemical precursors which is conjugated directly to the protein [33].

Table 17.1 Licensed meningococcal conjugate vaccines

	Proprietary name	Manufacturer	Presentation	Active constituents	Conjugation chemistry	Adjuvant	Other excipients	Date first licensed
Monovalent	Meningitec	Wyeth	Single dose, liquid-filled vial	10 μg *O*-acetylated group C oligosaccharide conjugated to CRM_{197} (∼15 μg)	Reductive amination	$AlPO_4$	NaCl	UK, October 1999
	Menjugate	Chiron	Single dose, freeze-dried vial and separate diluent	10 μg *O*-acetylated group C oligosaccharide conjugated to CRM_{197} (11–25 μg)	Active ester chemistry	$Al(OH)_3$	Mannitol and sodium phosphate buffer	UK, March 2000
	NeisVac-C	Baxter	Single dose, prefilled syringe	10 μg de-*O*-acetylated group C polysaccharide conjugated to tetanus toxoid (10–20 μg)	Reductive amination	$Al(OH)_3$	NaCl	UK, July 2000
Tetravalent	Menactra	Sanofi Pasteur	Single dose, liquid-filled vial	4 μg group A oligosaccharide, 4 μg group C oligosaccharide, 4 μg group W135 oligosaccharide, 4 μg group Y oligosaccharide, each conjugated separately to diphtheria toxoid (∼48 μg total)	Information not available	None	NaCl and sodium phosphate buffer	USA, January 2005 for 11–55 years of age

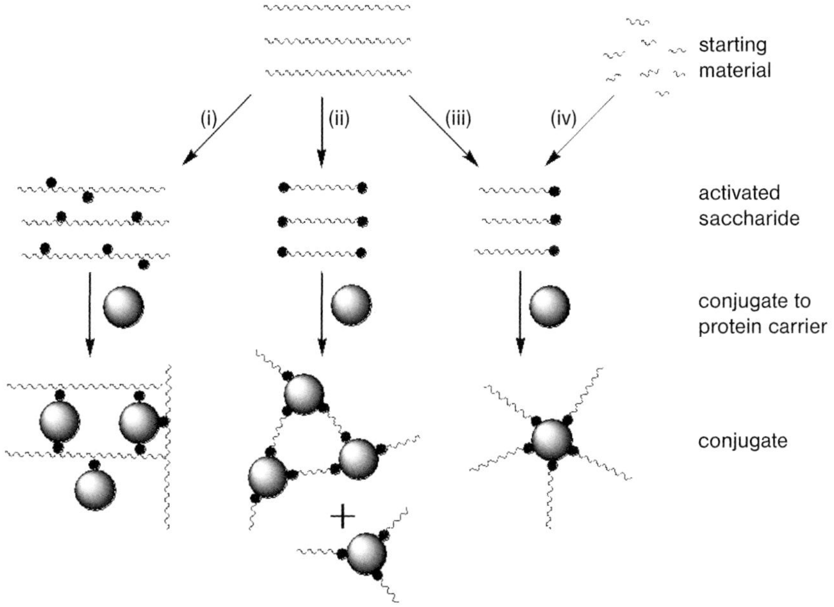

Fig. 17.1 Various approaches can be used in the preparation of meningococcal conjugate vaccines. The purified saccharide may be (i) randomly activated, (ii) partially degraded to form active functional groups at both terminals, or (iii) activated at only one terminal. The most recent approach (iv) involves the synthesis of a short saccharide chain which is conjugated directly to the protein. The final structure of the vaccine depends upon the approach adopted.

The carrier proteins used for licensed Hib conjugates are diphtheria toxoid (DT), tetanus toxoid (TT), CRM_{197} (a single amino acid variant of diphtheria toxin) and an outer membrane complex from *N. meningitidis* group B strain [34]. The structure and hence the immunogenicity of the derived conjugate depends on a number of factors: the size and loading of the antigen, the protein carrier and the conjugation chemistry employed. Polysaccharide-based conjugate vaccines use multiple attachment sites, resulting in a cross-linked lattice matrix, whereas oligosaccharide-based vaccines can either have a single terminal attachment site to give a simple "hairy ball" type of structure, or be attached through both terminals to form the type of cross-linked structures shown in Fig. 17.1. These structurally defined Hib conjugates and intermediates have been shown to be amenable to quality control by means of physicochemical methods of analysis [35–37] instead of bioassays, which are hampered by the lack of good animal models for evaluating Hib immunogenicity [38, 39]. Advances in bioanalytical technology and its application to saccharide-based vaccines, following the experience with Hib vaccines, has greatly facilitated the rapid development and characterization of the meningococcal conjugate vaccines described in this chapter.

The meningococcal conjugate vaccines licensed or currently in development against groups A, B, C, W135 and Y are based on the repeating unit of capsular polysaccharides, the specific conjugation approaches adopted depending on the chemical structure and size of the antigen, the protein carrier used and the proprietary technology and experience of the manufacturer. The first meningococcal conjugate vaccines to be licensed were three monovalent vaccines against group C disease: Meningitec (1999, by Wyeth Vaccines), Menjugate (2000, by Chiron Vaccines) and NeisVac-C (2000, by Baxter Immuno); and the corresponding WHO recommendations for group C conjugate vaccines were published in 2004 [40]. These recommendations serve as the basis for other novel meningococcal conjugates containing the other saccharides and for multivalent combinations.

17.2.2 Licensed Vaccines Against Group C Meningococci

Meningitec, Menjugate and NeisVac-C are oligosaccharide-based vaccines in which the saccharide is terminally activated using approaches (ii) and (iii) shown in Fig. 17.1. The starting material for each consists of the group C polysaccharide, which typically meets vaccine specifications with respect to purity, composition and size.

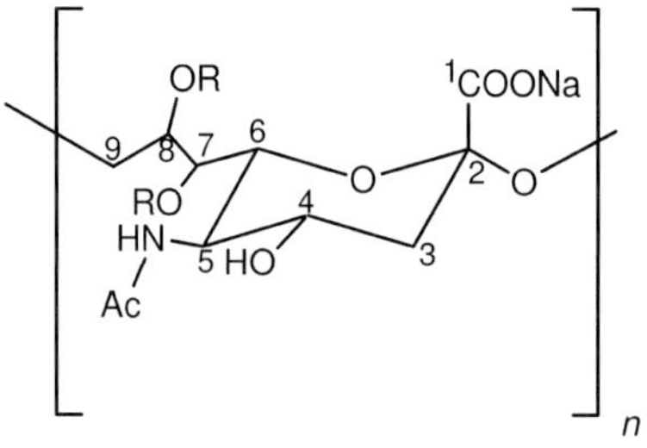

R = H or Ac

The Mn C polysaccharide is a homopolymer of partly *O*-acetylated 2,9-α-linked sialic acid; and the polysaccharide vaccine is required to have a minimal level of *O*-acetylation [41]. However, there is evidence that *O*-acetylation is not important for immunogenicity and, for NeisVac-C, the polysaccharide starting material is de-*O*-acetylated [42, 43].

The activated saccharide of both Meningitec and NeisVac-C is prepared by sodium periodate oxidation of the C7-C8 diol of de-*O*-acetylated sialic acid residues to generate oligosaccharides with reactive aldehyde groups at both terminals. In this approach (Fig. 17.1, ii), depolymerization and activation are achieved in a single step. The desired molecular mass distribution of the activated oligosaccharides is obtained by controlling the extent of oxidation and performing size fractionation (diafiltration) after the activation step. Finally, the aldehyde end-groups of the saccharide are directly coupled to amino groups of the protein carrier by reductive amination via the formation of Schiff bases, which are reduced to the stable secondary amine linkage with sodium cyanoborohydride. The protein carriers are CRM_{197} and tetanus toxoid for Meningitec and NeisVac-C, respectively. Estimations of the mean molecular masses of the conjugates by use of size exclusion chromatography with multiangle laser light scattering and refractive index detection (SEC/MALLS) suggest that Meningitec is largely comprised of conjugates containing three or four CRM_{197} molecules, whereas NeisVac-C is larger and contains some cross-linked complexes containing up to six TT molecules [44].

The Menjugate vaccine is prepared using approach (iii), in which single terminally activated oligosaccharides are generated by controlled acid hydrolysis. Following size fractionation by preparative ion exchange chromatography, reductive amination introduces an amino group at C2 of the reducing end sialic acid. Activation of the aminated oligosaccharide is achieved by covalent attachment to a bifunctional spacer molecule (the N-hydroxysuccinimidodiester of adipic acid). One end of this spacer is covalently attached to the oligosaccharide during activation, while the other end of the spacer (bearing the N-hydroxysuccinimide leaving group) provides for covalent attachment to the CRM_{197} carrier protein [45, 46]. Size analysis by SEC/MALLS confirms that this conjugate is monomeric in structure [44].

17.2.3 Meningococcal Conjugate Vaccine Developments

The efficacy of the group C conjugate vaccines introduced into routine vaccination demonstrated that a comprehensive conjugate vaccine against the five pathogenic serogroups would have the potential to eradicate meningococcal disease. However, the difficulties associated with a carbohydrate-based group B vaccine (Section 17.2.3.2) meant that most effort to date has focused on the development of conjugate vaccines against group A, C, Y and W135 meningococci [47].

17.2.3.1 Group A Conjugates

The meningococcal group A polysaccharide is a homopolymer of α-1,6-linked *N*-acetylmannosamine phosphate [$\rightarrow$6)-α-ManNAc-(1-$OPO_2$$\rightarrow$] with *O*-acetylation (70–95%) mainly at O-3 and a small amount at O-4 [48].

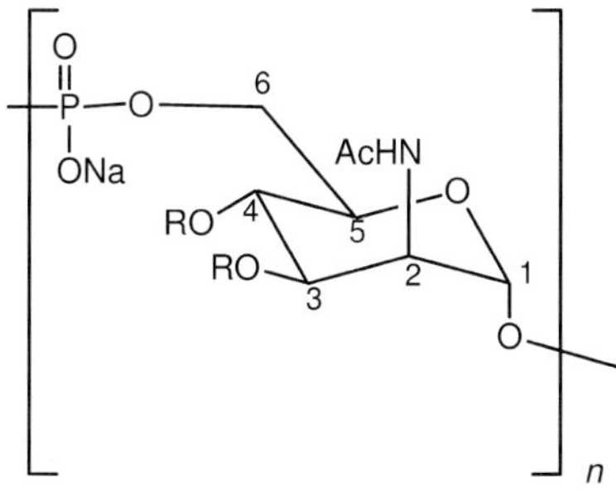

R=H or Ac

The extent of *O*-acetylation of the purified polysaccharide is determined by the strain used and the isolation and purification procedures employed. *O*-acetylation is important for the immunogenicity of the polysaccharide [49], but not for the antigenicity of small synthetic oligosaccharide conjugates [50]. The lability of the phosphodiester linkage which makes it the least stable of the meningococcal polysaccharides [51, 52], favored the development of polysaccharide-based conjugates. The structure of the Mn A saccharide permits random activation (i) of the polysaccharide through (a) derivatization of free hydroxyl groups with reagents such as cyanogen bromide (CNBr), 1-cyano-4(dimethylamino)-pyridinium tetrafluoroborate (CDAP) or carbonyldiimidazole (CDI) [53–57], (b) periodate oxidation of the C3-C4 diol of de-*O*-acetylated residues to generate aldehyde groups [58], or (c) treatment with base to deacetylate and generate amine groups at C2 [59]. The reactive intermediates formed can then be reacted with spacers or coupled directly to the carrier protein. Terminal activation (iii) can be achieved by acid hydrolysis to generate a reducing end group which can be reacted directly or with a spacer [45] or by reduction of the terminal reducing N-acetylmannosamine followed by controlled periodate oxidation to generate a reactive aldehyde at C5 [60]. Synthesis (iv) of short Mn A oligosaccharides containing an aminoethyl spacer which can be readily coupled to human serum albumin via Diels–Alder-type reactions has been described [50]. Chemical approaches to improve the hydrolytic stability of the Mn A saccharide component include modification of ring hydroxyl groups [61, 62] and synthesis of stabilized derivatives [63].

17.2.3.2 **Group B Conjugates**

The meningococcal group B polysaccharide is a homopolymer of *α*-2,8-*α*-linked sialic acid and conjugation reactions are hampered by the formation of stable lactones between the carboxyl at C1 and the hydroxyl on C9 of the adjacent residue [64].

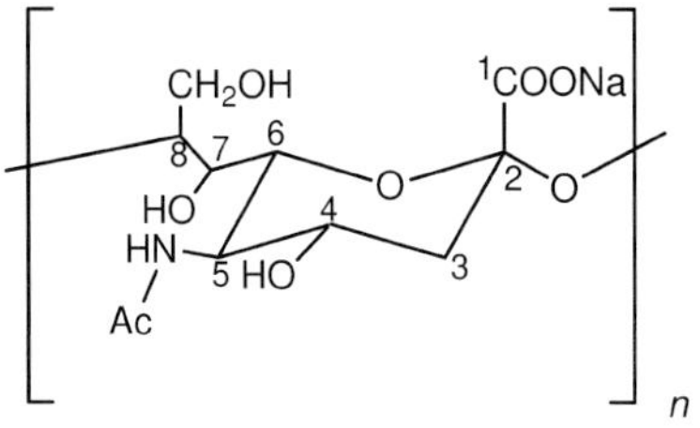

Random activation of the polysaccharide (i) may be achieved by reaction of the carboxyl groups with adipic acid dihydrazide (ADH)/carbodiimide [60]. Although there is no direct evidence for autoantibody activity in the immune response to group B capsular polysaccharide, the similarity of the group B polysaccharide to sialylated host glycopeptides and the poor immunogenicity of group B polysaccharide raises the theoretical possibility that a group B vaccine might induce an immune response that is cross-reactive with self antigens [65]. The notional risk associated with the use of vaccines based on group B polysaccharide has largely deterred the pharmaceutical industry from developing such products. However, one approach, which attempts to address these concerns, involves the modification of the group B polysaccharide by replacing the N-acetyl groups with N-propionyl groups prior to conjugation to either tetanus toxoid or a recombinant porin protein (rPorB) from *N. meningitidis* [66–68].

17.2.3.3 **Group C Conjugates**

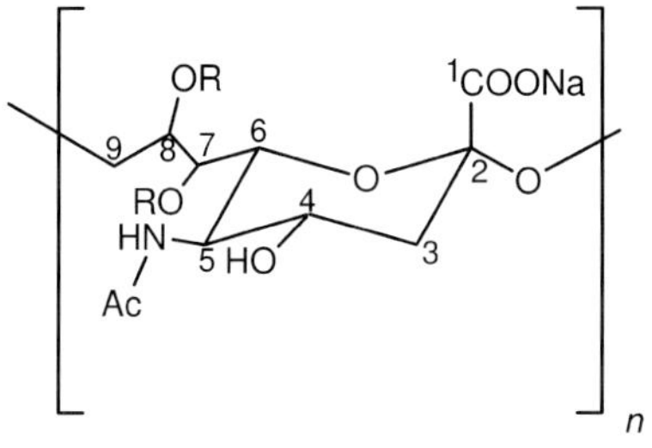

R = H or Ac

In addition to approaches used for the three licensed conjugate vaccines, other conjugation strategies have been described that involve random activation (i) of the polysaccharide by: (a) reaction of the carboxyl groups with adipic acid dihydrazide (ADH)/carbodiimide and (b) treatment with base to de-N-acetylate and generate amine groups at C5 [59] and terminal activation (iii) by use of hydrogen peroxide depolymerization [69].

17.2.3.4 **Group Y and W-135 Conjugates**

The capsular polysaccharides of group Y and W135 consist of a repeating unit of → 4-*O*-*α*-D-Glc*p*-(1 → 6)-*α*-D-NeuAc-(2 → and → 4-*O*-*α*-D-Gal*p*-(1 → 6)-*α*-D-NeuAc-(2 →, respectively [70].

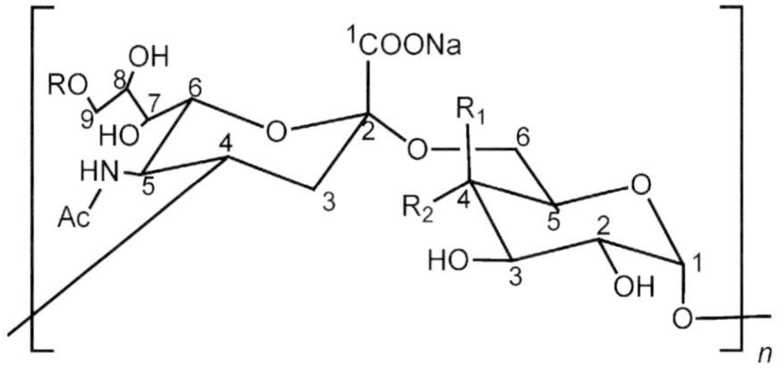

Serogroup W-135
(R_1 = OH, R_2 = H)
Serogroup Y
(R_1 = H, R_2 = OH)
R = H or Ac

Although both polysaccharide vaccines are required to be partly *O*-acetylated [71] at O7/O9 of sialic acid [48], preclinical studies in mice have indicated that *O*-acetylation may not be important for the immunogenicity of either group W-135 [72] or group Y [73] conjugates. A recent survey of meningococci isolated in the UK showed that only 8% of group W135 isolates but 79% of group Y were found to express *O*-acetylated capsules [74]. The conjugation strategies for both group Y and W-135 are identical and may involve random activation (i) of the polysaccharide by: (a) reaction of the carboxyl groups, (b) derivatization of free hydroxyl groups as previously described, or (c) selective periodate oxidation to generate an aldehyde in the exocyclic chain of the sialic acid residue [75]. Terminal activation (ii) can be achieved by acid hydrolysis to generate oligosaccharides with *N*-acetylneuraminic acid at the reducing end [76]; and the terminal keto group can be reacted directly or with a spacer.

17.2.4
Combination Meningococcal Conjugate Vaccines

Since 1992, bivalent conjugate vaccines (against groups A and C) – prepared using oligosaccharide-CRM_{197} [77, 78] and polysaccharide–diphtheria toxoid conjugates [79–81] – have been tested in clinical trials. Finally in 2005, the first tetravalent conjugate vaccine against groups A, C, Y and W-135 (Menactra, manufactured by Sanofi Pasteur) was licensed by the FDA [32]. The individual polysaccharides are depolymerized, derivatized and purified by diafiltration prior to conjugation to diphtheria toxoid, followed by further purification by serial diafiltration [82]. No additional details about the method of conjugation used for the different group saccharides are available in the public domain.

17.2.5
Lipo-oligosaccharide Conjugate Vaccines

The lipo-oligosaccharide (LOS) of *N. meningitidis* is a surface glycolipid and major outer membrane component important for the survival of the organism [83]. It plays a critical role in the immunopathology of meningococcal disease as an activator of inflammatory cytokines [84] and is involved in the immune response to natural infection, but its use in vaccines has been hampered by its toxicity, potential cross-reactivity with self antigens, antigenic diversity and phase variability. Two approaches have been adopted to prepare LOS-derived conjugate vaccines. The first is to conjugate the terminal variable oligosaccharide structure to a protein carrier. The majority of group B meningococcal disease isolates express the L3 or the L3,7 immunotype and Verheul et al. [85] produced a L3,7,9-tetanus conjugate that was immunogenic in both rabbits and mice. The alternative approach is to base a conjugate vaccine on the LOS inner core, which is more conserved among genetically diverse meningococci and elicits opsonic antibodies in humans [86, 87]. Although vaccines produced by either approach can induce the production of opsonic antibodies, neither has yet resulted in a vaccine capable of inducing bactericidal antibodies. In addition to the purification of LOS from wild-type meningococcal isolates, specific LOS antigen structures for use in prospective conjugate vaccines may be chemically synthesized [63, 88] or purified from genetically engineered meningococcal strains, in which the LOS biosynthetic genes are "locked" to express the desired immunotype [89].

17.2.6 Alternative Carrier Proteins for Meningococcal Vaccines

The increasing use of glycoconjugate vaccines that use the toxoids and CRM_{197} as carriers has led to concerns about carrier-induced immune suppression, particularly with multivalent conjugate vaccines in which the dose of carrier protein can be high. A recent clinical study, for example, showed that the immune response to a Mn C-CRM_{197} vaccine was significantly reduced when it was coadministered with a 9-valent pneumococcal CRM_{197} vaccine. These concerns have stimulated interest in new carrier proteins that may augment the immune response or provide additional protection against meningococcal or other diseases. Carriers for group C saccharide tested in preclinical studies include a recombinant membrane-associated P64 protein from *N. meningitidis* [90], N19, a string of human universal CD4 T-cell epitopes from various pathogen-derived antigens [91] and *Bordetella pertussis* fimbriae [92]. A recombinant porin protein (rPorB) from *N. meningitidis* was used as a group B carrier [68] and the immunogenicity and potency of a tetravalent meningococcal conjugate vaccine in development for infants was reported to be enhanced when diphtheria toxoid was substituted with a surface protein from pneumococci, PspA [93]. In addition, the potential of outer membrane protein D of *H. influenzae* as a carrier has been demonstrated in preclinical studies of Hib PRP conjugates [94].

17.2.7 New Formulations and Delivery of Meningococcal Conjugate Vaccines

At present, all licensed meningococcal conjugate vaccines are delivered parenterally in several doses; and aluminium salts are used as adjuvant for the monovalent group C vaccines, while the tetravalent vaccine (Menactra) is nonadjuvanted (Table 17.1). With the development of new combination vaccines, there is a need for novel adjuvants that are more potent than aluminium salts, which will permit less of each antigen to be used in vaccine formulations and also allow for the possibility of reducing the number of doses required. Another concern with the use of aluminium hydroxide for the liquid formulation of meningococcal vaccines, is its role in decreasing the potency of Hib conjugate vaccines by facilitating cleavage of the Hib phosphodiester linkage [95]; and a similar depolymerization reaction may be possible with the group A saccharide.

One approach is the use of lipid-based adjuvants which act as immunostimulants (e.g. monophosphoryl lipid A), as tested for pneumococcal conjugates [96]. Another route is the use of microspheres which permit the gradual release of antigen, thus obviating the need for multiple doses. This was demonstrated in mice, where a single injection of a group C polysaccharide–tetanus toxoid conjugate vaccine encapsulated within microspheres of biodegradable polymers of polylactide-co-glycolide resulted in a highly bactericidal and long-lasting antibody [97]. Most research in this area is directed at mucosal vaccination, which offers two major advantages: delivery is needle-free and it has the potential to mount an immune response at the portal of entry of meningococci. Bactericidal antibodies (serum, mucosal) were elicited by intranasal immunization of mice with group C conjugates adjuvanted with nontoxic *Escherichia coli* heat-labile enterotoxin (LT) mutants and nanoparticle- [98] or chitosan-based [99, 100] delivery systems.

17.3 Control Testing of Conjugate Vaccines

The successful use of any vaccine depends on the implementation of a strategy to ensure that it is manufactured consistently and is similar to the lots demonstrated to be protective in clinical studies [101, 102]. The quality of the conjugate vaccine is assured by the control of each step in the manufacturing process (shown in Fig. 17.1) and by analysis of the vaccine intermediates and final product. While each step of the process can be monitored by traditional methods of analysis, recent advances in bioanalytical technology permit the structure and integrity of the polysaccharide starting material, protein carrier, saccharide intermediates and the conjugate to be evaluated by physicochemical methods. These include chromatography, spectroscopy and hyphenated techniques that have been developed for the structural elucidation of biologicals.

The level of physicochemical characterization and understanding of the possible structures varies with the type of conjugate and carrier protein. The simple monomeric type of conjugate (iii) with CRM_{197} as carrier is the most amenable to structural characterization, whereas a cross-linked lattice conjugate (i), formed with a toxoid as carrier, presents the biggest challenge to structural characterization. Nevertheless, the spectra and chromatograms obtained throughout the process constitute structural fingerprints of the vaccine intermediates and final product and provide a sensitive probe of manufacturing consistency from lot to lot. This is important because of the lack of reliable animal models for predicting the potency of conjugates in humans and the added advantage that the introduction of conjugate vaccines has not significantly increased the number of animals used in control testing by the vaccine industry and control agencies [103]. The detailed structural information provided by these techniques means that they can reveal subtle changes in the conjugate such as O-acetyl migration, the nature and extent of cleavage of the saccharide antigen, or the unfolding of the carrier protein; and they can identify previously undetected traces of contaminants and residuals from the process. The physicochemical data can also provide substantial proof of equivalence between vaccine lots when changes in the manufacturing process have been implemented; and this greatly facilitates the rapid licensure of group C conjugate vaccines in the UK [31].

The control tests applied to meningococcal group C conjugate vaccines (Fig. 17.2) are described in recommendations recently published by the World Health Organization [40] and in a European Pharmacopoeia monograph [41]. The analysis regime is summarized in Fig. 17.2 and has been the subject of recent reviews [104, 105].

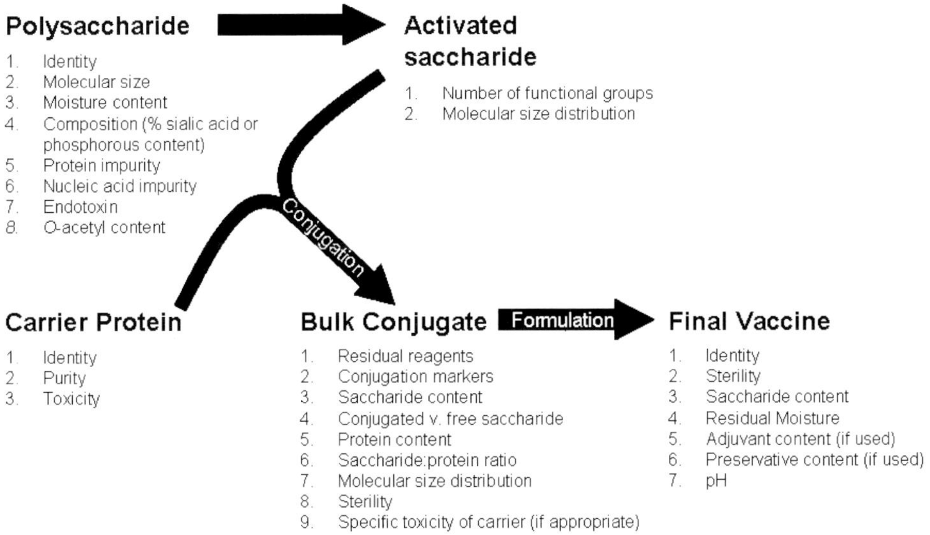

Fig. 17.2 Control tests applied to meningococcal conjugate vaccines. Control tests typically applied at each stage during the manufacture of the meningococcal group C conjugate vaccines are shown. Details are published in World Health Organization recommendations [40] and in a European Pharmacopoeia monograph [41]. This approach has been summarized in recent reviews [104, 105].

17.3.1 Polysaccharide

The polysaccharide starting material is tested for purity, identity and composition, typically determined using a combination of an immunological identity test and colorimetric assays for phosphorus (group A), sialic acid (groups C, W135, Y) and O-acetyl groups. The identity test can be replaced by the use of NMR spectroscopy. This technique yields spectra of magnetic sensitive nuclei (e.g. ^{1}H, ^{13}C, ^{31}P), which depend on the structural environment of the nuclei, and therefore provides a sensitive and nondestructive way of "fingerprinting" the molecular structure of organic molecules such as polysaccharides [106]. The position and degree of *O*-acetylation of the acetylated polysaccharide can be estimated from key signals in the ^{1}H NMR spectrum of the native polysaccharide, which may change with time due to acetyl migration [107]. The pattern of *O*-acetylation determined for different lots indicates the consistency of manufacture and, importantly, may be critical for the subsequent activation reaction, particularly if it is based upon the availability of hydroxyl groups for derivatization or periodate oxidation.

The saccharide may be quantified by the use of the colorimetric assays for phosphorus [108], sialic acid [109] and O-acetyl group content [110]. Newer analytical techniques employing chromatography offer greater specificity and sensitivity than colorimetric assays and can be applied to quantify saccharide and nonsugar components in combination vaccines. The approach involves acid or base depolymerization to monomers and their quantification by use of high-performance anion exchange chromatography with pulsed amperometric detection (HPAEC-PAD) for sugars or with conductivity detection (HPAEC-CD) for ions [111, 112]. For group B polysaccharide, problems associated with incomplete hydrolysis due to lactone formation can be circumvented by performing methanolysis. The stable methyl glycoside of sialic acid generated has been N-acetylated and quantified by use of HPAEC-PAD [113]. The O-acetyl content of meningococcal polysaccharides can be determined by HPAEC-CD after performing mild base hydrolysis to release O-acetyl groups selectively [112], while the total acetate content (both N- and O-linked) has been measured by HPAEC-CD after complete hydrolysis. In contrast, capillary zone electrophoresis has been shown to be a robust technique for the identification and quantification of a mixture of group A, C, Y and W135 polysaccharides without hydrolysis [114].

Although the activated saccharide is typically size-reduced, a consistent molecular size distribution of each lot of purified polysaccharide is required to achieve manufacturing consistency and permit control of the subsequent depolymerization/activation reactions. Soft gel filtration techniques have been largely replaced by high-performance size-exclusion chromatography (SEC-HPLC) equipped with ultraviolet (UV) [52], refractive index or light scattering/refractive index detectors [115] to determine the size of the polysaccharide. SEC-HPLC-UV provides a rapid indication of the quality of the polysaccharide and is sensitive to modifications in the molecular size distribution of the polysaccharide due to thermally induced hydrolysis.

17.3.2
Activated Saccharide

In addition to the tests applied to native polysaccharide, the degree of activation and the molecular size distribution of the activated saccharide should be analyzed, as this will determine the saccharide/protein ratio and size of the derived conjugate vaccine [116]. For randomly activated polysaccharides, the degree of activation can be determined by colorimetric assays for the reactive species introduced (amino group, active aldehyde, etc.). Chromatographic methods can also be used, but both approaches only provide information about the amount of activation and not its nature or position [117]. The molecular size distribution of the activated polysaccharide can be monitored by SEC-HPLC or determined accurately by size-exclusion chromatography (SEC) with detection by multiangle laser light-scattering photometry (MALLS) and differential refractometry (RI). The terminally activated saccharides generated by periodate oxidation, hydrogen peroxide or acid hydrolysis are generally of lower molecular weight and thus more amenable to detailed characterization than randomly activated polysaccharides [46, 48, 69, 76, 117].

17.3.3
Carrier Protein

Criteria for the control of proteins that have been used as carriers in meningococcal conjugate vaccines licensed to date (tetanus toxoid, CRM_{197}) are well established from experience in the control of Hib conjugate vaccines. In addition to biological tests, modern methods of protein characterization can also be applied. However, their applicability may be limited if the carrier protein has been chemically detoxified. The physicochemical techniques applied include SDS-PAGE, isoelectric focusing, HPLC, amino acid analysis, amino acid sequencing, circular dichroism, fluorescence spectroscopy, peptide mapping and mass spectrometry [118–120]. Prior hydrazide activation of the protein carrier has been reported to increase the yields of the conjugation reaction [75]. In this case, the degree of activation would need to be controlled.

17.3.4
Monovalent Conjugate Bulk

Vaccines formed from conjugation of randomly activated polysaccharides or terminally activated saccharides consist of a myriad of glycoforms, of which only the average properties can be measured. Strict control of the quality of the activated saccharide and carrier protein, as well as the conjugation conditions are therefore required to ensure consistent production of these structurally complex vaccines. Once the immunogenicity of a particular meningococcal conjugate vaccine has been demonstrated, then both the conjugation method and the control procedures used to ensure the reproducibility, stability and safety of the conjugate should be established [40].

Apart from assessing sterility, most of the control testing of the conjugate vaccine is product-specific and includes assays for: the absence of residual reagents, the absence of activated functional groups used for conjugation and, when toxoids are used, the specific toxicity of the carrier protein. Evidence for the covalent linkage between the saccharide and carrier protein is established and its extent determined. The molecular size distribution, the saccharide and protein content and the ratio of saccharide to protein are determined. The amount of free (unbound) saccharide present in the vaccine is also determined; and this serves as a key stability indicator for conjugate vaccines. The procedures used for the analysis and control of conjugate vaccines are based on the methods described for analysis of the carrier protein and the activated saccharide intermediate; and these are summarized in Fig. 17.2.

17.3.5
Final Product Conjugate

The range of control tests that might be carried out on the final product is largely governed by the formulation of the vaccine: in particular, the number of vaccine components included in the formulation and whether it contains an adjuvant. The identity of the saccharides and carrier can be demonstrated using a serological test and the saccharide content determined using sensitive HPAEC-PAD methods. If adjuvant is present, then the amount of adjuvant and the adsorption of the conjugate to the adjuvant should be controlled [40]. Determination of the amount of free saccharide and the size distribution of the conjugate (described in Section 17.3.4) have also been applied to the final formulated product [121, 122], but sample preparation is product-specific and may require the removal of adjuvant prior to analysis.

17.3.6 Stability and Potency of Conjugate Vaccines

The ability of a conjugate vaccine to elicit a T cell-dependent immune response depends on both the covalent attachment of the saccharide to the carrier protein and the maintenance of the structural integrity of saccharide antigen. Cleavage of bonds between the sugar units or at the position of attachment of the sugar chain to the carrier protein leads to loss of saccharide from the conjugate and decreased vaccine efficacy. Besides the loss in potency of the conjugate vaccine, excessive levels of unbound polysaccharide could theoretically result in immunological hyporesponsiveness. The stability of the vaccine is determined by the intrinsic structural features of the glycoconjugate as well as the formulation (buffer, adjuvant, other excipients), storage temperature and type of presentation. With the exception of group A vaccines, meningococcal conjugates are generally stable. Nevertheless, one of the licensed MnC conjugates (Menjugate) is lyophilized; and lyophilization may play a part in the stability of future meningococcal conjugate vaccines.

The degradation of conjugates under normal storage conditions is slow and therefore the development of appropriate physicochemical and bioassays to assess the integrity of conjugate vaccines is based on accelerated degradation studies. Such studies on the stability of group C conjugate vaccines with CRM_{197} [121, 123] and TT [122] carrier proteins have recently been reviewed [105]. All of the conjugate vaccines were stable when stored at the recommended temperatures, but differences in the structural stability and immunogenicity of the conjugates were observed at elevated temperatures and after cycles of freeze-thawing; these were attributed to differences in conjugate structure, the coupling chemistry employed, protein carrier and formulation. Saccharide integrity, as indicated by the free saccharide and size distribution assays, determines the immunogenicity of conjugate vaccines and is not affected by protein conformation. A similar study of group A, C, W135 and Y polysaccharides conjugated to diphtheria toxoid showed that, while all four were stable at 4 °C, each released different amounts of free saccharide after three weeks stored at 55 °C (degradation of A>C>W135>Y) [124]. The analytical challenges presented by multivalent meningococcal vaccines means that, as for pneumococcal conjugate vaccines, stability studies will be conducted on the monovalent bulk conjugate and testing of the final product may require the use of quantitative serological assays, such as rate nephelometry or ELISA inhibition [125, 126].

17.4 Immunogenicity of Meningococcal Conjugate Vaccines

The development of meningococcal conjugate vaccines, converting the saccharide antigen to T cell dependency, overcomes the principal immunobiological limitations that have precluded the use of polysaccharide vaccines in routine immunization programs. These vaccines have many properties that contribute to their effectiveness, including the ability to: elicit protective immunity in infants, induce immunological memory, provide herd immunity and overcome hyporesponsiveness. In terms of their higher avidity and bactericidal activity, the quality of antibody responses induced by conjugate vaccines is generally better than that induced by their unconjugated counterparts. The licensure of meningococcal conjugate vaccines has relied largely on immunogenicity data, as the low incidence of meningococcal disease generally limits the feasibility of randomized controlled trials to determine protective efficacy (see Chapter 16). The complement-mediated bactericidal antibody response, although often debated, continues to be widely accepted as the best serological correlate of protection for the evaluation of these vaccines (reviewed in Chapter 16).

17.4.1 Age-related Immunity

The three group C conjugates, first licensed in the UK and now widely used across Europe, are safe and highly immunogenic in all age groups [42, 43, 127–129]. In infants, two or three doses of vaccine given during the first six months of life have been shown to elicit a bactericidal antibody response of similar magnitude to that induced by unconjugated polysaccharide vaccine, and known to be protective in young adults [20]. In older children and adults, a single dose of vaccine is sufficient to elicit protective bactericidal antibody levels in the majority of immunized individuals [130]. Limited evidence suggests that NeisvacC may induce slightly higher bactericidal antibody responses than the other monovalent Mn C conjugates, but it remains unclear whether this can be attributed to the TT carrier protein, the de-*O*-acetylation of the conjugated saccharide, or a combination of the two [129].

The immune response has not yet been as extensively studied for other meningococcal conjugate vaccine formulations. In a study carried out in Niger, comparing a bivalent conjugate vaccine, consisting of A and C polysaccharides conjugated to diphtheria toxoid, with an unconjugated A and C polysaccharide vaccine showed that a higher proportion of the infants receiving the conjugate vaccine had elevated serum bactericidal activity against both groups of meningococci [79]. More recently, the prelicensure studies of Menactra demonstrated that the tetravalent formulation is safe and immunogenic in all age groups. In adults, it induced protective levels of bactericidal antibody against isolates of all four (A, C, W135, Y) meningococcal groups [131]. In children between two and ten years of age, the vaccine induced significantly higher and more persistent serum bactericidal antibody responses against meningococcal group A, C, Y and W-135 bacteria than the licensed tetravalent unconjugated polysaccharide vaccine [132]. In infants, however, the vaccine was only modestly immunogenic but there was evidence that it primed the immune system in the majority of infants who received three doses [133]. On the basis of its noninferiority to the licensed tetravalent polysaccharide vaccine, the FDA initially licensed Menactra for the 11–55 year age group [134]. The potential of this vaccine for younger age groups remains to be confirmed, but recent studies have demonstrated that a single dose given to two year old children elicits higher A, C, W135 and Y bactericidal titers than a licensed unconjugated tetravalent polysaccharide vaccine [135, 136].

Conjugate vaccines based on other meningococcal polysaccharide antigens have not yet been studied extensively in humans. The safety and immunogenicity of a group B vaccine, consisting of *N*-propionylated B capsular polysaccharide conjugated to tetanus toxoid, has been tested in a small number of adult male volunteers [137]. Although the vaccine was shown to be safe and immunogenic, the IgG response was specific for the *N*-propionylated form of the polysaccharide and was not bactericidal. Lipooligosaccharide conjugate vaccines remain to be tested in humans.

17.4.2 Antibody Persistence and Memory

Long-term protection against disease depends upon antibody persistence and immunological memory. Experience gained with the monovalent Mn C conjugates in the UK suggested that these vaccines initially elicit high bactericidal antibody concentrations, but for infants routinely immunized with three doses of vaccine early in life, antibody concentrations wane rapidly during the following 12 months [127, 138] with a corresponding decline in vaccine effectiveness (Section 17.4.3) [139]. In one study, bactericidal antibody titers had returned to preimmunization levels by four years of age [140].

Conjugate vaccines induce a population of memory B cells specific for the saccharide antigen, which can be stimulated by the corresponding unconjugated polysaccharide, resulting in an immunological memory response. Such a response is of greater magnitude than the primary response and is characterized by the production of higher avidity antibodies. Numerous studies have demonstrated the ability of monovalent Mn C conjugates to induce immunological memory [129, 138, 140, 141]. Similarly, immunization with bivalent formulations has been shown to result in immunological memory to both the A and C components [79, 142]. The recent studies of the immune reponse to the tetravalent conjugate, Menactra, provide evidence of avidity maturation to the C and W135 components, also indicating the induction of memory [136, 143].

17.4.3
Effectiveness

In the absence of randomized controlled trials to determine protective efficacy, the effectiveness of the monovalent group C conjugate vaccines was monitored post-licensure by an enhanced disease surveillance program [31]. Soon after the introduction of the vaccine in the UK, a marked reduction in group C disease was observed in the immunized age groups. Short-term estimates, using the screening method [144], showed that the effectiveness of the vaccines in England was 97% for teenagers and 92% for toddlers within one year of vaccination [145]. Similarly, the vaccines were 93% effective for infants routinely immunized with three doses of vaccine between the second and fourth month of life [139]. In this group, however, protection was short-lived and the vaccines confer little protection more than one year after the last scheduled dose. This reflects waning bactericidal antibody levels observed in clinical studies (Section 17.4.2) and suggests that, although these vaccines prime the infant immune system, immunological memory alone is insufficient to protect this age group. Although the rapid decline in vaccine effectiveness is worrying, there has not been an upsurge in infant cases of disease, largely because of the indirect effect of herd immunity (Section 17.4.6). These observations have prompted a review of the immunization schedule in the UK and provide the rationale for the development of a bivalent Hib/Mn C formulation for use as a single booster dose later in infancy.

17.4.4
Use of Conjugate Vaccines in the Immunocompromised

Individuals with asplenia or deficiencies in the terminal components of complement are known to be at increased risk of meningococcal infection. There is also concern that other immunocompromised individuals may not respond satisfactorily to vaccination. The magnitude of the bactericidal antibody response elicited by monovalent Mn C conjugate is significantly reduced in asplenic individuals, although the majority still have protective levels of antibody [146]. Evidence suggests that the nonresponders often attain protective levels of antibody following a second dose of vaccine. In the UK, the current advice is that, following the vaccination of patients with asplenia, either the level of functional antibody should be determined and a second dose of vaccine offered to nonresponders or two doses of vaccine should be offered routinely. A recent study has also shown that patients infected with human immunodeficiency virus (HIV) do not respond as well to Mn C conjugate vaccine as uninfected individuals. In the United States, the Advisory Committee on Immunization Practices (ACIP) recommends routine immunization with the tetravalent conjugate for patients with asplenia or terminal complement deficiency and suggests that individuals infected with HIV may elect to be vaccinated to reduce their risk of meningococcal disease [147].

The relative immaturity of the immune system of premature infants may explain their increased susceptibility to infection; and their response to vaccination with conjugates is, therefore, of particular interest. The limited available data suggest that the immune response of premature infants to Mn C conjugate is similar to that of full-term infants [148].

17.4.5 Hyporesponsiveness to Meningococcal Polysaccharides

Immunization with unconjugated meningococcal polysaccharide vaccine results in hyporesponsiveness to group C polysaccharide, so that the magnitude of the immune response to subsequent doses of vaccine is reduced (for a review, see [20]). Although there is no clinical evidence that individuals who have received more than one dose of polysaccharide vaccine have an increased risk of disease, this observation has implications for groups with an elevated risk of meningococcal disease, who tend to have multiple immunizations over a number of years. Several studies have demonstrated that vaccination with Mn C conjugate vaccine overcomes this hyporesponsiveness [149–151].

There are limited data to indicate whether other meningococcal polysaccharides induce hyporesponsiveness. A study in the Gambia, while demonstrating reduced bactericidal antibody responses to group C polysaccharide in infants who received multiple doses of bivalent polysaccharide vaccine, failed to provide any evidence of hyporesponsiveness to group A polysaccharide [152]. However, other studies provide conflicting, yet convincing, evidence that group A polysaccharide induces hyporesponsiveness in both infants [153] and adults [154].

17.4.6 Herd Immunity

Although the complement-mediated serum bactericidal antibody response is the accepted correlate of protection for meningococcal disease, conjugate vaccines also induce mucosal immunity, influencing carriage and transmission of the organism [155]. The highest rates of carriage of meningococci are found in teenagers and young adults, while the lowest rates are observed in infants, who are more likely to carry *N. lactamica* [156]. From the analysis of attack rates in children before and after vaccine introduction, it was inferred that herd immunity contributes to the control of group C infection, reducing the attack rate in the unvaccinated population by an estimated 67%. The introduction of the Mn C conjugate vaccine in the UK included a catch-up vaccination for everyone up to 18 years of age. Given the rapidly waning bactericidal antibody titers and the corresponding decline in the effectiveness of the vaccine in infants, the indirect protection afforded by the immunization of the older carrier population appears to have been crucial for the continued success of this program. It also has implications for the implementation of a booster program for those routinely immunized in infancy.

In 1999, a carriage study was initiated to assess the effects of the introduction of the Mn C conjugate vaccines on the meningococci circulating in the UK [157]. Meningococci were isolated from throat swabs prior to the mass vaccination program and then in the two subsequent years and were examined phenotypically for capsule expression and genotypically for both their sequence type and capsule operon [158]. The carriage study demonstrated that the implementation of the vaccination program resulted in a 67% reduction in the carriage of group C meningococci among teenagers. Before the introduction of the Mn C conjugate vaccine, ST-11 meningococci were the prevalent cause of group C disease and had higher rates of capsule expression than other organisms with the group C capsule gene. The implementation of the vaccination program had a significant impact on the carriage of ST-11 group C organisms but not other meningococci possessing the group C gene, suggesting that this epidemic genotype may be more dependent on the expression of its capsule for transmission than other group C genotypes and is consistent with the role of the capsule in meningococcal virulence.

17.5 Future Developments

17.5.1 Affordable Conjugate Vaccines for Developing Countries

Compared with most traditional vaccines, the research and development costs of novel conjugates are high and the decision to manufacture a particular vaccine is inevitably market-driven. The production of new drugs and vaccines for developing countries is often prohibitively expensive, despite significant incentives from governments and international organizations [159]. Even when vaccine might be produced profitably, an established manufacturer in an industrialized country may be deterred by the opportunity costs [160]. Although rarely a cause for concern in Europe and North America, group A meningococci are a major cause of recurrent epidemics in sub-Saharan Africa, with attack rates as high as 800 per 100 000 [161]. In 2001, the WHO and the Programme for Appropriate Technology for Health (PATH) established the Meningitis Vaccine Project (MVP), with a ten-year grant from the Bill and Melinda Gates Foundation, to eliminate meningococcal epidemics in sub-Saharan Africa [160]. The MVP opted for an approach based on the transfer of technology to a manufacturer in a developing country with finance, technical assistance and coordination provided by MVP. In partnership with the Serum Institute of India, MVP has developed a Mn A conjugate using TT as carrier and is on target to commence phase II clinical studies during 2006. This innovative model offers opportunities for the future development of multivalent meningococcal conjugates as well as other affordable orphan vaccines for use in developing countries.

17.5.2
Towards a Comprehensive Vaccine

The impact of mucosal immunity elicited by conjugate vaccines (Section 17.4.6) may prove to be double-edged: the advantages for the overall effectiveness of the vaccine have to be weighed against concerns that such immunoselective pressure might drive capsule-switching or strain replacement with nonvaccine serogroups [162]. *N. meningitidis* is a naturally transformable and highly recombinogenic bacterium [2] and there is ample evidence that capsule genes have been exchanged horizontally between different meningococcal genotypes in the absence of selective pressure imposed by vaccination programs. Immunoselection would not be a problem if the vaccine only induced systemic immunity as, for all practical purposes, meningococci are not transmissible once they have entered the vascular system; and any genetic variants selected would therefore be unlikely to persist. However, meningococcal variants selected during carriage are able to spread and have the potential to persist in the population.

Since almost all meningococcal disease is caused by one of five serogroups, the solution would be to produce a pentavalent conjugate (A, B, C, W135, Y), if it were not for the hypothetical concerns about the safety of a B component (Section 17.2.3.2). With the licensure of Menactra and the prospect of other tetravalent formulations, we are already four-fifths of the way towards a comprehensive vaccine. However, the reluctance to pursue a group B conjugate has inevitably shifted the search for a comprehensive vaccine towards other meningococcal antigens, such as lipooligosaccharide (Section 17.2.5) or cell surface proteins, which are discussed in subsequent chapters. In the long term, the development of a vaccine based on noncapsular antigens, if it were both effective and comprehensive, would probably lead to the redundancy of the capsular polysaccharide conjugates, but the licensure of such a vaccine is not imminent.

References

1 J. M. Griffiss **1982**, *Rev. Infect. Dis.* 4, 159–172.

2 M. C. J. Maiden **2002**, Population structure of *Neisseria meningitidis*, in *Emerging Strategies in the Fight Against Meningitis: Molecular and Cellular Aspects*, eds. C. Ferreirós, M. T. Criado, J. Vazques, Horizon Scientific Press, Wymondham.

3 S. L. Morley, A. J. Pollard **2001**, *Vaccine* 20, 666–687.

4 N. Steven, M. Wood **1995**, The clinical spectrum of meningococcal disease, in *Meningococcal Disease*, ed. K. Cartwright, John Wiley and Sons, Chichester.

5 S. Nadel, J. Britto, R. Booy, I. Maconochie, P. Habibi, M. Levin **1998**, *J. Accid. Emerg. Med.* 15, 298–303.

6 S. B. Welch, S. Nadel **2003**, *Arch. Dis. Child* 88, 608–614.

7 C. E. Frasch **1995**, Meningococcal vaccines: past, present and future, in *Meningococcal Disease*, ed. K. Cartwright, John Wiley and Sons.

8 I. M. Feavers **2001**, Meningococcal vaccines and vaccine developments, in *Meningococcal Vaccines: Methods and Protocols*, eds. A. J. Pollard, M. C. J. Maiden, Humana Press, Totowa, N.J.

9 E.A. Underwood **1940**, *Br. Med. J.* 1940 i, 757–763.

10 N.S. Ferry, A.H. Steele **1935**, *J. Am. Med. Assoc.* 104, 983–984.

11 D. Kuhns, P. Kisner, M.P. Williams, P.L. Moorman **1938**, *J. Am. Med. Assoc.* 110, 484–487.

12 I. Goldschneider, E.C. Gotschlich, M.S. Artenstein **1969**, *J. Exp. Med.* 129, 1307–1326.

13 I. Goldschneider, E.C. Gotschlich, M.S. Artenstein **1969**, *J. Exp. Med.* 129, 1327–1348.

14 E.C. Gotschlich, T.Y. Liu, M.S. Artenstein **1969**, *J. Exp. Med.* 129, 1349–1365.

15 E.C. Gotschlich, I. Goldschneider, M.S. Artenstein **1969**, *J. Exp. Med.* 129, 1367–1384.

16 M.S. Artenstein, R. Gold, J.G. Zimmerly, F.A. Wyle, H. Schneider, C. Harkins **1970**, *N. Engl. J. Med.* 282, 417–420.

17 R. Gold, M.S. Artenstein **1971**, *Bull. World Health Organ.* 45, 279–282.

18 P.H. Makela, H. Kayhty, P. Weckstrom, A. Sivonen, O.V. Renkonen **1975**, *Lancet* 2, 883–886.

19 J.T. Poolman, P.A. van der Ley, J. Tommassen **1995**, Surface structures and secreted products of meningococci, in *Meningococcal Disease*, ed. K. Cartwright, John Wiley, Chichester.

20 D.M. Granoff, I.M. Feavers, R. Borrow **2004**, Meningococcal vaccines, in *Vaccines*, eds. S.A. Plotkin, W.A. Orenstein, Saunders, Philadelphia.

21 K. Ahmad, *Lancet* **2004**, *363*, 1290.

22 J.J. Mond, A. Lees, C.M. Snapper **1995**, *Annu. Rev. Immunol.* 13, 655–692.

23 Q. Vos, A. Lees, Z.Q. Wu, C.M. Snapper, J.J. Mond **2000**, *Immunol. Rev.* 176, 154–170.

24 A. Weintraub **2003**, *Carbohydr. Res.* 338, 2539–2547.

25 E.A. Kabat, A.E. Bezer **1958**, *Arch. Biochem.* 78, 306–313.

26 F.S. Rosen **1989**, *Semin. Immunol.* 1, 87–91.

27 P.H. Makela, H. Kayhty **2002**, *Expert. Rev. Vaccines* 1, 399–410.

28 P.H. Makela **2003**, *Southeast Asian J. Trop. Med. Public Health* 34, 249–253.

29 D.C. Parker **1993**, *Annu. Rev. Immunol.* 11, 331–360.

30 J.B. Robbins, R. Schneerson, P. Anderson, D.H. Smith **1996**, *J. Am. Med. Assoc.* 276, 1181–1185.

31 E. Miller, D. Salisbury, M. Ramsay **2001**, *Vaccine* 20 [Suppl. 1], S58–S67.

32 M. Mitka **2005**, *J. Am. Med. Assoc.* 293, 1433–1434.

33 V. Verez-Bencomo, V. Fernandez-Santana, E. Hardy, M.E. Toledo, M.C. Rodriguez, L. Heynngnezz, A. Rodriguez, A. Baly, L. Herrera, M. Izquierdo, A. Villar, Y. Valdes, K. Cosme, M.L. Deler, M. Montane, E. Garcia, A. Ramos, A. Aguilar, E. Medina, G. Torano, I. Sosa, I. Hernandez, R. Martinez, A. Muzachio, A. Carmenates, L. Costa, F. Cardoso, C. Campa, M. Diaz, R. Roy **2004**, *Science* 305, 522–525.

34 A.A. Lindberg **1999**, *Vaccine* 17 [Suppl. 2], S28–S36.

35 M.R. Holliday, C. Jones **1999**, *Biologicals* 27, 51–53.

36 EDQM/European Pharmacopoeia Meeting **2000**, *Biologicals Beyond 2000, Challenges for Quality Standards in an Evolving Field*, European Department for the Quality of Medicines. Pharmeuropa BIO, Strasbourg.

37 F. Brown, M. Corbel, E. Griffiths **2000**, *Physico-chemical procedures for the characterization of vaccines*, Karger, Basel.

38 D.V. Madore, N. Strong, R. Eby **1999**, *Dev. Biol. Stand.* 101, 49–56.

39 X. Lemercinier, D. Crane, C. Gee, S. Austin, B. Bolgiano, C. Jones **1999**, *Dev. Biol. Stand.* 101, 177–183.

40 World Health Organization **2004**, Recommendations for the production and control of meningococcal group C conjugate vaccines (Technical report series, no. 924), World Health Organization, Geneva.

41 EDQM **2005**, Meningococcal group C conjugate vaccine, in *European Pharmacopoeia*, EDQM, Strasbourg.

42 P. Richmond, D. Goldblatt, P.C. Fusco, J.D. Fusco, I. Heron, S. Clark, R. Borrow, F. Michon **1999**, *Vaccine* 18, 641–646.

43 P. Richmond, R. Borrow, J. Findlow, S. Martin, C. Thornton, K. Cartwright, E. Miller **2001**, *Infect. Immun.* 69, 2378–2382.

44 K. Jumel, M.M. Ho, B. Bolgiano **2002**, *Biotechnol. Appl. Biochem.* 36, 219–226.
45 P. Costantino, F. Norelli, A. Giannozzi, S. D'Ascenzi, A. Bartoloni, S. Kaur, D. Tang, R. Seid, S. Viti, R. Paffetti, M. Bigio, C. Pennatini, G. Averani, V. Guarnieri, E. Gallo, N. Ravenscroft, C. Lazzeroni, R. Rappuoli, C. Ceccarini **1999**, *Vaccine* 17, 1251–1263.
46 N. Ravenscroft, G. Averani, A. Bartoloni, S. Berti, M. Bigio, V. Carinci, P. Costantino, S. D'Ascenzi, A. Giannozzi, F. Norelli, C. Pennatini, D. Proietti, C. Ceccarini, P. Cescutti **1999**, *Vaccine* 17, 2802–2816.
47 M. D. Snape, A. J. Pollard **2005**, *Lancet Infect. Dis.* 5, 21–30.
48 C. Jones, X. Lemercinier **2002**, *J. Pharm. Biomed. Anal.* 30, 1233–1247.
49 D.S. Berry, F. Lynn, C.H. Lee, C.E. Frasch, M.C. Bash **2002**, *Infect. Immun.* 70, 3707–3713.
50 A. Berkin, B. Coxon, V. Pozsgay **2002**, *Chemistry* 8, 4424–4433.
51 C.E. Frasch **1990**, *Adv. Biotechnol. Processes* 13, 123–145.
52 C. von Hunolstein, L. Parisi, D. Bottaro **2003**, *J. Biochem. Biophys. Methods* 56, 291–296.
53 E.C. Beuvery, K.A. vd, V. Kanhai, A.B. Leussink **1983**, *Vaccine* 1, 31–36.
54 E.C. Beuvery, F. Miedema, R.W. van Delft, J. Haverkamp, A.B. Leussink, B.J. te Pas, K.S. Teppema, R.H. Tiesjema **1983**, *Infect. Immun.* 40, 369–380.
55 G.T. Hermanson **1996**, *Bioconjugate Techniques*, Academic Press, San Diego.
56 Z. Jin, C. Chu, J.B. Robbins, R. Schneerson **2003**, *Infect. Immun.* 71, 5115–5120.
57 C.E. Frasch **2005**, *Expert. Opin. Biol. Ther.* 5, 273–280.
58 C.H. Lee, C.E. Frasch **2005**, Preparation of polysaccharide–protein conjugate for use as vaccines, *PCT Int. Appl.*
59 O. Cabrera, M. Cuello, C.R. Soto, M.E. Martinez, J.M. del Campo, O. Perez, J.F. Infanta, G. Sierra, G. **2005**, New method for obtaining conjugated vaccines, *Vaccine*, in press.
60 H.J. Jennings, C. Lugowski **1981**, *J. Immunol.* 127, 1011–1018.
61 P. Costantino, F. Berti, F. Norelli, A. Bartoloni **2003**, Modified saccharides having improved stability in water, *Patent* WO 03/080678 A1.
62 A. Giannozzi, G. Averani, F. Norelli, P. Costantino, P. **2004**, Modified saccharides and their protein conjugates, *Patent* WO 2004019992 A1
63 S. Oscarson **2001**, *Abstr. Nat. Meet. Am. Chem. Soc.* 222.
64 M.R. Lifely, A.S. Gilbert, C. Moreno **1981**, *Carbohydr. Res.* 94, 193–203.
65 J. Finne, M. Leinonen, P.H. Makela **1983**, *Lancet* 1983ii, 355–357.
66 H.J. Jennings, R. Roy, A. Gamian **1986**, *J. Immunol.* 137, 1708–1713.
67 R.A. Pon, M. Lussier, Q.L. Yang, H.J. Jennings **1997**, *J. Exp. Med.* 185, 1929–1938.
68 P.C. Fusco, F. Michon, J.Y. Tai, M.S. Blake **1997**, *J. Infect. Dis.* 175, 364–372.
69 X. Cai, Q.P. Lei, D.H. Lamb, A. Shannon, J. Jacoby, J. Kruk, R.D. Kensinger, R. Ryall, E. Zablackis, P. Cash **2004**, *Anal. Chem.* 76, 7387–7390.
70 A.K. Bhattacharjee, H.J. Jennings, C.P. Kenny, A. Martin, I.C.P. Smith **1975**, *J. Biol. Chem.* 250, 1926–1932.
71 EDQM **2005**, Meningococcal polysaccharide vaccine, in *European Pharmacopoeia*, EDQM, Strasbourg.
72 S.H. Doares, J.L. Cowell **2001**, *Abstr. Nat. Meet. Am. Chem. Soc.* 222.
73 F. Michon **2005**, Vaccines against group Y Neisseria meningitidis and meningococcal combinations thereof, *Patent.*
74 E. Longworth, P. Fernsten, T.L. Mininni, U. Vogel, H. Claus, S. Gray, E. Kaczmarski, R. Borrow **2002**, *FEMS Immunol. Med. Microbiol.* 32, 119–123.
75 C.E. Frasch, S. Kapre, S. Beri, D.M. Granoff, N. Bouveret, F.M. LaForce, C.H. Lee, **2004**, *Int. Pathog. Neisseria Conf.* 14.
76 A. Bardotti, G. Averani, F. Berti, S. Berti, C. Galli, S. Giannini, B. Fabbri, D. Proietti, N. Ravenscroft, S. Ricci **2005**, *Vaccine* 23, 1887–1899.
77 P. Costantino, S. Viti, A. Podda, M.A. Velmonte, L. Nencioni, R. Rappuoli **1992**, *Vaccine* 10, 691–698.
78 E.L. Anderson, T. Bowers, C.M. Mink, D.J. Kennedy, R.B. Belshe, H. Harakeh, L. Pais, P. Holder, G.M. Carlone **1994**, *Infect. Immun.* 62, 3391–3395.

79 G. Campagne, A. Garba, P. Fabre, A. Schuchat, R. Ryall, D. Boulanger, M. Bybel, G. Carlone, P. Briantais, B. Ivanoff, B. Xerri, J. P. Chippaux **2000**, *Pediatr. Infect. Dis. J.* 19, 144–150.

80 S.L. Harris, A. Finn, D.M. Granoff **2003**, *Infect. Immun.* 71, 3402–3408.

81 H. Joseph, R. Ryall, M. Bybel, T. Papa, J. Maclennan, J. Buttery, R. Borrow **2003**, *J. Infect. Dis.* 187, 1142–1146.

82 Aventis Pasteur **2005**, *Meningococcal (Groups A, C, Y and W-135) Polysaccharide Diphtheria Toxoid Conjugate Vaccine Menactra (Product Information)*, Aventis Pasteur, New York.

83 J.M. Griffiss, H. Schneider, R.E. Mandrell, R. Yamasaki, G.A. Jarvis, J.J. Kim, B.W. Gibson, R. Hamadeh, M.A. Apicella **1988**, *Rev. Infect. Dis* 10, S287–S295.

84 P. Brandtzaeg, A. Halstensen, P. Kierulf, T. Espevik, A. Waage **1992**, *Microb. Pathog.* 13, 423–431.

85 A.F.M. Verheul, H. Snippe, J.T. Poolman **1993**, *Microbiol. Rev.* 57, 34–45.

86 J.S. Plested, K. Makepeace, M.P. Jennings, M.A. Gidney, S. Lacelle, J. Brisson, A.D. Cox, A. Martin, A.G. Bird, C.M. Tang, F.M. Mackinnon, J.C. Richards, E.R. Moxon **1999**, *Infect. Immun.* 67, 5417–5426.

87 J.S. Plested, B.L. Ferry, P.A. Coull, K. Makepeace, A.K. Lehmann, F.G. Mackinnon, H.G. Griffiths, M.A. Herbert, J.C. Richards, E.R. Moxon **2001**, *Infect. Immun.* 69, 3203–3213.

88 E. Segerstedt, K. Mannerstyedt, M. Johansson, S. Oscarson **2004**, *J. Carbohydr. Chem.* 23, 443–452.

89 R. Biemans, P.A. Denoël, C. Feron, K.K. Goraj, M.P. Jennings, J. Poolman, V. Weynants **2004**, Meningococcal genetically engineered vaccine composition which has a fixed or locked lipooligosaccharide (LOS) immunotype, *Patent Int. Appl.* WO 2004015099.

90 T. Carmenate, M. Guirola, A. Alvarez, L. Canaan, S. Gonzalez, E. Caballero, T. Menendez, G. Guillen **2005**, *FEMS Immunol. Med. Microbiol.* 43, 133–140.

91 K. Baraldo, E. Mori, A. Bartoloni, R. Petracca, A. Giannozzi, F. Norelli, R. Rappuoli, G. Grandi, G. Del Giudice **2004**, *Infect. Immun.* 72, 4884–4887.

92 K.M. Reddin, A. Crowley-Luke, S.O. Clark, P.J. Vincent, A.R. Gorringe, M.J. Hudson, A. Robinson **2001**, *FEMS Immunol. Med. Microbiol.* 31, 153–162.

93 A. D'Ambra, F. Arnold, B.A. Clark, R.K. Coffman, S.K. Faust, J.S. Jacoby, J.R. Kruk, D.J.Pekala, M. Soika **2001**, *Abstr. Nat. Meet. Am. Chem. Soc.* 222.

94 M. Akkoyunlu, A. Melhus, C. Capiau, O. van Opstal, A. Forsgren **1997**, *Infect. Immun.* 65, 5010–5016.

95 A.W. Sturgess, K. Rush, R.J. Charbonneau, J.I. Lee, D.J. West, R.D. Sitrin, J.P. Hennessy, Jr. **1999**, *Vaccine* 17, 1169–1178.

96 L. Vernacchio, H. Bernstein, S. Pelton, C. Allen, K. MacDonald, J. Dunn, D. D. Duncan, G. Tsao, V. LaPosta, J. Eldridge, S. Laussucq, D.M. Ambrosino, D.C. Molrine **2002**, *Vaccine* 20, 3658–3667.

97 C.E. Frasch, C.H. Lee, J. Zhang **2003**, *Abstr. Am. Chem. Soc. Nat. Meet.* 225.

98 B.C. Baudner, O. Balland, M.M. Giuliani, P. Von Hoegen, R. Rappuoli, D. Betbeder, G. Del Giudice **2002**, *Infect. Immun.* 70, 4785–4790.

99 B.C. Baudner, M.M. Giuliani, J.C. Verhoef, R. Rappuoli, H.E. Junginger, G.D. Giudice **2003**, *Vaccine* 21, 3837–3844.

100 B.C. Baudner, M. Morandi, M.M. Giuliani, J.C. Verhoef, H.E. Junginger, P. Costantino, R. Rappuoli, G. Del Giudice **2004**, *J. Infect. Dis.* 189, 828–832.

101 J. Milstien, N. Dellepiane, S. Lambert, L. Belgharbi, C. Rolls, I. Knezevic, J. Fournier-Caruana, D. Wood, E. Griffiths **2002**, *Vaccine* 20, 1000–1003.

102 E. Griffiths, I. Knezevic **2003**, *Methods Mol. Med.* 87, 353–376.

103 B. Metz, C.F. Hendriksen, W. Jiskoot, G.F. Kersten **2002**, *Vaccine* 20, 2411–2430.

104 L. Jodar, E. Griffiths, I. Feavers **2004**, *Vaccine* 22, 1047–1053.

105 J. Suker, I.M. Feavers, M.J. Corbel, C. Jones, B. Bolgiano **2004**, *Expert. Rev. Vaccines* 3, 533–540.

106 C. Jones **2002**, *J. Pharm. Biomed. Anal.* 30, 1233–1247.

107 X. Lemercinier, C. Jones **1996**, *Carbohydr. Res.* 296, 83–96.
108 P.S. Chen, T.Y. Toribara, H. Warner **1956**, *Anal. Chem.* 28, 1756–1758.
109 L. Svennerholm **1957**, *Biochim. Biophys. Acta* 24, 604–611.
110 S. Hestrin **1949**, *J. Biol. Chem.* 180, 249–261.
111 S. Ricci, A. Bardotti, S. D'Ascenzi, N. Ravenscroft **2001**, *Vaccine* 19, 1989–1997.
112 G. Kao, C.M. Tsai **2004**, *Vaccine* 22, 335–344.
113 V.E. Turula, J. Kim, F. Michon, J. Pankratz, Y. Zhang, C. Yoo **2004**, *Anal. Biochem.* 327, 261–270.
114 D.H. Lamb, Q.P. Lei, N. Hakim, S. Rizzo, P. Cash **2005**, *Anal. Biochem.* 38, 263–269.
115 B. Bednar, J.P. Hennessey, Jr. **1993**, *Carbohydr. Res.* 243, 115–130.
116 N. Ravenscroft, S. D'Ascenzi, D. Proietti, F. Norelli, P. Costantino **2000**, *Dev. Biol.* 103, 35–47.
117 A. D'Ambra, J.E. Baugher, P.E. Concannon, R.A. Pon, F. Michon **1997**, *Anal. Biochem.* 250, 228–236.
118 C.L. Hsieh **2000**, *Dev. Biol.* 103, 93–104.
119 D.T. Crane, B. Bolgiano, C. Jones **1997**, *Eur. J. Biochem.* 246, 320–327.
120 A.B. Sasiak, B. Bolgiano, D.T. Crane, D.J. Hockley, M.J. Corbel, D. Sesardic **2000**, *Vaccine* 19, 694–705.
121 M.M. Ho, B. Bolgiano, M.J. Corbel **2000**, *Vaccine* 19, 716–725.
122 M.M. Ho, F. Mawas, B. Bolgiano, X. Lemercinier, D.T. Crane, R. Huskisson, M.J. Corbel **2002**, *Vaccine* 20, 3509–3522.
123 M.M. Ho, X. Lemercinier, B. Bolgiano, D. Crane, M.J. Corbel **2001**, *Biotechnol. Appl. Biochem.* 33, 91–98.
124 Q.P. Lei, A.G. Shannon, R.K. Heller, D.H. Lamb **2000**, *Dev. Biol.* 103, 259–264.
125 D.M. Katkocin **2000**, *Dev. Biol.* 103, 113–119.
126 C.J. Lee **2002**, *Biologicals* 30, 97–103.
127 J.M. MacLennan, F. Shackley, P.T. Heath, J.J. Deeks, C. Flamank, M. Herbert, H. Griffiths, E. Hatzmann, C. Goilav, E.R. Moxon **2000**, *J. Am. Med. Assoc.* 283, 2795–2801.
128 J.C. Bramley, T. Hall, A. Finn, R.B. Buttery, D. Elliman, S. Lockhart, R. Borrow, I.G. Jones **2001**, *Vaccine* 19, 2924–2931.
129 P. Richmond, R. Borrow, D. Goldblatt, J. Findlow, S. Martin, R. Morris, K. Cartwright, E. Miller **2001**, *J. Infect. Dis.* 183, 160–163.
130 R. Borrow, N. Andrews, D. Goldblatt, E. Miller **2001**, *Infect. Immun.* 69, 1568–1573.
131 J.D. Campbell, R. Edelman, J.C. King, Jr., T. Papa, R. Ryall, M.B. Rennels **2002**, *J. Infect. Dis.* 186, 1848–1851.
132 M. Pichichero, J. Casey, M. Blatter, E. Rothstein, R. Ryall, M. Bybel, G. Gilmet, T. Papa **2005**, *Pediatr. Infect. Dis. J.* 24, 57–62.
133 M. Rennels, J. King, Jr., R. Ryall, T. Papa, J. Froeschle **2004**, *Pediatr. Infect. Dis. J.* 23, 429–435.
134 C.M. Healy, C.J. Baker **2005**, *Pediatr. Infect. Dis. J.* 24, 175–176.
135 D.M. Granoff, S.L. Harris **2004**, *Pediatr. Infect. Dis. J.* 23, 490–497.
136 D.M. Granoff, A. Morgan, J.A. Welsch **2005**, *Vaccine*.
137 J. Bruge, N. Bouveret-Le Cam, B. Danve, G. Rougon, D. Schulz **2004**, *Vaccine* 22, 1087–1096.
138 P. Richmond, R. Borrow, E. Miller, S. Clark, F. Sadler, A. Fox, N. Begg, R. Morris, K. Cartwright **1999**, *J. Infect. Dis.* 179, 1569–1572.
139 C.L. Trotter, N.J. Andrews, E.B. Kaczmarski, E. Miller, M.E. Ramsay **2004**, *Lancet* 364, 365–367.
140 R. Borrow, D. Goldblatt, N. Andrews, J. Southern, L. Ashton, S. Deane, R. Morris, K. Cartwright, E. Miller **2002**, *J. Infect. Dis.* 186, 1353–1357.
141 N.E. MacDonald, S.A. Halperin, B.J. Law, B. Forrest, L.E. Danzig, D.M. Granoff **1998**, *J. Am. Med. Assoc.* 280, 1685–1689.
142 R. Borrow, A.J. Fox, P. Richmond, S. Clark, F. Sadler, J. Findlow, R. Morris, N.T. Begg, K.A. Cartwright **2000**, *Epidemiol. Infect.* 124, 427–432.
143 D.M. Granoff, A. Morgan, J.A. Welsch **2005**, *Pediatr. Infect. Dis. J.* 24, 132–136.
144 C.P. Farrington **1993**, *Int. J. Epidemiol.* 22, 742–746.

145 M.E. Ramsay, N. Andrews, E.B. Kaczmarski, E. Miller **2001**, *Lancet* 357, 195–196.

146 P. Balmer, M. Falconer, P. McDonald, N. Andrews, E. Fuller, C. Riley, E. Kaczmarski, R. Borrow **2004**, *Infect. Immun.* 72, 332–337.

147 O.O. Bilukha, N. Rosenstein **2005**, *Morbid. Mortal. Wkly Rep. Recomm. Rep.* 54, 1–21.

148 M.H. Slack, D. Schapira, R.J. Thwaites, M. Burrage, J. Southern, N. Andrews, R. Borrow, D. Goldblatt, E. Miller **2001**, *J. Infect. Dis.* 184, 1617–1620.

149 P. Richmond, E. Kaczmarski, R. Borrow, J. Findlow, S. Clark, R. McCann, J. Hill, M. Barker, E. Miller **2000**, *J. Infect. Dis.* 181, 761–764.

150 R. Borrow, J. Southern, N. Andrews, N. Peake, R. Rahim, M. Acuna, S. Martin, E. Miller, E. Kaczmarski **2001**, *Vaccine* 19, 3043–3050.

151 D.M. Granoff, R.K. Gupta, R.B. Belshe, E.L. Anderson **1998**, *J. Infect. Dis.* 178, 870–874.

152 A. Leach, P.A. Twumasi, S. Kumah, W.S. Banya, S. Jaffar, B.D. Forrest, D.M. Granoff, D.E. Libutti, G.M. Carlone, L.B. Pais, C.V. Broome, B.M. Greenwood **1997**, *J. Infect. Dis.* 175, 200–204.

153 J. Maclennan, S. Obaro, J. Deeks, D. Williams, L. Pais, G. Carlone, R. Moxon, B. Greenwood **1999**, *Vaccine* 17, 3086–3093.

154 R. Borrow, H. Joseph, N. Andrews, M. Acuna, E. Longworth, S. Martin, N. Peake, R. Rahim, P. Richmond, E. Kaczmarski, E. Miller **2000**, *Vaccine* 19, 1129–1132.

155 M.E. Ramsay, N.J. Andrews, C.L. Trotter, E.B. Kaczmarski, E. Miller **2003**, *Br. Med. J.* 326, 365–366.

156 R. Gold, I. Goldschneider, M.L. Lepow, T.F. Draper, M. Randolph **1978**, *J. Infect. Dis.* 137, 112–121.

157 M.C. Maiden, J.M. Stuart **2002**, *Lancet* 359, 1829–1831.

158 M.C.J. Maiden, A.-B. Ibarz-Pavon, R. Urwin, J.M. MacLennan, J.S.Bennet, J.C. Bramley, J.M. Stuart, Meningococcal Carriage Group **2004**, *Int. Pathog. Neisseria Conf.* 14.

159 J. Wenger **2001**, *Vaccine* 19, 1588–1591.

160 L. Jodar, F.M. LaForce, C. Ceccarini, T. Aguado, D.M. Granoff **2003**, *Lancet* 361, 1902–1904.

161 L. Jodar, I.M. Feavers, D. Salisbury, D. M. Granoff **2002**, *Lancet* 359, 1499–1508.

162 M.C. Maiden, B.G. Spratt **1999**, *Lancet* 354, 615–616.

18
Outer Membrane Vesicle-based Meningococcal Vaccines

Jan T. Poolman, Philippe Denoël, Christiane Feron, Karine Goraj and Vincent Weynants

18.1
Introduction

The availability of *H. influenzae* type b (Hib), meningococcal serogroup C (MenC), meningococcal serogroup A, C, W_{135} and Y (MenACWY) and multivalent pneumococcal conjugate vaccines will soon make serogroup B meningococci the remaining major cause of bacterial meningitis. The first candidate for a MenB vaccine is the capsular polysaccharide. Although the polysaccharide itself is not very immunogenic, attempts have been made to improve its immunogenicity via conjugation and/or chemical alteration [1]. However, clinical immunogenicity has demonstrated that no or low serum bactericidal antibodies (in the presence of human complement) can be induced with such improved capsular polysaccharide [2, 3] (H. J. Jennings, personal communication).

Serum bactericidal activity is the pivotal protective mechanism against invasive meningococcal (and invasive gonococcal) infectious diseases [4]. This is clearly demonstrated by the extreme susceptibility of late complement component (C6, C7, C8) deficient individuals who specifically suffer from recurrent invasive meningococcal (and gonococcal) infectious diseases [5]. Meningococcal sialic acid containing capsular polysaccharides (serogroups B, C, W, Y) protect the bacteria from complement attack (serum resistance) [6]. Sialylated lipopolysacharide (LPS) contributes to serum resistance [7]. Gonococci lacking a polysialic acid capsule have developed even further mechanisms of serum resistance, such as expression of complement-binding outer membrane proteins (OMP), but it also seems that gonococcal LPS reaches a higher level of sialylation [7]. Gonococci (and probably meningococci) are resistant to opsonophagocytotic killing mechanisms, which explains the extreme susceptibility of individuals with late complement component deficiency [8].

The meningococcal group B capsular polysaccharide (BPS) seems particularly capable to interact specifically with human complement in order to downregulate serum killing activity [9]. Animal complement in the presence of low avidity human antiBPS leads to strong bactericidal activity, whilst the use of human

Handbook of Meningococcal Disease. Infection Biology, Vaccination, Clinical Management.
Edited by M. Frosch and M. C. J. Maiden

ISBN: 3-527-31260-9

complement results in no or low activity [3]. This illustrates the pivotal role of BPS as a virulence factor and efforts are continuing to render this structure immunogenic [10, 11].

Alternative vaccine candidates have been sought since the early 1970s and research has been focussed on major OMPs and LPS [12–14]. The porin PorA and LPS came out as key candidate components [15] and optimization efforts to render these components strongly immunogenic are still ongoing [16, 17]. It became evident that: (a) PorA and LPS reveal significant heterogeneity amongst group B meningococci [18] and (b) the appropriate bactericidal immune responses can best be induced by using the natural outer membrane environment as a delivery vehicle [19]. Group B meningococci are subdivided into PorB:PorA:LPS typing systems, leading to the B:4:P1.15:L3 (example) nomenclature which is now in common use [18]. It was found possible to extract the outer membrane from the bacteria or culture supernatant in the form of outer membrane vesicles (OMV).

OMV vaccines have been developed by using detergent extraction mostly by deoxycholate (DOC) to reduce the LPS (endotoxin) content and hence the local and systemic reactogenicity [19]. In addition to OMV-based vaccine development, activities on subunit development have been initiated, which include OMP and LPS. LPS conjugate vaccine development is an active research area [20]. A few new OMP candidates were recently discovered via the availability of full genomic sequences [21, 22]. Announcements were made that the genomic work "within 18 months of the beginning of the sequencing of meningococcus B far surpassed 40 years of conventional vaccine work" [23]. The conventional vaccine work started approximately 30 years ago and will be discussed below. For the vaccine value of the genomic work, it is too early to come to meaningful conclusions.

The process development of OMV vaccines was described in detail recently [19]. A short schedule of the process is given in Fig. 18.1.

OMV vaccines made from single epidemic strains have been applied during two placebo-controlled efficacy studies, one conducted in Norway and one in Cuba [24, 25], both in teenagers. The efficacy with a 4:P1.15 OMV in Cuba (16-month follow-up) was found to be 83%. In Norway with a 15:P1.16 OMV, the efficacy was found to be 57% after a 29-month follow-up but was 87% after a 10-month observation period [24]. These studies were performed using a two-dose immunization schedule; and a third immunization dose resulted in an increased level and persistence of the antibody response [26]. Therefore, it seems feasible to induce a high level of protection with homologous OMV vaccines in teenagers, whereby a three-dose schedule is preferable, with a reasonable interval for the third dose. This principle could be developed further into bivalent or higher valency OMV vaccines. A hexavalent PorA-OMV vaccine has been developed and found to induce relevant bactericidal antibody levels in infants [17].

Two case-control studies have been performed in Brazil with the Cuban 4:P1.15 OMV vaccine in partly heterologous endemic settings [27, 28]. Both studies demonstrated an efficacy of approximately 70% in >4 year olds and little

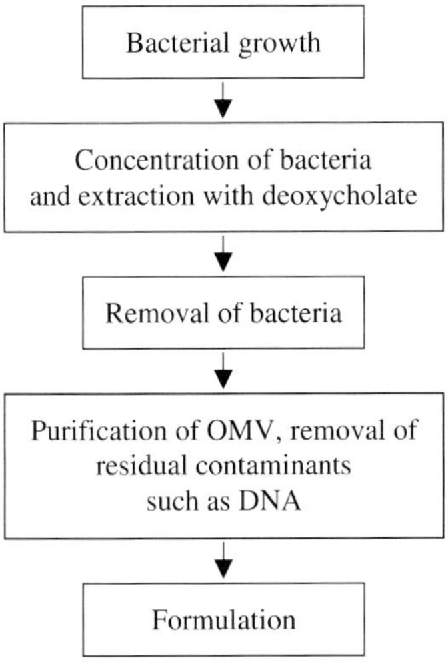

Fig. 18.1 OMV manufacturing process.

or no efficacy in <4 year olds after a two-dose immunization schedule and a 12-month follow-up period. The cross-protective efficacy/activity is related to the observed cross-bactericidal activity (see Table 18.1) [29]. The in vitro serum bactericidal activity (SBA) levels appear to underestimate the observed clinical efficacy after two doses of the Cuban OMV vaccines. SBA responses can be detected in 27–42% of subjects against the heterologous strains and in 53% against the homologous strain.

It is interesting to note that similar levels of cross-bactericidal activity can be observed in 2–4 year olds after three doses as compared to 17–30 year olds after two doses. Continuous efforts are being undertaken to develop even stronger cross-reactive vaccines, which can possibly be achieved via adapted OMVs, subunit OMP, subunit LPS and/or improved BPS. This chapter on OMV vaccines will further review the OMP and LPS literature and describe the development of recombinant technology to adapt OMV vaccines, process development and preclinical experiments.

Table 18.1 Serum bactericidal activity (SBA) response after OMV immunization.

Age group	SBA responders (%)					
	B:4:P1.15 homologous		B:15P:P1.16 heterologous		B:15:P1.3 heterologous	
	2-dose	3-dose	2-dose	3-dose	2-dose	3-dose
<1 year	56	90	16	31	2	10
2–4 years	38	78	22	41	14	31
17–30 years	53	67	42	56	27	37

18.2
Candidate Protein and LPS Immunogens

Various research groups have focussed most of their work on noncapsular surface antigens of *N. meningitidis* B. The outcome of this research has resulted into the recognition of three categories of candidate antigens:

1. Major OMPs. These have a high surface density; and they were found to be antigenically diverse/variable.
2. Minor OMPs. These can be conserved but not much proof exists about functional, bactericidal activity in relation to antibodies induced by infection and/or immunization in preclinical experiments.
3. LPS. The antigenic variability appears to be limited, but the immunogenicity is poor; and the molecule was shown to be toxic (lipid A).

18.2.1
Major OMPs

The porins (PorA and PorB) are the most abundant OMPs in the pathogenic *Neisseria* species. These trimeric β-barrel structured proteins function as pores for the exchange of ions and small molecules. In meningococci, they are named class 1 (Por A) and either class 2 or class 3 (PorB; mutually exclusive alleles) [18]. These porins are essential for bacterial survival, although PorA minus strains exist naturally and PorB mutant strains can be constructed.

PorB has the ability to activate B-cells via a TLR-2-dependent mechanism [30]. PorB is also an important target of the antibody response to *Neisseria* but the protective potential of antiPorB antibodies has been controversial [31]. It seems that anticlass 2 porB antibodies can be more protective as compared to anticlass 3 [15].

Bactericidal antibodies to PorA play an important role in protection against meningitis and sepsis caused by meningococci [15]. However, the antiPorA bactericidal antibodies are directed against the two longest external variable loops (loops 1, 4) of the protein [32] which indicate that the antiPorA protective immune response is serosubtype-specific. The number of serosubtypes is limited within a given geographical region but varies more extensively on a global basis.

18.2.2
The Opacity-associated Proteins

Opacity-associated (Opa) proteins are outer membrane proteins which play a critical role in the adhesion of pathogenic *Neisseria* spp to epithelial and endothelial cells and polymorphonuclear neutrophils. The adherence is mainly mediated by the CD66 epitope-containing members of the carcinoembryonic antigen family of human cell adhesion molecules (CEACAM) [33, 34]. Despite a high overall level of conservation, the immunodominant, surface-exposed regions of Opa proteins display sequence and antigenic variability as well as functional diversification among Opa variants. Up to 11 distinct Opa proteins are encoded in unlinked chromosomal loci in gonococci; and up to four can be expressed in the meningococci. Each variant locus is subject to phase variation, resulting in a heterogeneous population of bacteria expressing none, one or several Opa proteins [35].

18.2.3
Iron-restricted Proteins

Iron acquisition by *Neisseria* has been reviewed by Schryvers and Stojiljkovic [36]. Several proteins and receptors ensure availability of this essential element to *Neisseria*.

The FrpB protein (also named FetA) from *Neisseria* is an iron-regulated OMP that shows the characteristics of a TonB-dependent receptor. It has a molecular mass of around 77 kDa [37]. Although this protein is the target of bactericidal antibodies, it has been found that the variability of surface exposed regions prevents cross-reactivity of antibodies between strains [38]. Nevertheless, it was recently proposed that an OMP-based vaccine with as few as six PorA and five FrpB variant sequences could induce a protective immune response against most circulating *Neisseria* isolates [39].

In *N. meningitidis*, the transferrin receptor is composed of two proteins (Tbp1 and 2 or TbpA and B) of 95 kDa and 68–85 KDa depending on the strain [40]. Mutants defective in the synthesis of either TbpA or TbpB, but not defective in both, can bind transferrin, indicating that both proteins function in transferrin binding [41]. Tbp1 (TbpA) is produced as a precursor with a conventional secretion sequence and displays features of integral OMP. Tbp2 (TbpB) contains a 20-amino-acid sequence whose cleavage follows a lipidation step typical of lipoproteins [42]. The binding to transferrin by this receptor has been studied in detail and binding sites have been proposed [43–47].

Two major families of transferrin receptors have been identified among *N. meningitidis* strains, based on the reactivity of antiTbpB antibodies and gene sequence [48]. Both families share sequence similarities but differ substantially in size. TbpBs of family I have a molecular mass of around 68 kDa, whereas family II proteins are characterized by a molecular mass of 80–90 kDa. The genetic analysis of a collection of diverse *N. meningitidis* strains reveals that bacteria harboring a family II TbpB are more frequently found (82%) than family I-containing strains [49].

Sera from healthy individuals, asymtomatic carriers and cases of meningococcal diseases have been studied to determine the presence of antiTbp antibodies. Sera from carriers and cases of meningococcal diseases, but not from controls, had detectable antibodies to Tbp suggesting expression of Tbp by *Neisseria in vivo* [50].

Recombinant expression of TbpA has been achieved in *E. coli* and transferrin-binding activity has been demonstrated [51]. Also, affinity-isolated Tbps from *N. meningitidis* were found to induced protection against challenge in mice after passive or active immunization. Moreover, antiTbp-specific serum has been shown to be bactericidal against approximately 50% of the N. meningitidis strains tested [52, 53].

The safety and immunogenicity of TbpB has been evaluated in a phase I clinical trial. The recombinant lipoprotein purified from E. coli was used in a vaccine which was shown to be safe and immunogenic, although the bactericidal antibody levels induced were disappointing [54].

The main entry site of N. meningitidis into the human body is the nasopharynx, where lactoferrin is probably the main iron source [55]. Utilization of iron from lactoferrin involves a lactoferrin receptor composed of two proteins, Lbp1 and 2 (LbpA and B). Using an affinity isolation procedure, a single lactoferrin-binding protein was identified originally [56]. The structural gene for this protein, designated LbpA, has been characterized [57, 58] and a topology model for the protein in the outer membrane has been proposed [59]. The protein showed a high degree of similarity to TbpA. Part of an open reading frame was identified upstream of the lbpA gene; and the deduced amino acid sequence showed homology to TbpB [60]. This second protein (LbpB) has been identified and characterized [61, 62]. Variability in LbpB sequence (mostly in two regions) has been reported [63]. Moreover, it has been shown that LbpA does not induce a broadly cross-reactive antibody response in humans upon Neisseria infection, although the variability of LbpA is limited [64].

18.2.4
PilQ

Neisseria meningitidis expresses surface appendages called type IV pili. These pili confer adhesive properties and are known to mediate attachment to epithelial cells during host colonization. Moreover, type IV pili are involved in cellular agglutination [65], twitching motility [66] and DNA uptake [68]. PilQ is the only component of the type IV pilus that consists of an integral OMP. PilQ forms a complex that plays an essential role in pilus translocation across the outer membrane [67]. The gene product is essential for the biogenesis of type IV pili in N. gonorrhoeae [68]. The structure of the PilQ complex was recently elucidated, revealing that the complex is a homodecamer with a large central chamber that may not only allow translocation of the pilus through the outer membrane but could be also involved in pilus assembly [69–71]. The PilQ protein of N. gonorrhoeae, originally named Omc or OMP-macromolecular complex (OMP-MC) [72, 73], has been shown to be immunogenic in humans; and antibodies to this protein turned out to promote complement-mediated bactericidal killing of homologous and heterologous N. gonorrhoae strains [74]. Antibodies to OMP-MC are bactericidal for serum-resistant gonococci. More recently, native PilQ complexes from outer membranes of N. meningitidis and N. lactamica have been shown to induce protection against bacteremic meningococcal disease in a mouse model as well as the production of bactericidal and opsonic antibodies in mice [75].

18.2.5
OMP85

Using an antiserum raised against isolated gonococcal outer membranes to screen a *Neisseria* genomic library, the gene encoding OMP85 has been identified and was found to be similar to *H. influenzae* D15 and *P. multocida* Omp 87 [76, 77]. This protein is a minor antigen present in outer membrane vesicles of *N. meningitidis* [78]. The role of Omp85, which is highly conserved in all gram-negative bacteria [79], has been studied. This protein seems to have a function in the positioning and folding of other outer membrane proteins into the bacterial outer membrane [80–82]. However, it has also been proposed that OMP85 could play a role in lipid transport to the outer membrane [83].

18.2.6
Minor OMPs

Using classic immunological approaches, several research groups have identified minor surface-exposed proteins that are potential vaccine candidates.

18.2.7
Adhesins

An adhesion and penetration protein (App) [84] homologous to the *H. influenzae* Hap protein has been identified. This protein is highly conserved; and recombinant App has been shown to induce antibodies that cross-react with a panel of MenB strains. Recombinant expression in *E. coli* showed that App is expressed on the surface and autoprocessed by an endogenous serine protease activity which releases the passenger domain in the supernatant. App mediates adhesion to host cells [85].

A homologous protein to *H. influenzae* Hsf/Hia has been identified in *Neisseria*, referred to as Hsf. Hsf (or NhhA) has a structure that is common to autotransporter proteins [86]. Moreover, it has been proposed that a sequence motif present in this protein would mediate adhesion by mimicking a cell-recognition mechanism of the N-CAM proteins [87]. Western blot studies conducted with sera from patients or healthy carriers showed that at least one of the two autotransporter proteins Hap or Hsf was detected by these sera. This finding supports the wide distribution of Hap and Hsf amongst *Neisseria* circulating strains as well as their inclusion in a *N. meningitidis* vaccine [88].

Neisseria surface protein A (NspA) is the target of bactericidal antibodies and is present on the surface of 99% of the strains tested. Immunization of mice with NspA resulted in protection against *N. meningitidis* challenge [89]. The folding of this protein seems relevant as studies have demonstrated that an NspA-based vaccine prepared from OMV was more potent than the recombinant protein vaccine [90]. This makes NspA an interesting candidate for expression in an OMV vaccine. However, the accessibility of this protein could be reduced in strains with a strong expression of the capsular polysaccharide B resulting in resistance to serum bactericidal activity mediated by antiNspA [91]. In a lethal infant rat model, it has been suggested that NspA is not an essential virulence factor [92]. The crystal structure of NspA has now been published and will help in the design of new NspA-based vaccines [93].

18.2.8
Other Antigens

A study of sera from healthy volunteers and convalescent patients showed an interesting correlation between serum bactericidal activity and reaction of the serum against one of two high molecular weight proteins (162 kDa, 138 kDa). These two proteins induced bactericidal antibodies upon immunization of mice [94]. No further identification of these proteins has been reported yet.

lpdA encodes a 64-kDa protein named P64k which has been described as a dihydrolipoamide dehydrogenase [95]. P64k is well recognized by sera from patients convalescent after meningococcal disease or from vaccinees immunized with VA-MENGOC-BC. It has been suggested that this protein could be used as a carrier for serogroup C polysaccharide in the production of a conjugate vaccine that would protect against MenB and MenC disease [96]. The safety and immunogenicity of this protein has been evaluated in healthy volunteers but no SBA data have been reported [97].

18.2.9
In Silico Identified Antigens

Minor conserved proteins can be identified by *in silico* genome mining. The availability of the complete genome sequences of one serogroup A strain [98] and one serogroup B strain [99] provides a great opportunity for the identification of such proteins.

Our genome-mining effort started before the release of complete serogroup A, B and C meningococcal genome sequences (strain FAM 18, The Wellcome Trust Sanger Institute). The private genome of MenB ATCC13090 was primarily used as a template to search for vaccine candidate antigens. Using a combination of public and proprietary algorithms, MenB open reading frames (ORFs) were delineated and genes likely to encode surface-exposed proteins, such as sec-dependent secretion, integral outer membrane proteins and/or lipoproteins signatures, were selected. The following categories of MenB antigens were considered for vaccine development:
– high molecular weight adhesins
– piliation-related proteins/secretins
– iron-regulated proteins
– low molecular weight adhesins
– lipoproteins.

A total of ~100 candidate genes were selected for further characterization. At that stage, sequence variability was assessed by direct DNA sequencing or restriction fragment length polymorphism mapping in a subset of ten representative N. meningitidis strains. Genes likely to undergo phase variation, genes absent from some meningococcal strains as well as genes sharing less than 80% of sequence conservation were discarded. Approximately 50 genes were then selected for recombinant expression in E. coli. A similar approach has been followed by our colleagues at Chiron Vaccines [100] which has resulted in the identification of a number of vaccine candidates. We refer to Chapter 19 for a detailed description of genome derived vaccine antigens (see also [101–110]).

18.2.10
Lipopolysaccharide

The LPS of N. meningitidis is immunogenic in infants and children [111, 112]. The Norwegian serogroup B OMV vaccine induces antiLPS antibodies in humans [25]. After intranasal immunization with native OMV, most of the bactericidal antibodies are directed against PorA but also LPS [113]. Meningococcal LPS consists of a single oligosaccharide unit attached to the Heptose I of the inner core di-heptose backbone which is linked to two 2-keto-2-deoxyoctulosonic acid residues and anchored in the outer membrane by lipid A. Substitutions such as phosphoethanolamine and glucose at the heptose II also play a crucial role for antigenic specificity. LPS is highly variable and 12 distinct immunotypes can be identified [114]. Despite this relatively high variability, LPS has been proposed as a vaccine candidate but the presence of endotoxin lipid A and sialylated sugars on some immunotypes that mimic human antigens have raised concerns about its safety [115, 116]. Even if the inclusion of LPS in OMV clearly reduces its toxicity [117], the use of detergent during the process is required to reduce the LPS content. Approaches using genetic engineering allow a reduction in the endotoxic activity of lipid A by alteration of its acylation patterns [118]. Nevertheless, adjuvantation seems to be required due to a reduction of the immunogenicity of "detoxified" OMV [119]. In addition to the inter-strain immunotype variation, individual N. meningitidis strains exhibit extensive phase variation of the "outer core" LPS [120, 121]. The inner core is more conserved [122], with its biosynthetic genes lacking the homopolymeric tracts responsible of the phase variation of the outer core LPS [123]. The fact that the inner core is less variable than the outer core but accessible to antibodies, as demonstrated by the presence of antibodies in convalescent sera [124], makes the inner core LPS a potential vaccine candidate. Opsonic activity of inner core antibodies has been demonstrated [125]. However, the protection induced by anti-inner core antibodies seems to correlate with the expression of truncated glycoforms on the target strains [126].

Development of Adapted OMV Vaccines

Besides immunodominant and variable OMPs, such as PorA, Opas and Opc, the minor and conserved OMV proteins may induce cross-protective immune responses. It is expected that addition/upregulation/modification of key antigens in OMVs may provide an improved vaccine against *Men*B.

The publication of several *Neisseria* genomes highlighted the high intrinsic plasticity [127] of the bacterium via mechanisms such as phase variation [128], recombination [129, 130] and repeated sequences (e.g. Correia, IS, RS). The findings support the use of conserved antigens to overcome this intrinsic variability. Moreover, as detailed above, the availability of complete neisserial genome sequences has facilitated the identification of potential conserved and surface-exposed vaccine candidates involved in the metabolism of iron uptake [131], virulence [132], toxicity [133] and adhesion [86, 106].

18.3.1
Upregulation of Minor Conserved Proteins

18.3.1.1 Recombinant Technologies

Homologous Recombination Genetic methods are available to engineer chromosomal modifications, leading to the overexpression of selected proteins in neisserial OMVs. Vectors allowing homologous recombination and stable integration of genes, promoters, regulation elements, operons and/or expression cassettes in the genome of *N. meningitidis* have all been constructed at GlaxoSmithKline Biologicals. Based on the same features, pNLE1 v

Fig. 18.2 Upregulation of OMP85, Hsf and NspA expression in MenB OMVs by homologous recombination. OMVs purified from different strains were separated by SDS-PAGE and stained with Coomassie brillant blue R250. The strains used are: wild-type strain H44/76 (lanes 1, 5), H44/76 PorA knockout (KO; lane 2), H44/76 PorA KO, OMP85 upregulated (lane 3), H44/76 PorA KO, Hsf upregulated (lane 4) and H44/76 PorA KO, NspA upregulated (lane 6).

1. The gene delivery strategy consists in integration of a second copy of the gene of interest into the meningococcal B chromosome, placed under the control of a strong promoter.
2. The promoter replacement approach consists in delivering a strong promoter upstream from the native chromosomal sequence encoding the gene of interest [135].

In the examples proposed in Fig. 18.2, the overexpression of the genes coding for Omp85 [78, 136], Hsf/NhhA [87] and NspA [137] was realized via the strong PorA promoter.

Replicative Plasmids A limited number of plasmids replicating in *Neisseria* are available and have been used to overexpress the genes of interest. pFP10-derived plasmids [138] allow the overexpression of genes of interest under the control of the strong T7 promoter. pHT128-derived plasmids [139] utilize the Tac promoter. The advantages of both approaches are that more than one copy of the gene of interest is present in the bacterium and the overexpression is IPTG-inducible. However, such plasmids are relatively unstable. They are rapidly lost in the absence of the selection pressure, or integrated in the chromosome via homologous recombination. To avoid this latter problem, strains deleted in the corresponding gene have to be generated before plasmid transformation.

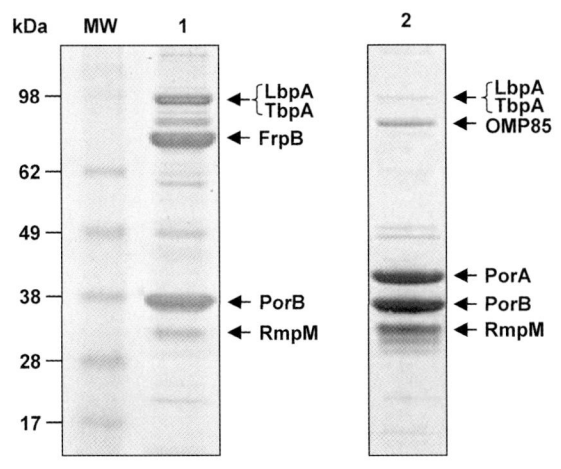

Fig. 18.3 Upregulation of iron-regulated proteins in *Men*B OMVs by culture in the presence of 25 μM Desferal. Purified OMVs were separated by SDS-PAGE and stained with Coomassie brillant blue R250. MW: molecular weight markers; lane 1: Iron depletion (PorA-strain); lane 2: wild type H44/76 blebs.

18.3.1.2 Iron Limitation Culture Conditions

Iron is limiting in the human host and bacterial pathogens respond to this environment by activating genes required for bacterial virulence. Such genes could be important vaccine targets. Using DNA microarray technology [140], the entire gene repertoire of *N. meningitidis* MC58 in response to iron was defined. Culture of *Neisseria* in iron depletion conditions has been used to overexpress iron-regulated proteins, such as LbpA [60], TbpA and FrpB [38], without any genetic modification. In the example presented in Fig. 18.3, several OMPs were upregulated in *Neisseria* grown in culture medium in the presence of 25 μM Desferal.

18.3.2
Downregulation of Major Immunodominant Proteins

Genes coding for strain-specific, variable antigens can be deleted in order to redirect the immune response to conserved, upregulated, minor components. Amongst those immunodominant and hypervariable antigens, PorA was successfully deleted from the chromosome by homologous recombination. Opc and Opa proteins of *Neisseria meningitidis* could also divert the immune system from minor conserved proteins. Their expression is phase variable [141]. Opc phase variation is the result of transcriptional regulation. The gene can easily be deleted by homologous recombination. Eventually, minus variants can be selected and used as recipient strain for recombinant OMV production. Opas exhibit translational phase variation via addition or deletion of repetitive coding repeat units within the DNA encoding the protein leader sequence. Four different genes coding for Opa proteins are known in N. meningitidis [142, 143]. Deletion of all four genes is fastidious and can be avoided by the selection of strains expressing naturally low levels of Opa [144].

In summary, combination of: (a) homologous recombination (to up- and downregulate the expression of target antigens), (b) selection of naturally low Opa and Opc Neisseria strains and (c) culture in iron depletion conditions, may allow the engineering of recombinant N. meningitidis strains presenting higher amounts of minor, conserved antigens at their surface and a low level of immunodominant but variable proteins.

18.4
Process for MenB OMV

Membrane blebs (or OMV), naturally formed by meningococcal cells during growth, contain mainly large amounts of outer membrane proteins, 25–50% of LOS and capsular B polysaccharide. The OMV purification concept is very simple: after culture inactivation by either phenol or detergent treatment, OMVs can be easily separated from cells by low-speed centrifugation and concentrated by ultracentrifugation. The B polysaccharide is depolymerized by neuraminidase treatment and eliminated during the subsequent purification of blebs. The LPS content can be reduced to about 5% by effective detergent treatment using DOC. DOC is added either directly to the resuspended cells (or broth), or to the extracted outer membranes. DOC-treated membranes are stabilized by the addition of sucrose (conventionally about 3%) in order to prevent aggregation during and after the purification procedure.

Several methods for producing LPS-depleted OMV have been published and reviewed by Frasch [19]. Wild-type OMVs produced by this method contain the major class 1, 2 or 3 proteins (porins), some minor high molecular weight components and, relative to protein, 5–9% of LPS [145]. The resulting OMV composition can be modulated. It has been demonstrated by several groups that N. meningitidis growing under iron restriction can induce expression of specific OMPs with an apparent molecular mass of 70–100 kDa [146–149]. These "enriched OMV" could maximize vaccine coverage.

Multivalent PorA strains (without expression of PorB and capsular polysaccharide) can also be produced using the conventional detergent extraction [150]. However, detergent-treated OMV could readily aggregate when pelleted by centrifugation. A way to prevent this aggregation is to apply other methods for OMV concentration/purification. Ultrafiltration and tangential flow filtration could help to concentrate OMV in suspension. Size exclusion chromatography is an effective method to purify OMV and eliminate membrane debris. A production method combining this type of alternative techniques was published recently [19].

As an alternative to the purification of LPS-depleted OMV, native OMV (NOMV) can be purified without any exposure to detergent [151]. At the Walter

Reed Army Institute of Research, methods for producing NOMV have been applied, in which the conventional ultracentrifugation steps were replaced by batchwise adsorption onto a DEAE ion exchange matrix, followed by an ultrafiltration step [152]. The soluble proteins, residual nucleic acid and soluble capsular polysaccharide pass through the membrane while vesicles are retained and can be easily concentrated. Time and cost of large-scale processes are decreased with these improvements.

In conclusion, several methods using genetically modified strains or particular culture conditions exist for the production of OMV, with the selected alternative depending on the OMV composition. Regarding the quality control (QC) of OMV vaccine production, no official guidelines have yet been published. Some clues are given by Frasch and coworkers [19] who describe quality data, including an example flow sheet with QC sampling points, QC methods and a proposal for specifications. The development of QC tests is crucial to assess the manufacturing robustness and consistency through the antigen content and purity, to evaluate OMV reactogenicity and to demonstrate OMV potency.

18.5
The Upregulation of Vaccine Candidates in OMV: Immunogenicity Data

The NhhA auto-transporter protein, homologous to the Hia/Hsf protein of *H. influenzae*, forms a multimeric complex and is expressed during infection and colonization [87]. Upregulation of NhhA by gene delivery enhances the immune response against this adhesin in mice immunized with upregulated blebs (Table 18.2). Indeed, mice immunized with control OMVs did not produce a detectable ELISA response against NhhA, while mice immunized with OMVs containing upregulated NhhA were shown to produce high levels of antiNhhA antibodies. A second example of upregulation by gene delivery technology is illustrated with NspA. The function of NspA is unknown but when properly folded this conserved membrane protein elicits protective antibody responses [153]. Presentation of NspA in OMVs avoids the potential issues linked to the folding of purified recombinant protein. Again, mice immunized with OMVs harboring high levels of NspA induce an immune response against NspA, as measured by ELISA, whilst no antiNspA antibodies are detected in mice immunized with the control blebs (Table 18.2). It was recently reported that the heterologous expression of NspA in commensal *Neisseriae* allows the production of OMVs which can induce a protective response in mice against lethal intraperitoneal challenge with *N. meningitidis* B [154]. This illustrates the correct folding of NspA when overexpressed in OMVs.

The promoter replacement strategy also allows an increased immune response against minor proteins. PilQ is one such example. Even if this protein is reasonably abundant at the surface of the outer membrane of *N. meningitidis*, the upregulation of PilQ by promoter replacement can enhance its immunogenicity in mice (Table 18.2). Another example of upregulation by promoter re-

Table 18.2 Impact of upregulation on the induction of antibodies in mice [a].

Upregulation Targeted proteins	Methodology	ELISA titers [a] after immunization with:		
		Upregulated blebs	Control blebs	AS04
NhhA	Gene delivery	51 200 (≥1024) [b]	<50	<50
NspA	Gene delivery	400 (≥8)	<50	<50
PilQ	Promoter replacement	6400 (64)	100	<50
OMP85	Promoter replacement	200 (≥4)	<50	<50
FrpB	Iron limitation	6400 (8)	800	<50

a) OF1 mice were immunized three times with 5 µg of OMVs in AS04 formulation (MPL+Al3$^+$ salts). Blood samples were taken 14 days after the third injection and pooled prior to serological analysis. Antibody titers were determined by ELISA on microtiter plates coated with purified native or recombinant proteins. Ig titers are expressed as the reciprocal of serum dilution equivalent to an absorption value (at 490 nm; A_{490}) of 0.5.
b) Increase of antibody response by upregulation.

placement is OMP85. Mice immunized with OMVs containing upregulated OMP85 produce detectable levels of antiOMP85 antibodies, compared to no response in mice immunized with control OMVs.

Finally, proteins such as the human transferrin receptor (TbpA/TbpB complex) or the lactoferrin receptor (LbpA/LbpB complex) or the FrpB protein can be easily upregulated when *N. meningitidis* strains are cultivated in iron-depleted media. Table 18.2 gives an example of the antiFrpB immune response induced in mice after immunization with OMVs obtained from cultures with and without iron chelator.

References

1 H. J. Jennings, R. Roy, A. Gamian **1986**, *J. Immunol.* 137, 1708–1713.
2 J. Bruge, N. Bouveret-Le Cam, B. Danve, G. Rougon, D. Schulz **2004**, *Vaccine* 22, 1087–1096.
3 E. Robert, F. H. Azmi, D. Granoff **1995**, *J. Infect. Dis.* 172, 1279–1289.
4 I. Goldschneider, E. C. Gotschlich, M. S. Artenstein **1969**, *J. Exp Med.* 129, 1307–1326.
5 P. Densen **1989**, *Clin. Microbiol. Rev.* 2, S11–S17.
6 Y.-L. Tzeng, A. K. Datta, C. A. Strole, M. A. Lobritz, R. W. Carlson, D. S. Stephens **2005**, *Inf. Immun.* 73, 1491–1505.
7 J. L. Edwards, M. A. Apicella **2004**, *Clin. Microbiol. Rev.* 17, 965–981
8 M. P. Simon, W. M. Naussef, M. A. Apicella **2005**, *Infect. Immun.* 73, 1971–1977.
9 U. Vogel, S. Hammerschmidt, M. Frosch **1996**, *Med. Microbiol.* 185, 81–87.
10 G. R. Moe, A. Dave, D. M. Granoff **2005**, *Infect. Immun.* 73, 2123–2128.
11 J. D. Berry, D. J. Boese, D. K. S. Law, W. D. Zollinger, R. S. W. Tsang **2005**, *Mol. Immun.* 42, 335–344.

12 C. E. Frasch, E. C. Gotschlich **1974**, *J. Exp. Med.* 140, 87–104.
13 W. D. Zollinger, D. L. Kasper, B. J. Veltri, M. S. Artenstein **1977**, *Infect. Immun.* 18, 424–433.
14 J. T. Poolman, C. T. P., Hopman, H. C. Zanen **1980**, *J. Gen. Microbiol.* 116, 465–473.
15 K. Saukkonen, M. Leinonen, H. Abdillahi, J. T. Poolman **1989**, *Vaccine* 7, 325–328.
16 J. C. Wright, D. W. Hood, G. A. Randle, K. Makepeace, A. D. Cox, J. Li, R. Chalmers, J. C. Richards, E. R. Moxon **2004**, *J. Bacteriol.* 186, 6970–6982.
17 K. Cartwright, R. Morris, H. Rumke, A. Fox, R. Borrow, N. Begg, P. Richmond, J. Poolman **1999**, *Vaccine* 17, 2612–2619.
18 C. E. Frasch, W. D. Zollinger, J. T. Poolman **1985**, *Rev. Infect. Dis.* 7, 504–510.
19 C. E. Frasch, L. van Alphen, J. Holst, J. T. Poolman, E. Rosenqvist **2001**, in: *Meningococcal Vaccines*, ed. A. J. Pollard, M. C. J. Maiden, Humana Press, New York, pp 81–107
20 M. Mieszala, G. Kogan, H. J. Jennings **2003**, *Carb. Res.* 338, 167–175.
21 M. M. Giuliani, L. Santini, B. Brunelli, A. Biolchi, B. Aric, F. Di Marcello, E. Cartocci, M. Comandicci, V. Masignani, L. Lozzi, S. Savino, M. Scarselli, R. Rappuoli, M. Pizza **2005**, *Infect. Immun.* 73, 1151–1160.
22 M. Comandicci, S. Bambini, D. A. Caugant, M. Mora, B. Brunelli, B. Capecchi, L. Ciucchi, R. Rappuoli, M. Pizza **2004**, *Infect. Immun.* 72, 4217–4223.
23 R. Rappuoli **2003**, *NSNBC*, October.
24 G. Bjune, J. K. Gronnesby, E. A. Hoiby, O. Closs, H. Nokleby **1991**, *NIPH Ann.* 14, 81–93.
25 G. V. G. Sierra, H. C. Campa, N. M. Varcacel, I. L. Garcia, P. L. Izquierdo, P. F. Sotolongo, G. V. Casanueva, C. O. Rico, C. R. Rodriguez, M. H. Terry **1991**, *NIPH Ann.* 14, 195–207.
26 E. Rosenqvist, E. A. Hoiby, E. Wedege, K. Bryn, J. Kolberg, A. Klem, E. Ronnild, G. Bjune, H. Nokleby **1995**, *Infect. Immun.* 63, 4642–4652.
27 J. C. de Moraes, B. A. Perkins, M. C. C. Camargo, R. N. T. Hidalgo, H. A. Barbosa, C. T. Sacchi, I. M. Land Gral, V. L. Gattas, H. de G. Vasconcelos, B. D. Plikaytis, J. D. Wenger, C. V. Broone **1992**, *Lancet* 340, 1074–1078.
28 C. P. Noronha, C. J. Struchiner, M. E. Hallooran **1995**, *Int. J. Epidemiol.* 24, 1050–1057.
29 J. W. Tappero, R. Lagos, A. M. Ballesteros, B. Plikaytis, D. Williams, J. Dykes, L. L. Gheesling, G. M. Carlone, E. A. Hoiby, J. Holst, H. Nokleby, E. Rosenqvist, G. Sierra, C. Campa, F. Sotolongo, J. Vega, J. Garcia, P. Herrera, J. T. Poolman, B. A. Perkins **1999**, *J. Am. Med. Assoc.* 281, 1520–1527.
30 P. Massari, P. Henneke, Y. Ho, E. Latz, D. T. Golenbock, L. M. Wetzler **2002**, *J. Immunol.* 168, 1533–1537.
31 T. E. Michaelsen, A. Aase, J. Kolberg, E. Wedge, E. Rosenqvist **2001**, *Vaccine* 19, 1526–1533.
32 B. McGuinness, A. K. Barlow, I. N. Clarke, J. E. Farley, A. Anilionis, J. T. Poolman, J. E. Heckels **1990**, *J. Exp. Med.* 171, 1871–1882.
33 M. Virji, S. M. Watt, S. Barker, K. Makepeace, R. Doyonnas **1996**, *Mol. Microbiol.* 22, 929–939.
34 M. Virji, D. Evans, A. Hadfield, F. Grunert, A. M. Teixeira, S. M. Watt **1999**, *Mol. Microbiol.* 34, 538–551.
35 M. Virji **2000**, *Trends Microbiol.* 8, 260–261.
36 A. B. Schryvers, Igor Stojiljkovic **1999**, *Mol. Microbiol.* 32, 1117–1123.
37 M. Beucher, P. Sparling **1995**, *J. Bacteriol.* 177, 2041–2049.
38 A. Petterson, B. Kuipers, M. Pelzer, E. P. M. Verhagen, R. H. Tiesjema, J. Tomassen, J. T. Poolman **1990**, *Infect. Immun.* 58, 3036–3041.
39 R. Urwin, J. E. Russell, E. A. L. Thompson, E. C. Holmes, I. M. Feavers, M. C. J. Maiden **2004**, *Infect. Immun.* 72, 5955–5962.
40 P. Stevenson, P. Williams, E. Griffiths **1992**, *Infect. Immun.* 60, 2391–2396.
41 M. Pintor, J. A. Gomez, L. Ferron, C. M. Ferreiros, M. T. Criado **1998**, *J. Med. Microbiol.* 47, 757–760.
42 M. Legrain, V. Mazarin, S. W. Irwin, B. Bouchon, M.-J. Quentin-Millet, E. Jacobs, A. B. Schryvers **1993**, *Gene* 130, 73–80.

43 J. S. Oakhill, B. J. Sutton, A. R. Gorringe, R. W. Evans **2005**, *Protein Eng. Des. Sel.* (epub ahead of print).

44 H. R. Stokes, J. S. Oakhill, C. L. Joannou, A. R. Gorringe, R. W. Evans **2005**, *Infect. Immun.* 73, 944–952.

45 G. Renauld-Mongénie, D. Poncet, M. Mignon, S. Fraysse, C. Chabanel, B. Danve, T. Krell, M-J. Quentin-Millet **2004**, *Infect. Immun.* 72, 3461–3470.

46 G. Renauld-Mongénie, L. Lins, T. Krell, L. Laffly, M. Mignon, M. Dupuy, R.-M. Delrue, F. Guinet-Morlot, R. Brasseur, L. Lissolo **2004**, *J. Bacteriol.* 186, 850–857.

47 C. A. Fuller, R. Yu, S. W. Irwin, A. B. Schryvers **1998**, *Microb. Pathog.* 24, 75–87.

48 B. Rokbi, V. Mazarin, G. Maitre-Wilmotte, M.-J. Quentin-Millet **1993**, *FEMS Microbiol. Lett.* 110, 51–57.

49 B. Rokbi, G. Renauld-Mongenie, M. Mignon, B. Danve, D. Poncet, C. Chabanel, D. A. Caugant, M.-J. Quentin-Millet **2000**, *Infect. Immun.* 68, 4938–4947.

50 A. R. Gorringe, R. Borrow, A. J. Fox, A. Robinson **1995**, *Vaccine* 13, 1207–1212.

51 H. M. Palmer, N. B. L. Powell, D. A. Ala'Aldeen, J. Wilton, S. P. Borriello **1993**, *FEMS Microbiol. Lett.* 110, 139–145.

52 B. Danve, L. Lissolo, M. Mignon, P. Dumas, S. Colombani, A. B. Schryvers, M.-J. Quentin-Millet **1993**, *Vaccine* 11, 1214–1220.

53 D. A. A. Ala'Aldeen, S. Peter Borriello **1993**, *Vaccine* 14, 49–53.

54 B. Danve, M. Cadoz, L. Lissolo, E. Boutry, F. Guinet, D. Speck, X. Nassif **1998**, *Abstr. Int. Path. Neisseira Conf.* 11, 53.

55 R. A. Finkelstein, C. V. Sciortino, M. A. McIntosh **1983**, *Rev. Infect. Dis.* 1983, S759–S777.

56 A. B. Schryvers, L. J. Morris **1988**, *Infect. Immun.* 56, 1144–1149.

57 A. Pettersson, P. van der Ley, J. T. Poolman, J. Tommassen **1993**, *Infect. Immun.* 61, 4724–4733.

58 G. D. Biswas, P. F. Sparling **1995**, *Infect. Immun.* 63: 2958–2967.

59 A. Pettersson, V. Klarenbeek, J. van Deurzen, J. T. Poolman, J. Tommassen **1994**, *Microb. Pathog.* 17, 395–408.

60 A.Pettersson, A. Maas, J. Tommassen **1994**, *J. Bacteriol.* 176, 1764–1766.

61 A. Pettersson, T. Prinz, A. Umar, J. van der Biezen, J. Tommassen **1998**, *Mol. Microbiol.* 27, 599–610.

62 L. A. Lewis, K. Rohde, M. Gipson, B. Behrens, E. Gray, S. I. Toth, B. A. Roe, D. W. Dyer **1998**, *Infect. Immun.* 66, 3017–3023.

63 A. Pettersson, J. van der Biezen, V. Joosten, J. Hendriksen, J. Tommassen **1999**, *Gene* 231, 105–110.

64 A. S. Johnson, A. R. Gorringe, F. G. Mackinnon, A. J. Fox, R. Borrow, A. Robinson **1999**, *FEMS Immunol. Med. Microbiol.* 25, 349–354.

65 H.-S. M. Park, M. Wolfgang, M. Koomey **2002**, *Infect. Immun.* 70, 3891–3903.

66 M. Wolfgang, H. S. Park, S. F. Hayes, J. P. van Putten, M. Koomey **1998**, *Proc. Natl Acad. Sci. USA* 95, 14973–14978.

67 F. E. Aas, M. Wolfgang, S. Frye, S. Dunham, C. Lovold, M. Koomey **2002**, *Mol. Microbiol.* 46, 749–760.

68 S. L. Drake, M. Koomey **1995**, *Mol. Microbiol.* 18, 975–986.

69 R. F. Collins, S. A. Frye, A. Kitmitto, R. C. Ford, T. Tonjum, J. P. Derrick **2004**, *J. Biol. Chem.* 279, 39750–39756.

70 R. F. Collins, R. C. Ford, A. Kitmitto, R. O. Olsen, T. Tonjum, J. P. Derrick **2003**, *J. Bacteriol.* 185, 2611–2617.

71 R. F. Collins, L.Davidsen, J. P. Derrick, R. C. Ford, T. Tonjum **2001**, *J. Bacteriol.* 183, 3825–3832.

72 W. M. Tsai, S. H. Larsen, C. E. Wilde **1989**, *Infect. Immun.* 57, 2653–2659.

73 J. T. Poolman, P. A. van der Ley, J. Tommassen **1995**, in: *Meningococcal Disease*, ed. K. Cartwright, John Wiley & Sons, Chichester.

74 M. J. Corbett, J. R. Black, C. E. Wilde **1988**, in: *Gonococci and Meningococci*, 3rd edn, ed. J. T. Poolman, H. C. Zanen, T. F. Meyer, J. E. Heckels, P. R. H. Makela, H. Smith, E. C. Beuvery, Kluwer Academic Publishers, Dordrecht, p. 685–691.

75 D. Halliwell, S. A. Frye, S.Taylor, A. Flockhart, M. Finney, K. Reddin, M. Hudson, T. Tonjum, A. Gorringe, H. Seifer, M. Apicella **2004**, *Abstr. Int. Pathog. Neisseria Conf.* 14.

76 S.M. Loosmore, Y.P. Yang, D.C. Coleman, J.M. Shortreed, D.M. England **1997**, *Infect. Immun.* 65, 3701–3707.

77 D.S. Manning, D.K. Reschke, R.C. Judd **1998**, *Microb. Pathog.* 25, 11–21.

78 G. Norheim, A. Aase, D.A. Caugant, E.A. Hoiby, E. Fritzsonn, T. Tangen, P. Kristiansen, U. Heggelund, E. Rosenqvist **2005**, *Vaccine* 23, 3762–3774.

79 D.A. Fitzpatrick, J.O. Mc Inerney **2005**, *J. Mol. Evol.* 60, 268–273.

80 M.P. Bos, J. Tommassen **2004**, *Curr. Opin. Microbiol.* 7, 610–616.

81 I. Gentle, K. Gabriel, P. Beech, R. Waller, T. Lithgow **2004**, *J. Cell Biol.* 164, 19–24.

82 R. Voulhoux, Ma.P. Bos, J. Geurtsen, M. Mols, J. Tommassen **2003**, *Science* 299, 262–265.

83 S. Genevrois, L. Steeghs, P. Roholl, J.-J. Letesson, P. van der Ley **2003**, *EMBO J.* 22, 1780–1789.

84 H.A. Hadi, K.G. Woolddridge, K. Robinson, D.A.A. Ala'Aldeen **2001**, *Mol. Microbiol.* 41, 611–623.

85 D. Serruto, J. Adu-Bobie, M. Scarselli, D. Veggi, M. Pizza, R. Rappuoli, B. Aric **2003**, *Mol. Microbiol.* 48, 323–334.

86 I.R.A. Peak, Y. Srikhanta, M. Dieckelmann, E.R. Moxon, M.P. Jennings **2000**, *FEMS Immunol. Med. Microbiol.* 28, 329–334.

87 M. Scarselli, R. Rappuoli, V. Scarlato **2001**, *Microbiology* 147, 250–252.

88 P. van Ulsen, L. van Alphen, C.Ph.P. Hopman, A. van der Ende, J. Tommassen **2001**, *FEMS Immunol. Med. Microbiol.* 32, 53–64.

89 D. Martin, N. Cadieux, J. Hamel, B.R. Brodeur **1997**, *J. Exp. Med.* 185, 1173–1183.

90 G.R. Moe, P. Zuno-Mitchell, S.N. Hammond, D.M. Granoff **2002**, *Infect. Immun.* 70, 6021–6031.

91 G.R. Moe, S. Tan, D.M. Granoff **1999**, *Infect. Immun.* 67, 5664–5675.

92 G.R. Moe, P. Zuno-Mitchell, S.S. Lee, A.H. Lucas, D.M. Granoff **2001**, *Infect. Immun.* 69, 3762–3771.

93 L. Vandeputte-Rutten, M.P. Bos, J. Tommassen, P. Gros **2003**, *J. Biol. Chem.* 278, 24825–24830.

94 S. Sánchez, G. Troncoso, M.T. Criado, C. Ferreirós **2002**, *Vaccine* 20, 2964–2971.

95 G. Guillén, A. Alvarez, R. Silva, V. Morera, S. González, A. Musacchio, V. Besada, E. Coizeau, E. Caballero, C. Nazabal, T. Carmenate, L.J. González, R. Estrada, Y. Támbara, G. Padrón, L. Herrera **1998**, *Biotechnol. Appl. Biochem.* 27, 189–196.

96 T. Carmenate, L. Canaán, A. Álvarez, M. Delgado, S. González, T. Menéndez, L. Rodés, G. Guillén **2004**, *FEMS Immunol. Med. Microbiol.* 40, 193–199.

97 A. Pérez, F. Dickinson, Z. Cinza, A. Ruíz, T. Serrano, J. Sosa, S. González, Y. Gutiérrez, C. Nazábal, O. Gutiérrez, D. Guzmán, M. Díaz, M. Delgado, E. Caballero, G. Sardias, A. Alvarez, A. Martín, G. Guillén, R. Silva **2001**, *Biotechnol. Appl. Biochem.* 34, 121–125.

98 J. Parkill, M. Achtam, K.D. James, S.D. Bentley, C. Churcher, S.R. Klee, G. Morelli, D. Basham, D. Brown, T. Chillingworth, R. M. Davies, P. Davis, K. Delvin, T. Feltwell, N. Hamlin, S. Holroyd, K. Jagels, S. Leather, S. Moule, K. Mungall, M.A. Quail, M.A. Rajandream, K.M. Rutherford, M. Simmonds, J. Skelton, S. Whitehead, B.G. Spratt, B.G. Barrell **2000**, *Nature* 404, 502–506.

99 H. Tettelin, N.J. Saunders, J. Heidelberg, A.C. Jeffries, K.E. Nelson, J.A. Eisen, K.A. Ketchum, D.W. Hood, J.F. Peden, R.J. Dodson, W.C. Nelson, M.L. Gwinn, R. DeBoy, J.D. Peterson, E.K. Hickey, D.H. Haft, S.L. Salzberg, O.White, R.D. Fleischmann, B.A. Dougherty, T. Mason, A. Ciecko, D.S. Parksey, E. Blair, H. Cittone, E.B. Clark, M.D. Cotton, T.R. Utterback, H. Khouri, H. Qin, J. Vamathevan, J. Gill, V. Scarlato, V. Masignani, M. Pizza, G. Grandi, L. Sun, H.O. Smith, C.M. Fraser, E.R. Moxon, R. Rappuoli, J.C. Venter **2000**, *Science* 287, 1809–1815.

100 M. Pizza, V. Scarlato, V. Masignani, M. M. Giuliani, B. Aric, M. Comanducci, G.T. Jennings, L. Baldi, E. Bartolini, B. Capecchi, C.L. Galeotti, E. Luzzi, R. Manetti, E. Marchetti, M. Mora, S. Nuti, G. Ratti, L. Santini, S. Savino, M. Scarselli, E. Storni, P. Zuo, M. Broeker, E. Hundt, B. Knapp,

E. Blair, T. Mason, H. Tettelin, D.W. Hood, A.C. Jeffries, N.J. Saunders, D.M. Granoff, J.C. Venter, E.R. Moxon, G. Grandi, R. Rappuoli **2000**, *Science* 287, 1816–1820.

101 G.T. Jennings, S. Savino, E. Marchetti, B. Arico, T. Kast, L. Baldi, A. Ursinus, J.V. Holtje, R.A. Nicholas, R. Rappuoli, G. Grandi **2002**, *Eur. J. Biochem.* 15, 3722–3731.

102 D.M. Granoff, G.R. Moe, M.M. Giuliani, J. Adu-Bobie, L. Santini, B. Brunelli, F. Piccinetti, P. Zuno-Mitchell, S.S. Lee, P. Neri, L. Bracci, L. Lozzi, R. Rappuoli **2001**, *J. Immunol.* 167, 6487–6496.

103 J.A.Welsch, G.R. Moe, R. Rossi, J. Adu-Bobie, R. Rappuoli, D.M. Granoff **2003**, J. *Infect. Dis.* 188, 1730–1740.

104 B. Capecchi, J. Adu-Bobie, F. Di Marcello, L. Ciucchi, V. Masignani, A. Taddei, R. Rappuoli, M. Pizza, B. Aric **2005**, *Mol. Microbiol.* 55, 687–698.

105 P. Martin, T. van de Ven, N. Mouchel, A.C. Jeffries, D.W. Hood, E.R. Moxon **2003**, *Mol. Microbiol.* 50, 245–257.

106 M. Comanducci, S. Bambini, B. Brunelli, J. Adu-Bobie, B. Aric, B. Capecchi, M.M. Giuliani, V. Masignani, L. Santini, S. Savino, D.M. Granoff, D.A. Caugant, M. Pizza, R. Rappuoli, M. Mora **2002**, *J. Exp. Med.* 195, 1445–1454.

107 V. Masignani, M. Comanducci, M.M. Giuliani, S. Bambini, J. Adu-Bobie, B. Aric, B. Brunelli, A. Pieri, L. Santini, S. Savino, D. Serruto, D. Litt, S. Kroll, J.A. Welsch, D.M. Granoff, R. Rappuoli, M. Pizza **2003**, *J. Exp. Med.* 197, 789–799.

108 J.A. Welsch, R. Rossi, M. Comanducci, D.M. Granoff **2004**, *J. Immunol.* 172, 5606–5615.

109 L.D. Fletcher, L. Bernfield, V. Barniak, J.E. Farley, A. Howell, M. Knauf, P. Ooi, R.P. Smith, P. Weise, M. Wetherell, X. Xie, R. Zagursky, Y. Zhang, G.W. Zlotnick **2004**, *Infect. Immun.* 72, 2088–2100.

110 V. Masignani, E. Balducci, F. Di Marcello, S. Savino, D. Serruto, D. Veggi, S. Bambini, M. Scarselli, B. Aric, M. Comanducci, J. Adu-Bobie, M. Giuliani, R. Rappuoli, M. Pizza **2003**, *Mol. Microbiol.* 50, 1055–1067.

111 M. Estabrook, C. J. Baker, Griffis J. M. **1993**, *J. Infect. Dis.* 167, 966–970.

112 J. M. Griffis, B.L. Brandt, D.D. Broud, D. K. Goroff, C. J. Baker **1984**, *J. Infect. Dis.* 150, 71–79.

113 J. J. Drabick, B. L. Brandt, E. E. Moran, N.B. Saunders, D.R. Shoemaker, W.D. Zollinger **2000**, *Vaccine* 18, 160–172.

114 R.J. Scholten, B. Kuipers, H.A.Valkenburg, J. Dankert, W.D. Zollinger, J.T. Poolman **1994**, *J. Med. Microbiol.* 41, 236–243.

115 A.F.M. Verheul, H. Snippe, J.T. Poolman **1993**, *Microbiol. Rev.* 57, 34–49.

116 M.M. Estabrook, J.M. Griffis, G.A. Jarvis **1997**, *Infect. Immun.* 65, 4436–4444.

117 E. Rosenqvist, E.A. Hoiby, G. Bjune, A. Aase, A. Halstensen, A.K. Lehmann, J. Paulsen, J. Holst., T.E. Michaelsen, H. Nokleby, L.O. Froholm, O. Closs **1998**, *Dev. Biol. Stand.* 92, 323–333.

118 L. Steeghs, J. Tommassen, J.H.W. Leusen, J.G.J. van de Winkel, P. van der Ley **2004**, *J. Endotox. Res.* 10, 113–119.

119 M. Fisseha, P. Chen, T.M. Kijek, B.L. Brandt, B. Ionin, W.D. Zollingert **2004**, IPNC 13, 263.

120 S.R. Andersen, J. Kolberg, E.A. Hoiby, E. Namork, D.A. Caugant, L.O. Froholm, E. Jantzen, G. Bjune **1997**, *Microb. Pathog.* 23, 139–155.

121 J.P. van Putten, B.D. Robertson **1995**, *Mol. Microbiol.* 16, 847–853.

122 M.A.J. Gidney, J.S. Plested, S. Lacelle, P.A. Coull, J.C. Wright, K. Makepeace, J.R. Brisson, A.D. Cox, E.R. Moxon, J.C. Richards **2004**, *Infect. Immun.* 72, 559–569.

123 M.P. Jennings, Y.N. Srikhanta, E.R. Moxon, M. Kramer, J.T. Poolman, B. Kuipers, P. van der Ley **1999**, *Microbiology* 145, 3013–3021.

124 J.S. Plested, M.A. Gidney, P.A. Coull, H.G. Griffiths, M.A. Herbert, A.G. Bird, J.C. Richards, E.R. Moxon **2000**, *J. Immunol. Methods* 237, 73–84.

125 J.S. Plested, B.L. Ferry, P.A. Coull, K. Makepeace, A.K. Lehmann, F.G. MacKinnon, H.G. Griffiths, M.A. Herbert, J.C. Richards,

E.R. Moxon **2001**, *Infect. Immun.* 69, 3203–3213.

126 J.S. Plested, S.L. Harris, J.C. Wright, P.A. Coull, K. Makepeace, M.-A. Gidney, J.R. Brisson, J.C. Richards, D.M. Granoff, E.R. Moxon **2003**, *J Infect Dis.* 187, 1223–1234.

127 U. Vogel, M. Frosch **2002**, *Curr. Top. Microbiol. Immunol.* 264, 23–45.

128 L. Snyder, S. Butcher, N. Saunders **2001**, *Microbiology* 147, 2321–2332.

129 E. Feil, M. Enright, B. Spratt **2000**, *Res. Microbiol.* 151, 465–469.

130 B. Linz, M. Schenker, P. Zhu, M. Achtman **2000**, *Mol. Microbiol.* 36, 1049–1058.

131 A. Schryvers, I. Stojiljkovic **1999**, *Mol. Microbiol.* 32, 1117–1123.

132 X. Nassif, C. Pujol, P. Morand, E. Eugene **1999**, *Mol. Microbiol.* 32, 1124–1132.

133 S. Thompson, P. Sparling **1993**, *Infect. Immun.* 61, 2906–2911.

134 P. Salvatore, G. Cantalupo, C. Pagliarulo, M. Tredici, A. Lavitola, C. Bucci, C. Bruni, P. Alifano **2000**, *Plasmid* 44, 275–279.

135 J. Poolman, C. Feron, G. Dequesnes, P. Denoel, S. Dessoy, K. Goraj, D. Janssens, S. Kummert, Y. Lobet, E. Mertens, D. Monnom, P. Momin, N. Pepin, J.-L. Ruelle, J. Thonnard, V. Verlant, P. Voet, F.-X. Berthet **2002**, *Emerging Strategies in the Fight Against Meningitis: Molecular and Cellular Aspects*, ISBN 1-898486-34-4, p. 135–149.

136 R. Voulhoux, J. Tommassen **2004**, *Res. Microbiol.* 155, 129–135.

137 D. Martin, B. Brodeur, J. Hamel, F. Couture, U. de Alwis, Z. Lian, S. Martin, D. Andrews, R. Ellis **2000**, *J. Biotechnol.* 83, 27–31.

138 F. Pagotto, H. Salimnia, P. Totten, J. Dillon **2000**, *Gene* 244, 13–19.

139 H. Takahashi, H. Watanabe **2002**, *Microbiology* 48, 229–236.

140 R. Grifantini, S. Sebastian, E. Frigimelica, M. Draghi, E. Bartolini, A. Muzzi, R. Rappuoli, G. Grandi, C. Genco **2003**, *Proc. Natl Acad. Sci. USA* 100, 9542–9547.

141 J. Sarkari, N. Pandit, E. Moxon, M. Achtman **1994**, *Mol Microbiol.* 13, 207–217.

142 M. Virji, K. Makepeace, D. Ferguson, M. Achtman, E. Moxon **1993**, *Mol. Microbiol.* 10, 499–510.

143 M. de Jonge, H. Hamstra, L. van Alphen, J. Dankert, P. van der Ley **2003**, *Mol. Microbiol.* 50, 1005–1015.

144 J.T. Poolman, C.T.P. Hopman, H.C. Zanen **1985**, *J. Med. Microbiol.* 119, 203–209.

145 J.H. Fredriksen, E. Rosenqvist, E. Wedege, K. Bryn, G. Bjune, L.O. Froholm, A.-K. Lindbak, B. Mogster, E. Namork, U. Rye, G. Stabbetorp, R. Winsnes, B. Aase, O. Closs **1991**, *NIPH Ann.* 14, 67–80.

146 L.M. Wetler, M.S.K. Blake Barry, E.C. Gotschlich **1992**, *J. Infect. Dis.* 166, 551–555.

147 M.C. Brandileone, R.C. Zanella, V.S. Vieira, V.T. Sacchi, L.C. Milagres, C.E. Frash **1994**, *Rev. Inst. Med. Trop. Sao Paulo* 36, 301–310.

148 C.M. Tsai, C.E. Frasch, E. Rivera, H.D. Hochstein **1989**, *J. Biol. Stand.* 17, 249–258.

149 C.E. Frasch, R.M. Mc Nelis, E.C. Gotschlich **1976**, *J. Bacteriol.* 127, 973–981.

150 P.A. Van der Ley, J. van der Biezen, J.T. Poolman **1995**, *Vaccine* 13, 401–407.

151 W.D. Zollinger, R.E. Mandrell, J.M. Griffiss, P. Altieri, S. Berman **1979**, *J. Clin. Invest.* 63, 836–848.

152 W.D. Zollinger **2004**, *Patent* US 6,558,677 B2.

153 V.C. Hou, G.R. Moe, Z. Raad, T. Wuorimaa, D.M. Granoff **2003**, *Infect. Immun.* 71, 6844–6849.

154 C.A. O'Dwyer, K. Reddin, D. Martin, S.C. Taylor, A.R. Gorringe, M.J. Hudson, B.R. Brodeur, P.R. Langford, J.S. Kroll **2004**, *Infect. Immun.* 72, 6511–6518.

19
Genome Mining and Reverse Vaccinology

Rosanna Leuzzi, Silvana Savino, Mariagrazia Pizza and Rino Rappuoli

19.1
Impact of Genomics on Vaccine Design: the Reverse Vaccinology Approach

Before the advent of the genomic era, the identification of bacterial components as a basis for vaccine development was based on their *in vivo* immunogenicity or on their role in virulence. Bacterial factors were therefore isolated and purified by direct isolation from cultivated microorganisms, or expressed in high amounts, taking advantage of recombinant DNA technologies, and tested for their ability to induce an immune response. Although this approach has been the basis for the development of existing vaccines, it has not always been successful and vaccines against many human pathogens are still unavailable.

The genomic revolution led to the possibility to approach the design of vaccines from a completely different perspective; the availability of complete genome sequences of an increasing number of microorganisms has defined a potential universal approach to discover novel antigens for any new vaccine.

Release of the genome sequence of a pathogen provides the opportunity to know the entire repertoire of proteins potentially expressed by bacteria at any time during their growth and in any phase of infection. In this context, every protein synthesized by the pathogen can be tested as a vaccine candidate without any prior selection based on their *in vitro* expression or their role in virulence and immunogenicity. This method based on the identification of vaccine candidates from a whole-genome sequence rather than from live microorganisms has been termed "reverse vaccinology" [1, 2] and is schematically represented in Fig. 19.1.

Serogroup B of *Neisseria meningitidis* was the first potential vaccine developed with the reverse vaccinology approach; this pioneer project led to the definition of a new paradigm of a more general use in developing the next generation of vaccines for which traditional studies had failed.

In fact, decades of research with conventional approaches have not been successful in discovering an efficacious universal vaccine against serogroup B of *N. meningitidis*. Outer membrane vesicle (OMV)-based vaccines, although effica-

Handbook of Meningococcal Disease. Infection Biology, Vaccination, Clinical Management.
Edited by M. Frosch and M. C. J. Maiden

ISBN: 3-527-31260-9

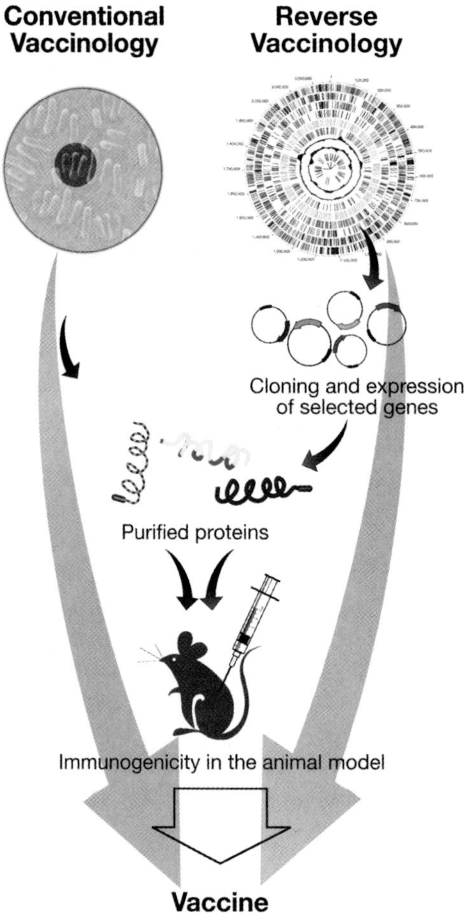

Fig. 19.1 Schematic representation of the conventional and "reverse" genome-based approaches to vaccine development. (This figure also appears with the color plates.)

cious, have the limitation that the major components show sequence and antigenic variability and consequently the protection induced is strictly serotype- or serosubtype-specific. In addition, the complex multiple-protein-based composition of these vaccines makes it difficult to manage them from the standardization and quality control points of view.

This problem could be overcome by developing a vaccine based on a small number of conserved and protective antigens.

To reach this goal and identify potential antigens, the complete genome sequence of the virulent strain MC58 of *N. meningiditis* was obtained using the random shotgun strategy (GenBank accession number AE002098) [3].

Genome contains 2 272 351 base pairs with an average G+C content of 53%. Using open reading frame (ORF) prediction algorithms and whole-genome homology searches, 2158 putative ORFs have been identified.

Biological roles have been assigned to 53.7% of the genes (1158 ORFs) on the basis of similarity to proteins of known function. The other ORFs are distributed between conserved hypothetical proteins sharing significant similarities to proteins present in several organisms without any putative function assigned (345 ORFs, corresponding to 16% of the predicted coding sequences) and hypothetical proteins (532 ORFs, corresponding to 24.7%) with no database match (considered unknown *Neisseria*-specific hypothetical proteins) [3].

In the next paragraphs, we show in more detail the methods used and the results obtained in developing a potential vaccine starting from genome analysis.

19.2 Candidate Antigen Prediction

The general criterion for selection of vaccine candidates is the necessary condition of their surface localization. In fact, surface-exposed and secreted proteins are the best immunological targets because of their accessibility to antibodies able to evoke a protective response. On these grounds, the selection of antigen candidates is based on computer predictions of secretion or surface localization. First, proteins homologous to surface-exposed proteins or virulence factors of other microorganisms, known by previous experimental characterizations, are selected. Then, predicted ORFs with no assigned function are analyzed by software (PSORT, SignalIP) which can identify classic signal peptide sequences pre-

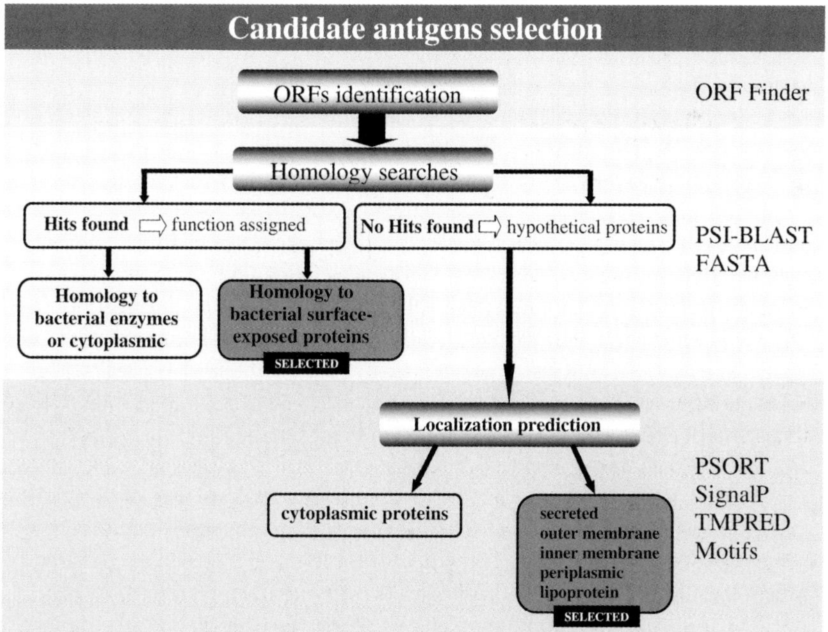

Fig. 19.2 Criteria and bioinformatic software used for *in silico* genome analysis and selection of putative vaccine candidates.

dictive of protein export or secretion. In addition, computer programs are used to search putative lipoproteins (by identification of lipo-box motifs) or predicted membrane spanning regions (TMPRED). Proteins carrying more than four predicted transmembrane domains are discarded because they are likely to be totally embedded in the cell membrane and therefore inaccessible to antibodies. Shorter motifs, such as host integrin-binding domain (RGD) and choline-binding domain (WYY), are also searched by classic pattern matching. Criteria and bioinformatic software used for *in silico* vaccine candidates screening are summarized in Fig. 19.2.

The list of potential vaccine candidates identified by concomitant use of these computer analyses contained 570 genes coding for predicted surface-exposed or membrane-associated proteins [4]: the higher proportion of putative candidates was represented by integral membrane proteins (characterized by multiple hydrophobic domains), followed by periplasmic proteins, lipoproteins and outer membrane and secreted proteins, which represented less than 15% of the total.

19.3
Antigen Screening

Once all the possible vaccine candidates had been identified, the next step was to test their ability to confer protective immunity against *N. meningitidis* infection. Complement-mediated bactericidal activity of antibodies against *N. meningitidis* is the accepted correlate of protection in humans [5]; thus, the strategy used was the screening of all the sera raised against the putative antigens by bactericidal assay.

In order to screen this large number of candidate antigens, it was necessary to use a simple procedure for the cloning and purification of antigens. To this end, selected ORFs were amplified by PCR, using primers that exclude the signal peptide sequences in order to produce a cytoplasmic form of each protein. To achieve the highest level of expression and the easiest purification procedure, amplified genes were cloned in parallel into vectors containing the necessary promoters and sequences coding for either a C-terminal histidine tag, or an N-terminal glutathione S-transferase (GST) fusion protein. These constructs permitted the rapid purification of soluble recombinant proteins by simple column chromatography. Of the 570 selected candidates, 344 were successfully cloned in *E. coli* and soluble recombinant proteins were purified [4]. Each purified recombinant protein was used to immunize mice and sera against each antigen were used in a series of assays. First, immunoblot analysis was performed on total cell extracts and on purified OMVs in order to demonstrate that the protein is expressed by the bacteria and to get an indication of the cellular localization. Surface localization was then confirmed by enzyme-linked immunosorbent assay (ELISA) and fluorescence-activated cell sorter (FACS). Using this approach, 91 novel surface-exposed proteins were identified. All sera were analyzed by complement-mediated bactericidal activity assay and 28 recombinant proteins were identified as able to induce a protective immune response [4]. This was a very significant result, given that in the past four decades of research only a dozen bactericidal antibodies eliciting proteins had been identified. Furthermore, whereas the proteins identified by conventional approaches were highly variable among the different isolates, many of the proteins identified by reverse vaccinology were expressed in a lower amount, but nevertheless able to induce high titers of bactericidal activity.

Once the first prerogative of a vaccine candidate was established, i.e. the ability to evoke an immune response, the second necessary condition was the evaluation of the degree of sequence conservation among different pathogenic strains. N. meningitidis has evolved many tools to evade the human immune response, like phase variation and antigenic variability. Therefore, the evaluation of the sequence conservation of the selected antigens is an important issue in its consideration as a wide protective vaccine. Therefore, the most promising antigens displaying the higher bactericidal titers were evaluated for their sequence conservation in a high number of N. meningitidis strains representative of the genetic and geographic diversity. In addition, strains of N. cinerea, N. lactamica and N. gonorrhoeae were also included in this analysis. The sequences were compared for their degree of diversity; unexpectedly, although surface-exposed proteins are generally variable because of selective pressure induced by the human immune system, most of the novel antigens identified were well conserved and cross-protective.

The identified antigens have been further characterized from the immunological and functional points of view. We will show here an example of immunological characterization.

19.4
GNA1870 as an Example of Immunological Characterization

GNA1870 is a surface-exposed lipoprotein of 255 of residues, with a signal peptide of 19 amino acids and a predicted molecular mass of 26 964 Da.

Sequencing of the gene in 71 strains, representative of the genetic and geographic diversity of the N. meningitidis population, showed that the protein is present as three variants [6]. Conservation within each variant ranges between 91.6% and 100%, while conservation among the three variants can be as low as 62.8%. Bactericidal activity is variant-specific and antibodies against a recombinant form of the protein elicit complement-mediated killing of strains that carry the same variant, whereas the activity against strains carrying a different variant is very low or absent [6].

In order to map the immunological regions and to identify the functional epitopes, overlapping dodecapeptides designed on GNA1870 variant 1 sequence were synthesized and tested for binding to polyclonal antibodies, using the PepScan system [7]. Immunogenic peptides were present only in the region spanning residues 8–164, whereas no linear peptides were recognized in the C-terminal region, at residues 164–255. Similar results were obtained using antivariant 2 and antivariant 3 polyclonal antisera.

On the basis of these data, three different domains, A, B and C, were identified and expressed as recombinant fragments in *E. coli*, either individually, or as AB and BC domains. The purified domains were used for the immunization of mice. Antisera were analyzed by Western blot, FACS analysis and for bactericidal activity. Results indicated that bactericidal antibodies were directed against conformational epitopes located in the BC domain, which included the residues 100–255. These data have also been confirmed by using the bactericidal mouse monoclonal antibody mAb502, specific for GNA1870 variant 1. mAb502 does not bind the A, B and C domains individually, but binds the BC domain and the combination of the B and C domains, suggesting that the related epitope is conformational. Arginine in position 204 has been identified as a key residue involved in the formation of the bactericidal epitope and in binding to the monoclonal antibody [7].

Recent studies have confirmed the importance of this protein in inducing bactericidal antibodies against *N. meningitidis* [8]. Moreover, protection in the infant rat model using monoclonal antibodies against GNA1870 can also be achieved in the absence of measurable bactericidal activity [9].

19.5
Exploring the Genome: Functional Characterization of Vaccine Candidates

Besides the identification of new potential vaccine candidates, an ambitious goal of the genomic analysis of *N. meningitidis* is to explore the functional role of meningococcal proteins.

The availability of the genome sequences of *Neisseria* species, together with a large number of other bacterial genomes, has generated a massive amount of data; a challenge for bioinformatics is to explore this disparate data from the point of view of comparative analyses and to uncover biologically relevant functions of meningococcal proteins.

The most common approach to attribute a functional role to unknown proteins is the use of conventional methods of homology search.

Searching for sequence homologies to known virulence factors, a number of meningococcal proteins have been identified and further characterized. Among them, NMB1985/App showed 55% homology with Hap, a protein of *Haemophilus influenzae* involved in attachment and internalization in epithelial cells [10] and GNA33/MltA shows 41% homology to MltA of *E. coli*, a membrane-bound lytic transglycosylase [11]. These two proteins are typical examples of sequences sharing high levels of homology to known bacterial proteins and for which the simple sequence alignment has been the starting point for functional characterization.

In the presence of low homology to known proteins, or in the total absence of sequence conservation, homology criteria can be inadequate or insufficient to reveal possible functions. In this case, the search for common folding and structural similarities can reveal a potential attribution to an existing bacterial family.

NMB1994/NadA is a protein identified by concomitant analysis of sequence homology and structural modeling. NadA displays a low level of sequence identity to YadA of *Yersinia* spp and UspA1 and UspA2 of *Moraxella catarrhalis*, two nonfimbrial adhesins belonging to the Oca family (oligomeric coiled-coil adhesin) [12]. Despite the weak sequence conservation, NadA and its corresponding homologs have substantial structural similarity converging to similar functions. NadA, similarly to the other members of the Oca family, shows a typical structural organization with three major domains: (a) an outer membrane anchor domain that shares sequence identity to the corresponding domain of other Oca members, (b) an intermediate coiled-coil domain stalk containing a leucine zipper and (c) an N-terminal globular head region. Extending the overview to the viral and eukaryotic world, this tripartite structural architecture is reminiscent of the molecular motifs of both viral spike proteins and eukaryotic SNAREs. This recurrence of architectural domains across species leads to the fascinating hypothesis that evolutionary pressure selected a common mechanism of cell membrane translocation to provide an efficient solution to penetrate host barriers [13].

For some proteins, the assignment of a putative function is acquired by multiple bioinformatic tools. NMB1343/NarE is a paradigm of proteins with a non-conserved primary structure, for which a more complex *in silico* analysis successfully allowed the identification of an undiscovered putative toxin. NMB1343 is an ADP-ribosyltransferase identified by a two-pattern-based computational approach flanked by secondary structure prediction [14]. In the first step, two sequence patterns, comprising the consensus motifs of the CT and DT groups of toxins, were used to screen the complete genome of *N. meningitidis*. This analysis allowed the detection of three hits subsequently analyzed for secondary structure prediction. Only the protein NMB1343 revealed good conservation of a typical secondary structure topology of bacterial ADP ribosyltransferase. In particular, the protein included the conserved catalytic residues, their relative distance along the protein and all the secondary structure elements contributing to the scaffold of the active site.

In the following paragraphs, we give a brief overview of the functional characterization of meningococcal proteins, selected by the described preliminary computer analysis.

19.5.1
NMB1985-App

Sequence analysis of NMB1985 showed high degree of homology with Hap (*H*aemophilus *a*dhesion and *p*enetration protein) of *H. influenzae*, a protein promoting bacterial attachment and internalization in epithelial cells [10]; on the basis of sequence similarity it was named App [15]. App is a member of the autotransporter family containing a serine protease motif, which mediates autoproteolytic cleavage. When expressed in *E. coli*, App is correctly exported on the bacterial surface and undergoes an autoproteolytic process, resulting in cleavage of an internal passenger domain and in its secretion [16]. Importantly, *E. coli* expressing App on the bacterial surface acquires the ability to adhere to epithelial cells. These results suggest that the *E. coli* system can be used to establish the structural and biological relevance of meningococcal proteins. This adhesive property highlighted in *E. coli* has been confirmed in *N. meningitidis,* since disruption of the *app* gene in a capsulated virulent strain significantly reduces its adherence to epithelial cells compared to the wild type. Moreover, purified App protein binds epithelial cells *in vitro,* supporting the possibility of a direct interaction to a putative cellular receptor [16].

19.5.2 **NMB1994-NadA**

Sequence analysis and structural prediction revealed that NMB1994 belongs to the family of putative nonfimbrial adhesins, defined as Oca (oligomeric coiled-coil adhesin) [12]; the protein was named NadA (*N*eisseria *ad*hesin *A*) [17].

NadA forms high molecular weight oligomers on the meningococcal surface and the oligomerization domain is likely to be mediated by the stalk domain. Recombinant NadA protein expressed in *E. coli* is able to be correctly processed and exposed to the outer membrane as stable oligomers [18]. Expression of NadA contributes to the adhesion and invasion of *N. meningitidis* on epithelial cells: inactivation of the *nadA* gene causes an approximately three-fold reduction in the adhesion and invasion capability of meningococcal strains [18]. The functional properties of NadA are emphasized when the protein is expressed in a heterologous system: expression of NadA confers to *E. coli* the ability to adhere to epithelial cells. The adhesive property resides in the N-terminal head domain, since the recombinant protein devoid of the head domain loses the ability to bind to epithelial cells. The purified NadA protein is able to bind to epithelial cells *in vitro* and binding is prevented by treatment with pronase, suggesting that a protein receptor could mediate the binding [18]. Moreover, it is confirmed that NadA is involved in cellular internalization: transmission electron microscopy (TEM) analysis and gentamicin protection assay revealed that an *E. coli* strain expressing NadA enters epithelial cells concomitantly with cytoskeletal rearrangements.

Analysis of sequence conservation reveals that the gene is present in about 50% of *N. meningitidis* strains, including hypervirulent lineages, whereas it is absent in other *Neisseria* species [17], supporting the hypothesis that NadA is a disease-related gene essential for full meningococcal virulence. Furthermore, from a study performed on 154 carrier strains of *N. meningitidis,* NadA segregated differently in strains isolated from healthy individuals (carriers) and in strains isolated from patients (clinical isolates). Only 5.1% of the genuine carrier population harbors the NadA gene. This form, named NadA4, has the same overall features of other NadA forms. It is also able to form high molecular weight aggregates, is exposed on the surface, is able to bind to epithelial cells and is bactericidal [19]. These data could confirm NadA as a potential cofactor of *Neisseria* pathogenicity.

19.5.3
GNA33-MltA

GNA33 encodes a predicted lipoprotein homologous to the membrane-bound lytic transglycosylase (MltA) of *E. coli*, an enzyme involved in murein enlargement during bacterial growth and division. The purified GNA33 protein of *N. meningitidis* displays the predicted muramidase and transglycosylase activity *in vitro* [20]. Studies on a strain of *N. meningitidis* deficient in the GNA33 gene indicate a relevant role of the corresponding protein in meningococcal growth and shaping: the GNA33 mutant exhibits a marked decreased in viability, an abnormal cellular morphology and a perturbed membrane profile [21], suggesting an important contribution of this protein in meningococcal membrane architecture and in replication. These alterations cause a virulence-attenuated phenotype, since the GNA33 mutant is unable to cause bacteremia in an infant rat animal model [21].

The deletion in the *gna33* gene seems to affect the correct topological organization of the *N. meningitidis* membrane, resulting in the spontaneous release of outer membrane vesicles. These vesicles are constituted mainly by OMVs and this phenotype can be the basis for the design of new effective vaccines [21].

19.5.4
NMB1343-NarE

In silico analysis identified NMB1343 as a possible ADP ribosyltransferase. Confirmation of this prediction was experimentally given by *in vitro* assay, showing that purified NarE has ADP ribosylation and NAD glycohydrolase activities and is able to transfer the ADP ribose moiety to an arginine residue on small guanidine compounds [14]. This novel ADP ribosyltransferase of *N. meningitidis* was named NarE. The *narE* gene is present in a subset of hypervirulent lineages of *N. meningitidis* and, when present, the gene sequence is 100% conserved. Together with evidence of an unusual low GC content, this perfect conservation in a restricted number of meningococcal strains sustains the hypothesis of a recent acquisition by horizontal transfer.

Despite the *narE* gene not having a canonic secretory signal, the protein is able to cross the inner membrane and to localize in the periplasmic space [14]. However, it is not clear how the protein crosses the outer membrane to exert its demonstrated toxic activity on possible host cell targets.

19.6
Advantages of Multiple-genome Analysis in Vaccine Design: the Example of GBS

The "reverse vaccinology" approach described for serogroup B of *N. meningitidis* has also been successfully applied to group B *Streptococcus* (GBS). In this case, an extensive comparative genome analysis has been carried out on eight GBS strains representative of the most important disease-causing serotypes [22].

This approach represents an advance in the use of reverse vaccinology, since it has highlighted the potential of looking at more than one genome for the same bacterial species to overcome the problems represented by gene presence and variability. This analysis has allowed the identification of two "subgenomes" for each genome sequenced: a "core genome" composed by 80% of the total gene numbers and a "variable portion" constituted by genes not present in all strains. The 20% of genes included in the "variable portion" are absent from at least one of the other strains [23]. By this approach, four proteins derived from the "core" and the "variable" portion of the GBS genomes have been identified and proposed as components of a vaccine against GBS.

One of these antigens, GBS322, was previously described as a Sip protein and is part of the core genome. The other three antigens, GBS67, GBS80 and GBS104, are encoded by genes contained in the variable portion. Each antigen elicits protection in the mouse model against more than one GBS strain, but not against all strains sequenced. The genes encoding these three antigens are included in two genomic islands, which have been named "adhesin islands" because of their homology to genes encoding for known adhesins. The *gbs80* and *gbs104* genes are located in adhesin island 1 (AI-1), while the *gbs67* gene is located in the adhesin island 2 (AI-2). Four of the eight strains sequenced contain both AI-1 and AI-2, whereas two strains contain only AI-1 and two strains contain only AI-2. Five genes are present in each island, three of which code for the LPXTG motif, known to be the requisite in Gram-positive bacteria for covalent attachment of proteins to the peptidoglycan cell wall. The other two genes present in each island code for sortase enzymes that catalyze this covalent coupling [24]. GBS80 contains a pilin motif similar to that found in the *Corynebacterium diphtheriae* pilin subunit [25], suggesting that it may also code for pilus-like structures.

These antigens are covalently linked in high molecular weight structures. These oligomers have been visualized on the surface of intact bacteria by immunogold staining and TEM as a pilus-like structure, which protrudes beyond the cell wall and the polysaccharide capsule. These pili structures have never before been described for GBS [26].

In conclusion, the "reverse vaccinology" approach applied to more than one genome, has allowed the identification, in a very short period of time, of four cross-protective antigens which can form the basis of a multicomponent vaccine against GBS. Moreover, the sequence comparison between various bacterial species has hugely helped in understanding their functional role.

References

1 Rappuoli R **2000**, Reverse vaccinology, *Curr. Opin. Microbiol.* 3, 445–450.

2 Rappuoli R **2001**, Conjugates and reverse vaccinology to eliminate bacterial meningitis, *Vaccine* 19, 2319–2322.

3 Tettelin H, Saunders NJ, Heidelberg J, Jeffries AC, Nelson KE, Eisen JA, Ketchum KA, Hood DW, Peden JF, Dodson RJ, et al. **2000**, Complete genome sequence of Neisseria meningitidis serogroup B strain MC58, *Science* 287, 1809–1815.

4 Pizza M, Scarlato V, Masignani V, Giuliani MM, Arico B, Comanducci M, Jennings GT, Baldi L, Bartolini E, Capecchi B, et al. **2000**, Identification of vaccine candidates against serogroup B meningococcus by whole-genome sequencing, *Science* 287, 1816–1820.

5 Goldschneider I, Gotschlich EC, Artenstein MS **1969**, Human immunity to the meningococcus. I. The role of humoral antibodies, *J. Exp. Med.* 129, 1307–1326.

6 Masignani V, Comanducci M, Giuliani MM, Bambini S, Adu-Bobie J, Arico B, Brunelli B, Pieri A, Santini L, Savino S, et al. **2003**, Vaccination against *Neisseria meningitidis* using three variants of the lipoprotein GNA1870, *J. Exp. Med.* 197, 789–799.

7 Giuliani MM, Santini L, Brunelli B, Biolchi A, Arico B, Di Marcello F, Cartocci E, Comanducci M, Masignani V, Lozzi L, et al. **2005**, The region comprising amino acids 100 to 255 of *Neisseria meningitidis* lipoprotein GNA 1870 elicits bactericidal antibodies, *Infect. Immun.* 73, 1151–1160.

8 Fletcher LD, Bernfield L, Barniak V, Farley JE, Howell A, Knauf M, Ooi P, Smith RP, Weise P, Wetherell M, et al. **2004**, Vaccine potential of the *Neisseria meningitidis* 2086 lipoprotein, *Infect. Immun.* 72, 2088–2100.

9 Welsch JA, Rossi R, Comanducci M, Granoff DM **2004**, Protective activity of monoclonal antibodies to genome-derived neisserial antigen 1870, a *Neisseria meningitidis* candidate vaccine, *J. Immunol.* 172, 5606–5615.

10 St Geme JW, 3rd, de la Morena ML, Falkow S **1994**, A *Haemophilus influenzae* IgA protease-like protein promotes intimate interaction with human epithelial cells, *Mol. Microbiol.* 14, 217–233.

11 Holtje JV **1998**, Growth of the stress-bearing and shape-maintaining murein sacculus of *Escherichia coli, Microbiol. Mol. Biol. Rev.* 62, 181–203.

12 Desvaux M, Parham NJ, Henderson IR **2004**, The autotransporter secretion system, *Res. Microbiol.* 155, 53–60.

13 Barocchi MA, Masignani V, Rappuoli R **2005**, Cell entry machines: a common theme in nature? *Nat. Rev. Microbiol.* 3, 349–358.

14 Masignani V, Balducci E, Di Marcello F, Savino S, Serruto D, Veggi D, Bambini S, Scarselli M, Arico B, Comanducci M, et al. **2003**, NarE: a novel ADP-ribosyltransferase from *Neisseria meningitidis, Mol. Microbiol.* 50, 1055–1067.

15 Hadi HA, Wooldridge KG, Robinson K, Ala'Aldeen DA **2001**, Identification and characterization of App: an immunogenic autotransporter protein of *Neisseria meningitidis, Mol. Microbiol.* 41, 611–623.

16 Serruto D, Adu-Bobie J, Scarselli M, Veggi D, Pizza M, Rappuoli R, Arico B **2003**, *Neisseria meningitidis* App, a new adhesin with autocatalytic serine protease activity, *Mol. Microbiol.* 48, 323–334.

17 Comanducci M, Bambini S, Brunelli B, Adu-Bobie J, Arico B, Capecchi B, Giuliani MM, Masignani V, Santini L, Savino S, et al. **2002**, NadA, a novel vaccine candidate of *Neisseria meningitidis, J. Exp. Med.* 195, 1445–1454.

18 Capecchi B, Adu-Bobie J, Di Marcello F, Ciucchi L, Masignani V, Taddei A, Rappuoli R, Pizza M, Arico B **2005**, *Neisseria meningitidis* NadA is a new invasin which promotes bacterial adhesion to and penetration into human epithelial cells, *Mol. Microbiol.* 55, 687–698.

19 Comanducci M, Bambini S, Caugant DA, Mora M, Brunelli B, Capecchi B, Ciucchi L, Rappuoli R, Pizza M **2004**, NadA diversity and carriage in Neisseria meningitidis, *Infect. Immun.* 72, 4217–4223.

20 Jennings GT, Savino S, Marchetti E, Arico B, Kast T, Baldi L, Ursinus A, Holtje

JV, Nicholas RA, Rappuoli R, et al. **2002**, GNA33 from *Neisseria meningitidis* serogroup B encodes a membrane-bound lytic transglycosylase (MltA), *Eur. J. Biochem.* 269, 3722–3731.

21 Adu-Bobie J, Lupetti P, Brunelli B, Granoff D, Norais N, Ferrari G, Grandi G, Rappuoli R, Pizza M **2004**, GNA33 of Neisseria meningitidis is a lipoprotein required for cell separation, membrane architecture, and virulence, *Infect. Immun.* 72, 1914–1919.

22 Maione D, Rinaudo CD, Masignani V, Mora M, Scarselli M, Tettelin H, Brettoni C, Iacobini ET, Rosini R, D'Agostino N, et al. **2005**, Identification of a universal group B streptococcus vaccine by multiple genome screen, *Science* 309, 148–150.

23 Tettelin H, Masignani V, Cieslewicz MJ, Donati C, Medini D, Ward NL, Angiuoli SV, Crabtree J, Jones AL, Durkin AS, et al. **2005**, Genome analysis of multiple pathogenic isolates of *Streptococcus agalactiae*: implications for the microbial "pan-genome", *Proc. Natl. Acad. Sci.* 102, 13950–13955.

24 Navarre WW, Schneewind O **1999**, Surface proteins of gram-positive bacteria and mechanisms of their targeting to the cell wall envelope, *Microbiol. Mol. Biol. Rev.* 63, 174–229.

25 Ton-That H, Marraffini LA, Schneewind O **2004**, Sortases and pilin elements involved in pilus assembly of *Corynebacterium diphtheriae, Mol. Microbiol.* 53, 251–261.

26 Lauer P, Rinaudo CD, Soriani M, Margarit I, Maione D, Rosini R, Taddei AR, Mora M, Rappuoli R, Grandi G, Telford JL **2005**, Genome analysis reveals pili in group B streptococcus, *Science* 309, 105.

20
Vaccination for the Control of Meningococcal Disease: the Use of Meningococcal Vaccines from the Public Health Perspective

Elizabeth Miller, Mary Ramsay and Helen Campbell

20.1
Considerations Before the Introduction of New Vaccines or Revised Immunization Programs

Different vaccines are available to protect against meningococcal disease. As with any vaccine, it is important to develop the most appropriate immunization strategy to best target the national or regional situation. This may include a selective vaccination program for those identified to be at high risk. Alternatively, a decision may be made to provide mass vaccination to everyone in a certain age group in the population. Before a new or revised immunization program can be considered, high-quality epidemiological data on vaccine-preventable disease and characteristics of the disease organism are essential. In order to develop appropriate policy, a surveillance system needs to identify which groups are at particular risk of infection within the population in terms of acute illness, mortality and longer-term morbidity. It also needs to distinguish which organisms, and which serogroups and serotypes of these organisms, are important for these clinical outcomes.

There is usually an established framework for making and implementing national policy decisions on mass vaccination. This often takes the form of independent expert national advisory committees such as the National Advisory Committee on Immunization (NACI) in Canada, the Joint Committee on Vaccination and Immunization (JCVI) in the United Kingdom, the Advisory Committee on Immunization Practices (ACIP) in the USA and the Ständige Impfkommission (standing committee on vaccination, STIKO) in Germany. These expert committees should consider all of the available evidence before advising ministers.

There is a need to balance the benefits of proposed vaccine programs against possible other uses of the same resources within the health systems that are in place. Therefore many developed countries require economic analyses to be conducted before a vaccine can be introduced. Such analyses may be performed from the perspective of the health care sector; that is by attempting to assess

Handbook of Meningococcal Disease. Infection Biology, Vaccination, Clinical Management.
Edited by M. Frosch and M.C.J. Maiden

ISBN: 3-527-31260-9

the balance between the costs of providing vaccination against the potential savings from the reduced health care costs associated with disease. In this respect, many of the widely used vaccines are considered to be cost-saving, whereas others compare favorably with currently available therapeutic interventions. Some analyses may choose to consider the wider benefits to society of providing vaccination by also estimating the costs incurred by families and individuals, for example through loss of work days [1]. Such considerations may be relatively more important with the arrival of vaccines against diseases that are common but rarely severe, such as rotavirus in a developed country.

Estimating the potential benefits of vaccination requires accurate data on the burden and costs of disease; and this will often be obtained from population-based studies or from enhanced surveillance. The costs of the vaccination program will include both the costs of vaccine and of administration and must also consider the potential costs of adverse events. The reduction in disease burden can be assessed from large clinical trials or from predictions based upon knowledge of the efficacy of the vaccine. Where large-scale trials are not feasible, mathematical models have become an important tool for these analyses and can also be used to predict potential indirect effects of mass vaccination.

The aim of mathematical models is to simulate the key processes that determine the interaction between the organism and an individual and that influence the characteristics of the disease at a population level [2]. Mathematical models have enabled a more quantified and consistent approach to the prediction of the impact of vaccines or vaccine schedules. These can take into account many complex issues, such as reduction in disease transmission, increased average age at infection, differences in vaccine or disease induced immunity, heterogeneous mixing within and between different age groups and herd immunity effects [3]. Models may also need to be developed to help predict the impact of vaccination on antigenically variable agents [4]. This follows the concern that high levels of population immunity to one antigen may lead to the emergence of other strains of the same agent, thus reducing or reversing the impact of the vaccine program.

Once a mass immunization program is in place, measurement of the implementation of the program (vaccine coverage) and the outcome, based on pre- and post-vaccine disease epidemiology, is required. The surveillance needs to include the facility for monitoring vaccine safety. In developed countries, different disease surveillance mechanisms are in place to monitor communicable diseases and mass immunization programs at a national level (Table 20.1).

Vaccines are usually licensed on the basis of efficacy measured in controlled clinical trials. After implementation, however, vaccines are not necessarily used under the same ideal conditions and may be given to individuals with clinical conditions that could interfere with the response of the vaccine. Therefore it may be necessary to assess the effectiveness [5] of a vaccine under routine use. Vaccine effectiveness can be estimated using surveillance data (such as laboratory reports) in populations who have been vaccinated as part of a routine program using cohort, case-control or case-cohort studies.

Table 20.1 A summary of sources of epidemiological data for communicable diseases.

Data source	Description of data
Statutory notifications	A legal requirement for certain diseases to be reported. This information is usually compiled nationally and based on clinical diagnosis.
Laboratory reports	Central and/or regional reporting of laboratory confirmed cases of certain diseases.
Enhanced surveillance	Reconciliation of laboratory confirmed cases with clinically confirmed cases. There may also be detailed follow-up of individual cases. This is useful for monitoring vaccine failures as information on immunization history, etc. can be obtained.
Serological surveys	Based on blood samples taken from the population for other diagnostic or disease management purposes. This can provide information on levels of protection against individual diseases within the population.
Death data	Usually compiled nationally and based on recorded causes of death on death certificates. Enhanced surveillance can also be a useful source of information on outcome of individual laboratory-confirmed cases.
Special registries or surveillance schemes	These may be established to provide information on certain (usually rare) conditions that may be associated with particular communicable diseases.
Hospital episode statistics	Provide summary statistics on disease cases that have resulted in hospitalization and may be a useful source of information on long-term morbidity.
Sentinel reporting	By recruited general practitioners, can provide useful data on patient consultations and referrals.
Carriage studies	For certain communicable diseases, like *Neisseria meningitidis*, information on carriage of the disease organism within the population can be useful. Such information may be obtained through specific studies.
Vaccine coverage	In many countries there is routine collection of national immunization coverage levels for all antigens included in the childhood program. Other countries collect representative data through surveys and other studies.
Vaccine safety	There may be active or passive surveillance systems in place to monitor adverse reactions to new or existing vaccines. If passive reporting is suggestive of a previously unrecognized risk linked to the vaccine then a hypothesis can be generated for investigation by more robust scientific methods.

This chapter considers in detail the public health perspective concerning the first introduction of meningococcal C conjugate (MCC) vaccine for mass immunization in the UK. Experiences with immunization against meningococcal disease in other developed countries are then discussed.

20.2
The UK Example of the Introduction of Meningococcal C Conjugate Vaccine

20.2.1
Epidemiology of Meningococcal Disease in England and Wales Before the Introduction of MCC Vaccines

Since the 1980s, the majority of cases of meningococcal infection in England and Wales were due to serogroup B disease. Approximately 25–30% of all confirmed meningococcal disease was caused by meningococcal C infection. During the 1990s, the incidence of laboratory-confirmed meningococcal infection of all serogroups increased in England and Wales (Fig. 20.1). The rise was partly explained by improved ascertainment, with the introduction of more sensitive polymerase chain reaction (PCR) methods for the identification and serogrouping of meningococci [6, 7]. However cases of serogroup C disease increased proportionately more than other serogroups, signifying a genuine rise in the level of endemic serogroup C infection. This increase was thought to be due to the emergence of a "hypervirulent" strain of serogroup C. Such increases had occurred in Canada and the Czech Republic, and were associated with strains of the ST-11 complex [8–10]. In the UK, these strains were usually associated with serotype 2a.

In 1998 enhanced surveillance was carried out in five regions in England [11]. This showed a sizeable number of cases of meningococcal infection were clinically diagnosed but not confirmed by culture or PCR methods.

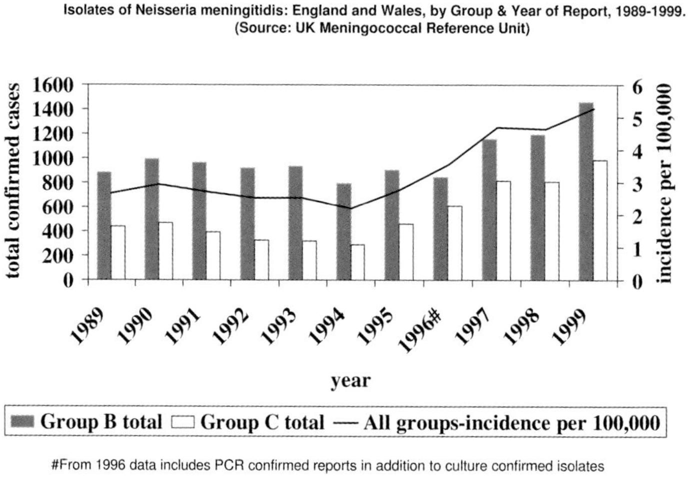

Fig. 20.1 Isolates of *N. meningitidis*: England and Wales, by serogroup and year of report, 1989–1999 (source: UK Meningococcal Reference Unit).

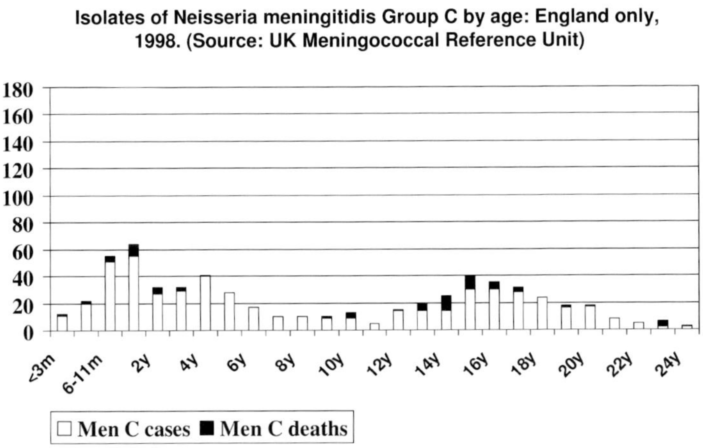

Fig. 20.2 Isolates of *N. meningitidis* serogroup C by age: England only, 1998 (source: UK Meningococcal Reference Unit).

In the 1990s in England and Wales, rates of serogroup B and C meningococcal infection were highest in the under 5 years age group with a peak in children under 1 year of age (Figs. 20.2, 20.3). Both serogroups had a secondary peak in adolescents and teenagers, but serogroup C was proportionately more common in this age group. Case fatality rates increased with age but were higher overall for serogroup C (around 12% overall) than serogroup B disease (around 5% overall). So in 1998, whilst serogroup B disease accounted for more confirmed cases of meningococcal disease than serogroup C, the latter caused more deaths.

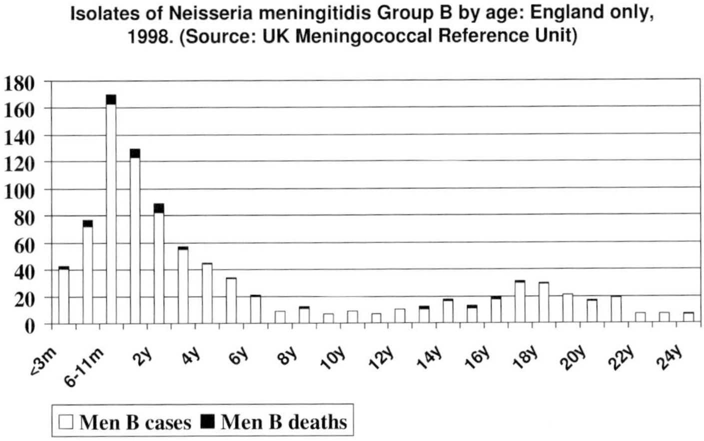

Fig. 20.3 Isolates of *N. meningitidis* serogroup B by age: England only, 1998 (source: UK Meningococcal Reference Unit).

20.2.2 Choice of Strategy

20.2.2.1 Vaccine Development in the UK

The early indications of an increase in serogroup C meningococcal disease were first noticed in 1995. At this time, a plain polysaccharide vaccine against serogroup C meningococcal disease was available (combined with serogroups A, C, Y, W-135). However, good progress had also been made towards the development of meningococcal A and C conjugate vaccines.

Polysaccharide vaccines have a number of limitations and there were uncertainties around its use for mass vaccination in the UK at that time. Protection from polysaccharide vaccines is short-term and they are ineffective in individuals under 2 years of age, who are at most risk of disease. This is because T-cell-independent immunity is elicited by the purified capsular polysaccharides from which the vaccine is derived (see Chapter 17). There were concerns that two major interventions would be required in a relatively short time-frame if polysaccharide vaccine was used initially, as conjugate vaccines were likely to be available in the near future. These concerns were compounded by the possibility that immunization with conjugate vaccine, after polysaccharide vaccine had already been given, could induce immunologic hyporesponsiveness to C polysaccharide, as had been observed after a second dose of polysaccharide vaccine [12].

This knowledge informed the vaccine research program of the National Vaccine Evaluation Consortium (NVEC), a collaborative group largely funded by the Department of Health and consisting of different bodies within the Health Protection Agency (a publicly funded organization), the National Institute for Biological Standards and Control and an academic immunobiology unit. Vaccine manufacturers also collaborated on the meningococcal C conjugate (MCC) vaccine development program [13]. The objective of the research program was to generate the safety and immunogenicity data needed to support the licensure of MCC vaccines and to inform policy decisions about their use in the UK population. This portfolio of research was therefore specific to the UK situation and provided information on MCC vaccine safety and efficacy when administered as part of the UK routine schedule at 2, 3 and 4 months of age with the other antigens that would be administered concomitantly. Research also provided data to inform the use of a catch-up campaign in children aged 4 months to 18 years and the development of pre-clinical tests for controlling the quality of the vaccine batches once it was licensed.

The resultant clinical trials of MCC vaccines showed that they were immunogenic in all age groups and that their reactogenicity profiles were similar to other routinely recommended vaccines with no serious adverse events identified [14–18]. The vaccines also induced immunological memory, which lasted at least 4 years after infant immunization; and they were therefore expected to provide long-term immunity against meningococcal C disease [19]. The first MCC vaccine was licensed in the UK in September 1999. This was on the basis that there was a putative correlate of protection and that the low incidence of meningococcal serogroup C disease would have required a lengthy and expensive Phase III trial [5] (see Chapter 22).

20.2.2.2 **The UK Immunization Strategy**

Projected vaccine supplies, combined with knowledge about the age profile of meningococcal serogroup C disease incidence and deaths drove the MCC vaccine strategy that was adopted in the UK. It was decided to introduce routine immunization for all infants (three doses), together with a catch-up campaign for all children aged 4 months to 17 years. Twelve million children were offered the vaccine in England and Wales. Based on data generated by the NVEC research program, babies aged 5–12 months were offered two doses of vaccine whilst those over 12 months of age required a single dose of MCC vaccine. Each age group was assigned a priority within the schedule according to the risk of disease in children of that age. Immunization of each age group began as enough vaccine became available.

On 1 November 1999, the UK became the first country to introduce MCC vaccine with the vaccine being offered to all children aged 15–17 years. The vaccine was introduced into the routine primary immunization schedule from the end of November 1999, with catch-up for those aged 12–15 months introduced simultaneously. The intention was to immunize the highest risk age groups before the 1999/2000 winter season got underway. The 5–8 year age group was the last to be offered MCC vaccine and was scheduled to complete immunization by the end of October 2000. From early January 2002, the use of MCC vaccine was extended so that it could be offered to all individuals up to 25 years of age.

Cost effectiveness analysis in the UK indicated that, under most assumptions, MCC vaccination was likely to be highly cost-effective in comparison with most health care interventions even without a herd immunity effect [20]. Because of the need to provide more doses to those immunized in infancy, infant immunization was less cost-effective than vaccination of school-age children or of preschool children in primary care.

20.2.2.3 **The UK Surveillance Strategy**

The decision to introduce MCC vaccine in the UK was undertaken at a time when there were still a number of uncertainties surrounding the use of the vaccine. Firstly, licensure was based on a correlate of protection. There was also the possibility that future boosting with MCC vaccine might be necessary if vaccine efficacy declined in the longer term. The impact of the vaccine on carriage was unknown. A reduction in carriage might lead to the positive outcome of herd immunity. However, there was also the theoretical possibility that the removal of the carriage of certain meningococcal serogroup C vaccine serotypes within the population might, with capsular switching, allow the expansion of more virulent non-serogroup C (in particular B) strains [21].

Table 20.2 Summary of the objectives of the UK surveillance strategy.

Objectives
To monitor the impact of MCC vaccine on the epidemiology of meningococcal disease
To measure age specific vaccine coverage
To measure age-specific effectiveness of MCC vaccines
To identify risk factors and mechanisms of MCC and meningococcal A/C polysaccharide vaccine failure
To monitor the effect of MCC introduction on the phenotypic and genetic characteristics of invasive meningococci
To establish an active system for monitoring vaccine-associated adverse events

Recognition of such uncertainties led to the establishment of a detailed and comprehensive surveillance program to monitor the impact of the new vaccine [22]. The objectives of this surveillance strategy are summarized in Table 20.2.

Generation of these data have enabled validation of the correlates of protection [23]. A cross-sectional nasopharyngeal carriage study was also set up to assess meningococcal strains carried in students aged 15–17 years before and after the introduction of MCC vaccine [24]. To investigate whether capsular switching from serogroup C to B might be occurring, a subcapsular marker for the serogroup C ET37 (ST11) complex strains was identified as PorB serotype 2a (B:2a) and the number of B:2a cases are being monitored by the Meningococcal Reference Unit. Regulatory monitoring of MCC vaccine safety is undertaken through the national voluntary reporting scheme (the "Yellow Card scheme") [25, 26]. This system is useful for generating signals which can then be investigated through established record linkage systems [27].

20.2.3 Impact of the MCC Immunization Campaign in England and Wales

20.2.3.1 Immunization Coverage

Overall coverage achieved through the schools based program, for children aged 5–17 years inclusive, was at least 85%. Standard collection of coverage data for MCC vaccine at 1, 2 and 5 years of age showed that the level of coverage achieved within each of these age groups rapidly became comparable to other vaccines offered at the same age. Uptake of the primary course of MCC vaccine (at 2, 3, 4 months) very quickly exceeded 90% by first birthday. This indicated good acceptance of MCC vaccine by parents. This had been anticipated from the attitudinal surveys conducted on behalf of the Department of Health that had consistently shown the disease that was almost universally considered by mothers of young children to be very serious was meningitis.

20.2.3.2 Disease Epidemiology

Total cases of serogroup C disease fell progressively from 1999, when MCC vaccine became available. In 2004 the total number of cases of serogroup C disease fell to its lowest since the introduction of the vaccine. The breakdown of cases by age and calendar year in England is given in Table 20.3 for meningococcal C disease from 1998. Large sustained reductions in the level of C disease have been observed for each age group subsequent to the introduction of the vaccine within that cohort. Deaths have similarly been reduced (Fig. 20.4).

MCC vaccine was also offered to those aged 20–24 years from January 2002. As well as a significant decrease in the number of cases in this age group there has been an impact on those aged 25 years and over, most of whom would be too old to have been offered the vaccine. This is one piece of evidence that points to a herd immunity effect (see Section 20.2.3.4).

Cases of serogroup B disease in England continued to increase after cases of serogroup C disease had peaked, reaching the highest recorded levels in 2001 (Table 20.4). Total cases of serogroup B disease then fell to levels similar to those in 1998. The changes have been inconsistent between age groups. Deaths from meningococcal B disease have shown a high level of stability with very similar percentages of cases dying in each age group through time.

These general observations are consistent, with reductions in serogroup C disease in immunized age groups under 20 years of age being largely due to the introduction of MCC vaccine. Consistent marked reductions in the number of serogroup C cases have occurred in all immunized cohorts under 20 years, whereas changes in serogroup B disease have been smaller and less consistent. The changes in the level of serogroup B disease are likely to reflect natural variation and are independent of the changes observed in serogroup C disease.

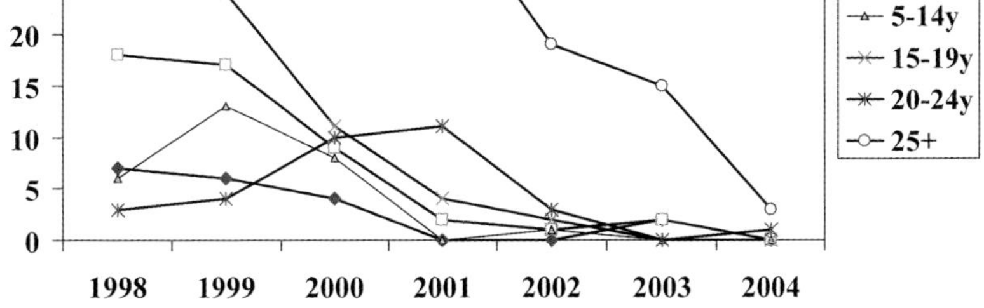

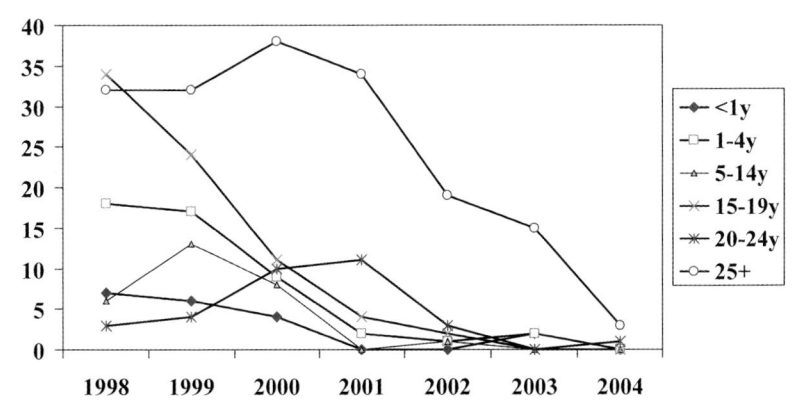

Fig. 20.4 Total deaths recorded as due to meningococcal C infection in England by year (ONS data only).

Table 20.3 All cases of meningococcal C disease by age and year (provisional, England only).

Age (years)	1998	1999		2000		2001		2002		2003		2004	
	Total	Total	% change from 1998	Total	% change from 1998	Total	% change from 1998	Total	% change from 1998	Total	% change from 1998	Total	% change from 1998
<1	89	95	7	26	–71	18	–80	4	–96	2	–98	2	–98
1	64	75	17	36	–44	7	–89	4	–94	5	–92	2	–97
2	32	45	41	39	22	13	–59	2	–94	3	–91	1	–97
3–4	73	89	22	85	16	9	–88	6	–92	9	–88	6	–92
5–8	65	92	42	71	9	4	–94	5	–92	5	–92	1	–98
9–10	18	20	11	14	–22	1	–94	1	–94	0	–100	1	–94
11–14	53	73	38	50	–6	6	–89	3	–94	0	–100	1	–98
15–19	162	178	10	65	–60	24	–85	14	–91	4	–98	3	–98
20–24	37	48	30	64	73	42	14	24	–35	11	–70	3	–92
≥25	170	184	8	226	33	174	2	92	–46	55	–68	36	–79
<20	556	667	20	386	–31	82	–85	39	–93	28	–95	17	–97
≥20	207	232	12	290	40	216	4	116	–44	66	–68	39	–81
Unknown	5	11	120	0	–100	1	–80	0	–100	0	–100	0	–100
Total	768	910	18	676	–12	299	–61	155	–80	94	–88	56	–93

Table 20.4 All cases of meningococcal B disease by age and year (provisional, England only).

Age (years)	1998	1999		2000		2001		2002		2003		2004	
	Total	Total	% change from 1998	Total	% change from 1998	Total	% change from 1998	Total	% change from 1998	Total	% change from 1998	Total	% change from 1998
<1	290	303	4	355	22	373	29	297	2	319	10	280	−3
1	130	154	18	171	32	208	60	184	42	200	54	153	18
2	89	112	26	141	58	122	37	111	25	105	18	93	4
3–4	102	129	26	150	47	151	48	140	37	130	27	98	−4
5–8	76	111	46	102	34	119	57	97	28	80	5	74	−3
9–10	16	26	63	23	44	26	63	41	156	29	81	13	−19
11–14	45	49	9	61	36	92	104	56	24	63	40	49	9
15–19	117	162	38	175	50	181	55	129	10	135	15	108	−8
20–24	57	55	−4	63	11	68	19	49	−14	46	−19	40	−30
≥25	179	220	23	284	59	266	49	196	9	197	10	188	5
<20	865	1046	21	1178	36	1272	47	1055	22	1061	23	868	0
≥20	236	275	17	347	47	334	42	245	4	243	3	228	−3
Unknown	9	17	89	5	−44	4	−56	3	−67	5	−44	1	−89
Total	1110	1338	21	1530	38	1610	45	1303	17	1309	18	1097	−1

20.2.3.3 **Efficacy of MCC Vaccine**

All cases of confirmed and probable serogroup C disease in individuals under 20 years of age are being followed up to obtain immunization history. These cases are then categorized according to whether they meet the criteria for a true vaccine failure. A true MCC vaccine failure is defined as confirmed invasive meningococcal serogroup C disease with onset at least 10 days after the last dose of a completed course of MCC vaccine in that individual. Available information on vaccine coverage in different age cohorts, details of true vaccine failures and cases of meningococcal C disease in individuals who were eligible for the vaccine but did not receive it are used to calculate vaccine effectiveness.

Efficacy estimates [28] using the screening method, have shown high vaccine effectiveness (≥83%) in all children who had received MCC vaccines between the ages of 5 months and 18 years in the catch-up campaign. Overall, routine infant immunization was estimated to be 66% effective, but there were clear differences based on time since vaccination. Within one year of scheduled vaccination, vaccine effectiveness was high and comparable with cohorts vaccinated at older ages. However, MCC vaccines appeared to confer little protection more than 1 year after the last scheduled dose in infants and vaccine effectiveness was significantly lower compared to catch-up cohorts in the same period. Vaccine effectiveness also declined with time since immunization in the catch-up cohorts. When these cohorts were combined there was a significant decline in effectiveness after 1 year of vaccination. Updated estimates of effectiveness in all older age cohorts have remained reasonably stable and high, whilst the apparent decline in infants has continued (Table 20.5).

Such reductions in vaccine effectiveness with time have subsequently been shown for conjugate vaccines against *Haemophilus influenzae* type b (Hib) when given at 2, 3 and 4 months of age without a booster [29, 30].

20.2.3.4 **Herd Immunity and Carriage**

The observed waning of MCC vaccine effectiveness in routinely vaccinated infants is of concern, but the actual number of cases in these cohorts has remained low due to high levels of indirect protection [31]. The decline in the catch-up cohorts is considered less worrying because overall effectiveness remains high after 4 years.

There is some evidence of a herd immunity effect in unimmunized individuals who would have been offered MCC vaccine [31]. This was investigated by comparison of the meningococcal C attack rate in all unimmunized individuals in age groups targeted by the MCC campaign in one complete epidemiological year before and after the introduction of MCC vaccine. These data (Table 20.6) indicated considerable reductions in the attack rates in unimmunized individuals in all targeted age groups after the introduction of MCC vaccine that became progressively more marked with time (Health Protection Agency, unpublished data).

The herd immunity effect following MCC vaccination resulted from a reduction in the prevalence of serogroup C carriage and is likely to persist for several years

Table 20.5 MCC vaccine effectiveness in immunized cohorts to end of December 2004, England only (Health Protection Agency, unpublished data).

Cohort	Age at MCC vaccine	Doses scheduled [a]	Period of observation (by quarter and year)	Cases of confirmed serogroup C disease (vaccinated)			% vaccine effectiveness (95% CI) [a]			
				Total	Time since scheduled vaccination [b, c]		Overall	Time since scheduled vaccination [b, c]		Difference between ≤1 year and >1 year since MCC vaccine
					Within 1 year	>1 year		Within 1 year	>1 year	
Routine	2, 3, 4 months	3	Q1 2000–Q4 2004	34 (26)	12 (5)	22 (21)	65 (10, 84)	90 (63, 97)	–90 (–7761,69)	$P < 0.01$
Infant catch-up	5 to 11 months	2	Q3 2000–Q4 2004	14 (5)	4 (1)	10 (4)	86 (54, 96)	91 (–8, 100)	84 (31, 97)	$P = 0.63$
Toddlers catch-up	1 to 2 years	1	Q3 2000–Q4 2004	25 (10)			83 (60, 93)			
Pre-school catch-up	3 to 4 years	1	Q3 2000–Q4 2004	37 (2)			98 (91, 100)			
Infant school catch-up	4 to 6 years	1	Q3 2000–Q4 2004	16 (0)	105 (10)	66 (17)	100 (68, 100)	95 (90, 98)	89 (80, 94)	P = 0.03
Junior school catch-up	7 to 10 years	1	Q3 2000–Q4 2004	8 (3)			88 (38, 98)			
Secondary school catch-up	11 to 16 years	1	Q2 2000–Q4 2004	40 (8)			96 (90, 98)			
Sixth form catch-up	17 to 18 years	1	Q1 2000–Q4 2004	45 (4)			94 (82, 98)			
Total				219 (58)	121 (16)	98 (42)				

a) Vaccine effectiveness compares children eligible for complete vaccination who had received all scheduled doses versus 0 doses. Partially vaccinated children were excluded.
b) Unvaccinated cases are based on the date of birth cohort to which each individual belongs.
c) For the time change analysis, cohorts aged 1–18 years were combined.

Table 20.6 Reduction in meningococcal serogroup C incidence in unvaccinated groups by age in pre- and post-vaccine periods (adapted from [31]).

Age scheduled for MCC (years)	Rate per 10^5 pre-MCC campaign	Rate per 10^5 post-MCC campaign	% reduction (95% CI)
15 to 17	5.30	1.79	66 (37 to 82)
11 to 14	5.54	1.11	80 (46 to 93)
9 to 10	1.69	1.30	23 (−228 to 82)
5 to 8	2.07	0.87	58 (−35 to 87)
2 to 4	3.94	1.20	70 (30 to 87)
1	6.82	2.05	70 (−24 to 93)
Infant catch-up	7.49	1.56	79 (−54 to 97)
Overall	4.08	1.36	67 (52 to 77)

[20]. The introduction of the *H. influenzae* b (Hib) vaccine similarly reduced the attack rate in those too young or too old to be directly protected by immunization [32–34]. A rapid, indirect protective effect in young infants was realized with Hib vaccine probably because the organism carriage rates were highest in the preschool population with whom infants have a relatively high level of interaction. The potential for such a protective effect in infants is less with meningococcal C disease as carriage rates are highest in those aged 15–24 years [35]. The potential for reduction is affected by the level of mixing of those age groups targeted for immunization both within and without that age group.

Before the experience with MCC vaccine in the UK, it was widely believed that conjugate vaccines were effective largely through the direct protection that they offered individuals and that this protection endured even without a booster. The experience with Hib vaccine, together with close monitoring of true effectiveness of MCC vaccine, suggested that the impact of conjugate vaccines on interruption of carriage was more important than previously understood [20]. Efficacy and antibodies rapidly wane after a 2/3/4 month infant course and persist better after a single dose in older age groups.

Presence of immune memory (as currently measured by avidity maturation and booster response) is not predictive of long-term protection and there are currently no clear correlates of long term protection against disease. Protection against carriage induced by the MCC catch-up campaign is the major determinant of program outcome and cost-effectiveness [20]. MCC immunization has been shown to significantly reduce carriage of meningococcal serogroup C organisms in the short term in immunized cohorts [24].

20.2.3.5 Meningococcal Diversity

Concerns have been raised about the possibility that, as a result of capsular switching arising from selection pressure by MCC vaccine, the hypervirulent strain responsible for the increase in incidence in the UK may emerge as another serogroup. It has also been suggested that new virulent meningococcal clones may appear, to fill the ecological niche. The monitoring conducted by the Health Protection Agency Meningococcal Reference Unit has detected no such changes to date. In particular, the number of B:2a cases has not risen above previously seen levels since the introduction of the MCC vaccines.

20.3 Other Examples of the Introduction of Meningococcal Vaccines

20.3.1 Meningococcal C Conjugate Vaccine

European Countries

In Europe, the reported incidence of meningococcal infection, and the relative contribution of different serogroups vary markedly. For example, in 1999, the proportion of meningococcal disease due to serogroup C ranged from 14 to 48% [36]. A high incidence of meningococcal disease and a high proportion of serogroup C disease were reported from Ireland, Spain and Iceland. Both Ireland and Spain had experienced increases in incidence in the mid 1990s [37, 38].

In Spain, 14 of the 17 autonomous regions had chosen to implement a mass campaign with meningococcal AC polysaccharide vaccination in 1997 [37]. Because of the continued high incidence of serogroup C disease in young children and following on from the introduction of MCC vaccine in the UK in 1999, MCC was included in the Spanish routine infant schedule from 2000. A catch-up campaign was also implemented nationally for all children under 6 years of age and extended to those under 19 years in three autonomous regions. MCC vaccine was also introduced in Ireland during 2000 [39]; and the incidence of infection has subsequently fallen in all regions of Spain [37, 39] and in Ireland [40]. Iceland also introduced MCC vaccine in 2002 [36].

Between 1999 and 2001–2, the incidence of serogroup C meningococcal infection in the Netherlands and Belgium increased. Based upon a detailed comparison of the economic benefits of various strategies, the decision was made to implement a mass catch-up campaign with addition of a routine single dose of vaccine in the second year of life in late 2002 [41]. The demonstration of a major herd immunity effect in the UK was used as evidence to justify the decision to leave younger infants unvaccinated. A major impact on the incidence of serogroup C infection has already been demonstrated in the Netherlands [42].

Countries Outside Europe

In Canada, an increase in serogroup C meningococcal disease in the early 1990s led to mass campaigns using polysaccharide serogroup A and C vaccine in many areas [43, 44]. Disease rates in those targeted for vaccination declined markedly, whilst staying high in older age groups [44]. Evidence of declining protection [45, 46], was followed by a further increase in disease rates in 2001. On this occasion, a mass campaign with MCC vaccine was used to control the epidemic and high levels of protection have been demonstrated [47]. Routine vaccination with MCC has been shown to be more cost-effective than the implementation of MCC as an outbreak control measure [48], and routine immunization with MCC is now recommended [49], although the choice of schedule varies by state [50].

Between 1999 and 2002, the incidence of meningococcal disease increased in Australia [51] and the proportion due to serogroup C infection rose to 41% [52]. Serogroup C disease was observed to be more common in adolescents and young adults and was associated with a high case-fatality rate. Cost-effectiveness analysis had indicated that adolescent vaccination was the most cost-effective option [53]. The Australian Technical Advisory Group on Immunization (ATAGI) recommended routine immunization at 12 months of age and 15 years, with a catch-up program for 15–17 year olds [54]. However, the Australian government eventually decided to offer the vaccine to everyone up to the age of 19 years.

20.4 Other Meningococcal Vaccines

20.4.1 United States of America

In the United States, the main serogroups are B, C and Y, with each being responsible for approximately one-third of the cases of meningococcal disease [55]. The proportion of cases caused by each serogroup varies by age. The public health strategy adopted needed to target the relatively high level of serogroup Y disease and therefore polyvalent conjugate vaccine was felt to be appropriate for the population of the United States. In January 2005, a tetravalent meningococcal polysaccharide–protein conjugate vaccine (MCV4) was licensed for use in individuals aged between 11 and 55 years. The vaccine contains capsular polysaccharide from serogroups A, C, Y and W-135.

Analysis in the United States suggested that routine immunization with MCV4 in adolescents would be more cost-effective than vaccination of toddlers or infants [56]. This was due to the higher disease rates and the high level of carriage in adolescents. However, because of the relatively low incidence of disease in the USA, the cost-effectiveness ratio would be high. Despite this, routine vaccination of young adolescents (aged 11–12 years) has now been recommended with MCV4 at the preadolescent health care visit [55]. For those adolescents who have not previously received MCV4, vaccination before high school entry (at approximately age 15 years) is recommended as an effective strategy to reduce meningococcal disease incidence among adolescents and young adults.

20.4.2
New Zealand

New Zealand has been experiencing an epidemic of invasive meningococcal disease for about a decade, with approximately 80% of all meningococcal disease was being caused by a single strain of *Neisseria meningitidis* serogroup B with the P1.7b, 4 PorA protein [57]. As in other countries, meningococcal disease disproportionately affected children and young people, with more than 80% of cases occurring in those aged 0–19 years. Maori and Pacific Island children, and those living in deprived areas, carried a disproportionately high risk of meningococcal disease.

The meningococcal vaccine strategy in New Zealand aimed to control the specific epidemic strain of serogroup B *N. meningitidis* by implementing a mass immunization program. A New Zealand meningococcal B vaccine, MeNZB, was manufactured using the same processes as, but a different strain to, the meningococcal B vaccine developed by the Norwegian Institute of Public Health, which was shown to be efficacious after two doses in adolescents [58]. It is an outer membrane vesicle (OMV) vaccine that is strain-specific to New Zealand.

In New Zealand, clinical trials were undertaken to generate immunogenicity and reactogenicity data for the 0–19 age group. Enhanced methods, including hospital surveillance, to monitor vaccine safety were put in place before the vaccine was introduced and an Independent Safety Monitoring Board was established to review the information collected.

The meningococcal B immunization program began on 19 July 2004. Given the disproportionate rates of disease suffered by Maori and Pacific children and children who were socially and economically disadvantaged, and the difficulty of reaching these groups, it was recognized that the program needed to prioritize delivery to these communities. Similar to the situation in the UK, the introduction of the immunization program was staggered in accordance with vaccine production. Implementation took into account the risk and burden of disease with the need to prioritize the highest risk group (those aged under 5 years) and the need to go to areas with high numbers of cases first. The roll-out was organized geographically to take into account the differential geographical burden of disease and targeted the majority of Maori and Pacific children in the early part of the program. Experience with OMV vaccines in Norway showed that efficacy declined markedly over time as serum bactericidal assay titer levels declined [59]. If protection is short-term and the vaccine has no effect on carriage, it may be that the population impact of OMP vaccines will be limited.

20.5
Future Direction for Meningococcal Vaccines

Much has been learnt from the introduction of MCC vaccines in the UK. The UK research collaboration between the public health sector and manufacturers focused the development on the meningococcal C conjugate vaccine. As there was a greater need for a serogroup A vaccine for sub-Saharan Africa, this was the subject of some criticism because it initially appeared to stall progress with the combined serogroup A and C vaccine. In the longer term, this public/private collaboration in the UK has generated high-quality data that facilitated better understanding of conjugate vaccines, in particular their impact on carriage and the validation of correlates of protection. This has informed meningococcal immunization strategies adopted in other countries and helped the establishment of The Meningitis Vaccine Project in 2001. This is a partnership between the World Health Organization and the Program for Appropriate Technology in Health. The Meningitis Vaccine Project's mission is to eliminate meningitis as a public health problem in sub-Saharan Africa through the development, testing, introduction and widespread use of meningococcal conjugate vaccines. The ability of these vaccines to provide high levels of indirect protection offers, at last, the possibility of a longer-term solution to serogroup A disease in Africa.

References

1 Ess SM, Szucs TD. **2002**, Economic evaluation of immunization strategies, *Clin. Infect. Dis.* 35, 294–297.

2 Miller E. 1 Part C. Potential and existing impact of vaccines on disease epidemiology. In Bloom BR, Lambert P-H, eds. The Vaccine Book. San Diego, California; Academic Press, **2003**, 37–50.

3 Nokes DJ, Anderson RM. **1988**, The use of mathematical models in the epidemiological study of infectious diseases and in the design of mass immunization programs, *Epidemiol. Infect.* 101, 1–20.

4 Anderson RM, Donnelly CA, Gupta S. **1997**, Vaccine design, evaluation, and community-based use for antigenically variable infectious agents, *Lancet* 350, 1466–1470.

5 Farrington P, Miller E. **2001**, Meningococcal vaccine trials, in: *Meningococcal Vaccines: Methods and Protocols*, ed. Pollard AJ, Maiden MCJ, Humana Press, Totowa, N.J., p. 23–40.

6 Guiver M, Borrow R, Marsh J, Gray SJ, Kaczmarski EB, Howells D, Boseley P, Fox AJ. **2000**, Evaluation of the Applied Biosystems automated Taqman PCR system for the detection of meningococcal DNA, *FEMS Immunol. Med. Microbiol.* 20, 173–179.

7 Kaczmarski E, Cartwright K. **1995**, Control of meningococcal disease: guidance for microbiologists, *Commun. Dis. Rep. CDR Rev.* 5, R196–R198.

8 Ashton FE, Ryan JA, Borczyk A, et al. **1991**, Emergence of a virulent clone of *Neisseria meningitidis* serotype 2a that is associated with meningococcal group C disease in Canada, *J. Clin. Microbiol.* 29, 2489–2493.

9 Whalen CM, Hockin JC, Ryan A, Ashton F. **1995**, The changing epidemiology of invasive meningococcal disease in Canada, 1985 through 1992, Emergence of a virulent clone of *Neisseria meningitidis*, *J. Am. Med. Assoc.* 273, 390–394.

10 Krizova P, Musilek M. **1995**, Changing epidemiology of meningococcal invasive disease in the Czech republic caused by a new clone of *Neisseria meningitidis* C:2a:P1.2(P1.5), ET-15/37, *Cent. Eur. J. Public Health* 3, 189–194.

11 Anon. **1998**, Enhanced surveillance of suspected meningococcal disease, *Commun. Dis. Rep. CDR Wkly* 8, 1.

12 Southern J, Deane S, Ashton L, et al. **2004**, Effects of prior polysaccharide vaccination on magnitude, duration and quality of immune responses to and safety profile of a meningococcal serogroup C tetanus toxoid conjugate vacci-

nation in adults, *Clin. Diagn. Lab. Immunol.* 11, 1100–1104.
13 Miller E, Salisbury D, Ramsay M. **2002**, Planning, registration, and implementation of an immunization campaign against meningococcal serogroup C disease in the UK: a success story, *Vaccine* 20, s58–s67.
14 Fairley CK, Begg N, Borrow R, Fox AJ, Jones DM, Cartwright KAV. **1996**, Reactogenicity and immunogenicity of conjugate meningococcal serogroup A and C vaccine in UK infants, *J. Infect. Dis.* 174, 1360–1363.
15 Richmond PC, Miller E, Borrow R, Clark S, Sadler F, Fox AJ, Begg NT, Morris R, Cartwright KAV. **1999**, Meningococcal serogroup C conjugate vaccine is immunogenic in infancy and primes for memory, *J. Infect. Dis.* 179, 1569–1572.
16 Richmond P, Borrow R, Goldblatt D, Findlow J, Martin S, Morris R, Cartwright K, Miller E. **2001**, Ability of three different meningococcal C conjugate vaccines to induce immunologic memory after a single dose in UK toddlers, *J. Infect. Dis.* 183, 160–163.
17 MacLennan JM, Shackley F, Heath PT, Deeks JJ, Flamank C, Herbert M, Griffiths H, Hatzmann E, Goilav C, Moxon ER. **2000**, Safety, immunogenicity and induction of immunologic memory by a serogroup C meningococcal conjugate vaccine in infants, *J. Am. Med. Assoc.* 283, 2795–2801.
18 Borrow R, Fox AJ, Richmond PC, Clark S, Sadler F, Findlow J, Morris R, Begg NT, Cartwright KAV. **2000**, Induction of immunological memory in UK infants by a meningococcal A/C conjugate vaccine, *Epidemiol. Infect.* 124, 427–432.
19 Borrow R, Goldblatt D, Andrews N et al. **2002**, Antibody persistence and immunological memory 4 years following meningococcal C conjugate vaccination in UK children, *J. Infect. Dis.* 186, 1353–1357.
20 Trotter CL, Edmunds WJ. **2002**, The cost-effectiveness of the meningococcal group C conjugate vaccination campaign in England and Wales, *Br. Med. J.* 324, 809.
21 Maiden MCJ, Spratt BG. **1999**, Meningococcal conjugate vaccines: new opportunities and new challenges, *Lancet* 354, 615–616.
22 http://www.hpa.org.uk/infections/topics-az/meningo/advice/mensurvw99.pdf.
23 Balmer P, Borrow R. **2004**, Serologic correlates of protection for evaluating the response to meningococcal vaccines, *Expert Rev. Vaccines* 3, 77–87.
24 Maiden MC, Stuart JM, Meningococcal Carriage Group **2002**, Carriage of serogroup C meningococci 1 year after meningococcal C conjugate polysaccharide vaccine, *Lancet* 359, 1829–1831.
25 Anon. **2000**, Safety of meningococcal group C conjugate vaccines, *Curr. Prob. Pharmacovigil.* 26, 14.
26 Medicines Control Agency **2002**, Report of the committee on safety of medicines expert working group on meningococcal group C conjugate vaccines, http://medicines.mhra.gov.uk/ourwork/monitorsafequalmed/safetymessages/mencwgreport.pdf.
27 Miller E, Waight P, Farrington P. **1998**, Safety assessment post licensure, *Dev. Biol. Stand.* 95, 235–243.
28 Trotter CL, Andrews NA, Kaczmarski EB et al. **2004**, Effectiveness of meningococcal serogroup C conjugate vaccines four years after the introduction of mass immunization in England, *Lancet* 364, 365.
29 Ramsay ME, McVernon J, Andrews NJ, Heath PT, Slack MP. **2003**, Estimating Haemophilus influenzae Type b vaccine effectiveness in England and Wales by use of the screening method, *J. Infect. Dis.* 188, 481–485.
30 Ramsay M, Miller E, Andrews N, Slack M, Heath P. **2004**, Epidemiological data are essential (rapid response to Heikki Peltola, Eeva Salo, and Harri Saxén. Incidence of Haemophilus influenzae type b meningitis during 18 years of vaccine use: observational study using routine hospital data, bmj.38301.657014.79v1). *Br. Med. J.* 79 (online).
31 Ramsay ME, Andrews NJ, Trotter CL, Kaczmarski EB, Miller E. **2003**, Herd immunity from meningococcal serogroup C conjugate vaccination in England, *Br. Med. J.* 326, 365–366.
32 Booy R et al. **1997**, Vaccine failures after primary immunization with Haemophi-

lus influenzae type b conjugate vaccine without booster, *Lancet* 349, 1197–1202.
33 Eskala J, Kayhty H. **1996**, Ten years experience with Haemophilus influenzae type b (Hib) conjugate vaccine in Finland, *Rev. Med. Microbiol.* 7, 231–241.
34 Teare E, et al. **1994**, Efficacy of Hib vaccine (letter), *Lancet* 344, 828–829.
35 Cartwright KA, Stuart JM, Jones DM, Noah ND. **1987**, The Stonehouse survey: nasopharyngeal carriage of meningococci and *Neisseria lactamica*, *Epidemiol. Infect.* 99, 591–601.
36 http://www.euibis.org/documents/19992000_meningo.pdf.
37 Salleras L, Dominguez A, Cardenosa N. **2003**, Impact of mass vaccination with polysaccharide conjugate vaccine against serogroup C meningococcal disease in Spain, *Vaccine* 21, 725–728.
38 Fogarty J. **1997**, Trends in serogroup C meningococcal disease in the Republic of Ireland, Eurosurv. Mon. 2, 75–76 (http://www.euibis.org/meningo/vacc_sched_meningo.htm).
39 Cano R, Larrauri A, Mateo S et al. **2004**, Impact of the meningococcal C conjugate vaccine in Spain: an epidemiological and microbiological decision. *Eurosurv. Mon.* 9, 5–6.
40 http://www.eurosurveillance.org/ew/2004/040129.asp#3.
41 Welte R, van den Dobbelsteen G, Bos JM, de Melker H, van Alphen L, Spanjaard L, Rumke HC, Postma MJ. **2004**, Economic evaluation of meningococcal serogroup C conjugate vaccination programs in the Netherlands and its impact on decision-making, *Vaccine* 23, 470–479.
42 de Greeff SC, de Melker HE, Spanjaard L, van den Hof S, Dankert J. **2003**, The first effect of the national vaccination campaign against meningococcal-C disease: a rapid and sharp decrease in the number of patients, *Ned. Tijdschr. Geneeskd.* 147, 1132–1135.
43 De Wals P. **2004**, Meningococcal C vaccines: the Canadian experience, *Pediatr. Infect. Dis. J.* 23[Suppl], S280–S284.
44 De Wals P, Dionne M, Douville-Fradet M, Boulianne N, Drapeau J, De Serres G. **1996**, Impact of a mass immunization campaign against serogroup C meningococcus in the Province of Quebec, Canada, *Bull. WHO* 74, 407–411.
45 De Wals P, Deceuninck G, De Serres G, Boivin JF, Duval B, Remis R, Masse R. **2005**, Effectiveness of serogroup C meningococcal polysaccharide vaccine: results from a case-control study in Quebec, *Clin. Infect. Dis.* 40, 1116–1122.
46 De Wals P, De Serres G, Niyonsenga T. **2001**, Effectiveness of a mass immunization campaign against serogroup C meningococcal disease in Quebec, *J. Am. Med. Assoc.* 285, 177–181.
47 De Wals P, Deceuninck G, Boulianne N, De Serres G. **2004**, Effectiveness of a mass immunization campaign using serogroup C meningococcal conjugate vaccine, *J. Am. Med. Assoc.* 292, 2491–2494.
48 De Wals P, Nguyen VH, Erickson LJ, Guay M, Drapeau J, St-Laurent J. **2004**, Cost-effectiveness of immunization strategies for the control of serogroup C meningococcal disease, *Vaccine* 22, 1233–1240.
49 Advisory Committee Statement **2001**, National Advisory Committee on Immunization (NACI) statement on recommended use of meningococcal vaccines. *Can. Commun. Dis. Rep.* 27, ACS6 (http://www.phac-aspc.gc.ca/publicat/ccdr-rmtc/01vol27/27sup/acs6.html).
50 http://www.phac-aspc.gc.ca/im/ptimprog-progimpt/table-1_e.html.
51 Cohen N. **2003**, Introduction of the national meningococcal C vaccination program, *Commun. Dis. Intel.* 27, 161–162.
52 http://www.seniors.gov.au./internet/wcms/publishing.nsf/Content/cda-pubs-cdi-2003-cdi2702-htm-cdi2 702f.htm#results.
53 Skull SA, Butler JR, Robinson P, Carnie J. **2001**, Should programs for community-level meningococcal vaccination be considered in Australia? An economic evaluation, *Int. J. Epidemiol.* 30, 571–579.
54 Welte R, Trotter C, Edmunds J, Postma M, Beutels P. **2005**, The role of economic evaluation on vaccine decision making: focus on meningococcal C vaccination, *Pharmacoeconomics* 23(9), 855–874.

55 Bilukha OO, Rosenstein N. **2005**, Prevention and control of meningococcal disease: recommendation of the advisory committee on immunization practices (ACIP), *Morbid. Mortal. Wkly Rep.* 54, 1–21.

56 Shepard CW, Ortega-Sanchez IR, Scott RD 2nd, Rosenstein NE **2005**, ABCs team, Cost-effectiveness of conjugate meningococcal vaccination strategies in the United States, *Pediatrics* 115, 1220–1232.

57 Ministry of Health **2004**, The meningococcal B immunization program: a response to an epidemic: national implementation strategy, working for a healthy future, Ministry of Health, Wellington.

58 Bjune G, Hoiby EA, Gronnesby JK, Arnesen O, Fredriksen JH. **1991**, Effect of outer membrane vesicle vaccine against group B meningococcal disease in Norway, *Lancet* 338, 1093–1096.

59 Holst J, Feiring B, Fuglesang JE, et al. **2003**, Serum bactericidal activity correlates with the vaccine efficacy of outer membrane vesicle vaccines against *Neisseria meningitidis* serogroup B disease, *Vaccine* 21, 734–737.

Part V
Clinical and Public Health Management

Handbook of Meningococcal Disease. Infection Biology, Vaccination, Clinical Management.
Edited by M. Frosch and M. C. J. Maiden

ISBN: 3-527-31260-9

21
Pathogenesis and Pathophysiology of Invasive Meningococcal Disease

Petter Brandtzaeg

21.1
Introduction

During the past 10 years, two seminal discoveries have increased our understanding of the molecular pathophysiology of meningococcal infections. The elucidation of the Toll-like receptor (TLR) system as a major molecular pattern recognition receptor complex has enabled us to understand the complexity and specificity of the innate immune system better than before [1]. It is a key defense mechanism protecting us from invasive pathogens but also a mechanism that destructs the host in the most fulminating infections. The TLR system is activated in a dose-dependent manner by different molecules harbored in the cell wall of *Neisseria meningitidis* [2, 3]. The result is a differentiated production of inflammatory mediators which may defend or harm the host depending on their levels. The production of key inflammatory mediators is closely associated with organ dysfunction and outcome in patients with meningococcemia [2, 4]. The second important discovery was the creation of a knock-out mutant of *N. meningitidis* completely lacking lipopolysaccharides (LPS) in the outer membrane [5]. Both discoveries have been utilized to probe new aspects of the bacterium–host interaction, leading to disease symptoms and organ dysfunction. The ability of the LPS-deficient mutant to elicit a cytokine response in different immune cells documents that nonLPS components in the outer membrane may contribute to the inflammatory reaction in man. Meningococcal LPS are still considered to be the most potent group of molecule in the outer membrane that induces inflammation. However, bacterial lipoproteins and fragments of peptidoglycan may contribute to and broaden the inflammatory response. Furthermore, genetic polymorphism contributes to a differentiated host's response. Still, the basic concept of how meningococci cause the different clinical presentations is unchanged. There is a close association between the load of meningococci, being alive or dead, in plasma and cerebrospinal fluid (CSF) and the magnitude of the inflammatory response of the patients. The ability of the meningococcus to survive in the circulation, to multiply slowly or rapidly and

Handbook of Meningococcal Disease. Infection Biology, Vaccination, Clinical Management.
Edited by M. Frosch and M. C. J. Maiden

ISBN: 3-527-31260-9

the propensity to penetrate into the subarachnoid space causing meningitis are the major determinants of the different clinical syndromes.

21.2 Classification of the Clinical Presentations

N. meningitidis causes a range of different clinical presentations, ranging from rapidly progressing septicemia to transient bacteremia. However, the meningococcus has the propensity to invade the meninges and the majority of the patients develop distinct clinical signs of meningitis.

To classify the different disease presentations accurately for scientific studies, a system was developed in the early 1980s, based on the two characteristic clinical features of meningococcal infections that determine the outcome: (a) the presence or absence of persistent septic shock and (b) the presence or absence of clinical symptoms and laboratory signs of distinct meningitis [6]. The patients were classified into four different clinical groups:

1. *Fulminant meningococcal septicemia.* Patients with severe, persistent septic shock lasting >24 h or until death and minimal pleocytosis ($<10^8$ leukocytes l^{-1} CSF) or lack of distinct clinical signs of meningitis.
2. *Distinct meningitis.* Patients with marked pleocytosis ($\geq 10^8$ leukocytes l^{-1} CSF) or distinct clinical signs of meningism, i.e. nuchal and back rigidity and positive Kernig's sign.
3. *Distinct meningitis and persistent septic shock.* Patients with marked pleocytosis ($\geq 10^8$ leukocytes l^{-1} CSF) or distinct clinical signs of meningitis and severe, persistent septic shock.
4. *Mild systemic meningococcal infection.* Patients with mild meningococcemia, without developing persistent septic shock or distinct meningitis.

By applying these definitions rigorously to patients admitted to hospitals, it has been possible to elucidate and describe the underlying pathophysiology at a molecular level [2, 4, 6–20]. The case fatality rate is closely associated with the pathophysiology. It varies from 25% to 55% in patients with fulminant meningococcal septicemia, 10–25% in patients with meningitis and shock, <5% in patients with distinct meningitis and 0% in patients with mild systemic meningococcal infections [2, 4].

Table 21.1 shows the percentage of positive blood cultures among 157 patients with documented meningococcal infection and classified into one of the four clinical categories. None of the patients received antibiotics before the specimen was drawn. The percentage of positive CNS cultures among 119 of the same patients is also given in Table 21.1. The data clearly document the tendency of pathogenic meningococci to invade the meninges in all clinical presentations. However, to understand the relationship between intruding meningococci, the clinical pictures and outcome, quantitative data related to bacterial proliferation and the host's inflammatory response in the different compartments are required.

Table 21.1 The percentage of positive cultures of *N. meningitidis* drawn from blood and CSF in relation to the clinical presentation. (*n*) denotes the number of patients from which specimens were collected.

Clinical presentation	Blood, % (*n*)	CSF, % (*n*)
Fulminant septicemia	93 (56)	59 (34)
Distinct meningitis	50 (65)	84 (64)
Septic shock and meningitis	87 (6)	83 (6)
Mild systemic meningococcal disease	77 (30)	47 (15)

21.3 Localized Oropharyngeal Infection

21.3.1 The Initial Stage of Colonization

We assume that invasive meningococci, transmitted in droplets, are expressing type IV pili which attach to specific receptor sites such as CD46 and other proteins expressed on epithelial cells in the oropharynx [21]. Subsequently other molecules, including different group 5 opacity proteins, in the outer membrane contribute to a firmer contact between the meningococci and the host epithelial cells. *Ex vivo* models employing intact surface epithelium from the nasal cavity suggest that meningococci initially adhere to nonciliated epithelial cells [22]. The epithelium undergoes marked changes during the first 24 h. The meningococci start to multiply locally and influence the physical appearance of the epithelium cells [22, 23]. Some of the patients developing systemic meningococcal infections feel pharyngeal discomfort starting 24–72 h before developing symptoms of the invasive infection (P. Brandtzaeg, unpublished data). This may be the clinical correlate to the initial focal meningococcal infection.

21.3.2 Passage Through the Mucosal Barrier in Oropharynx

After a certain time of adaptation and proliferation, the meningococci initiate a parasite-directed endocytosis, passing through the epithelial cells [22, 23]. In adenoid tissue covered with intact epithelium, meningococci are gradually engulfed by the epithelial cells. The epithelium overlying the tonsils and the adenoids are relatively sparsely ciliated, which may facilitate adherence of meningococci [23]. After adherence, adaptation and initial proliferation, the meningococci gradually move through the cytoplasma to the basal membrane. Virulent meningococci expressing capsule polysaccharide are carried in vacuoles, whereas uncapsulated variants are transported through the cytoplasm without vacuoles [22]. When biopsies from other parts of the nasal cavity are studied, few meningococci are transported across the epithelium by parasite-directed endocytosis at these sites [23]. It is presently not known whether these observations indicate that meningococci are transported at different rate across the mucosal lining depending on the site in the oropharyngeal cavity or just reflect differences in the experimental conditions. The attachment of meningococci to epithelial cells induces specific structural changes as a consequence of altered gene expression in the cells [24]. It is not known whether release of outer membrane vesicles (OMV), in addition to attachment of virulent *N. meningitidis*, plays a role in altering the epithelial cells.

21.3.3 Passage into the Circulation

Studies of *ex vivo* transplants of oropharyngeal tissue have not clearly documented how meningococci pass through the basal membrane. They have been observed after the passage, while they are dividing within macrophages in submucosa [23]. How they gain access to the circulation is unknown. Meningococci located in the extracellular space may penetrate between or through capillary endothelial cells into the lumen. Since meningococci have been observed intracellularly in mononuclear phagocytes, one may speculate whether neutrophils and monocytes may carry them as "Trojan horses" into the bloodstream without killing them. The ability to survive and multiply in the circulation is a basic requirement for causing a systemic infection.

21.3.4 *N. meningitidis* IgA1 Protease

IgA1 protease is secreted by pathogenic meningococci and splits IgA1 but not IgA2 in the hinge region [25]. *In vitro* studies using high concentrations of purified meningococcal IgA1 proteases have documented the ability to induce proinflammatory cytokines when applied to responsive cells [26]. Interestingly, no IL-10 was produced in these experiments whereas IL-10 is secreted in high concentrations by patients with meningococcal septicemia [15, 27]. The pathogenetic role of IgA1 protease at the early stage of invasive meningococcal disease is still unclear. It may neutralize secretory IgA on the mucosal surface and thereby circumvent a first-line defense mechanism, facilitating the attachment of meningococci to the mucosal epithelial cells. Although high levels of IgA1 protease may induce the production of proinflammatory cytokines *in vitro*, its contribution to the generalized inflammatory response in patients is less certain. The cytokine response in patients appears primarily to be triggered by LPS [7]. The levels and biological activity of meningococcal IgA1 protease in patient plasma or CSF have never been reported.

21.4
Generalized Infection

21.4.1
The Initial Meningococcemia

The first clinical manifestations of systemic meningococcal infection are caused by *N. meningitidis* multiplying in the circulation. A prerequisite for causing clinical disease is the ability of *N. meningitidis* to resist the bactericidal capacity of the blood caused by the combined action of antibodies and complement and to circumvent rapid phagocytosis by stationary and circulating phagocytes. Subsequently, meningococci are seeded in specific areas of the body, primarily the skin and the meninges. Metastatic focal infections may also occur in the pericardium, large joints, eyes and more rarely in other tissues. Studies during the past 20 years have fully supported the conclusion of W. W. Herrick from 1918: "The disease with which we were dealing was not a primary meningitis but a meningococcic sepsis with secondary meningeal localization" [28]. The early symptoms of meningococcemia, including general malaise, fever and sometimes muscle ache, are recognized by the patient and relatives when the number of multiplying bacteria in the blood surpasses a certain threshold. Vascular cells in the preoptic area of anterior hypothalamus in the brain are expressing TLR4, possibly TLR2 and receptors for the three fever-causing cytokines: tumor necrosis factor α (TNF-α), interleukin 1β (IL-1β) and interleukin-6 (IL-6) [29]. These different agonists activate cyclooxygenase 2, increase the production of prostaglandin E2 and activate the hypothalamic prostaglandin E2 receptors as a common pathway. The temperature set point in the hypothalamic thermoregulatory centre is upregulated, leading to increased muscle work, altered skin perfusion and raised body core temperature.

21.4.2
Markers of Proliferation of Meningococci in the Circulation

It was assumed since early 1900 that endotoxin, defined as heat-resistant molecules in the bacterium itself, caused the clinical symptoms in patients with meningococcal infections [14]. No heat-labile exotoxins had been isolated. Up to the early 1980s, little direct evidence existed to support this assumption. Meningococci were isolated from blood and CSF from patients with acute lethal infections as well as very mild clinical manifestations such as transient meningococcemia in infants. Quantitative blood culture was a cumbersome though direct method to quantify the number of living bacteria in the circulation. The results from the few studies performed with this method suggested that the highest number of meningococci were found among patients developing distinct meningitis [30–33]. However, since the early 1980s, quantitative measurements of meningococcal LPS in plasma and CSF have clarified important quantitative aspects of meningococcal infection, explaining the different clinical manifestations

[2, 8–11, 14, 16]. In the past few years, quantitative determination of *N. meningitidis* DNA by polymerase chain reaction (PCR) has completed the picture and documented the close association between clinical manifestations and compartmentalized growth of meningococci [34, 35]. We can now, to a large extent, explain the different clinical presentations and the marked differences in survival and development of sequelae in patients with SMD.

21.4.3
Meningococcal LPS as a Marker of Bacterial Growth

The magnitude of bacterial growth, as estimated by the content of meningococcal LPS, differs markedly between the different patients developing meningococcal infections. Most patients have a relatively low-graded meningococcemia, resulting in a LPS plasma level below 7 endotoxin units (EU) ml^{-1}, where 1 EU ml^{-1} is equal to the activity of 100 pg ml^{-1} of purified LPS extracted from a reference strain of *Escherichia coli*. These patients present with the clinical picture of either distinct meningitis or mild systemic meningococcal disease without serious circulatory disturbance (Table 21.2) [2, 9]. However, in 10–20% of the patients *N. meningitidis* multiplies much faster in the circulation resulting in 10- to 1000-fold higher levels of LPS in plasma on hospital admission [2]. These patients have a much shorter duration of the disease before they arrive at the hospital due to the serious symptoms which are recognized early. Patients with LPS >7 EU ml^{-1} in plasma usually present with persistent septic shock and multiple organ failure (Table 21.2) [2]. They have rarely marked symptoms of distinct meningitis, although meningococci can be isolated in CSF in >50% of the patients.

Table 21.2 The relationship between clinical presentation and LPS in the circulation in 150 patients. EU ml^{-1} denotes endotoxin units per milliliter heparin plasma or occasionally serum.

LPS (EU ml^{-1})	Fulminant septicemia	Meningitis	Meningitis and septicemia	Mild systemic meningococcal disease
>150	13	0	0	1 a)
150–50	13	0	0	0
50–10	21	1 b)	2	0
10–0.5	6 c)	13	3 c)	8
<0.5	1 c)	46	2 c)	20

a) Boy, 27 months, LPS 214 EU ml^{-1}, *N. meningitidis* DNA 4.2×10^{7} ml^{-1} plasma, shock-resistant.
b) Boy, 25 months, LPS 16 EU ml^{-1}, *N. meningitidis* DNA 7.4×10^{5} ml^{-1} plasma, shock-resistant.
c) First sample collected 3–18 h after antibiotic treatment was started.

21.4.4
Quantitative Detection of *N. meningitidis* DNA in Plasma and Cerebrospinal Fluid

Recently, quantitative measurement of meningococcal DNA in plasma and CSF has become feasible by using real-time PCR. The number of DNA copies reflects the true bacterial load which is defined as the sum of live and dead meningococci. The numbers of *N. meningitidis* DNA copies are closely correlated to the level of meningococcal LPS ($r=0.91$), indicating that the number of *N. meningitidis* is the crucial determinant of the levels of LPS in the blood and CSF of the patients (Fig. 21.1) [35]. The results from two different studies show that the clinical presentation and severity are positively correlated to the levels of meningococcal DNA in the blood [34, 35]. It has been speculated whether different strains of meningococci may release different quantities of outer membrane vesicles which could explain the difference in clinical presentation [36]. Avirulent meningococci carried in the oropharynx may release less outer membrane blebs than invasive strains when assayed *in vitro* [36]. However, when virulent meningococci cause clinical disease, the magnitude of bacterial growth in the circulation and the subarachnoid space is the major factor determining the clinical presentation [35].

21.4.5
The True Load of Meningococci Versus Colony-forming Units in the Blood

Using real-time PCR, it was for the first time possible to compare the true load of meningococci, as compared with the number of live bacteria detectable in quantitative blood culture. For each live meningococcus that was able to form a

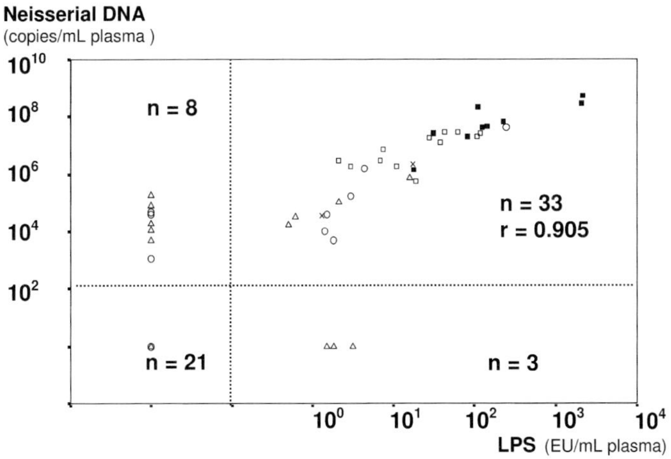

Fig. 21.1 The relationship between *N. meningitidis* DNA and LPS in plasma samples from patients with systemic meningococcal disease at admission to hospital. The dotted lines separate samples as either positive or negative for *N. meningitidis* DNA or LPS. Reproduced from [35] with permission from the American Society for Microbiology.

new colony by direct plating on chocolate agar, 10^3–10^4 copies of meningococcal DNA were present. This observation, which was consistent among different patients, indicates that 1000- to 10 000-fold higher levels of biologically active outer membrane molecules are present in the blood than can be accounted for by measuring colony-forming units by direct plating on growth media [35]. Interestingly, this discrepancy was observed when systematic measurements of LPS in patient plasmas were initiated and the results were compared with the results of quantitative blood cultures [9]. Quantitative blood culture technique has significantly underestimated the true bacterial load and the amount of bacterial molecules that trigger the innate immune system in meningococcal patients [9, 30, 31, 33].

21.4.6 Variable Growth During the Bacteremic Phase and the Clinical Presentation

Patients with meningococcal infections can be divided in patients with or without persistent septic shock. This dichotomy is crucial to predict patient survival. Patients with persistent shock have a much higher case fatality rate than patients without shock (Table 21.3) [2, 4, 9]. Previously, we defined a LPS level of 7 EU ml^{-1} in plasma as a septic shock threshold [2, 9, 14]. Patients with LPS levels <7 EU ml^{-1} very rarely develop a persistent septic shock, whereas most but not all patients with LPS in plasma ≥ 7 EU ml^{-1} develop long-lasting hypotension, coagulopathy and impaired tissue perfusion (Table 21.1). The case fatality rate increases sharply with increasing levels of LPS in plasma (Table 21.3) [2].

21.4.7 Identification of Two Shock-resistant Patients

We identified two young children among 161 patients that tolerated higher levels of LPS (16 EU ml^{-1} and 214 EU ml^{-1}) and higher loads of meningococci (7.4×10^5 copies ml^{-1} and 4.2×10^7 copies ml^{-1}) than most patients do without

Table 21.3 The relationship between plasma and serum levels of LPS and case fatality rate caused by septic shock and multiple organ failure in 150 patients.

LPS (EU ml^{-1})	Number	Number dead	Case fatality rate (%)
>250	7	7	100
250–50	20	17	85
50–10	24	6	25
10–0.5	31	1 a)	3
<0.5	68	0	0

a) The sample was collected 12 h after the initiation of antibiotic treatment.

developing persistent septic shock (P. Brandtzaeg, unpublished data). Interestingly, the child with 214 EU ml^{-1} of LPS and 4.2×10^7 ml^{-1} copies of *N. meningitidis* DNA had levels of cytokines in plasma otherwise only found in patients with lethal meningococcal septic shock. TNF-α, interleukin 1β, IL-6, IL-10, macrophage inflammatory protein 1α (MIP-1α), monocyte chemoattractant protein 1 (MCP-1) and granulocyte colony-stimulating protein (G-CSF) were excessively high. These observations suggest that the patient had a normal functioning TLR system. What protected him from an irreversible circulatory collapse is presently not known. The underlying mechanism is clearly different from the endotoxin resistant mice with mutations in the TLR4 gene [37].

21.4.8 The Duration of Symptoms Related to the Clinical Presentation

The time span between the onset of the clinical symptoms and admission to hospital (onset/admission time) has been studied prospectively during the meningococcal epidemics in Norway caused by serogroup B *N. meningitidis* (B:15:P1,7,16:L3,7,9) in a population that comprised 4.3 million inhabitants [38]. Two subsequent studies from Norway and the Netherlands, respectively, have also reported the onset/admission time of patients [8, 11]. The median onset/admission times for patients with distinct meningitis were 29, 26 and 24 h, respectively. For patients developing fulminant meningococcal septicemia, the median onset admission times were 13, 12 and 12 h in the three studies [8, 11, 38]. Thus, patients developing meningococcal septic shock and massive disseminated intravascular coagulation (DIC) generated 10- to 1000-fold higher levels of LPS and meningococcal DNA copies in plasma within half of the time used by patients developing characteristic symptoms of meningitis.

21.4.9 Meningococcemia Leading to Meningitis

Approximately 50–60% of patients developing a systemic meningococcal infection present with clinical symptoms of distinct meningitis. The classic symptoms are headache, nuchal and back rigidity and a positive Kernig's symptom. The hemorrhagic skin rash is characterized by petechiae [39]. The diameter of the hemorrhagic lesions is usually <10 mm [39]. *N. meningitidis* grows gradually in the circulation. Most patients (69%) with meningococcal meningitis have <1000 DNA copies ml^{-1} and <0.5 EU ml^{-1} LPS plasma [35]. Nine of 29 patients with distinct meningitis had DNA copies varying from 1×10^3 to 7.4×10^5 DNA copies ml^{-1}, whereas only one of 66 patients had LPS in plasma >3.2 EU ml^{-1} [35] (P. Brandtzaeg, unpublished data). The median time required to build up this level of meningococcal DNA and LPS is in the range of 24–29 h. During this gradual proliferation phase, meningococci transverse the blood–brain barrier and invade the subarachnoid space. The blood culture is positive in approximately 50% of the patients (P. Brandtzaeg, unpublished data). Some of the patients may have a persistent low-graded meningococcemia. Others may have a transient meningococcemia seeding the meninges and then disappearing from the circulation. After extensive proliferation in the subarachnoid space, the meningococci may reseed the blood.

21.4.10 Meningococcemia Leading to Fulminant Septicemia

N. meningitidis multiplies much more rapidly in patients developing septic shock than in patients with distinct meningitis or mild systemic meningococcal disease. Within 12 h, the number of meningococcal DNA copies has reached a median number of 2.0×10^7 ml^{-1} and a median LPS level equal to 31 EU ml^{-1} [35]. The highest levels of DNA copies (5.4×10^8 ml^{-1}) and LPS (1505 EU ml^{-1}) were detected in a 6-month-old girl dying shortly after admission [35].

When grown *in vitro*, meningococci may multiply every 30 min, if the conditions are optimal. In a group of 17 patients with fulminant meningococcal septicemia studied consecutively, the median time span from the recognition of the first symptoms to hospital admission was 12 h, with a range of 8–20 h [9]. The median level of meningococcal LPS among the same 17 patients was 28 EU ml^{-1}, which equalled 3×10^6 copies of meningococcal DNA [9, 35]. Assuming that approximately 10 meningococci ml^{-1} are present in the circulation at time the patient develops the first recognized symptoms, a doubling time of 35 min would result in 3×10^6 bacteria ml^{-1} within 12 h. In reality the doubling time may be even shorter, given the continuous clearance of meningococci, LPS and meningococcal DNA from the circulation [9, 14, 35]. What causes this massive bacterial proliferation in persons with no previous signs of immune deficiency is presently not understood. Lack of specific bactericidal and opsonizing antibodies is an important cause since the large-scale vaccination campaigns in the UK and the Netherlands in recent years have virtually eliminated such cases caused by *N. meningitidis* serogroup C.

21.4.11 Meningococcemia Associated with Mild Systemic Meningococcal Disease

Patients with meningococcal infections develop fever and petechial rash, often with marked cutaneous infiltrates around the hemorrhagic center. The circulation is not severely compromised and the patients have no distinct signs of meningitis. Twenty-nine of 30 patients studied had initial LPS in plasma $\leq$6 EU ml^{-1}. One patient had an initial plasma level of 214 EU ml^{-1}, as described above, without developing shock. Nine of 14 patients had *N. meningitidis* DNA levels $>10^3$ copies ml^{-1} plasma with a median level of 4×10^4 copies ml^{-1} [35]. This was a composite group. Patients with symptoms lasting only a few hours before treatment starts might develop fulminant meningococcal septicemia or distinct meningitis if left untreated. In other patients, the bacterial growth is low-graded and balanced, with a continuous clearance of LPS never reaching the endotoxin shock level of >7 EU ml^{-1} [2, 9, 35]. Moreover, the innate immune system adapts to LPS over time. It becomes "tolerant" to LPS and downregulates the production of inflammatory mediators triggered by LPS [40, 41]. There is a "reprograming" of circulating leukocytes and other LPS-responsive cells as a consequence of continuous LPS stimulation [42–44]. The mild meningoococcemia may last from days to weeks or even months in the rare cases of chronic meningococcemia.

21.4.12 Clearance of Bacteria From the Circulation

The liver is the largest organ in the body and contains more phagocytic cells, primarily Kupffer cells, than any other organ. The Kupffer cells represent approximately 15% of all liver cells [45]. The liver receives 30% of the cardiac output, as compared with the spleen which receives 5%. In his classic animal study, Benacerraf documented that *Escherichia coli* and *Staphylococcus aureus* were removed from the circulation primarily by the Kupffer cells in the liver [46]. A minor fraction was removed by the spleen macrophages. These results have subsequently been confirmed by others [47–49]. The bacteria have to be opsonized by antibodies and complement and bind to the cell surface to be cleared effectively by the Kupffer cells [46, 48]. If the animals lacked opsonins, the bacteria were primarily cleared by the spleen macrophages. Circulating neutrophils and monocytes contribute little to the total bacterial clearance capacity of the body [46].

Recent studies support the idea that neutrophils may cooperate with the Kupffer cells in killing bacteria in the liver [50]. Furthermore, in a rat model, the liver played an important role in regulating the number of neutrophils in the circulation during endotoxinemia. The Kupffer cells removed apoptotic granulocytes more effectively after upregulation of P-selectin in the liver sinusoids [51]. Different subpopulations of Kupffer cells appear to exist. The function is related to the anatomical position of the cells in the liver tissue. Periportal Kupffer cells from rats phagocytose zymosan more effectively than Kupffer cells derived from the perivenous acinar region of rat liver. However, the latter cell type produce significantly more inflammatory mediators after 24 h priming with LPS [52]. High levels of IL-10 produced by the Kupffer cells may depress the phagocytic capacity and removal of *E. coli* in animals [53]. It is not known whether the high levels of IL-10 in patients with fulminant meningococcal septicemia depress the phagocytic capacity in the liver and thereby contribute to the escalating levels of circulating meningococci. LPS containing bacterial fragments are cleared from the circulation as rapidly in patients with high levels of IL-10 as in those with 100- to 1000-fold lower levels [9].

Assuming that these observations are valid for other pathogenic bacteria and in different mammals, one may speculate as to the role of the Kupffer cells and the spleen macrophages in meningococcal infections. The massive proliferation of meningococci within the vasculature in patients with fulminant meningococcal septicemia indicates that the combined action of the Kupffer cells and the endothelial cells in the liver and the spleen macrophages is insufficient. The reason could be a lack of specific antibodies, resulting in ineffective microbial killing and opsonization. The question then arises whether the comparatively low-graded meningococcemia observed in patients with distinct meningitis and mild systemic meningococcal disease is related to partial functioning of one of the two systems protecting these patients from developing overwhelming meningococcemia and shock within 12–24 h.

21.4.13
Clearance of *N. meningitidis* LPS from the Circulation in Patients

In patients with meningococcal infections, the clearance of bioactive LPS appears to be fairly constant. LPS activity, as measured by the limulus amoebocyte lysate (LAL) assay, was reduced by 50% within 1–3 h (mean 2 h) after the initiation of antibiotic treatment [9, 14, 35]. Subsequently, the clearance decreased to 4–9 h (mean 6 h) in some patients [9]. The clearance was the same in patients with 1000-fold difference in initial plasma LPS level and differed little from patient to patient [9]. It appeared to be independent of age [9]. Ultracentrifugation studies of septic shock plasma containing high levels of meningococcal LPS indicate that the LPS molecules are bound to large structures with high sedimentation constant [54]. These structures have been visualized as whole- and disintegrated meningococci and outer membrane vesicles [54, 55]. The observations indicate that LPS are cleared as effectively in patients with fulminant meningococcal septicemia as in patients with mild systemic meningococcal disease and meningitis. The main difference between these categories of patients is the rate of multiplication during the log phase growth and not a difference in the capacity of clearance.

21.4.14
Clearance of *N. meningitidis* DNA from the Circulation in Patients

The level of meningococcal DNA declines after antibiotic treatment is initiated. In a few patients, a slight increase is present from the first to the second sample before the level declines. The half-life was 3–4 h among seven patients studied with serial samples [35]. These results are in accordance with the results obtained by Hackett et al. [34].

21.4.15
The Scavenger Receptors that Clear Bacteria, LPS and Proteins

The Kupffer cells and endothelial cells in the liver remove whole bacteria, bacterial fragments and specific molecules. The scavenger receptor system comprises a complex of different receptor molecules. Purified LPS are removed by scavenger receptors class A [56]. Other scavenger receptors contribute significantly to the large clearance capacity of the liver [57, 58].

Meningococcal LPS, although abundantly present on the bacterial surface, may not be the major molecule recognized by different scavenger receptors in the sinusoids of the liver. In a mouse model using bone marrow-derived macrophages, nonopsonized *N. meningitidis* were almost exclusively phagocytosed by a scavenger receptor type A [59]. The phagocytosis of meningococci was independent of meningococcal LPS as ligand. The receptor recognized a certain amino acid motif consisting of a minimum of 11 amino acids. Activation of the receptor did not lead to the production of inflammatory mediators, such as TNF-α. It is presently not known whether the same type scavenger receptor A is expressed on human Kupffer cells and liver endothelial cells.

21.5 Lipopolysaccharides Triggering the Innate Immune System

21.5.1 Structure of *N. meningitidis* LPS

LPS, the endotoxin of *N. meningitidis,* are often referred to as lipooligosaccharides (LOS) owing to the short polysaccharide side chains (Fig. 21.2). The molecule consists of lipid A embedded in the outer membrane with three fatty acids symmetrically attached to each of two D-glycosamine molecules. The inner part of the side chain consists of two 2-keto-3-deoxy-octulosonic acid (KDO) and two L-glycero-D-manno-heptopyranoside (heptoses) substituted with short polysaccharide side-chains [60–62]. Lipid A has for a long time been regarded as the toxic center of LPS [62, 63]. Three fatty acids and one phosphate group are symmetrically attached to each of the two D-glycosamine molecules which form the backbone structure of lipid A (Fig. 21.2). The fatty acids contain 12 or 14 carbon atoms [60]. The symmetric lipid A of *N. meningitidis* differs from the asymmetric lipid A derived from *E. coli, Salmonella* and *Shigella* species but is equally biologically potent on a molar basis. The short LOS structure is common among human pathogens residing in the upper airways, including *Haemophilus influenzae* and *Bordetella pertussis* [64]. The synthetic pathway of meningococcal LPS has recently been characterized in detail [64, 65].

21.5.2 Heterogeneity of Lipid A

Heterogeneity of the lipid A fraction exists. Strains of meningococci may harbor minor fractions of lipid A with five (penta-acylated) or four (tetra-acylated) fatty acids and lipid A with an altered degree of phosphorylation. These structures are biologically less potent than the six fatty chain (hexa-acylated) lipid A [66]. By using the ability to activate the limulus amebocyte lysate (LAL) assay, it has been shown that different strains of *N. meningitidis* reveal quite a variable capacity to activate this primitive coagulation system [67]. The variability in potency is

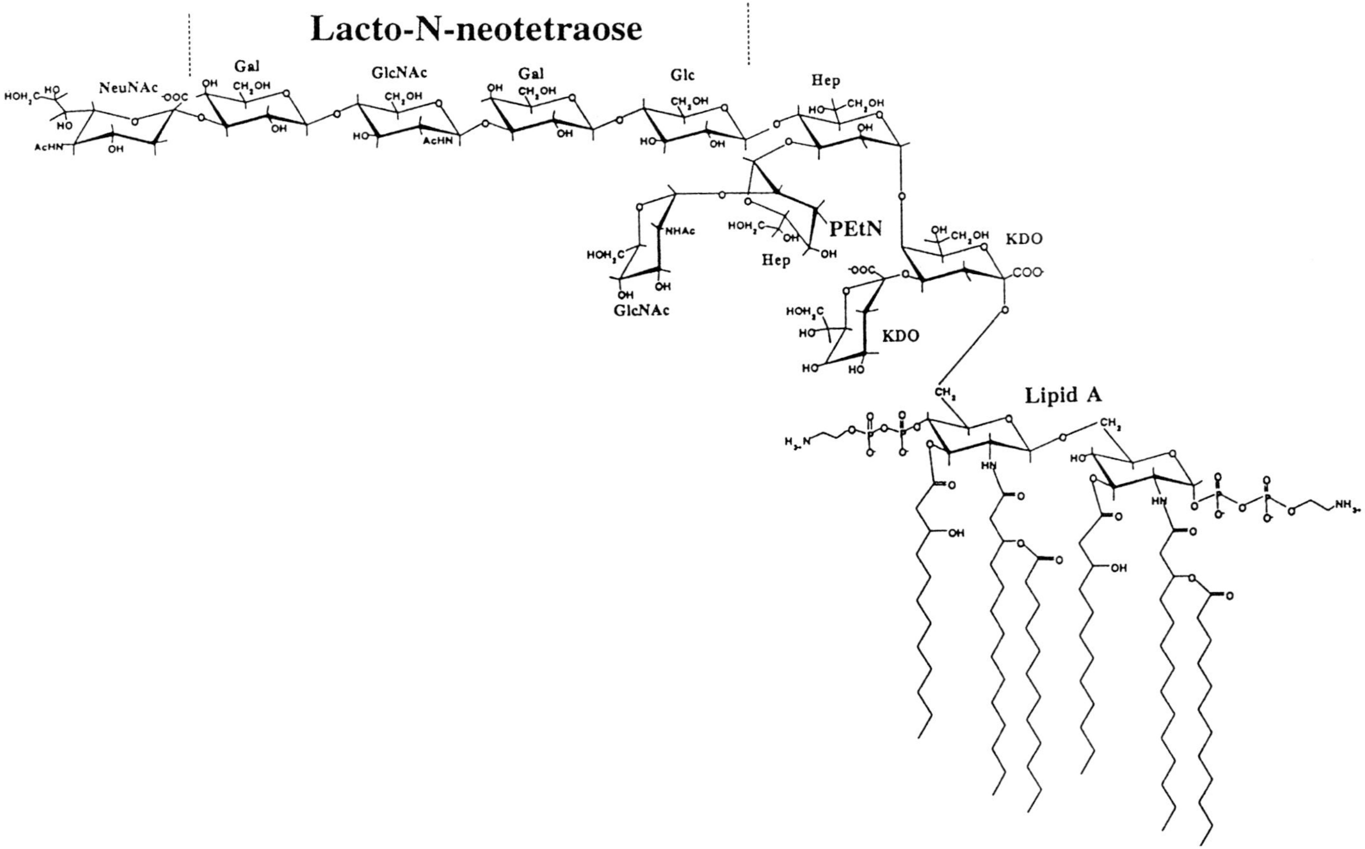

Fig. 21.2 Structure of *N. meningitidis* LPS, immunotype L3. NeuNAc, sialic acid; Gal, galactose; GlcNac, N-acetylglucosamine; Glc, glucose; Hep, heptose, KDO, 3-deoxy-D-manno-2-octulosonic acid; PEN phosphoethanolamine. Reproduced from [61, 62] with permission from the American Society for Biochemistry and Molecular Biology and the American Society for Microbiology.

related to small differences in the structure of lipid A. Although lipid A has been considered to be the "toxic center" of LPS, studies of a series of meningococcal mutants with different lengths of side-chains attached to lipid A have documented that the minimal requirement of the LPS molecule for optimal cell activation is a hexacylated lipid A to which two KDO molecules are attached [68]. A mutant expressing only lipid A was significantly less active than mutants expressing lipid A and two KDOs [68].

21.5.3
Immunotypes of Meningococcal LPS, Biological Activity and Clinical Disease

The substitution of the two heptoses is variable and 12 different immunotypes (L1–L12) have been described, using a panel of monoclonal antibodies. Strains from hyperinvasive clones of meningococci usually produce L3, L7, L9, whereas carrier strains often express the shorter L8 as the dominant immunotype [69]. Strains with L3, L7, L9 immunotypes induced higher levels of TNF-α in a monocyte-like cell line than other immunotypes associated with noninvasive strains [70]. Thus, the polysaccharide side-chains in *N. meningitidis* may influence the biological activity which primarily is exerted through the lipid A moiety. Although one major immunotype was initially associated with a single strain, many disease-causing meningococci harbor several immunotypes at the same time [71]. Furthermore, in a detailed study, Kahler et al. [72] were able to show that the meningococcal strain NMB had the capacity to express epitopes of all known immunotypes. Other invasive strains lack enzymes for this complete synthesis [72].

21.6
Molecular Mimicry Between Meningococcus and Man

21.6.1
Capsule Polysaccharide of Serogroup B

Pathogenic bacteria may express multiple epitopes on the surface that are identical to those found on human cells, a phenomenon denoted molecular mimicry [73, 74]. The serogroup B capsule polysaccharide and LPS are two chemical structures where molecular mimicry is present and may contribute to the pathogenicity. The serogroup B polysaccharide consists of long chains of N-acetylneuraminic acid (sialic acid) in $2 \rightarrow 8$ linkage with epitopes identical to the polysialic acid which is part of neural cell adhesion molecules. These adhesion molecules are present in different tissues and organs in the body. Serogroup B polysaccharide induces only a transient increase in specific IgM and no lasting IgG response in man. The phenomenon is explained as immune tolerance. Certain clones of immune cells reacting with these epitopes are possibly deleted during early fetal life to avoid the development of autoimmune reactions.

21.6.2
Lipopolysaccharides

The terminal four-sugar moiety lacto-N-neotetraose consisting of Galβ1 → 4GlcNAcβ1 → 3Galβ1 → 4Glc connected to the first heptose (α-chain) in the meningococcal LPS is identical to the glycosphingolipid paragloboside on mammalian cells (Fig. 21.2). The terminal galactose of this four-sugar unit functions as an acceptor unit for sialic acid, which covers human cells. The combined action of the capsule polysaccharide and LPS avoids proper insertion of the membrane attack complex of complement in the outer membrane, which is required to induce lysis of the bacterium [75]. If sialic acid is attached to the terminal LPS, the meningcocci become more resistant to bactericidal antibodies, but this does not impair the invasive potential when tested in a rat model [76, 77]. *In vitro* studies suggest that the terminal sialic acid may impair the ability of meningococci to penetrate into epithelial cells [76]. The trisaccharide structure galactose–glucosamine–galactose expresses the same epitopes on pathogenic *N. meningitidis* as are found on human cells. Meningococci may possibly alter the structure of LPS and other molecules many times through phase variation during their invasion of the human body.

Given the abundance of capsule polysaccharide and LPS molecules covering the surface of meningococci, bacterial epitopes mimicking human epitopes are presumably of importance, disguising meningococci from being recognized by the human immune system. Human erythrocytes, monocytes and neutrophils expose epitopes on the cell surface which are identical to epitopes formed by

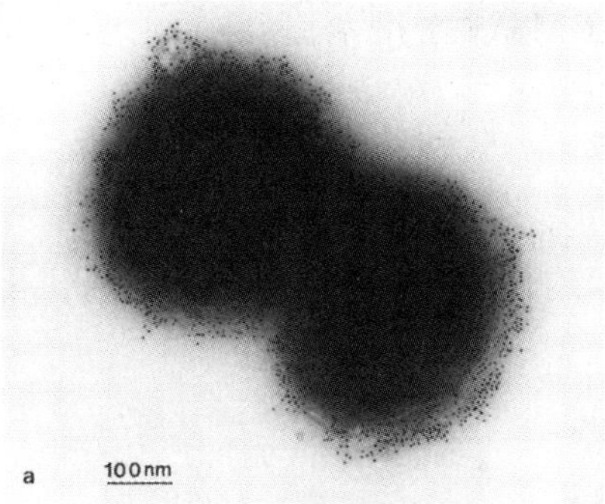

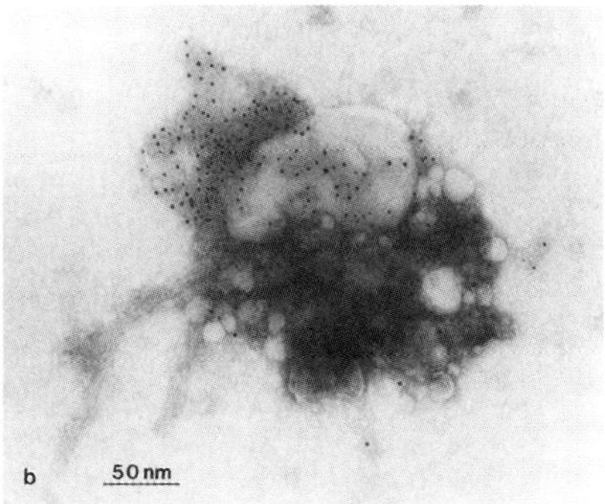

Fig. 21.3 Transmission electron micrographs. (a) *N. meningitidis* serogroup B (ET-5) isolated from a young man with distinct meningitis, stained with mouse Mab 3F11 reacting with the distal part of the lacto-N-neotetraose of LPS and a secondary gold-labeled gout antimouse Ab (diam. 10 nm). (b) A fragment, most likely from a leukocyte, in the CSF collected from a patient with distinct meningitis caused by *N. meningitidis* serogroup B (ET-5) stained with mouse Mab 3F11 and a secondary gold-labeled gout antimouse Ab (diam. 5 nm). The mouse Mab 3F11 was kindly provided by Professor M. Apicella (University of Iowa, Iowa City, USA). The micrographs were prepared by Ellen Namork (National Public Health Institute, Oslo, Norway).

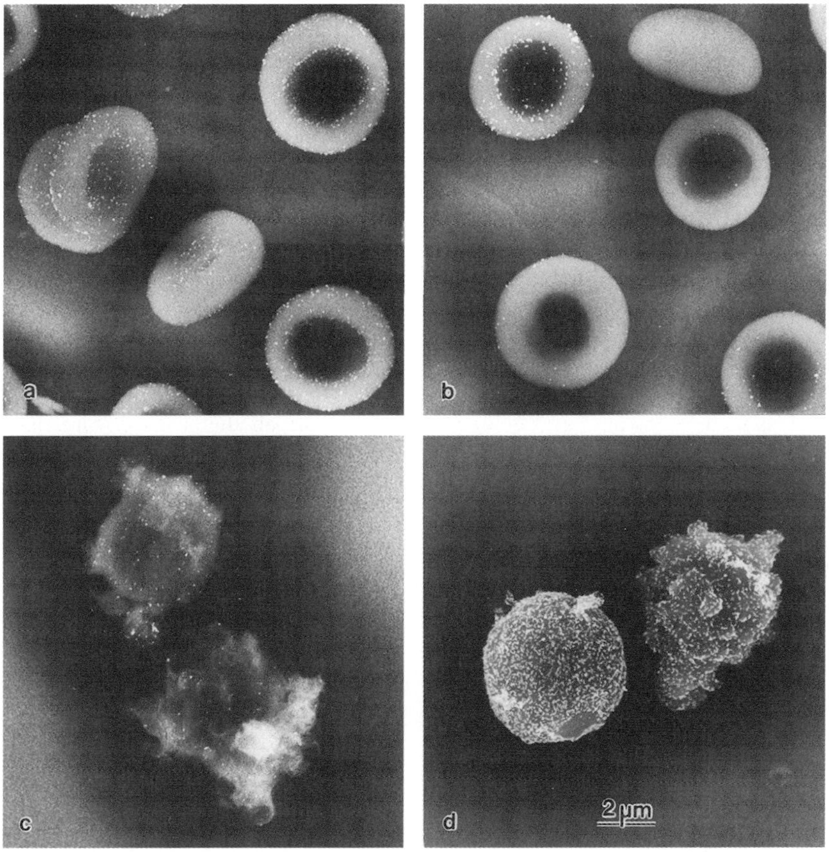

Fig. 21.4 Scanning electron micrographs of: (a) papain-treated red blood cells type A1 stained with antiA003 and gold labels (diam. 30 nm) goat–antimouse IgM (positive control), (b) papain-treated red blood cells strained with mouse Mab 3F11 reacting with the distal part of the lacto-N-neotetraose of LPS and a secondary gold-labeled goat–antimouse IgM (diam. 30 nm), (c) human monocytes and (d) human neutrophils stained with 3F11 and gold-labeled goat–antimouse IgM (diam. 30 nm). The mouse Mab 3F11 was kindly provided by Professor Michael Apicella (University of Iowa, Iowa City, USA). The micrographs were prepared by Ellen Namork (National Public Health Institute, Oslo, Norway).

Galβ1 $\rightarrow$ 4GlcNAcβ1 in the terminal part of the lacto-N-neotetraose of meningococcal LPS (Figs. 21.3, 21.4).

21.6.3
Molecular Mimicry Versus Clinical Presentation

Patients developing fulminant meningococcal septicemia give the impression of a profound immune deficiency towards the intruding meningococcus. However, the role of molecular mimicry in meningococcal disease is presently not clearly defined. Observations during the serogroup B epidemics in Norway showed that isolates from the ET-5 clone of meningococci (B:15:P1.7,16:L3,7,9) expressing lacto-N-neotetraose as the terminal sugar unit caused the whole spectrum of clinical presentations [2, 6]. Furthermore, >99% of the persons carrying this hypervirulent clone in the upper airways never developed clinical disease [78].

21.7 *N. meningitidis* LPS Reacting with the Innate Immune System

21.7.1 *N. meningitidis* and Cell Activation

LPS are a very potent activators of the innate immune system. Lipid A interacts with the LPS receptor complex on cells belonging to the mononuclear phagocytosis system, primarily monocytes and tissue macrophages. A few picograms per milliliter of purified *N. meningitidis* LPS trigger human monocytes to produce TNF-α and a variety of other inflammatory mediators and to upregulate tissue factor, which initiates blood coagulation. When restricted to a localized area, this immune reaction is beneficial to the body, limiting a potential spreading infection. However, in case of a massive growth of meningococci in the circulation or subarachnoid space, the immune reaction becomes toxic and detrimental to the body, ultimately killing the host if not treated.

21.7.2 LPS-binding Protein

LPS-binding protein (LBP), a 60-kDa acute phase protein, is present in plasma at concentrations of 3–7 $\mu g\ ml^{-1}$. During acute inflammation, it may increase 100-fold [79]. It is primarily synthesized in the hepatocytes, but a small fraction may also be produced in other tissues [79]. LBP has been described as a lipid “shuttle”, transporting different lipid molecules to lipoprotein complexes in plasma. In experiments with purified LPS, it dissociates aggregates of LPS into monomers and then catalyzes the transfer to CD14 on myeloid cells. How LBP functions during infection with LPS located in Gram-negative bacteria is not known in detail. In meningococcal infection, the small LPS molecules of *N. meningitidis* (approx. 4 kDa) are possibly detached from the outer leaflet of the bacterial outer membrane and associated with LBP in plasma. LBP presumably associates with LPS molecules in whole or fragmented bacteria and with outer membrane vesicles released during log phase growth. The meningococcal LPS-LBP monomer complex is then transported to myeloid cells expressing membrane-bound CD14 and endothelial cells to which soluble CD14 is attached.

21.7.3
CD14

CD14 is a 55-kDa glycerophosphorylinositol (GPI) anchored glycoprotein found on myelomonocytic cells, including monocytes, macrophages and, less abundantly (1:30), on neutrophils. It consists of 356 amino acids and exists in two forms: membrane-bound CD14 (mCD14) and soluble CD14 (sCD14) circulating in plasma. The main function of mCD14 is to convey the lipid A moiety of LPS to the Toll-like receptor 4 (TLR4). Only the first 152 amino acids at the N-terminal part of CD14 are required for the receptor function. Most of mCD14 resides in lipid rafts in the cell membrane. To generate a transmembrane signal initiated by LPS, mCD14 has to make physical contact with TLR4 and myeloid differentiation protein 2 (MD2), a plasma protein, which is not present in the lipid rafts [80].

mCD14 is essential for activation of human monocytes by purified *N. meningitidis* LPS or meningococcal LPS bound to the outer membrane. If the mCD14 receptor site is blocked with a monoclonal antibody, TNF-α production in human monocytes is reduced by >95% [81]. sCD14 contributes to the activation of endothelial cells which lack mCD14 [82]. Proinflammatory cytokines such as TNF-α and IL-1β together with albumin and hemoglobin may enhance this activation [83–85].

21.7.4
Toll-like Receptors

The Toll-like receptors (TLRs) are transmembrane glycoproteins recognizing conserved molecular structures which are essential for conducting signals from the surface to the interior of cells belonging to the innate immune system [1, 86, 87]. The surface-exposed parts of the TLR contain leucine-rich repeats and the cytoplasmatic tails are homologous to the intracellular part of the interleukin 1 receptor and denoted TLR/IL-1R (TIR) domain [1]. Eleven TLRs have been described in mammals [1]. The receptors recognize certain molecular structures which are conserved among different pathogens. TLR1 and TLR2 recognize lipoproteins in the bacterial cell wall and TLR2 is stimulated by fragments of peptidoglycan [1]. Using the LPS-deficient mutant of *N. meningitidis*, it has been documented with certainty that the human innate immune system recognizes nonLPS components in meningococci [88–93]. The cell activation is induced through the activation of TLR2 [88–91]. TLR4 is not activated by these nonLPS molecules.

21.7.5
TLR4 is Part of the LPS Receptor Complex

TLR4 was the first discovered mammalian homolog of the *Drosophilia* Toll protein. It recognizes LPS. Mice with a mutation leading to a truncated intracellular form of TLR4 are hyporesponsive to LPS [37]. Monomeric LPS is transferred from LBP to mCD14. The lipid A moiety of LPS makes physical contact with the extracellular domain of TLR4 [94]. The soluble plasma protein denoted myeloid differentiation protein 2 (MD2) interacts with lipid A and TLR4, forming a third essential component in the LPS receptor complex [95]. Genetically modified mice lacking MD2 are hyporesponsive to LPS stimuli. It is presently not known whether MD2 first associate with the acylated fatty acids of lipid A and then associate with TLR4, or modify TLR4 stereometrically. A close physical association between lipid A, MD2 and TLR4 appears to be essential for transmembrane signaling [95]. Together, mCD14-TLR4-MD2 forms the complete LPS receptor complex which initiates transmembrane and intracellular signaling [1, 80, 86, 87].

21.7.6
TLR4 and TLR2 on Leukocytes and Endothelial Cells

TLR2 and TLR4 are expressed on human monocytes, macrophages and, at lower concentrations, on neutrophils [1]. TLR4 and a little TLR2 are normally expressed on human endothelial cells [96, 97]. LPS and proinflammatory cytokines in plasma may upregulate both TLR4 and TLR2. In patients with sepsis, both TLR4 and TLR2 on circulating leukocytes are upregulated as compared with normal controls [98]. Still, leukocytes collected from patients with fulminant meningococcal septicemia are not responsive to further LPS stimuli, a phenomenon which is ascribed to "reprograming" of human leukocytes during sepsis [42–44].

21.7.7
The Intracellular Receptors for Peptidoglycan Fragments from Gram-negative Bacteria

The chemical structure of the thin peptidoglycan layer residing underneath the outer membrane of N. meningitidis has recently been published [99]. Peptidoglycan from Gram-negative bacteria are recognized by the nucleotide-binding oligomerization domain (NOD) molecules NOD1 and NOD2, two cytoplasmic surveillance proteins. They bind short fragments of peptidoglycan and initiate intracellular signaling and activation of nuclear factor (NF) κB [100, 101]. If the peptidoglycan layer in N. meningitidis really plays a role in the pathogenesis of meningococcal infections, it may trigger the innate immune system via the extracellular CD14-TLR2 and the intracellular NOD1 and NOD2 receptor systems.

21.7.8
Intracellular Signaling Through Nuclear Factor κB

Binding of ligands to different TLRs leads to dimerization of the receptor molecules and transmembrane signaling. Transmembrane signals induce a conformational change in the intracellular TIR domain. A variety of adapter molecules and kinases known by acronyms (MyD88, IRAK1-4, TRAF, TAK1, TAB1-2, TIRAP, TRAM) are then activated [1]. N. meningitidis LPS is a potent TLR4 agonist activating different cell types in a MyD88-dependent and MyD88-independent pathway [102]. Ultimately this leads to transcription of a large number of genes coding for inflammatory mediators [1]. Activation of the interleukin 1 receptor (IL-1R) is conveyed through the same chain of molecules. NFκB is a key transcription factor that is activated through different intracellular signal pathways. After release from its inhibitor, it migrates into the nucleus and initiates transcription of a large number of genes coding for inflammatory mediators [1].

21.7.9
Wild-type *N. meningitidis* Activates the Human Innate Immune System Through TLR4

Wild-type meningococci and outer membrane vesicles activate different cell types primarily through the CD14-TLR4-MD2 pathway [68, 81, 89–91]. This observation suggests that LPS is the dominant class of molecules in the outer membrane that trigger the human innate immune system when invasive meningococci gain access to the human circulation. Outer membrane vesicles, prepared for serogroup B vaccine, are depleted of 80–90% of the LPS molecules in the outer membrane. This preparation, which contains relatively more nonLPS molecules than outer membrane from wild-type meningococci, activates both TLR4 and, to a lesser extent, TLR2 [103]. A monoclonal antibody blocking TLR4 resulted in 78% inhibition of TNF-α production in human monocytes, whereas blocking TLR2 caused 43% inhibition [103]. PorB, one of the two major porins in *N. meningitidis*, activates B-lymphocytes and dendritic cells but not T-lymphocytes through the TLR2 signaling pathway [104, 105].

21.8
LPS Activates Human Cells During Meningococcal Infection

21.8.1
A Bioassay to Document the Effect of LPS in Human Disease

Plasma and CSF collected from patients with meningococcal infections, containing high levels of LPS, have been assayed using the activity of purified human monocytes to monitor the effects. The secretion of TNF-α and upregulation of tissue factor, measured as procoagulant activity, were used as indicators of cell activation [7]. The test system was built on a previously established functional assay and endogenous IL-10, a strong inhibitor of the monocytes in this system, was removed by immune precipitation [15]. The LPS levels in plasma were closely correlated to the secreted levels of TNF-α by the monocytes ($r=0.82$) [7]. This observation suggests that a close quantitative association exists between the levels of LPS generated during infection and the activation of human monocytes.

21.8.2
Blocking mCD14 in Normal Monocytes

When heparin plasma collected from patients with fulminant meningococcal septicemia was combined with human monocytes pretreated with an antiCD14 monoclonal antibody (60bca) to block parts of the LPS receptor complex, the secretion of TNF-α was reduced to median 5% and procoagulant activity to median 10% of the levels in unblocked monocytes. Plasma from patients with low or undetectable levels of LPS did not activate the monocytes [7].

21.8.3
Selective Blocking of TLR4 with the Lipid A Antagonist RsDPLA

When TLR4 was selectively blocked by pretreating the human monocytes with the lipid A antagonist RsDPLA derived from *Rhodobacter spheroides*, the secretion of TNF-α induced by meningococcal shock plasma was reduced to median 12% and the procoagulant activity to median 32% of the values generated by normal control monocytes. The secretion of TNF-α induced by CSF from patients with meningococcal meningitis was reduced to median 31% of the values generated by the monocytes before pretreatment with RsDPLA [7]. So far, this is the first direct specific proof that meningococcal LPS is the major contributor to the massive activation of the mononuclear phagocytosis system in patients with meningococcal infections.

21.9
The Biological Effect of Outer Membrane Vesicles

N. meningitidis forms large quantities of outer membrane vesicles (OMV) during log phase growth *in vitro* [106]. OMV are present in plasma and CSF collected from patients with fulminant septicemia and distinct meningitis [54, 55, 107]. They induce a strong cytokine response and potently activate the coagulation system [81]. Ninety-five percent of monocyte-mediated activity can be blocked by an antiCD14 monoclonal antibody [81]. OMV activate the limulus amebocyte lysate system more actively than purified meningococcal LPS [81].

If piglets are injected with meningococcal OMV, they develop septic shock. Two different doses of OMV (containing 10 µg kg^{-1} and 1 µg kg^{-1} LPS) resulted in 44% and 6% mortality, respectively [108]. In OMV developed for use in the Norwegian serogroup B vaccine, 80–90% of the LPS molecules were removed from the outer membrane by detergents. Much higher doses are required to induce inflammatory responses, activation of the coagulation system, burst reactions of leukocytes and leukocyte platelet interactions [81, 109–112]. The wild-type OMV activate primarily TLR4 (A. Bjerre, unpublished data). The LPS-depleted vaccine vesicles activate TLR4 and TLR2 [103].

The LPS-deficient *N. meningitidis* Mutant

21.10.1
The Creation of LPS-deficient Mutant

The creation of the mutant meningococcus H

91]. At a concentration of 10^8, the LPS-deficient mutant elicited as much cytokines as the wild-type strain. Looking at interferon-γ, the LPS-deficient mutant induced the same level as the LPS-containing parent strain [92]. High concentrations of the LPS-deficient strain are able to kill mice [92].

21.10.4
The Effect of LPS-deficient Mutant on Human Dendritic Cells

Using *in vitro*-generated human dendritic cells, the LPS-deficient mutant elicits less TNF-α and IL-6 than wild-type meningococci and completely lacks the ability to induce IL-12 [115]. Interleukin-12 is required for proper stimulation of T-helper (Th1) lymphocytes and subsequently interferon-γ production by the T-cells. Thus, for proper dendritic cell function, LPS integrated in the outer membrane of *N. meningitidis* is necessary [115]. LPS is also required for a normal function of pili and defensin-enhanced adherence to epithelial cells in the upper respiratory tract of man, since in the LPS-deficient mutant these functions are severely reduced [116, 117].

21.10.5
What is the Contribution of nonLPS Molecules in the Inflammatory Response of Patients?

The contribution of the nonLPS molecules to the inflammatory response in patients with meningococcal infections is presently not known. Wild-type meningococci with LPS are significantly more potent than the LPS-deficient mutant in eliciting cytokines at concentrations $<10^8$ meningococci ml^{-1} [88, 92]. In one *in vitro* study the nonLPS components had a marked additive effect on the production of TNF-α, IL-1β and interferon-γ [92]. This was not confirmed in a second study [90]. The only cytokine identified, so far, which was induced as readily with the LPS-deficient mutant as with the wild-type strain is interferon-γ [92]. Interestingly, patients with a massive load of meningococci developing lethal fulminant septicemia have very low plasma levels of interferon-γ [12, 118]. The nonLPS components may play a more important role in activating other parts of the immune system. The complement system and possibly other parts of the plasma contact system are primarily activated by nonLPS molecules of meningococci [119–121].

21.11
Distinct Differences Between Meningococcal and Pneumococcal Lethal Septic Shock Plasma

Some patients with septic shock caused by the Gram-positive *Streptococcus pneumoniae* reveal a clinical presentation similar to fulminant meningococcal septicemia. These patients develop septic shock, large hemorrhagic skin lesions and multiple organ failure. Plasmas from such patients completely lack detectable LPS [12]. The levels of cytokines differ from patients with meningococcal sepsis since they have relatively higher levels of interferon-γ and lower levels of IL-10 [12]. When pneumococcal shock plasma was added to normal human monocytes after removal of IL-10, the monocytes were not stimulated to produce any TNF-α or tissue factor [12]. The results differed completely from what had previously been observed with plasmas from patients with fulminant meningococcemia [7, 15]. We assume that plasmas from pneumococcal septic shock contain molecules derived from the cell wall of pneumococci, including lipoteichoid acid and peptidoglycan fragments which have the capacity to activate human monocytes through CD14-TLR2, but no activation was observed. Thus, in this bioassay, plasma from patients with lethal pneumococcal septic shock differed completely from meningococcal septic shock, indicating major differences in activation of the human innate system by these two important invasive human pathogens.

21.12 Plasma Systems Neutralizing *N. meningitidis* LPS

21.12.1 Lipoproteins May Contribute Little to Neutralization of Meningococcal LPS in Plasma

Different classes of lipoproteins, including high density lipoprotein (HDL), low density lipoprotein (LDL) and very low density lipoprotein (VLDL), may reduce the biological activity of purified *E. coli* LPS by incorporating lipid A into the complex lipoprotein structure [122]. However, when purified *N. meningitidis* LPS are used in the same type of experiments, the neutralizing capacity of the lipoproteins is much less than for *E. coli* LPS [123]. Meningococcal LPS is less hydrophilic owing to the short side-chain, as compared with *E. coli* LPS; and it may behave differently in plasma. Most importantly, the different fractions of the lipoproteins constituting a buffer system for LPS in plasma, neutralize very little of the biological activity induced by whole and fragmented meningococci [123]. The LPS activity in patient plasmas is caused by structures with a high sedimentation coefficient, indicating the presence of large fragments [54]. Fragments of meningococci and outer membrane vesicles have been visualized in electron micrographs after ultracentrifugation of patient plasma [54, 55].

21.12.2 Antibodies in Plasma Reduce the Activity of Meningococcal LPS

Antibodies detected in human plasma may contribute in the LPS buffer system since they neutralize the biological activity of different immunotypes of meningococcal LPS [70]. These antibodies, which recognize epitopes in the side-chain, appear indirectly to influence the cell activating property of lipid A.

21.13
Compartmentalized Inflammatory Response in the Vasculature Versus Subarachnoid Space

21.13.1
Bacterial Components and Inflammatory Mediators as Indicators

The magnitude of proliferation of meningococci in the circulation of cerebrospinal fluid is reflected in the host's inflammatory response, i.e. the production of pro- and anti-inflammatory mediators [2, 4, 8]. The infection and the host's inflammatory response is compartmentalized. Patients with fulminant septicemia with massive microbial proliferation in the circulation are characterized by extraordinarily high levels of inflammatory mediators in plasma and very low levels of meningococci and mediators, if detectable at all, in CSF [2, 4, 8, 17]. In patients with meningococcal meningitis, the opposite pattern is present. High levels of meningococci and inflammatory mediators are present in the subarachnoid space, whereas low levels are present in plasma [2, 4, 8, 17]. This reflects that the mediators are produced separately in each compartment and are closely associated with the number of bacteria, as determined by *N. meningitidis* DNA and LPS levels [2, 4, 35].

21.13.2
The Cytokine Profile in Patients with Fulminant Meningococcal Septicemia

The magnitude of the inflammatory response in the cardiovascular system or in the subarachnoid space is reflected in the upregulation of key pro- and anti-inflammatory cytokines. The cytokines appear to be gradually upregulated as the proliferation of the meningococci proceeds. The levels of the different cytokines studied are closely associated with the levels of LPS in plasma or CSF [2]. TNF-α was the first cytokine identified in severe meningococcemia [124]. Increased bioactivity of TNF-α was associated with death due to septic shock. Shortly thereafter, the complex cytokine pattern was identified [2, 4, 12, 13, 16, 125]. The major proinflammatory cytokines which are massively upregulated in fulminant meningococcal septicemia are TNF-α, IL-1β, IL-6, IL-8, MCP-1, MCP-1α and G-CSF. The levels of all these cytokines are closely correlated to the plasma levels of LPS [2, 13]. TNF-α, IL-1β, IL-6, IL-10 and G-CSF are present in a bioactive form [15, 17, 124] (P. Brandtzaeg, unpublished data). The levels of the different cytokines have usually been determined by immunological methods. The biological activity may be considerably lower than estimated by ELISA techniques, since many of the cytokines circulate in complex with their soluble receptor(s) [11, 18, 19]. The major anti-inflammatory cytokines are IL-10 and interleukin-1 receptor antagonist (IL-1Ra). IL-2, IL-4, IL-12, interferon γ (IFN-γ) and transforming growth factor β are undetectable or present at very low, i.e. at the level of a few picograms [2, 12].

21.13.3
The Net Inflammatory Effect of Septic Shock Plasma on Human Monocytes

Plasmas from patients with fulminant meningococcal septicemia containing high levels of LPS and the key inflammatory cytokines deactivate normal human monocytes [15]. The net inhibitory effect observed in this bioassay is related to high levels of bioactive IL-10. Removal of IL-10 by immunoprecipitation leads to massive activation of the normal monocytes [15]. In this experiment the net inflammatory capacity of meningococcal septic shock plasma was inhibitory on monocyte activation owing to the high levels of IL-10 in spite of high levels of bioactive LPS, TNF-α, IL-1β and IL-6. In a few patients with shock plasma containing LPS levels >250 EU ml^{-1}, the monocytes were activated in spite of high levels (>10 ng ml^{-1}) of IL-10 [7] (P. Brandtzaeg, unpublished results). Monocytes represent a key cell line in the mononuclear phagocytosis system. They "home" in different tissues and are transformed and reprogramed to macrophages, revealing a different reaction pattern to LPS and other stimuli than monocytes recently released from the bone marrow. The highest levels of LPS and cytokines in plasma are found in patients with lethal septic shock, dying shortly after hospital admission [2, 4].

21.13.4
Where are the Circulating Cytokines Produced?

The different cytokines are probably produced at multiple sites in the body and released to the circulation. The liver, spleen, endothelial cells and circulating leukocytes all have the capacity to produce inflammatory mediators. The relative contribution of different organs and cell types is presently unknown. The liver consists of 15% Kupffer cells; and these exert a dual function [45]. They remove bacteria and bacterial molecules from the circulation; and simultaneously they produce key inflammatory cytokines. Isolated human and bovine Kupffer cells produce TNF-α, IL-1β, IL-6 and prostaglandin E2 (PGE2) after stimulation with LPS, peptidoglycan and lipoteichoid [126, 127]. Furthermore, if a low dose (2 ng kg^{-1}) of purified *E. coli* LPS is injected intravenously into healthy human volunteers, a major part of TNF-α in plasma is produced in the liver [128]. We know little about how the Kupffer cells are regulated when they are present in the normal liver tissue as compared with isolated Kupffer cells and human monocytes. The anatomical position in the liver sinusoids may influence cytokine production. Kupffer cells from the perivenous acinar region of rat livers produce more inflammatory mediators than Kupffer cells located in the periportal area [45, 52, 127].

Macrophages in the spleen and possibly other organs adjacent to the circulation may contribute to the release of cytokines. Endothelial cells can produce a variety of cytokines when triggered by LPS through circulating sCD14 interacting with the TLR4-MD2 receptor complex [129, 130]. Furthermore, the endothelial cells are activated by many different circulating cytokines, inducing phenotypical changes and altering the surface structures [130].

Circulating leukocytes collected from healthy persons synthesize cytokines in a dose-dependent manner when combined with wild-type and LPS-deficient meningococci, outer membrane vesicle and purified LPS [42, 81, 88, 92]. Mononuclear leukocytes in peripheral blood produce 100-fold more proinflammatory cytokines per cell than neutrophils do during LPS stimulation [131]. However, when wild-type invasive meningococci are added to whole blood, the levels of TNF-α are 10-fold higher and levels of IL-10 are 10-fold lower than observed in plasmas from patients with fulminant meningococcemia [42] (P. Brandtzaeg, unpublished data). This observation indicates that bioactive IL-10, leading to the strong anti-inflammatory effect of meningococcal shock plasma, is produced by cells than other circulating leukocytes.

21.13.5
Downregulation of Human Leukocytes in Shock Patients

Leukocytes collected during the acute phase of meningococcal septic shock hardly produce any cytokine upon LPS stimulation [42]. The production of TNF-α appears to be downregulated at a posttranscriptional level whereas IL-1β is regulated at mRNA and posttranscriptional levels [43]. During the subsequent 6–14 days, the capacity to produce cytokines gradually returned to a normal level. The reduced cytokine production was independent of circulating inhibitory factors [43]. This phenomenon is regarded as a downregulation of the cytokine-producing machinery to protect the host from cytokine overstimulation. It is part of the complex reaction pattern of the mammalian innate immune system, leading to LPS tolerance and reprograming of circulating leukocytes during sepsis [40, 41, 44].

21.14
Dysfunction of the Cardiovascular System

Fulminant meningococcal septicemia is characterized by a profound cardiovascular dysfunction, leading to circulatory collapse. The septic shock is caused by: (a) an altered vascular tone, (b) a reduced cardiac performance, (c) an altered endothelial function and (d) a reduced circulating blood volume. The development of meningococcal septic shock is closely related to LPS in plasma >7 EU ml^{-1}, which reflects the number of circulating meningococci $>5\times10^5$ ml^{-1} plasma and the host's inflammatory response to the bacteria [2, 9, 35]. A plethora of mediators may contribute to the altered circulation [2, 4, 14]. Hardly any patients with LPS levels above 120 EU ml^{-1} survive [2]. Circulatory collapse is the most common cause of death in patients contracting meningococcal infections in economically developed countries. Fifty percent of the nonsurviving patients die within 12 h after admission [4].

In young healthy volunteers 4 ng kg^{-1} of *E. coli* LPS injected intravenously induce a reduced cardiac function which lasts for 8 days [132]. In patients with sepsis and septic shock a biventricular dilation of the heart occurs. The increased volume of the heart, which is prominent after fluid resuscitation, is regarded as a compensatory mechanism [133]. It is presently regularly monitored by ultrasonographic examination of the heart in septic patients. The contractility and the ejection fraction are reduced [14, 133]. The clinical deterioration can be monitored by a continuously decline in the ejected blood volume.

21.14.1 The Circulatory Pattern in Meningococcal Septic Shock

Initially the circulation is hyperdynamic, with increased cardiac index and a high peripheral resistance [134]. The extremities are cold and sometimes cyanotic, although the blood pressure is maintained within the normal range for a certain period. After fluid loading and as the disease progresses, the peripheral resistance decreases to very low levels, in spite of the infusion of high doses of adrenalin or noradrenalin (P. Brandtzaeg, unpublished data). This functional state has been denoted vasoplegia. The circulation remains hyperdynamic. In nonsurvivors, the cardiac performance gradually decreases and the cardiac index declines. The circulation becomes hypodynamic [14]; and the ejection fraction declines. The terminal phase is characterized by a very low cardiac index and peripheral resistance, which does not react to vasoactive drugs. Ultrasonographic examination shows a very dilated left ventricular and a hardly contracting myocardium. Often a terminal arrhythmia leads to cardiac arrest.

21.14.2 The Vasculature in the Progressing Shock

As the septic shock progresses, the net effect of vasodilatating principles prevails over compensatory vasoconstricting mediators [14]. In the past 10 years, it has been assumed that nitric oxide (NO) generated by inducible nitric oxide synthase (iNOS) in the endothelial and smooth muscle cells plays a cardinal role in relaxing the tonus in the vasculature, leading to vasodilatation in septic shock. However, the exact role of iNOS and NO in septic shock is still unclear. Continuous generation of high levels of anaphylatoxins, mainly C3a and C5a, and bradykinin through activation of the plasma contact system may contribute to the persistent dilatation of the resistance vessels [135–137].

21.14.3 Cardiac Dysfunction

The deteriorating cardiac function has been related to structural changes in the heart muscles, including signs of myocarditis and structural changes in the myofibrils [138]. These structural changes may vary with the prevailing epidemic strain. In a large postmortem study with 200 autopsies, 78% had signs of myocarditis [138]. During the recent serogroup B epidemic in Norway, macroscopic and microscopic changes of the myocardium have been virtually absent, indicating that severe cardiac dysfunction, confirmed by ultrasonographic examination, may occur without major or even minor structural changes. The myocardial dysfunction is associated with increased circulating levels of cardiac troponin I levels and ECG abnormalities [139, 140].

Three inflammatory mediators identified as TNF-α, IL-1β and NO have myocardial depressant activity [133]. TNF-α synergizes with IL-1β in reducing the contractility of single myocytes [133]. NO is generated from L-arginine. Increased NO production in the heart, through upregulation of myocardial iNOS, may reduce the contractility of the myocardium. Recently, IL-6 has been proposed as an additional cytokine with cardiodepressive effect in MSS [141]. This observation requires further confirmation.

21.14.4
The Endothelial Cells

The altered function of the endothelium can be documented by: (a) increased release of molecules from the surface of the endothelial cells, (b) reduced antithrombotic properties and (c) reduced barrier function leading to capillary leak syndrome. Plasminogen activator inhibitor 1 (PAI-1), tissue factor pathway inhibitor (TFPI) and thrombomodulin levels in plasma are increased [20, 142–144]. In biopsies from hemorrhagic skin lesions, the expression of thrombomodulin and endothelial cell protein C receptor are lower than normal controls, suggesting a release and/or downregulation of these important surface receptors [144]. The reduced antithrombotic effect of the epithelial lining results in thrombotic lesions in peripheral vessels in the extremities and typical skin lesions. The capillary leak syndrome is a consequence of the altered barrier function, resulting in leakage of albumin and other plasma proteins into the interstitial tissue.

In vitro studies using endothelial cells in culture suggest that meningococci alone do not damage the endothelial lining. However, when meningococci and neutrophils interact, the neutrophils cause structural changes in the endothelial cells [145]. Using *in vitro* systems and looking at the expression of tissue factor on endothelial cells, noncapsulated meningococci adhered more readily to the endothelial cells and induced more tissue factor than isogenic encapsulated variants [146]. Close contact between meningococci and endothelial cell brings LPS and other bacterial outer membrane components into close contact with TLR4 and TLR2 and activates NF-κB, thereby triggering tissue factor production. This may facilitate local formation of fibrin thrombi observed in skin biopsies [147]. However, invasive strains in the blood are encapsulated. Moreover, it has never been documented with certainty that tissue factor really is upregulated on the abluminal side of the vasculature in sepsis. The intercellular adhesion molecule 1 (ICAM-1) and vascular cellular adhesion molecule 1 (VCAM-1) are upregulated by wild-type meningococci and purified meningococcal LPS [115]. The endothelial type selectin (CD62E) appears to be induced by nonLPS molecules via a nonNF-κB pathway [115]. LPS and nonLPS components of meningococci appear to interact with the endothelial cells, activating different pathways. Meningococci "docking" on the endothelial cells may alter the surface locally, whereas bioactive cytokines, anaphylatoxins, bradykinin and other inflammatory mediators may exert a more generalized influence on the large endothelial surface of the vasculature.

21.15 Capillary Leak Syndrome

This syndrome is caused by an altered barrier function of the endothelial lining of the vascular bed, leading to an increased flux of H_2O and proteins, primarily albumin, across the capillary wall. It is prominent among patients with fulminant meningococcal septicemia and is caused by the marked inflammatory reaction in the vasculature. The severity of the leakage is associated with the levels of circulating meningococci, LPS, proinflammatory cytokines and complement activation products [2, 4, 137]. It is assumed that LPS, TNF-α, IL-1β, NO, bradykinin and the effect of proteolytic enzymes and oxygen radicals, released by marginated neutrophils, decrease the barrier function. The close quantitative correlation between the ongoing complement activation and persistant meningococcal shock with increasing capillary leakage during the first days of treatment suggests a cause effect relationship [135, 137].

21.16 Renal Failure

Reduced kidney function is closely associated with reduced renal circulation and severe coagulopathy in meningococcal septic shock. In patients with LPS levels >8 EU ml^{-1}, hypotension and disseminated coagulopathy, combined with reduced fibrinolysis, lead to reduced kidney function [9, 20]. The cardinal changes are reduced blood flow to the tubuli and thrombotic lesions in the glomerular capillaries [14, 138, 148, 149]. Proinflammatory cytokines and other mediators may possibly induce apoptosis of the tubular cells and thereby contribute to the reduced function of the tubuli. This renal failure is reversible in most cases, although a permanent reduced kidney function may persist in some patients surviving fulminant meningococcal septicemia.

21.17 Altered Adrenal Function

Lethal meningococcemia has for almost a century been associated with hemorrhagic adrenals and known as Waterhouse-Friderichsen syndrome [138, 150, 151]. The hemorrhagic lesions are associated with fibrin clots in the adrenal vessels and a bleeding tendency. The hemorrhage starts in the inner zona reticulosa and expands outwards. The cortex may escape hemorrhagic destruction [14]. Acute adrenal insufficiency was for a long time regarded as the cause of the circulatory collapse. Previous measurements of circulating cortisol were conflicting [14]. In a large study recently conducted, the group of 12 nonsurviving patients with meningococcal shock had lower median levels of cortisol (654 nmol l^{-1}) and higher median levels of ACTH (equal to 1271 ng l^{-1}) than the 38 patients surviving the septic shock (with median cortisol of 2184 nmol l^{-1} and ACTH median of 85 ng l^{-1}) [152]. The results suggest that the nonsurvivors had a relatively insufficient cortisol response to the high ACTH levels. Currently, most clinicians treat these patients with a low dose of cortisol [44]. The regeneration capacity must be considerable, since very few patients surviving meningococcal septic shock develop Addison's disease.

21.18 Other Endocrine Reactions Associated with Meningococcal Septic Shock

The median level of growth hormone is approximately 20-fold higher in nonsurvivors than survivors with meningococcal septic shock [153]. Total and free fractions of insulin-like growth factor I are reduced 2- to 4-fold in the nonsurvivors. The ratio of growth hormone to insulin-like growth factor I indicates great differences between the two groups. Thyroid-stimulating hormone (TSH) is 3-fold higher, whereas the thyroid hormone reverse T3 is half of the value of the survivors. Nonesterified fatty acids are reduced to one-third of the levels found among survivors and lactate levels are doubled [154]. The observations are in line with many previous observations, suggesting that patients with fatal meningococcal septicemia are sicker as a group than those surviving the shock.

21.19 Coagulopathy in Meningococcal Disease

21.19.1 Hemorrhagic Skin Lesions

Hemorrhagic skin lesions are the hallmark of invasive meningococcal disease, although not pathognomonic. The size of these lesions is associated with the clinical presentation, the severity of the ongoing disseminated intravascular coagulation (DIC) and the development of multiple organ failure [39]. The lesions have been described as a hemorrhagic vasculitis with swollen epithelium protruding into the lumen of the blood vessels and fibrin thrombi or platelet thrombi plugging the lumen [14, 147, 155]. The vessel walls are often but not always infiltrated with neutrophils. Meningococci are present in endothelial cells, leukocytes and the perivascular interstitium [147]. They are located in clusters of microcolonies varying from 20 to 100 in a 4 μm section and express capsule polysaccharide and pilin, indicating the formation of type 4 pili as well as PorA when located in the lumen and in and around the vessel wall. These observations indicate that invasive meningococci are not downregulating the polysaccharide capsule and pili when passing from the blood through the endothelial cells to the extravascular interstitium. This may influence activation of the endothelial cells [146]. The perivascular leukocytes express specific markers of neutrophils and monocytes [147].

21.19.2 Thrombus Formation of Larger Vessels

Patients with fulminant meningococcal septicemia tend to develop thromboses in the extremities, leading to muscle necrosis, i.e. rhabdomyolysis and gangrene [14, 156]. Thrombosis and hemorrhage are most commonly observed in the adrenals, in the glomeruli of the kidneys and in the choroid plexus in the lateral ventricles of the brain [138, 150, 151]. Occasionally, microthrombi are seen in the lungs. Also, intracoccular hemorrhages and massive bleeding in the ovaries occur [157] (P. Brandtzaeg, unpublished data). The intestines, liver and heart are usually without massive thrombotic and hemorrhagic changes, even in the most fulminating cases, although ischemic lesion of the bowels has been described [158].

21.19.3 Activation of the Coagulation System Leading to Disseminated Intravascular Coagulation

Patients with fulminant meningococcal disease develop DIC characterized by consumption of coagulation factors and platelets. The plasma levels of coagulation factors V, VIII and fibrinogen and, to a lesser extent, coagulation factors IX and X are subnormal [143]. The activation is initiated by increased synthesis and exposure of tissue factor in monocytes [159, 160]. A widespread expression of tissue factor on the abluminal side of blood vessels as a reaction to the high levels of LPS and cytokines has not been documented in these patients or in primate septic shock studies [161]. The surface of the endothelial cells appears to be less antithrombotic than normal. Release of glycosamineglycan-like molecules, plasminogen activator inhibitor 1 (PAI-1), thrombomodulin and downregulation protein C endothelial receptor, combined with reduced flow, could all contribute to thrombus formation in certain parts of the vasculature [20, 143–145, 162, 163].

Cells exposing tissue factor are normally not in direct contact with circulating plasma. Human monocytes, the only circulating leukocyte with the capacity to synthesize tissue factor, are presently regarded as key cells in triggering the coagulation cascade during sepsis [164, 165]. Purified meningococcal LPS, meningococcal outer membrane vesicles and whole meningococci all activate human monocytes to synthesize tissue factor [81, 166]. This results in a dose-dependent increase in procoagulant activity when assayed in a plasma system [81]. After upregulation and exposure to plasma, tissue factor interacts with coagulation factor VIIa. The complex of tissue factor with factor VIIa activates coagulation factor VII and X to Xa. If chimpanzees or baboons are pretreated with a monoclonal antibody reacting with tissue factor or the coagulation factors VII/VIIa, activation of the coagulation system and development of shock can be avoided [167, 168]. Whole and fragmented monocytes, isolated from patients with meningococcal septic shock, reveal increased levels of tissue factor activity [159, 160]. Coagulation factor XII (Hageman factor) and XI are activated in fulminant meningococcal septicemia but do not contribute much to the coagulopathy [4, 136].

21.20 The Natural Coagulation Inhibitors

The natural coagulation inhibitory system consists of three different proteins working in concert with other molecules. Antithrombin (AT), protein C (PC) and tissue factor pathway inhibitor (TFPI) inhibit different steps in the coagulation cascade, leading to the consumption of these proteins through the formation of coagulation factor-inhibitor complexes.

21.20.1 Protein C

Activated protein C inhibits factor Va and factor VIIIa, dampens inflammation and increased the fibrinolysis. The functional level of protein C is reduced to 10–25% of normal levels (>75%) in lethal cases of fulminant meningococcal septicemia [142, 143, 169, 170]. In meningococcal patients with less severe coagulopathy, the protein C levels are subnormal but higher than in shock patients. Low levels of protein C are associated with the development of diffuse thrombosis in dermal vessels, a clinical manifestation seen in newborns with homocygote protein C deficiency. Protein C is converted to activated protein C by the thrombomodulin–thrombin complex on the surface of endothelial cells. The endothelial surface is also altered by activation of the protein C endothelial cell receptor. In patients with meningococcal septicemia, thrombomodulin is released into the circulation and the number of protein C endothelial cell receptors is reduced [144]. This makes the endothelial lining more thrombogenic. However, patients with fulminant meningococcal septicemia still have the capacity to convert endogenous protein C to activated protein C, which is elevated on hospital admission [171]. Moreover, if purified protein C is infused, the level of activated protein C increases significantly in patients with fulminant meningococcemia. This indicates that the thrombomodulin–thrombin complex on the endothelial cells works, although the capacity may be reduced in specific areas of the vasculature [171]. It remains to be documented whether early treatment with purified protein C or recombinant human activated protein C can reduce the massive thrombotic complications observed in the skin, adrenals, kidneys and extremities. Recombinant human activated protein C has reduced the case fatality rate in patients with severe sepsis and septic shock, but has not been specifically tested in patients with meningococcal shock and coagulopathy.

21.20.2
Antithrombin

Antithrombin neutralizes the effect of thrombin and inhibits activation of tissue factor VIIa, factor X and factor XI. The antithrombin levels are subnormal, i.e. 50–67% of normal values (>75%) in patients with fulminant meningococcal septicemia, but less reduced than protein C [142, 143]. Low levels of antithrombin impair the physiological effect of heparin. Supplementation with recombinant human antithrombin do not increase survival in patients with various types of sepsis.

21.20.3
Tissue Factor Pathway Inhibitor

Tissue factor pathway inhibitor (TFPI) inhibits the formation of tissue factor and factor VIIa, which initiates the coagulation cascade in sepsis. It also reduces the conversion of coagulation factor X to Xa. Longitudinal studies of patients with fulminant meningococcal septicemia reveal that TFPI initially is consumed, resulting in subnormal functional levels [142]. As the septic shock proceeds, TFPI is released from the endothelial cells and the functional level in plasma increases [142, 172]. The anticoagulant effect of TFPI is associated with the basic carboxy-terminal tail located in the released fraction; and TFPI contributes to the anticoagulant effect of heparin. Recombinant human tissue factor pathway inhibitor does not reduce the mortality in sepsis of various causes.

21.20.4
Thrombin Activation

The final step in the coagulation cascade is the conversion of fibrinogen to fibrin by thrombin. Fibrinopeptide A, a short peptide split-off from fibrinogen during fibrin formation, has a half-life of 2–3 min in the circulation. The plasma levels of fibrinopeptide A are direct measures of thrombin activity. The levels of fibrinopeptide A decline rapidly after antibiotic and volume treatment is started [142]. Thus, activation of the coagulation system is gradually downregulated and the levels of fibrinopeptide A are reduced by 50% within 12 h, whereas the observable thrombotic process in the skin and peripheral parts of the extremities seemingly increases. In patients with purpura fulminans, hemorrhagic skin lesions rapidly increase in number and size and the toes and fingers become cold and discolored blueish, indicating severely reduced perfusion.

Trapping of platelets may explain the diffuse ongoing thrombotic process in spite of the reduced activity of the coagulation system.

21.21 The Fibrinolytic System

21.21.1 Plasminogen Activator Inhibitor 1

When LPS are injected into the human circulation, tissue plasminogen activator (tPA) is released. It converts plasminogen to plasmin, counteracting the formation of a fibrin plug. Subsequently, plasminogen activator inhibitor 1 (PAI-1) is released from the endothelial cells and platelets, inactivating the effect of tPA [173]. This occurs at an early stage during meningococcemia [20, 163]. On admission, the plasma levels of tPA are moderately, i.e. 2- to 4-fold, increased and do not differ significantly between nonsurvivors and survivors of meningococcal septic shock [163]. The levels of PAI-1, inhibiting tPA, are 50-fold increased in nonsurvivors and 20-fold elevated in survivors of meningococcal shock [20, 163]. Genetic polymorphism in the promoter region of the PAI-1 gene influences the chances of survival. Patients with 4G/4G alleles reveal an increased chance of developing shock and dying [163, 174, 175]. However, the plasma levels of PAI-1 are closely correlated to the levels of LPS [20]. This indicates that the plasma levels of PAI-1 are determined by the load of meningococci and LPS and a particular genetic polymorphism (4G/4G) coding for the production of high levels of PAI-1.

21.21.2 Alpha-2-antiplasmin

Plasmin in plasma is inactivated by alpha-2-antiplasmin. In patients with fulminant meningococcal septicemia, the median functional level of alpha-2-antiplasmin for nonsurvivors is 26%, as compared with 54% surviving shock patients, 83% in patients with meningitis and 89% in those with mild systemic meningococcemia in the first collected sample on admission [20]. Serial measurements reveal a further decline in alpha-2-antiplasmin to $<12.5\%$ in half of the nonsurvivors, whereas the levels gradually increase in the survivors [20]. The low levels are presumably caused by complex formation with plasmin and other proteases. Leakage caused by the profound capillary leak syndrome in the most severely ill patients may also contribute to the low levels. The plasma levels of plasmin-antiplasmin (PAP) complexes are doubled in nonsurvivors as compared with surviving patients with shock [163].

21.21.3 Balance Between Coagulation and Fibrinolysis

The ratio between tPA/PAI-1 continuously decreases with increasing disease severity in meningococcal infections. The declining ratio parallels the increasing plasma levels of LPS and a variety of other inflammatory mediators. The balance between thrombus formation and endogenous thrombolysis tilts towards coagulation. High levels of monocyte-produced tissue factor, decreased levels of coagulation inhibitors (in particular protein C), high levels of PAI-1, low levels of alpha-2-antiplasmin and decreased antithrombotic properties of the endothelium all favor the formation of thrombi in certain parts of the vascular system.

21.22 The Complement System

21.22.1 The Effect of Bactericidal and Opsonophagocytic Antibodies and a Normal Complement System

The complement system is the effector system that makes antimeningococcal antibodies bactericidal. It plays a crucial role in protecting man from invasive *N. meningitidis*. If intruding meningococci circumvent the local defense mechanisms on the mucosal surface and submucosal tissue and enter the circulation, the number of bacteria is presumably low. In the majority of the population, the combined effect of bactericidal and opsonizing antibodies rapidly eliminates the bacteria, avoiding further multiplication in the blood. The activation of the complement system at this stage is effective, balanced and low-graded. The host is not harmed by the activation.

21.22.2 The Complement System in Patients with Invasive Meningococcal Disease

In patients lacking the necessary protective antibodies or with deficiencies or defects in the complement system, rapid proliferation of pathogenic meningococci results in an intense activation that becomes harmful to the patient and contributes to organ dysfunction. Primate models of septic shock have documented that the complement system induces hypotension through the production of anaphylatoxins, primarily C5a [176]. The activation of C3 and generation of the macromolecule C5b-C9 are closely associated with the levels of LPS in patients with invasive meningococcal infections [135]. Nonsurviving shock patients reveal the most intense complement activation and consumption of lysis inhibitors [135, 137, 177]. Based on *in vitro* experiments, the massive complement activation observed in fulminant meningococcal septicemia is primarily induced by nonLPS molecules. Mutant meningococci completely lacking LPS trigger the complement system as actively as the wild-type parent strain covered with LPS when assayed in whole-blood experiments [119, 121]. Antibodies to Por A and Por B, representing 70% of the outer membrane proteins, are assumed to be the major activators of complement in these experiments. In the most severely ill patients, the surface of the endothelial cells may be damaged, owing to increased levels of bioactive TNF-α, IL-1β, C5a, toxic oxygen species and different proteases released by adherent neutrophils. The endothelial cells are thought to be denuded of protective molecules. The septic plasma may alter the morphology of the endothelial cells and increase the distance between individual cells and thereby expose subendothelial structures possibly interacting with alternative pathways of complement.

21.22.3
Persistent Complement Activation

Serial studies show that the complement activation remains high or increases during the first 12–15 h after the initiation of antibiotic and volume therapy [135, 137]. The persistent activation of complement, in spite of declining levels of meningococci, LPS and cytokines, clearly suggests that a nonbacterial mechanism perpetuates the activation. The activation pattern of complement in these shock patients differs markedly from the kinetics of pro- and anti-inflammatory cytokines, which decline immediately after the initiation of antibiotic treatment in parallel with plasma levels of LPS [2, 4, 14].

21.22.4
C5a

C5a is a key anaphylotoxin that activates circulating neutrophils and monocytes, causing a burst reaction and release of toxic oxygen radicals and proteases [120, 121, 178]. C5a triggers "marginated" leukocytes adhering to the endothelium during the leukopenic period in patients with fulminant meningococcal septicemia. This is the time of maximum release of leukocyte proteases [179]. Interestingly, it is presently possible to manipulate the complement system with a monoclonal antibody that interacts with complement factor C5 and neutralizes the C5a moiety before it is split off. This prevents augmented cell activation without interfering with the formation of C5b-C9 and the bactericidal capacity of plasma [120].

21.22.5
Activation Pathways of Complement

Persons with bactericidal antimeningococcal antibodies activate the classic pathway of complement. However, in nonimmune persons developing invasive meningococcal infections, activation of the alternative pathway plays a more prominent role, particularly in patients with fulminant meningococcal septicemia

[180]. It is presently not known whether the massive activation of the alternative pathway is a direct activation or part of the amplification loop initiated by the mannose binding lectin (MBL) pathway. In children, but not in young adults, subnormal levels of MBL predisposes for meningococcal infections [181]. The contribution of MBL to the complement activation in patients has still not been clearly defined. Conflicting results exist as to the contribution of MBL to the opsonophagocytosis of encapsulated meningococci with sialylated LPS [182–184]. Recent studies suggest that MBL binds to outer membrane proteins, including PorB and opacity protein a (opa) of group B and C meningococci, but not to LPS [185]. In one study, very low concentrations of meningococci activate the complement system via the MBL pathway, an observation that was related to the ability of the outer membrane vesicles to activate complement [186]. MBL appears to participate in the regulation of the cytokine response to meningococci [187, 188]. Outer membrane vesicles may possibly function as decoys for specific antibodies and complement factors.

21.23 Activation of Neutrophils Related to Disease Severity

The levels of leukocytes on hospital admission are associated with the disease severity. Patients with meningococcal meningitis and mild systemic meningococcal disease with a comparatively low-graded meningococcemia reveal a marked leukocytosis on hospital admission, whereas patients with fulminant meningococcemia are usually leukopenic. The leukopenia is explained by the upregulation of various adhesion molecules on the leukocytes and endothelial cells, causing the leukocytes to adhere to the endothelial lining ("marginate") in the peripheral vasculature. A large proportion of the neutrophils in patients with septicemia are band forms, newly released from the bone marrow. They are directed to the periphery of the cardiovascular system by exceptionally high levels of IL-8, MCP-1 and MIP-1α [13]. During this "marginated state", the neutrophils are triggered by high levels of C5a and release multiple proteases, which is reflected in high levels of the neutrophil elastase–antiprotease complex in plasma [2, 121]. Simultaneously, they release different oxygen radicals in close proximity to endothelial cells. The combined effect of proteases and reactive oxygen metabolites on the endothelium may damage the cell surface. It is noteworthy that high levels of bioactive cytidine deaminase are present in meningococcal septic shock plasma [189]. Cytidine deaminase may counteract the effects of high levels of the different colony-stimulating factors, particularly G-CSF and neutralize reactive oxygen metabolites. The levels increase or remain high during the first 24–48 h after hospital admission [189]. The leukocytes are driven by high levels of complement activation products, primarily C5a [121]. The complement system continues to generate high levels of anaphylatoxins for 12–15 h before declining [135, 137].

21.24
Meningitis

21.24.1
Meningococci and the Meninges

Pathogenic strains of *N. meningitidis* have the propensity to invade the meninges. Meningitis, characterized by headache, vomiting, nuchal and back rigidity, is the most common clinical presentation of invasive *N. meningitidis*. The symptoms of meningitis are always preceded by a bacteremic phase without CNS symptoms. The meninges are seeded during this bacteremic phase. On hospital admission, the CSF is characterized by marked pleocytosis, i.e. a leukocyte count $> 10^8\ l^{-1}$. The time span between the debute of the symptoms and the admission to hospital was median 29, 26 and 24 h in three studies, as compared with 13, 12 and 12 h for patients developing fulminant meningococcal septicemia [8, 11, 38]. The longer time span between onset of the symptoms and hospital admission is explained by the fact that meningococci seed two different compartments, first the vascular system and then, subsequently, the meninges. Contrary to previous belief, the meningococcemia at this stage is comparatively low-graded (median $<10^3$ DNA ml^{-1}, LPS <0.5 EU ml^{-1}), explaining why patients with meningococcal meningitis seldom develop septic shock and severe coagulopathy, although petechial rash is common [2, 16, 30, 31, 35].

21.24.2
Where do Meningococci Enter the Subarachnoid Space?

The choroid plexus in both lateral ventricles of the brain are the production sites of the CSF. The blood flow through each choroid plexus is high. They have long since been regarded as a possible site of entrance of meningococci into the subarachnoid space [14]. Recently, it was documented that *N. meningitidis* indeed adheres to endothelium in the choroid plexus but also to endothelial cells in vessels of the meninges [190]. Meningococci may thus possibly enter at several places simultaneously if they express pili and, in particular, if the pili contain high levels of PilC, which facilitates adherence to the endothelial cells [190].

21.24.3
Molecules Regulating the Influx of Leukocytes

Gradually, while the meningococci grow in the subarachnoid space, LPS, other outer membrane products and pili induce an inflammatory reaction, with the release of TNF-α, IL-1β, IL-6, IL-8, MCP-1, MIP-α and G-CSF [191–194]. Based on experiences with meningioma cells, *N. meningitidis* induces higher levels of the cytokines than the same number of *S. pneumoniae, H. influenzae* and K1 capsule-type *E. coli* do. Interestingly, the meningioma cells were stimulated by a receptor system which is different from the TLRs [195].

The coordinated release of cytokines alters the vasculature of the meninges. Different complementary adhesion molecules on the endothelial cells and circulating leukocytes are upregulated, including selectins, intercellular adhesion molecules (ICAMs) and vascular endothelial adhesion molecules (VECAMs). Circulating leukocytes, primarily neutrophils, are attracted by IL-8 and pass between the activated endothelial cells entering the subarachnoid space. In parallel, proteins (mainly albumin, but also immunoglobulins and complement factors) leak into the CSF. TNF-α, IL-1β are produced early in the process and are found in a bioactive form in approximately 50% of the patients on hospital admission [191]. In half of the patients, they are already downregulated or inactivated when the diagnostic spinal puncture is done. The production of IL-6, IL-8, MCP-1 and MIP-1α appears to continue for a longer time or are upregulated to a higher level than TNF-α and IL-1β. They can be detected with sensitive immunoassays in the majority of the patients on admission [125, 191].

21.24.4
Proliferation of *N. meningitidis* in the Subarachnoid Space

Once the meningococci have penetrated into the subarachnoid space, the human body can mount little immediate resistance to *N. meningitidis*. The levels of antibodies and complement are very low and few mobile phagocytic cells are initially present in the CSF. Gradually, the neutrophils increase in number. A massive growth in bacteria without a marked accompanying pleocytosis, a phenomenon regularly observed in pneumococcal meningitis, is very uncommon in meningococcal meningitis.

21.24.5
The Compartmentalized Inflammatory Response

The bacterial proliferation and inflammatory response is compartmentalized between the subarachnoid space and the vasculature. A massive bacterial growth, high levels of LPS and inflammatory mediators are detected in CSF, whereas comparatively low levels of LPS and inflammatory mediators are present in plasma [4, 8, 16]. The meningococci are clearly not able to proliferate as rapidly in the circulation in patients with meningitis as they are in patients developing fulminant septicemia. This comparatively slow growth rate protects most patients with meningitis from developing septic shock.

Before serum therapy and antibiotics were available, patients with both clinical presentations died. However, the mechanisms leading to death differed. Currently, few patients (<5%) receiving adequate antibiotic treatment die of meningococcal meningitis [2, 4]. Patients dying of meningitis develop an irreversible brain edema, leading to herniation of the cerebellum. An altered function of the aquaporins, the water channels, in neural tissue may contribute to the edema formation [196].

21.25
Chronic Meningococcemia

Certain strains of *N. meningitidis* may circulate for many days or weeks and occasionally months, without causing meningitis. The symptoms observed in patients with chronic intermittent meningococcemia, including fever, skin rash and arthralgia or arthritis of the large joints, are related to the formation of circulating immune complexes. Since the symptoms are intermittent and blood cultures are regularly negative, one may speculate whether the meningococci survive intracellularly in endothelial cells or other cell types and enter the circulation from time to time. Why these meningococci do not pass into the subarachnoid space is not known. One hypothetical explanation could be phenotypical changes, including downregulation of pili or other adherence mechanisms, while they circulate in the blood [197].

21.26
Conclusion and Future Aspects

In the past 20 years, we have been able to quantify the bacterial invasion in the circulation and the subarachnoid space more accurately than previously. We have learned that the inflammatory responses in the patients with meningococcal infections are compartmentalized and closely related to the number of meningococci. The inflammatory response is induced by bacterial cell wall molecules, LPS and others, through activation of different arms of the innate immune system. Currently, we do not understand what enables the intruding meningococci to multiply very rapidly in 10–20% of patients, whereas growth is comparatively low-graded in the other presentations. The development of septic shock is presently the primary cause of death in the industrialized countries. The case fatality rate has not changed much since the introduction of sulfonamides 70 years ago. In developing countries, meningitis and septic shock remain deadly threats to the population. It is a paradox that virulent *N. meningitidis* is a peaceful inhabitant of the oropharyngeal mucosa in >99% of carriers, but causes life-threatening septicemia in 10–20% of those becoming ill. No other common invasive bacterium causes such a high percentage of septic shock as the meningococcus. This propensity to cause unimpeded growth in the vascular system remains an unexplained feature of *N. meningitidis*.

Future research should focus on what limits the meningococcus from rapid proliferation in the blood of patients developing distinct meningitis and mild meningococcemia, as compared with those developing a septic shock. We need more detailed knowledge of the very complex inflammatory reaction induced by this Gram-negative bacterium when gaining access to the vascular system and the subarachnoid space. Particularly intriguing is the recent observation that meningeoma cells may harbor a transmembrane signaling system which is different from the TLR [195]. Is this system also present in other cell types? Will we be able to modulate the activation state of the different arms of the innate immune system in the future to the benefit of our patients? How important is the continuous activation of the complement system in those developing shock? Will therapy blocking the excessive and long-lasting activation of C3 and C5 increase the chances of survival? Hopefully, this insight will provide us with better tools to modify and control the consequences of the exacerbated immune reaction. However, the only final solution of the meningococcal "problem" is to develop a vaccine covering all major classes of invasive meningococci and apply them to coming cohorts of infants, children and young adolescents.

References

1 Akira, S., K. Takeda. **2004**, Toll-like receptor signalling, *Nat. Rev. Immunol.* 4, 499–511.

2 Brandtzaeg, P., A. Bjerre, R. Ovstebo, B. Brusletto, G. B. Joø, P. Kierulf. **2001**, Neisseria meningitidis lipopolysaccharides in human pathology, *J. Endotoxin Res.* 7, 401–420.

3 Brandtzaeg, P. **2003**, Host response to Neisseria meningitidis lacking lipopolysaccharides, *Expert Rev. Anti Infect. Ther.* 1, 589–596.

4 van Deuren, M., P. Brandtzaeg, J. W. van der Meer. **2000**, Update on meningococcal disease with emphasis on pathogenesis and clinical management, *Clin. Microbiol. Rev.* 13, 144–166.

5 Steeghs, L., R. den Hartog, A. den Boer, B.Zomer, P. Roholl, P. van der Ley. **1998**, Meningitis bacterium is viable without endotoxin, *Nature* 392, 449–450.

6 Gedde-Dahl T. W., E. A. Høiby, A. Schillinger, A. Lystad, K. Bøvre. **1983**, An epidemiological, clinical and microbiological follow-up study of incident meningococcal disease cases in Norway, winter 1981–1982, *Nat. Inst. Public Health Ann.* 6, 155–181.

7 Bjerre, A., B. Brusletto, R. Øvstebø, G.B. Joø, P. Kierulf, P. Brandtzaeg. **2003**, Identification of meningococcal LPS as a major monocyte activator in IL-10 depleted shock plasmas and CSF by blocking the CD14-TLR4 receptor complex, *J. Endotoxin Res.* 9, 155–163.

8 Brandtzaeg, P., R. Øvstebø, P. Kierulf. **1992**, Compartmentalization of lipopolysaccharide production correlates with clinical presentation in meningococcal disease, *J. Infect. Dis.* 166, 650–652.

9 Brandtzaeg, P., P. Kierulf, P. Gaustad, A. Skulberg, J. N. Bruun, S. Halvorsen, E. Sørensen. **1989**, Plasma endotoxin as a predictor of multiple organ failure and death in systemic meningococcal disease, *J. Infect. Dis.* 159, 195–204.

10 Brandtzaeg, P., R. Øvstebø, P. Kierulf. **1995**, Bacteremia and compartmentalization of LPS in meningococcal disease, *Prog. Clin. Biol. Res.* 392, 219–233.

11 van Deuren, M., J. van der Ven-Jongekrij, A. K. Bartelink, R. van Dalen, R. W. Sauerwein, J. W. van der Meer. **1995**, Correlation between proinflammatory cytokines and antiinflammatory mediators and the severity of disease in meningococcal infections, *J. Infect. Dis.* 172, 433–439.

12 Bjerre, A., B. Brusletto, E. A. Høiby, P. Kierulf, P. Brandtzaeg. **2004**, Plasma interferon-gamma and interleukin-10 concentrations in systemic meningococcal disease compared with severe systemic Gram-positive septic shock, *Crit. Care Med.* 32, 433–438.

13 Møller, A. S., A. Bjerre, B. Brusletto, G. B. Joø, P. Brandtzaeg, P. Kierulf. **2005**, Chemokine patterns in meningococcal disease, *J. Infect. Dis.* 191, 768–775.

14 Brandtzaeg P. **1995**, Pathogenesis of meningococcal infections, in *Meningococcal Disease*, ed. Cartwright K., Wiley, Chichester, p. 71–114.

15 Brandtzaeg P., L. Osnes, R. Øvstebø, G. B. Joø, A. B.Westvik, P. Kierulf. **1996**,

Net inflammatory capacity of human septic shock plasma evaluated by a monocyte-based target cell assay: identification of interleukin-10 as a major functional deactivator of human monocytes, *J. Exp. Med.* 184, 51–60.

16 Brandtzaeg, P., A. Halstensen, P. Kierulf, T. Espevik, A. Waage. **1992**, Molecular mechanisms in the compartmentalized inflammatory response presenting as meningococcal meningitis or septic shock, *Microb. Pathog.* 13, 423–431.

17 Waage, A., P. Brandtzaeg, A. Halstensen, P. Kierulf, T. Espevik. **1989**, The complex pattern of cytokines in serum from patients with meningococcal septic shock, Association between interleukin 6, interleukin 1, and fatal outcome, *J. Exp. Med.* 169, 333–338.

18 Frieling, J.T., M. van Deuren, J. Wijdenes, D.R. van Dalen, A.K. Bartelink, C.J. van der Linden, et al. **1996**, Interleukin-6 and its soluble receptor during acute meningococcal infections: effect of plasma or whole blood exchange, *Crit. Care Med.* 24, 1801–1805.

19 van Deuren, M., J. van der Ven-Jongekrij, E. Vannier, R. van Dalen, G. Pesman, A.K. Bartelink, et al. **1997**, The pattern of interleukin-1beta (IL-1beta) and its modulating agents IL-1 receptor antagonist and IL-1 soluble receptor type II in acute meningococcal infections, *Blood* 90, 1101–1108.

20 Brandtzaeg, P., G.B. Joø, B. Brusletto, P. Kierulf. **1990**, Plasminogen activator inhibitor 1 and 2, alpha-2-antiplasmin, plasminogen, and endotoxin levels in systemic meningococcal disease, *Thromb. Res.* 57, 271–278.

21 Johansson, L., A. Rytkonen, P. Bergman, B. Albiger, H. Kallstrom, T. Hokfelt, B. Agerberth, R. Cattaneo, A.B. Jonsson. **2003**, CD46 in meningococcal disease, *Science* 301, 373–375.

22 Stephens, D.S., M.M. Farley. **1991**, Pathogenic events during infection of the human nasopharynx with Neisseria meningitidis and Haemophilus influenzae, *Rev. Infect. Dis.* 13, 22–33.

23 Read, R.C., L. Goodwin. **2001**, Experimental nasopharyngeal colonization by Neisseria meningitidis using explant organ culture, in *Methods in Molecular Medicine; Meningococcal Disease*, eds. Pollard, A.J., Maiden, M.C.J., Humana Press, Totowa, N.J., p. 621–633.

24 Plant, L., V. Asp, L. Lovkvist, J. Sundqvist, A.B. Jonsson. **2004**, Epithelial cell responses induced upon adherence of pathogenic Neisseria, *Cell Microbiol.* 6, 663–670.

25 Parsons, H.K., S. Vitovski, J.R. Sayers. **2004**, Immunoglobulin A1 proteases: a structure-function update, *Biochem. Soc. Trans.* 32, 1130–1132.

26 Lorenzen, D.R., F. Dux, U. Wolk, A. Tsirpouchtsidis, G. Haas, T.F. Meyer. **1999**, Immunoglobulin A1 protease, an exoenzyme of pathogenic Neisseriae, is a potent inducer of proinflammatory cytokines, *J. Exp. Med.* 190, 1049–1058.

27 Derkx, B., A. Marchant, M. Goldman, R. Bijlmer, S. van Deventer. **1995**, High levels of interleukin-10 during the initial phase of fulminant meningococcal septic shock, *J. Infect. Dis.* 171, 229–232.

28 Herrick, W.W. **1918**, Early diagnosis and intravenous serum treatment of epidemic cerebrospinal meningitis, *J. Am. Med. Assoc.* 71, 612–618.

29 Dinarello, C.A. **2004**, Infection, fever, and exogenous and endogenous pyrogens: some concepts have changed, *J. Endotoxin Res.* 10, 201–222.

30 La Scolea, L., D. Dryja, T.D. Sullivan, L. Mosovich, N. Ellerstein, E. Neter. **1981**, Diagnosis of bacteremia in children by quantitative direct plating and a radiometric procedure, *J. Clin. Microbiol.* 13, 478–482.

31 La Scolea, L., D. Dryja. **1984**, Quantitation of bacteria in cerebrospinal fluid and blood of children with meningitis and its diagnostic significance, *J. Clin. Microbiol.* 19, 187–190.

32 Zwahlen, A., F.A. Waldvogel. **1984**, Magnitude of bacteremia and complement activation during Neisseria meningitidis infection: study of two co-primary cases with different clinical presentations, *Eur. J. Clin. Microbiol.* 3, 439–441.

33 Sullivan, T.D., L.J. La Scolea. **1987**, Neisseria meningitidis bacteremia in children: quantitation of bacteremia and

spontaneous clinical recovery without antibiotic therapy, *Pediatrics* 80, 63–67.

34 Hackett, S. J., M. Guiver, J. Marsh, J. A. Sills, A. P. Thomson, E. B. Kaczmarski, et al. **2002**, Meningococcal bacterial DNA load at presentation correlates with disease severity, *Arch. Dis. Child.* 86, 44–46.

35 Ovstebo, R., P. Brandtzaeg, B. Brusletto, K. B. Haug, K. Lande, E. A. Høiby, et al. **2004**, Use of robotized DNA isolation and real-time PCR to quantify and identify close correlation between levels of Neisseria meningitidis DNA and lipopolysaccharides in plasma and cerebrospinal fluid from patients with systemic meningococcal disease, *J. Clin. Microbiol.* 42, 2980–2987.

36 Andersen, B. M., O. Solberg, K. Bryn, L. O. Froholm, P. Gaustad, E. A. Høiby, B. E. Kristiansen, K. Bovre. **1987**, Endotoxin liberation from Neisseria meningitidis isolated from carriers and clinical cases, *Scand. J. Infect. Dis.* 19, 409–419.

37 Poltorak, A., X. He, I. Smirnova, M. Y. Liu, C. Van Huffel, X. Du, et al. **1998**, Defective LPS signaling in C3H/HeJ and C57BL/10ScCr mice: mutations in Tlr4 gene, *Science* 282, 2085–2088.

38 Bøvre, K., E. A. Høiby. **1989**, Meningococcal disease in Norway 1981–1982, with focus on severe septicemia and death, Epidemiological trends and relation of cases to some health service factors, *Nat. Inst. Public Health Ann.* 12, 13–20.

39 Brandtzaeg, P., J. S. Dahle, E. A. Høiby. **1983**, The occurrence and features of hemorrhagic skin lesions in 115 cases of systemic meningococcal disease, *Nat. Inst. Public Health Ann.* 6, 183–190.

40 Cross, A. S. **2002**, Endotoxin tolerance-current concepts in historical perspective, *J Endotoxin Res.* 8, 83–98.

41 Fan, H., J. A. Cook. **2004**, Molecular mechanisms of endotoxin tolerance, *J. Endotoxin. Res.* 10, 71–84.

42 van Deuren M., J. van der Ven-Jongekrijg, M. Keuter, P. M. N. Demacker, J. W. M. van der Meer. **1993**, Cytokine production in whole blood cultures, *J. Int. Fed. Clin. Chem.* 5, 216–221.

43 van Deuren, M., M. G. Netea, A. Hijmans, P. N. Demacker, C. Neeleman, R. W. Sauerwein, et al. **1998**, Posttranscriptional down-regulation of tumor necrosis factor-alpha and interleukin-1beta production in acute meningococcal infections, *J. Infect. Dis.* 177, 1401–1405.

44 Annane, D., E. Bellissant, J. M. Cavaillon. **2005**, Septic shock, *Lancet* 365, 63–78.

45 Naito, M., G. Hasegawa, Y. Ebe, T. Yamamoto. **2004**, Differentiation and function of Kupffer cells, *Med. Electron Microsc.* 37, 16–28.

46 Benacerraf, B., M. M. Sebestyen, S. Schlossman. **1959**, A quantitative study of the kinetics of blood clearance of P32-labelled Escherichia coli and Staphylococci by the reticuloendothelial system, *J. Exp. Med.* 110, 27–48.

47 Andersson, R., A. Foss. **1991**, Abdominal sepsis following liver resection in the rat, *Hepatogastroenterology* 38, 547–549.

48 Hirakata, Y., K. Tomono, K. Tateda, T. Matsumoto, N. Furuya, K. Shimoguchi, et al. **1991**, Role of bacterial association with Kupffer cells in occurrence of endogenous systemic bacteremia, *Infect. Immun.* 59, 289–294.

49 Klein, A., M. Zhadkewich, J. Margolick, J. Winkelstein, G. Bulkley. **1994**, Quantitative discrimination of hepatic reticuloendothelial clearance and phagocytic killing, *J. Leukoc. Biol.* 55, 248–252.

50 Gregory, S. H., E. J. Wing. **2002**, Neutrophil-Kupffer cell interaction: a critical component of host defenses to systemic bacterial infections, *J. Leukoc. Biol.* 72, 239–248.

51 Shi, J., G. E. Gilbert, Y. Kokubo, T. Ohashi. **2001**, Role of the liver in regulating numbers of circulating neutrophils, *Blood* 98, 1226–1230.

52 Bykov, I., P. Ylipaasto, L. Eerola, K. O. Lindros. **2003**, Phagocytosis and LPS-stimulated production of cytokines and prostaglandin E2 is different in Kupffer cells isolated from the periportal or perivenous liver region, *Scand. J. Gastroenterol.* 38, 1256–1261.

53 Abe, T., T. Arai, A. Ogawa, T. Hiromatsu, A. Masuda, T. Matsuguchi, et al. **2004**, Kupffer cell-derived interleukin 10 is responsible for impaired bacterial clearance in bile duct-ligated mice, *Hepatology* 40, 414–423.

54 Brandtzaeg, P., K. Bryn, P. Kierulf, R. Øvstebø, E. Namork, B. Aase, et al. **1992**, Meningococcal endotoxin in lethal septic shock plasma studied by gas chromatography, mass-spectrometry, ultracentrifugation, and electron microscopy, *J. Clin. Invest.* 89, 816–823.

55 Namork, E., P. Brandtzaeg. **2002**, Fatal meningococcal septicaemia with "blebbing" meningococcus, *Lancet* 360, 1741.

56 Shnyra, A., A.A. Lindberg. **1995**, Scavenger receptor pathway for lipopolysaccharide binding to Kupffer and endothelial liver cells in vitro, *Infect. Immun.* 63, 865–873.

57 van Oosten, M., E.S. van Amersfoort, T.J. van Berkel, J. Kuiper. **2001**, Scavenger receptor-like receptors for the binding of lipopolysaccharide and lipoteichoic acid to liver endothelial and Kupffer cells, *J. Endotoxin Res.* 7, 381–384.

58 Vishnyakova, T.G., A.V. Bocharov, I.N. Baranova, Z. Chen, A.T. Remaley, G. Csako, et al. **2003**, Binding and internalization of lipopolysaccharide by Cla-1, a human orthologue of rodent scavenger receptor B1, *J. Biol. Chem.* 278, 22771–22780.

59 Peiser, L., M.P. De Winther, K. Makepeace, M. Hollinshead, P. Coull, J. Plested, et al. **2002**, The class A macrophage scavenger receptor is a major pattern recognition receptor for Neisseria meningitidis which is independent of lipopolysaccharide and not required for secretory responses, *Infect. Immun.* 70, 5346–5354.

60 Kulshin, V.A., U. Zähringer, B. Lindner, C.E. Frasch, C.M. Tsai, B.A. Dmitriev, et al. **1992**, Structural characterization of the lipid A component of pathogenic Neisseria meningitidis, *J. Bacteriol.* 174, 1793–1800.

61 Pavliak, V., J.R .Brisson, F. Michon, D. Uhrin, H.J. Jennings. **1993**, Structure of the sialylated L3 lipopolysaccharide of Neisseria meningitidis, *J. Biol. Chem.* 268, 14146–14152.

62 Diaz, R.J., I.M. Outschoorn. **1994**, Current status of meningococcal group B vaccine candidates: capsular or noncapsular? *Clin. Microbiol. Rev.* 7, 559–575.

63 Zähringer, U., et al. **1999**, Chemical structure of lipid A: recent advances in structural analysis of biologically active molecules, in *Endotoxin in Health and Disease*, eds. H. Brade, S.M. Opal, S.N. Vogel, D.C. Morrison, Marcel Dekker, New York, p. 93–114.

64 McLeod Griffiss J, S.H. **1999**, The chemistry and biology of lipooligosaccharides: the endotoxins of bacteria of the respiratory and genital mucosa, in *Endotoxin in Health and Disease*, ed. H. Brade, S.M. Opal, S.N. Vogel, D.C. Morrison, Marcel Dekker, New York, p. 179–194.

65 Kahler, C.M., D.S. Stephens. **1998**, Genetic basis for biosynthesis, structure, and function of meningococcal lipooligosaccharide (endotoxin), *Crit. Rev. Microbiol.* 24, 281–334.

66 van der Ley, P., L. Steeghs, H.J. Hamstra, J. ten Hove, B. Zomer, L. van Alphen. **2001**, Modification of lipid A biosynthesis in Neisseria meningitidis lpxL mutants: influence on lipopolysaccharide structure, toxicity, and adjuvant activity, *Infect. Immun.* 69, 5981–5990.

67 Roth, R.I., R. Yamasaki, R.E. Mandrell, J.M. Griffiss. **1992**, Ability of gonococcal and meningococcal lipooligosaccharides to clot Limulus amebocyte lysate, *Infect. Immun.* 60, 762–767.

68 Zughaier, S.M., Y.L. Tzeng, S.M. Zimmer, A. Datta, R.W. Carlson, D.S. Stephens. **2004**, Neisseria meningitidis lipooligosaccharide structure-dependent activation of the macrophage CD14/Toll-like receptor 4 pathway, *Infect. Immun.* 72, 371–380.

69 Jones, D.M., R. Borrow, A.J. Fox, S. Gray, K.A. Cartwright, J.T. Poolman. **1992**, The lipooligosaccharide immunotype as a virulence determinant in Neisseria meningitidis, *Microb. Pathog.* 13, 219–224.

70 Braun, J.M., C.C. Blackwell, I.R. Poxton, O.E. Ahmer, A.E. Gordon, O.M. Madani, et al. **2002**, Proinflammatory responses to lipo-oligosaccharide of Neisseria meningitidis immunotype strains in relation to virulence and disease, *J. Infect. Dis.* 185, 1431–1438.

71 Scholten R.J., B. Kuipers, H.A. Valkenburg, J. Dankert, W.D. Zollinger, J.T.

Poolman. **1994**, Lipooligosaccharide immunotyping of Neisseria meningitidis by a whole-cell ELISA with monoclonal antibodies, *J. Med. Microbiol.* 41, 236–243.

72 Kahler, C.M., A. Datta, Y.L. Tzeng, R.W. Carlson, D.S. Stephens. **2005**, Inner core assembly and structure of the lipooligosaccharide of Neisseria meningitidis: capacity of strain NMB to express all known immunotype epitopes, *Glycobiology* 15, 409–419.

73 Giardina P.C, M.Apicella. **1999**, Antigenic mimicry in Neisseria species, in *Endotoxin in Health and Disease*, ed. H. Brade, S.M. Opal, S.N. Vogel, D.C. Morrison, Marcel Dekker, New York, p. 55–65.

74 Tsai, C.M. **2001**, Molecular mimicry of host structures by lipooligosaccharides of Neisseria meningitidis: characterization of sialylated and nonsialylated lacto-N-neotetraose (Galbeta1-4GlcNAcbeta1-3Galbeta1-4Glc) structures in lipooligosaccharides using monoclonal antibodies and specific lectins, *Adv. Exp. Med. Biol.* 491, 525–542.

75 Ram, S., F.G. Mackinnon, S. Gulati, D.P. McQuillen, U. Vogel, M. Frosch, et al. **1999**, The contrasting mechanisms of serum resistance of Neisseria gonorrhoeae and group B Neisseria meningitidis, *Mol. Immunol.* 36, 915–928.

76 de Vries, F.P., E.A. van der Ende, J.P. van Putten, J. Dankert. **1996**, Invasion of primary nasopharyngeal epithelial cells by Neisseria meningitidis is controlled by phase variation of multiple surface antigens, *Infect. Immun.* 64, 2998–3006.

77 Vogel, U., H. Claus, G. Heinze, M. Frosch. **1999**, Role of lipopolysaccharide sialylation in serum resistance of serogroup B and C meningococcal disease isolates, *Infect. Immun.* 67, 954–957.

78 Yazdankhah, S.P., D.A. Caugant. **2004**, Neisseria meningitidis: an overview of the carriage state, *J Med. Microbiol.* 53, 821–832.

79 Tobias, P.S., R.I. Tapping, J.A. Gegner. **1999**, Endotoxin interactions with lipopolysaccharide-responsive cells, *Clin. Infect. Dis.* 28, 476–481.

80 Miyake, K. **2004**, Endotoxin recognition molecules, Toll-like receptor 4-MD-2, *Semin. Immunol.* 16, 11–16.

81 Bjerre, A., B. Brusletto, E. Rosenqvist, E. Namork, P. Kierulf, R. Ovstebo, et al. **2000**, Cellular activating properties and morphology of membrane-bound and purified meningococcal lipopolysaccharide, *J. Endotoxin Res.* 6, 437–445.

82 Frey, E.A., D.S. Miller, T.G. Jahr, A. Sundan, V. Bazil, T. Espevik, et al. **1992**, Soluble CD14 participates in the response of cells to lipopolysaccharide, *J. Exp. Med.* 176, 1665–1671.

83 Pugin, J., R.J. Ulevitch, P.S. Tobias. **1995**, Activation of endothelial cells by endotoxin: direct versus indirect pathways and the role of CD14, *Prog. Clin. Biol. Res.* 392, 369–373.

84 Gioannini, T.L., D. Zhang, A. Teghanemt, J.P. Weiss. **2002**, An essential role for albumin in the interaction of endotoxin with lipopolysaccharide-binding protein and sCD14 and resultant cell activation, *J. Biol. Chem.* 277, 47818–47825.

85 Roth, R.I. **1996**, Hemoglobin enhances the binding of bacterial endotoxin to human endothelial cells, *Thromb. Haemost.* 76, 258–262.

86 Dobrovolskaia, M.A., S.N. Vogel. **2002**, Toll receptors, CD14, and macrophage activation and deactivation by LPS, *Microbes Infect.* 4, 903–914.

87 Miller, S.I., R.K. Ernst, M.W. Bader. **2005**, LPS, TLR4 and infectious disease diversity, *Nat. Rev. Microbiol.* 3, 36–46.

88 Uronen, H., A.J. Williams, G. Dixon, S.R. Andersen, P. van der Ley, M. van Deuren, et al. **2000**, Gram-negative bacteria induce proinflammatory cytokine production by monocytes in the absence of lipopolysaccharide (LPS), *Clin. Exp. Immunol.* 122, 312–315.

89 Ingalls, R.R., E. Lien, D.T. Golenbock. **2000**, Differential roles of TLR2 and TLR4 in the host response to Gram-negative bacteria: lessons from a lipopolysaccharide-deficient mutant of Neisseria meningitidis, *J. Endotoxin. Res.* 6, 411–415.

90 Ingalls, R.R., E. Lien, D.T. Golenbock. **2001**, Membrane-associated proteins of a lipopolysaccharide-deficient mutant of Neisseria meningitidis activate the inflammatory response through toll-like receptor 2, *Infect. Immun.* 69, 2230–2236.

91 Pridmore, A.C., D.H. Wyllie, F. Abdillahi, L. Steeghs, P. van der Ley, S.K. Dower, et al. **2001**, A lipopolysaccharide-deficient mutant of Neisseria meningitidis elicits attenuated cytokine release by human macrophages and signals via toll-like receptor (TLR) 2 but not via TLR4/MD2, *J. Infect. Dis.* 183, 89–96.

92 Sprong, T., N. Stikkelbroeck, P. van der Ley, L. Steeghs, L. van Alphen, N. Klein, et al. **2001**, Contributions of Neisseria meningitidis LPS and non-LPS to proinflammatory cytokine response, *J. Leukoc. Biol.* 70, 283–288.

93 Al-Bader, T., M. Christodoulides, J.E. Heckels, J. Holloway, A.E. Semper, P.S. Friedmann. **2003**, Activation of human dendritic cells is modulated by components of the outer membranes of Neisseria meningitidis, *Infect. Immun.* 71, 5590–5597.

94 Shimazu, R., S. Akashi, H. Ogata, Y. Nagai, K. Fukudome, K. Miyake et al. **1999**, MD-2, a molecule that confers lipopolysaccharide responsiveness on Toll-like receptor 4, *J. Exp. Med.* 189, 1777–1782.

95 Poltorak, A., P. Ricciardi-Castagnoli, S. Citterio, B. Beutler. **2000**, Physical contact between lipopolysaccharide and toll-like receptor 4 revealed by genetic complementation, *Proc. Natl Acad. Sci. USA* 97, 2163–2167.

96 Faure, E., L. Thomas, H. Xu, A. Medvedev, O. Equils, M. Arditi. **2001**, Bacterial lipopolysaccharide and IFN-gamma induce Toll-like receptor 2 and Toll-like receptor 4 expression in human endothelial cells: role of NF-kappa B activation, *J. Immunol.* 166, 2018–2024.

97 Zhang, F.X., C.J. Kirschning, R. Mancinelli, X.P. Xu, Y. Jin, E. Faure, et al. **1999**, Bacterial lipopolysaccharide activates nuclear factor-kappa B through interleukin-1 signaling mediators in cultured human dermal endothelial cells and mononuclear phagocytes, *J. Biol. Chem.* 274, 7611–7614.

98 Harter, L., L. Mica, R. Stocker, O. Trentz, M. Keel. **2004**, Increased expression of toll-like receptor-2 and -4 on leukocytes from patients with sepsis, *Shock* 22, 403–409.

99 Antignac, A., J.C. Rousselle, A. Namane, A. Labigne, M.K. Taha, I.G. Boneca. **2003**, Detailed structural analysis of the peptidoglycan of the human pathogen Neisseria meningitidis, *J. Biol. Chem.* 278, 31521–31528.

100 Girardin, S.E., L.H. Travassos, M. Herve, D. Blanot, I.G. Boneca, D.J. Philpott, et al. **2003**, Peptidoglycan molecular requirements allowing detection by Nod1 and Nod2, *J Biol. Chem* 278, 41702–41708.

101 Philpott, D.J., S.E. Girardin. **2004**, The role of Toll-like receptors and Nod proteins in bacterial infection, *Mol. Immunol.* 41, 1099–1108.

102 Zughaier, S.M., S.M.Zimmer, A. Datta, R.W. Carlson, D.S. Stephens. **2005**, Differential induction of the toll-like receptor 4-MyD88-dependent and -independent signaling pathways by endotoxins, *Infect. Immun.* 73, 2940–2950.

103 Mirlashari, M.R., T. Lyberg. **2003**, Expression and involvement of Toll-like receptors (TLR)2, TLR4, and CD14 in monocyte TNF-alpha production induced by lipopolysaccharides from Neisseria meningitidis, *Med. Sci. Monit.* 9, BR316–BR324.

104 Massari, P., S. Ram, H. Macleod, L.M. Wetzler. **2003**, The role of porins in neisserial pathogenesis and immunity, *Trends Microbiol.* 11, 87–93.

105 Singleton, T.E., P. Massari, L.M. Wetzler. **2005**, Neisserial porin-induced dendritic cell activation is MyD88 and TLR2 dependent, *J. Immunol.* 174, 3545–3550.

106 DeVoe, I.W., J.E. Gilchrist. **1973**, Release of endotoxin in the form of cell wall blebs during in vitro growth of Neisseria meningitidis, *J. Exp. Med.* 138, 1156–1167.

107 Stephens, D.S., K.M.Edwards, F. Morris, Z.A. McGee. **1982**, Pili and outer membrane appendages on Neisseria meningitidis in the cerebrospinal fluid of an infant, *J. Infect. Dis.* 146, 568.

108 Hazelzet, J.A., R. Stubenitsky, A.B. Petrov, G.W. van Wieringen, E. van der Voort, V, J. Hess, et al. **1999**, Cardiovascular aspects of experimental meningococcal sepsis in young and older awake

piglets: age-related differences, *Shock* 12, 145–154.
109 Mirlashari, M.R., E.A. Høiby, J. Holst, T. Lyberg. **2001**, Outer membrane vesicles from Neisseria meningitidis: effects on tissue factor and plasminogen activator inhibitor-2 production in human monocytes, *Thromb. Res.* 102, 375–380.
110 Mirlashari, M.R., E.A. Høiby, J. Holst, T. Lyberg. **2001**, Outer membrane vesicles from Neisseria meningitidis: effects on cytokine production in human whole blood, *Cytokine* 13, 91–97.
111 Mirlashari, M.R., E.A. Høiby, J. Holst, T. Lyberg. **2002**, Outer membrane vesicles from Neisseria meningitidis, *APMIS* 110, 193–204.
112 Mirlashari, M.R., I.A. Hagberg, T. Lyberg. **2002**, Platelet-platelet and platelet-leukocyte interactions induced by outer membrane vesicles from N. meningitidis, *Platelets* 13, 91–99.
113 Steeghs, L., H. de Cock, E. Evers, B. Zomer, J. Tommassen, P. van der Ley. **2001**, Outer membrane composition of a lipopolysaccharide-deficient Neisseria meningitidis mutant, *EMBO J.* 20, 6937–6945.
114 van der Ley, P., L. Steeghs. **2003**, Lessons from an LPS-deficient Neisseria meningitidis mutant, *J. Endotoxin. Res.* 9, 124–128.
115 Dixon, G.L., R.S. Heyderman, P. van der Ley, N.J. Klein. **2004**, High-level endothelial E-selectin (CD62E) cell adhesion molecule expression by a lipopolysaccharide-deficient strain of Neisseria meningitidis despite poor activation of NF-kappaB transcription factor, *Clin. Exp. Immunol.* 135, 85–93.
116 Gorter, A.D., J. Oostrik, P. van der Ley, P.S. Hiemstra, J. Dankert, L. van Alphen **2003**, Involvement of lipooligosaccharides of Haemophilus influenzae and Neisseria meningitidis in defensin-enhanced bacterial adherence to epithelial cells, *Microb. Pathog.* 34, 121–130.
117 Albiger, B., L. Johansson, A.B. Jonsson. **2003**, Lipooligosaccharide-deficient Neisseria meningitidis shows altered pilus-associated characteristics, *Infect. Immun.* 71, 155–162.
118 Hazelzet, J.A., R.F. Kornelisse, van der Pouw Kraan TC, K.F. Joosten, E. van der Voort, G. van Mierlo, et al. **1997**, Interleukin 12 levels during the initial phase of septic shock with purpura in children: relation to severity of disease, *Cytokine* 9, 711–716.
119 Bjerre, A., B. Brusletto, T.E. Mollnes, E. Fritzsonn, E. Rosenqvist, E. Wedege, et al. **2002**, Complement activation induced by purified Neisseria meningitidis lipopolysaccharide (LPS), outer membrane vesicles, whole bacteria, and an LPS-free mutant, *J. Infect. Dis.* 185, 220–228.
120 Sprong, T., P. Brandtzaeg, M. Fung, A.M. Pharo, E.A. Høiby, T.E. Michaelsen, et al. **2003**, Inhibition of C5a-induced inflammation with preserved C5b-9-mediated bactericidal activity in a human whole blood model of meningococcal sepsis, *Blood* 102, 3702–3710.
121 Sprong, T., A.S. Møller, A. Bjerre, E. Wedege, P. Kierulf, J.W. van der Meer, et al. **2004**, Complement activation and complement-dependent inflammation by Neisseria meningitidis are independent of lipopolysaccharide, *Infect. Immun.* 72, 3344–3349.
122 Harris, H.W., J.E. Gosnell, Z.L. Kumwenda. **2000**, The lipemia of sepsis: triglyceride-rich lipoproteins as agents of innate immunity, *J. Endotoxin. Res.* 6, 421–430.
123 Sprong, T., M.G. Netea, P. van der Ley, T.J. Verver-Jansen, L.E. Jacobs, A. Stalenhoef, et al. **2004**, Human lipoproteins have divergent neutralizing effects on E. coli LPS, N. meningitidis LPS, and complete Gram-negative bacteria, *J. Lipid Res.* 45, 742–749.
124 Waage, A., A. Halstensen, T. Espevik. **1987**, Association between tumour necrosis factor in serum and fatal outcome in patients with meningococcal disease, *Lancet* 1, 355–357.
125 Hackett, S.J., A.P. Thomson, C.A. Hart. **2001**, Cytokines, chemokines and other effector molecules involved in meningococcal disease, *J. Med. Microbiol.* 50, 847–859.

126 Yoshioka, M., T. Ito, S. Miyazaki, Y. Nakajima. **1998**, The release of tumor necrosis factor-alpha, interleukin-1, interleukin-6 and prostaglandin E2 in bovine Kupffer cells stimulated with bacterial lipopolysaccharide, *Vet. Immunol. Immunopathol.* 66, 301–307.

127 Øverland, G., S. Morath, A. Yndestad, T. Hartung, C. Thiemermann, S. J. Foster, et al. **2003**, Lipoteichoic acid is a potent inducer of cytokine production in rat and human Kupffer cells in vitro, *Surg. Infect.* 4, 181–191.

128 Fong, Y. M., M. A. Marano, L. L. Moldawer, H. Wei, S. E. Calvano, J. S. Kenney, et al. **1990**, The acute splanchnic and peripheral tissue metabolic response to endotoxin in humans, *J. Clin. Invest.* 85, 1896–1904.

129 Krishnaswamy, G., J. Kelley, L. Yerra, J. K. Smith, D. S. Chi. **1999**, Human endothelium as a source of multifunctional cytokines: molecular regulation and possible role in human disease, *J. Interferon Cytokine Res.* 19, 91–104.

130 Kofler, S., T. Nickel, M. Weis. **2005**, Role of cytokines in cardiovascular diseases: a focus on endothelial responses to inflammation, *Clin. Sci.* 108, 205–213.

131 Xing, L., D. G. Remick. **2003**, Relative cytokine and cytokine inhibitor production by mononuclear cells and neutrophils, *Shock* 20, 10–16.

132 Suffredini, A. F., R. E. Fromm, M. M. Parker, M. Brenner, J. A. Kovacs, R. A. Wesley, et al. **1989**, The cardiovascular response of normal humans to the administration of endotoxin, *N. Engl. J. Med.* 321, 280–287.

133 Krishnagopalan, S., A. Kumar, J. E. Parrillo, A. Kumar. **2002**, Myocardial dysfunction in the patient with sepsis, *Curr. Opin. Crit. Care* 8, 376–388.

134 Mercier, J. C., F. Beaufils, J. F. Hartmann, D. Azema. **1988**, Hemodynamic patterns of meningococcal shock in children, *Crit. Care Med.* 16, 27–33.

135 Brandtzaeg, P., T. E. Mollnes, P. Kierulf. **1989**, Complement activation and endotoxin levels in systemic meningococcal disease, *J. Infect. Dis.* 160, 58–65.

136 Wuillemin, W. A., K. Fijnvandraat, B. H. Derkx, M. Peters, W. Vreede, H. ten Cate, et al. **1995**, Activation of the intrinsic pathway of coagulation in children with meningococcal septic shock, *Thromb. Haemost.* 74, 1436–1441.

137 Hazelzet, J. A., R. de Groot, G. van Mierlo, K. F. Joosten, E. van der Voort, A. Eerenberg, et al. **1998**, Complement activation in relation to capillary leakage in children with septic shock and purpura, *Infect. Immun.* 66, 5350–5356.

138 Hardman, J. M. **1968**, Fatal meningococcal infections: the changing pathologic picture in the '60s, *Mil. Med.* 133, 951–964.

139 Thiru, Y., N. Pathan, S. Bignall, P. Habibi, M. Levin. **2000**, A myocardial cytotoxic process is involved in the cardiac dysfunction of meningococcal septic shock, *Crit. Care Med.* 28, 2979–2983.

140 Briassoulis, G., P. Kalabalikis, V. Thanopoulos, T. Hatzis. **2000**, Non-Q wave acute myocardial infarction in acute meningococcemia in a 10-year-old girl, *Pediatr. Emerg. Care* 16, 33–38.

141 Pathan, N., C. A. Hemingway, A. A. Alizadeh, A. C. Stephens, J. C. Boldrick, E. E. Oragui, et al. **2004**, Role of interleukin 6 in myocardial dysfunction of meningococcal septic shock, *Lancet* 363, 203–209.

142 Brandtzaeg, P., P. M. Sandset, G. B. Joø, R. Ovstebo, U. Abildgaard, P. Kierulf. **1989**, The quantitative association of plasma endotoxin, antithrombin, protein C, extrinsic pathway inhibitor and fibrinopeptide A in systemic meningococcal disease, *Thromb. Res.* 55, 459–470.

143 Hazelzet, J. A., I. M. Risseeuw-Appel, R. F. Kornelisse, W. C. Hop, I. Dekker, K. F. Joosten, et al. **1996**, Age-related differences in outcome and severity of DIC in children with septic shock and purpura, *Thromb. Haemost.* 76, 932–938.

144 Faust, S. N., M. Levin, O. B. Harrison, R. D. Goldin, M. S. Lockhart, S. Kondaveeti, et al. **2001**, Dysfunction of endothelial protein C activation in severe

meningococcal sepsis, *N. Engl. J Med.* 345, 408–416.
145 Klein, N.J., G.I. Shennan, R.S. Heyderman, M. Levin. **1992**, Alteration in glycosaminoglycan metabolism and surface charge on human umbilical vein endothelial cells induced by cytokines, endotoxin and neutrophils, *J. Cell Sci.* 102, 821–832.
146 Heyderman, R.S., N.J. Klein, O.A. Daramola, S. Hammerschmidt, M. Frosch, B.D. Robertson, et al. **1997**, Induction of human endothelial tissue factor expression by Neisseria meningitidis: the influence of bacterial killing and adherence to the endothelium, *Microb. Pathog.* 22, 265–274.
147 Harrison, O.B., B.D. Robertson, S.N. Faust, M.A. Jepson, R.D. Goldin, M. Levin, et al. **2002**, Analysis of pathogen–host cell interactions in purpura fulminans: expression of capsule, type IV pili, and PorA by Neisseria meningitidis in vivo, *Infect. Immun.* 70, 5193–5201.
148 De Vriese, A.S., M. Bourgeois. **2003**, Pharmacologic treatment of acute renal failure in sepsis. *Curr. Opin. Crit. Care* 9, 474–480.
149 Lameire, N., W. Van Biesen, R. Vanholder. **2005**, Acute renal failure, *Lancet* 365, 417–430.
150 Ferguson, J.H., et al. **1948**, Fulminating meningococcic infections and the so-called Waterhouse-Friderichsen syndrome, *Am. J. Pathol.* 24, 763–795.
151 Guarner, J., P.W. Greer, A. Whitney, W.J. Shieh, M. Fischer, E.H. White, et al. **2004**, Pathogenesis and diagnosis of human meningococcal disease using immunohistochemical and PCR assays, *Am. J. Clin Pathol.* 122, 754–764.
152 de Kleijn, E.D., K.F. Joosten, B. van Rijn, M. Westerterp, R. de Groot, A.C. Hokken-Koelega, et al. **2002**, Low serum cortisol in combination with high adrenocorticotrophic hormone concentrations are associated with poor outcome in children with severe meningococcal disease, *Pediatr. Infect. Dis. J.* 21, 330–336.
153 de Groof. F., K.F. Joosten, J.A. Janssen, E.D. de Kleijn, J.A. Hazelzet, W.C. Hop, et al. **2002**, Acute stress response in children with meningococcal sepsis: important differences in the growth hormone/insulin-like growth factor I axis between nonsurvivors and survivors, *J. Clin. Endocrinol. Metab.* 87, 3118–3124.
154 Joosten, K.F., E.D. de Kleijn, M. Westerterp, M. de Hoog, F.C. Eijck, W.C.J. Hop, et al. **2000**, Endocrine and metabolic responses in children with meningoccocal sepsis: striking differences between survivors and nonsurvivors, *J. Clin. Endocrinol. Metab.* 85, 3746–3753.
155 Ramesh, V., A. Mukherjee, M. Chandra, S.K. Sehgal, U. Saxena, A.K. Jain, et al. **1990**, Clinical, histopathologic & immunologic features of cutaneous lesions in acute meningococcaemia, *Indian J. Med. Res.* 91, 27–32.
156 van Deuren, M., C. Neeleman, K.J. Assmann, J.F. Wetzels, J.W. van der Meer. **1998**, Rhabdomyolysis during the subacute stage of meningococcal sepsis, *Clin Infect. Dis.* 26, 214–215.
157 Shappell, K.K., K.M. Gehrs, R.V. Keech, T.C. Cannon, R. Folberg. **1999**, Meningococcemia with vitreous opacities: endophthalmitis or vitreous hemorrhage? *Arch. Ophthalmol.* 117, 268–269.
158 Britto, J., S. Nadel, P. Habibi, M. Levin. **1995**, Gastrointestinal perforation complicating meningococcal disease, *Pediatr. Infect. Dis. J.* 14, 393–394.
159 Østerud, B., T. Flaegstad. **1983**, Increased tissue thromboplastin activity in monocytes of patients with meningococcal infection: related to an unfavourable prognosis, *Thromb. Haemost.* 49, 5–7.
160 Nieuwland, R., R.J. Berckmans, S. McGregor, A.N. Boing, F.P. Romijn, R.G. Westendorp, et al. **2000**, Cellular origin and procoagulant properties of microparticles in meningococcal sepsis, *Blood* 95, 930–935.
161 Drake, T.A., J. Cheng, A. Chang, F.B. Taylor. **1993**, Expression of tissue factor, thrombomodulin, and E-selectin in baboons with lethal Escherichia coli sepsis, *Am. J. Pathol.* 142, 1458–1470.

162 Oragui, E.E., S. Nadel, P. Kyd, M. Levin. **2000**, Increased excretion of urinary glycosaminoglycans in meningococcal septicemia and their relationship to proteinuria, *Crit. Care Med.* 28, 3002–3008.

163 Kornelisse, R.F., J.A. Hazelzet, H.F. Savelkoul, W.C. Hop, M.H. Suur, A.N. Borsboom, et al. **1996**, The relationship between plasminogen activator inhibitor-1 and proinflammatory and counterinflammatory mediators in children with meningococcal septic shock, *J. Infect. Dis.* 173, 1148–1156.

164 Franco, R.F., E. de Jonge, P.E. Dekkers, J.J. Timmerman, C.A. Spek, S.J. van Deventer, et al. **2000**, The in vivo kinetics of tissue factor messenger RNA expression during human endotoxemia: relationship with activation of coagulation, *Blood* 96, 554–559.

165 Eilertsen, K.E., B. Østerud. **2004**, Tissue factor: (patho)physiology and cellular biology, *Blood Coagul. Fibrinolysis* 15, 521–538.

166 Schlichting, E., T. Lyberg, O. Solberg, B.M. Andersen. **1993**, Endotoxin liberation from Neisseria meningitidis correlates to their ability to induce procoagulant and fibrinolytic factors in human monocytes, *Scand. J Infect. Dis.* 25, 585–594.

167 Taylor, F.B., A. Chang, W. Ruf, J.H. Morrissey, L. Hinshaw, R. Catlett, et al. **1991**, Lethal E. coli septic shock is prevented by blocking tissue factor with monoclonal antibody, *Circ. Shock* 33, 127–134.

168 Biemond, B.J., M. Levi, H. ten Cate, H.R. Soule, L.D. Morris, D.L. Foster, et al. **1995**, Complete inhibition of endotoxin-induced coagulation activation in chimpanzees with a monoclonal Fab fragment against factor VII/VIIa, *Thromb. Haemost.* 73, 223–230.

169 Powars, D.R., Z.R. Rogers, M.J. Patch, W.G. McGehee, R.B. Francis. **1987**, Purpura fulminans in meningococcemia: association with acquired deficiencies of proteins C and S, *N. Engl. J Med.* 317, 571–572.

170 Fijnvandraat, K., B. Derkx, M. Peters, R. Bijlmer, A. Sturk, M.H. Prins, et al. **1995**, Coagulation activation and tissue necrosis in meningococcal septic shock: severely reduced protein C levels predict a high mortality, *Thromb. Haemost.* 73, 15–20.

171 de Kleijn, E.D., R. de Groot, C.E. Hack, P.G. Mulder, W. Engl, B. Moritz, et al. **2003**, Activation of protein C following infusion of protein C concentrate in children with severe meningococcal sepsis and purpura fulminans: a randomized, double-blinded, placebo-controlled, dose-finding study, *Crit. Care Med.* 31, 1839–1847.

172 Iversen, N., P. Brandtzaeg, P.M. Sandset, P. Kierulf, U. Abildgaard. **2002**, TFPI fractions in plasma from patients with systemic meningococcal disease, *Thromb. Res.* 108, 347–353.

173 Suffredini, A.F., P.C. Harpel, J.E. Parrillo. **1989**, Promotion and subsequent inhibition of plasminogen activation after administration of intravenous endotoxin to normal subjects, *N. Engl. J. Med.* 320, 1165–1172.

174 Westendorp, R.G., J.J. Hottenga, P.E. Slagboom. **1999**, Variation in plasminogen-activator-inhibitor-1 gene and risk of meningococcal septic shock, *Lancet* 354, 561–563.

175 Hermans, P.W., M.L. Hibberd, R. Booy, O. Daramola, J.A. Hazelzet, R. de Groot, et al. **1999**, 4G/5G promoter polymorphism in the plasminogen-activator-inhibitor-1 gene and outcome of meningococcal disease, Meningococcal Research Group, *Lancet* 354, 556–560.

176 Hangen, D.H., J.H. Stevens, P.S. Satoh, E.W. Hall, P.T. O'Hanley, T.A. Raffin. **1989**, Complement levels in septic primates treated with anti-C5a antibodies, *J. Surg. Res.* 46, 195–199.

177 Hogasen, K., T.E. Mollnes, P. Brandtzaeg. **1994**, Low levels of vitronectin and clusterin in acute meningococcal disease are closely associated with formation of the terminal-complement complex and the vitronectin-thrombin-antithrombin complex, *Infect. Immun.* 62, 4874–4880.

178 Ward, P.A. **2004**, The dark side of C5a in sepsis, *Nat. Rev. Immunol.* 4, 133–142.

179 Brandtzaeg P, P. Kierulf. **1992**, Endotoxin and meningococcemia, Intravascular inflammation induced by native endotoxin in man, in *Bacterial Endotoxic Lipopolysaccharides (Immunopharmacology and Pathophysiology*, vol. 2), eds. Ryan J.L., Morrison, M.D., CRC Press, Boca Raton, p. 327–346.

180 Brandtzaeg, P., K. Hogasen, P. Kierulf, T.E. Mollnes. **1996**, The excessive complement activation in fulminant meningococcal septicemia is predominantly caused by alternative pathway activation, *J. Infect. Dis.* 173, 647–655.

181 Hibberd, M.L., M. Sumiya, J.A. Summerfield, R. Booy, M. Levin. **1999**, Association of variants of the gene for mannose-binding lectin with susceptibility to meningococcal disease, Meningococcal Research Group, *Lancet* 353, 1049–1053.

182 Drogari-Apiranthitou, M., C.A. Fijen, S. Thiel, A. Platonov, L. Jensen, J. Dankert, et al. **1997**, The effect of mannan-binding lectin on opsonophagocytosis of Neisseria meningitidis, *Immunopharmacology* 38, 93–99.

183 Jack, D.L., A.W. Dodds, N. Anwar, C.A. Ison, A. Law, M. Frosch, et al. **1998**, Activation of complement by mannose-binding lectin on isogenic mutants of Neisseria meningitidis serogroup B, *J. Immunol.* 160, 1346–1353.

184 Jack, D.L., M.E. Lee, M.W. Turner, N.J. Klein, R.C. Read. **2005**, Mannose-binding lectin enhances phagocytosis and killing of Neisseria meningitidis by human macrophages, *J. Leukoc. Biol.* 77, 328–336.

185 Estabrook, M.M., D.L. Jack, N.J. Klein, G.A. Jarvis. **2004**, Mannose-binding lectin binds to two major outer membrane proteins, opacity protein and porin, of Neisseria meningitidis, *J. Immunol.* 172, 3784–3792.

186 Kuipers, S., P.C. Aerts, H. van Dijk. **2003**, Differential microorganism-induced mannose-binding lectin activation, *FEMS Immunol. Med. Microbiol.* 36, 33–39.

187 Jack, D.L., R.C. Read, A.J. Tenner, M. Frosch, M.W. Turner, N.J. Klein. **2001**, Mannose-binding lectin regulates the inflammatory response of human professional phagocytes to Neisseria meningitidis serogroup B, *J. Infect. Dis.* 184, 1152–1162.

188 Sprong, T., D.L. Jack, N.J. Klein, M.W. Turner, P. van der Ley, L. Steeghs, et al. **2004**, Mannose binding lectin enhances IL-1beta and IL-10 induction by non-lipopolysaccharide (LPS) components of Neisseria meningitidis, *Cytokine* 28, 59–66.

189 Boyum, A., V.A. Tennfjord, C. Gran, D. Lovhaug, O. Øktedalen, P. Brandtzaeg. **2000**, Bioactive cytidine deaminase, an inhibitor of granulocyte-macrophage colony-forming cells, is massively released in fulminant meningococcal sepsis, *J. Infect. Dis.* 182, 1784–1787.

190 Pron, B., M.K. Taha, C. Rambaud, J.C. Fournet, N. Pattey, J.P. Monnet, et al. **1997**, Interaction of Neisseria meningitidis with the components of the blood–brain barrier correlates with an increased expression of PilC, *J. Infect. Dis.* 176, 1285–1292.

191 Waage, A., A. Halstensen, R. Shalaby, P. Brandtzaeg, P. Kierulf, T. Espevik. **1989**, Local production of tumor necrosis factor alpha, interleukin 1, and interleukin 6 in meningococcal meningitis. Relation to the inflammatory response, *J. Exp. Med.* 170, 1859–1867.

192 Halstensen, A., M. Ceska, P. Brandtzaeg, H. Redl, A. Naess, A. Waage. **1993**, Interleukin-8 in serum and cerebrospinal fluid from patients with meningococcal disease, *J. Infect. Dis.* 167, 471–475.

193 Spanaus, K.S., D. Nadal, H.W. Pfister, J. Seebach, U. Widmer, K. Frei, et al. **1997**, C-X-C and C-C chemokines are expressed in the cerebrospinal fluid in bacterial meningitis and mediate chemotactic activity on peripheral blood-derived polymorphonuclear and mononuclear cells in vitro, *J. Immunol.* 158, 1956–1964.

194 Christodoulides, M., B.L. Makepeace, K.A. Partridge, D. Kaur, M.I. Fowler,

R. O. Weller, et al. **2002**, Interaction of Neisseria meningitidis with human meningeal cells induces the secretion of a distinct group of chemotactic, proinflammatory, and growth-factor cytokines, *Infect. Immun.* 70, 4035–4044.

195 Humphries, H. E., M. Triantafilou, B. L. Makepeace, J. E. Heckels, K. Triantafilou, M. Christodoulides. **2005**, Activation of human meningeal cells is modulated by lipopolysaccharide (LPS) and non-LPS components of Neisseria meningitidis and is independent of Toll-like receptor (TLR)4 and TLR2 signalling, *Cell Microbiol.* 7, 415–430.

196 Amiry-Moghaddam, M., O.P. Ottersen. **2003**, The molecular basis of water transport in the brain, *Nat. Rev. Neurosci.* 4, 991–1001.

197 Kristiansen, B. E., B. Sørensen, T. Simonsen, O. Spanne, V. Lund, B. Bjorvatn. **1984**, Isolates of Neisseria meningitidis from different sites in the same patient: phenotypic and genomic studies, with special reference to adherence, piliation, and DNA restriction endonuclease pattern, *J Infect. Dis.* 150, 389–396.

22
Course of Disease and Clinical Management

Andrew J. Pollard and Simon Nadel

22.1
Introduction

Since the first described meningococcal epidemic in Geneva in the Spring of 1805 [1], physicians on all continents have been faced with the devastating effects of invasive disease caused by this organism. The clinical features of an individual case of severe meningococcal septicemia are profound and shocking, but the true horror of meningococcal disease was experienced in the 19th century, long before antibiotics and intensive care units, as epidemics swept across Europe and North America, destroying families and communities [2].

Outbreaks and epidemics of meningococcal disease have been the usual epidemiological pattern until the past few decades and, even today, large epidemics in sub-Saharan Africa are associated with poor social circumstances, population movements during conflict and crowding [3–6]. In 2005, the experience of most clinicians in developed countries is of endemic meningococcal disease, consisting of occasional and sporadic cases. Improving the delivery of early medical care to these individuals is a surprisingly difficult task [7] but can have a profound impact on outcome [8, 9].

22.2
Disease Burden

Globally, infectious diseases account for 54% of the 10.6 million deaths in children each year [10]. However, meningococcal infection accounts for only about 50 000 of these deaths, with a global annual burden of disease of about 0.5 million cases [11]. By contrast, over 1.0 million deaths annually have been attributed to disease caused by *Streptococcus pneumoniae* [12].

Although in some industrialized nations the media have generated the perception of a high burden of meningococcal infection and mortality among children, the disease remains rare in this setting. In children under the age of 2 years in the

Handbook of Meningococcal Disease. Infection Biology, Vaccination, Clinical Management.
Edited by M. Frosch and M.C.J. Maiden

ISBN: 3-527-31260-9

United States, there are up to ten cases of meningococcal infection per 100 000 population [13, 14], a far lower rate of infection than that caused by a single serotype of *S. pneumoniae* prior to the introduction of a pneumococcal vaccine prevention programme (invasive disease rates ranging over 10–45 per 100 000 population) [14, 15].

The incidence of meningococcal disease varies considerably in different countries and in the same country at different times. Over the past several decades, rates of meningococcal disease in the United States have remained relatively stable, with an annual incidence of 0.9–1.5 cases per 100 000 population [13, 16], but disease rates may exceed 200 cases per 100 000 population in sub-Saharan Africa during an epidemic [4]. In Europe, during the mid 1990s, the overall annual incidence of meningococcal disease was estimated at about 1.3–1.7 cases per 100 000 population [17], with rates reported at 0.3 cases per 100 000 in Italy, 0.6 cases per 100 000 in France and 3.6 cases per 100 000 in England and Wales [17].

Although population rates of disease in industrialized countries are low, the age-dependent rates indicate a much higher burden of disease in early life. Children suffer the highest rates of invasive meningococcal disease, although infants under 6 months of age do appear to have some protection, presumably from persisting maternal antibodies [18]. There is a peak in cases at 6–24 months of age, with a steady decline in incidence with age until the teenage years, when there is a further increase in disease rates [13, 17]. During epidemics, the age-dependent incidence may change with more older children developing disease, probably due to lack of preexisting immunity to the epidemic clone [19, 20]. Despite the low overall burden of disease caused by meningococcal infection, mortality amongst cases remains as high as 10%. Thus, in countries with very low all-cause mortality in childhood, meningococcal infection is one of the leading infectious causes of death in children.

22.3
Susceptibility to Infection and Severity of Disease

Risk factors for meningococcal disease include young age [13, 21], winter or dry season [22], close contact with a carrier or case [23], overcrowding [24, 25], moving into new communities [26, 27], active or passive smoking [28, 29] and exposure to respiratory infection [24, 30].

Whilst many individuals are exposed to meningocococi, very few suffer disease; and the severity varies considerably amongst those in whom bacteremia occurs. These observations suggest that host genetic factors may exist which relate to susceptibility to infection or severity of disease. In support of the importance of host factors, complement deficiency [31, 32], hypogammaglobulinemia [33] and hyposplenism [34] all predispose to invasive meningococcal disease. These observations have led to extensive investigation directed at identifying genetic associations in meningococcal disease.

Table 22.1 Genetic polymorphisms associated with meningococcal infection. LBP and BPI polymorphisms have not been analyzed in meningococcal infection, only in sepsis, without further specification. Su = effect on susceptibility, Se = effect on severity, Ou = effect on outcome – relative risk (RR) for death given. NA = not available. MD = meningococcal disease. OR = odds ratio – any number >1 indicates more severe disease to be associated with the rare allele, unless stated otherwise. Reprinted from [35] with permission from Elsevier.

Pathway	Gene	Polymorphism	Su/Se/Ou	Odds ratio (OR)	Ref.	Comments
Innate immunity						
	TLR4	Asp299Gly	Su	No association	170	
			Su	OR 1.14 (0.86–1.52)	171	
			Se	OR 1.55 (0.70–3.44)		
		Rare polymorphisms combined	Su	OR 27	170	
	TLR2	P631H	Su	No association	170	
		R753Q	Su	No association	170	
		Multiple SNPs (no aa change)	Su	No association	170	
	LBP	Cys98Gly	Su	Only in male patients	172	No MD, sepsis in general
			Ou	Trend (low patient numbers)		
		Pro436Leu	Su	No association	172	No MD, sepsis in general
			Ou	Trend (low patient numbers)		
	BPI	A645G	Su	No association	172	No MD, sepsis in general
		G545C	Su	No association	172	No MD, sepsis in general
		*Pst*I in intron 5	Su	No association	172	No MD, sepsis in general
	ACE	284-bp insertion/dele tion	Se	>in DD	173	
			Ou	14% >risk of mortality		
	MBL[a)]	Codon 52 (Arg/Cys)	Su	OR 6.5 (2.0–27.2; homozygous)	174	
		Codon 54 (Gly/Asp)	Se	OR 4.5 (0.9–29.1; homozygous)		
		Codon 57 (Gly/Glu)		OR 1.7 (1.1–2.6; heterozygous)		
				OR 2.2 (1.1–4.3; heterozygous)		
				OR 2.0 (1.3–3.0; he+ho)		
				OR 2.4 (1.2–4.6; he+ho)		

Table 22.1 (continued)

Pathway	Gene	Polymorphism	Su/Se/Ou	Odds ratio (OR)	Ref.	Comments
				Trend to less severe disease	174	
	Properdin[b)]	C2061T (stop exon 4) type I	Su	RR 250	175	
		C2726T (stop exon 5) type I	Se	RR 4.7–15.0	175	
		C3041G (stop exon 6) type I	Ou	Increased mortality	175	
		C2124T (Arg/Trp) type II				
		G827A type II				
		Codon 387 (Tyr/Asp) type III				
	Factor D	Ser42 stop			176	Case report
	C3		Su	Increased		
	LCCD	Different defects	Su	Increased (57–71%)	175	
			Se	Decreased		
Acquired immunity						
	Fc RIIa	His131Arg	Se	His: sepsis Arg: meningitis	177	
			Su	No association	178	
			Se	Arg: OR 3.9 (1.0–16.0)	178	
			Su	OR 2.67 (1.09–6.53)	179	Only 25 survivors of MD studied
			Se	Arg: OR 14	180	LCCD patients
	Fc RIIIa	Val158Phe	Se	Val: meningitis	177	Relatives of patient
	Fc RIIIb	NA1/NA2 (codon 65 and 82)	Su	No association	179	
	Combination	RR-FF-NA2/2	Su	OR 2.6 (1.1–6.3)	177	Relatives of patient
		RR-NA2/2	Su	OR 13.9	181, 182	LCCD patients
			Su	No association	182	Properdin deficient individuals
Coagulation/fibrinolysis						
	tPA	Alu repeat insertion/deletion	Su	No association	183	
			Se	No association	183	
	PAI1	4G/5G insertion/deletion	Su	No association	184, 185	
			Ou	RR 4/4G 2.0 (1.0–3.8)	184, 185	
			Se	OR 4/4G 5.9 (1.9–18.0)	185	Relatives of patient

Table 22.1 (continued)

Pathway	Gene	Polymorphism	Su/Se/Ou	Odds ratio (OR)	Ref.	Comments
			Ou	No association	186	Relatives of patient
			Su	No association	186	
			Se	4/4G two-fold increase	186	Predicted mortality
			Se	R/R 4/4G 2.4	186	Vascular complications in survivors
			Ou	RR 2.7		In meningococcal sepsis patients
	Factor V	FV^L G1691A	Su	No association	187	
			Se	RR 3.1 (1.2–7.9; heterozygous)	187	
			Ou	No association	187	
Cytokines						
	TNFα	G-308A	Su	No association	188	No MD, sepsis in general
			Se	RR 1.6 (1.1–2.3)	188	
			Ou	RR 2.5 (1.1–5.7)	188	Relatives of patients
			Ou	No association	189	
			Ou	No association	190	
		G-238A	Ou	No association	189	Relatives of patients
	TNFβ	NcoI B1+, B2–	Ou	B2 increased mortality	191	No MD, sepsis in general
			Ou	OR 3.47	192	No MD, sepsis in general
	IL10	A-1082G	Su	Nonrandom distribution	177	In combination with Fc RIIa
	IL6	G-174C	Su	No association	193	
			Se	OR 3.06 (1.25–7.49) GG vs GC or CC	193	
			Ou	OR 2.64 (1.12–6.22) GG vs GC and CC	193	
			Su	No association	194	No MD, sepsis in general
			Se	No association OR 0.73 (0.32–1.71)	194	No MD, sepsis in general
			Ou	OR 0.11 (0.02–0.57) GG vs GC and CC	194	No MD, sepsis in general
		3-promoter polymorphisms	NA			
	IL1RN	86-bp repeat in intron 2/A2 or T2018C	Su (A2)	No association	195	

Table 22.1 (continued)

Pathway	Gene	Polymorphism	Su/Se/Ou	Odds ratio (OR)	Ref.	Comments
			Se	No association OR 1.0 (0.69–1.47)	195	
			Ou	No association OR 1.01 (0.49–2.09) Increased in A2	195	
			Su	No association	192	No MD, sepsis in general
			Ou		192	No MD, sepsis in general
	IL1B	C–511T	Ou	1/1 vs 1/2 OR 3.39 (1.39–8.29) 2/2 vs 1/2 OR 7.35 (2.51–21.45)	190	
			Su	No association	196	
			Survival	OR 2.05 (1.1–3.79) in model	196	
	IL1B and ILRN	–511 C/T+2018T	Survival	OR 7.78 (1.05–59.05)	190	
		–511 C or C/T+2018C or C/T	Survival	OR 0.61 (0.38–0.99)	196	

a) MBL variants were combined because of the effect of compound heterozygous individuals. Homozygous (ho): variant allele at two MBL loci. Heterozygous (he): a variant allele at one position and the common allele for both other loci.
b) Effects of properdin deficiencies are combined for all variants.

Invasion of *N. meningitidis* through the nasopharyngeal mucosa into the blood stream triggers a cascade of mediators in an inflammatory process that is mediated by endotoxin (lipopolysaccharide). A wide variety of genes are involved in these responses and various polymorphisms have been associated with susceptibility to meningococcal infection or severity of disease (see Table 22.1) [35].

22.4 Carriage

Asymptomatic nasopharyngeal carriage of *N. meningitidis* is universal. About 10% of the population carry meningococci in the upper respiratory tract at any point in time, with much higher rates amongst teenagers and young adults [36, 37]. By contrast, less than 1% of children under 4 years of age are colonized with *N. meningitidis* [38]. The duration of colonization after infection is variable and probably dependent on the host and bacterial genotype [39].

The cause of progression from carriage to invasive disease is unclear but probably depends on characteristics of both the host and the infecting organism. Disease usually occurs less than 10 days after colonization with a pathogenic strain in a susceptible individual but carriage prior to disease may be longer in some instances [40].

22.5 Presentation and Clinical Features

Meningococcal disease usually presents with fever and features of meningitis and/or septicemia and a characteristic nonblanching rash [41] with a wide variation in severity. Occult bacteremia with *N. meningitidis* may occur [42]. Thirty to fifty percent of cases have meningitis alone (mortality 5%), 7–10% have features of septicemia alone (mortality 5–40%) and 40% present a mixed picture of meningitis with septicemia [43, 44]. In the United Kingdom, there is some evidence that mortality rates have fallen over the past 15 years and, in specialist intensive care units, mortality in the most severe cases was less than 5% [8]. Mortality is highest in those with a rapidly progressive purpuric rash, absence of meningism, coma, temperature ≤38 °C, hypotension (mean arterial blood pressure ≤2SD below mean for age), low white cell count in peripheral blood ($\leq 10 \times 10^9\,l^{-1}$), low platelet count ($\leq 100 \times 10^9\,l^{-1}$) and young age [45].

In patients with meningococcal meningitis, the following symptoms predominate: headache, fever, vomiting, photophobia, neck stiffness, positive Kernig's sign and lethargy. Twenty percent may have seizures. In younger children, misery may be the dominant clinical feature and in infants, poor feeding, irritability, a high pitched cry and a bulging fontanelle are typical findings.

Patients with meningococcemia (meningococcal septicemia) may present with fever, rash, headache, flu-like symptoms (especially myalgia), vomiting and abdominal pain. Clinical signs of shock including tachycardia, poor peripheral perfusion, tachypnea, oliguria, confusion and finally hypotension may be present.

Rarely, invasive disease may take the form of arthritis, pneumonia, conjunctivitis, pericarditis or endophthalmitis [13, 46–48].

22.5.1 Rash

Eighty percent of bacteriologically proven cases of meningococcal disease develop purpura or petechiae, indicating that the disease should be considered in any individual who presents with fever and a nonblanching rash [41]. Unfortunately, some cases present with either a maculopapular rash (13%) or no rash (7%) and their initial presentation is indistinguishable from nonspecific viral illnesses. Despite the nonspecific presentation, some children without the characteristic rash will develop severe disease. In addition to the characteristic rash, features of meningitis or septicemia may be present in many cases [43, 49, 50].

Whilst the presentation of a fulminant case of meningococcal disease leaves no doubt about the clinical diagnosis, many children present for medical attention with petechiae that cannot be attributed to invasive meniongococcal disease. Most children with fever and petechiae have viral illnesses, but 2–11% of children in various studies had meningococcal infection [51–53]. In most studies, enterovirus infections account for the majority of cases of petechiae in children with fever. The differential diagnoses for petechiae or purpura are wide but include coagulation disorders (notably protein C or S deficiency), platelet disorders (idiopathic thrombocytopaenic purpura, drug effects, bone marrow infiltration, etc.), Henoch Schonlein purpura, connective tissue disorders, trauma (including nonaccidental injury in children), viral infections (enteroviruses, influenza and other respiratory viruses, parvovirus, Epstein Barr virus, cytomegalovirus, measles, etc.) and bacterial sepsis (streptococcal, staphylococcal or Gram-negative sepsis).

A large survey of deaths from meningococcal disease in the UK has starkly demonstrated that suboptimal health care delivery significantly reduces the likelihood of survival in children with meningococcal disease [7]. In particular, children with this disease should be managed by an experienced pediatrician. Meningococcal disease may progress rapidly even after admission to hospital and commencement of appropriate treatment [54]; and all children admitted to hospital with suspected menignococal disease should be closely monitored for signs of deterioration.

The clinical imperative in initial management and monitoring in the hospital depends whether shock or raised intracranial pressure predominate. These two clinical problems are discussed in detail below but they may coexist in some cases, whilst others with mild disease have neither shock nor raised intracranial pressure.

22.5.2 Laboratory Features

The suspicion of meningococcal disease should be clinical and not reliant on laboratory investigations. Initial management should not be delayed whilst waiting for the results of laboratory investigations. Elevated white cell count and C reactive protein levels are common features of invasive bacterial diseases. However, these markers of an acute phase response may take 12–24 h to occur after onset of invasive meningococcal infection and are commonly at normal levels early in the course of the disease, especially in severe or rapidly progressive cases [55, 56]. In severe cases, biochemical and hematological derangements are common; and these are discussed below.

Although the diagnosis of meningococcal disease should rely on clinical suspicion, microbiological confirmation is important to guide public health management and exclude alternate causes. Cultures of blood, throat, CSF (in the absence of contraindications) and skin aspirates may provide useful microbiological confirmation and allow antibiotic sensitivity testing. Where meningococcal infection is confused with pneumococcal disease, which can have an identical presentation, antibiotic sensitivity testing is especially important to identify strains of pneumococci that are penicillin- or cephalosporin-resistant. Latex agglutination tests on blood, CSF or urine have been used as adjunctive diagnostic tests but have poor sensitivity and specificity [57]. In many countries, molecular diagnosis from samples of blood or CSF are now used to detect meningococcal DNA. This is particularly used for confirmation of diagnosis in patients in whom antibiotics have been preadministered [58–60].

Among children with suspected meningococcal disease in the UK, PCR is more sensitive than blood culture (47 vs 31%) and both were 100% specific [61]. A combination of both culture and PCR increases the proportion of laboratory-confirmed cases by 31–60% [60, 62–65].

Several different methods and bacterial gene targets for PCR diagnosis have been described. Insertion sequence (IS)*1106*, a novel meningococcal insertion sequence [66], detects meningococcal DNA in CSF and blood samples [63, 64, 67]. For both blood and CSF, sensitivity and specificity were greater than 90% for laboratory-confirmed cases [63, 64] but unfortunately this assay is no longer widely used since the insertion sequence is present in some other non-meningococcal bacteria, leading to false positive results [64, 68]. Another approach has been to use broad-range bacterial PCR, based on amplification of genes encoding 16S and/or 23S ribosomal RNA followed by either a further species-specific amplification or sequencing of the amplified product [69–74] with sensitivity and specificity of this method for meningococcal disease reported as >90% when applied to cerebrospinal fluid [71]. Reagent contamination has been a problem with use of this assay [65]. Several other gene targets have been selected for diagnostic PCR, including dihydropteroate [75] PorA (followed by sequencing to identify the subtype) [72, 76–78] and nspA [79].

An intial screening PCR for a conserved meningococcal gene followed by a serogroup-specific PCR to amplify the *siaD* gene when the first round is positive allows serogroup-specific diagnosis [60, 64, 65, 80, 81]. Real-time PCR for detection of the meningococcal capsular transferase gene, *ctrA*, in clinical specimens has greater than 90% sensitivity with optimized DNA extraction methods [64, 82] and specificity is 100% for B, C, Y and W135 meningococci. The nonsialic acid containing serogroups (A, X, 29E) are not detected [64] because of nucleotide variation at the 5′ end [83]. Taha developed a screening PCR based on a gene involved in adhesion to host cells, the *crgA* gene, and also found greater than 90% sensitivity and specificity in clinical specimens using a multiplex PCR that also determined serogroup [65]. DNA from serogroup A meningococci has been amplified using a specific PCR for an open reading frame, *orf-3*, [84], between the *ctrA* gene and the *galE* gene that is not found in other meningococci [85]. Taha similarly used *orf-2* as the target for amplification [65].

22.6 Lumbar Puncture

Lumbar puncture (LP) is a useful investigation for microbiological confirmation of meningococcal infection and exclusion of other causes of the clinical features. However, the procedure coincides with deterioration in some patients with meningococcal disease; and in patients with shock it may further compromise cardiovascular function [54, 86, 87]. The following are contraindications to LP: cardiorespiratory insufficiency, raised ICP (evidence of raised ICP includes: fluctuating or deteriorating level of consciousness, normal or high blood pressure in the presence of a slow or normal heart rate, unequal, dilated or poorly reacting pupils, focal neurological signs or abnormal posturing, seizures, papilledema) and coagulopathy [88–90]; and, in view of the rapid and unpredictable progression of the disease in some children, we have previously argued that LP should be avoided or deferred in the initial assessment of all patients with clinically obvious meningococcal disease because the additional information provided by LP adds little to the diagnosis [91]. Some authors have argued that microbiological confirmation is important, especially where an alternative etiology is possible [92, 93]. However, in the age of molecular diagnostics with a high pick-up rate, it is unlikely that LP will add any more to microbiological diagnosis.

Computed tomography (CT) brain imaging is frequently used in patients with meningococcal disease with a depressed conscious level and is particularly recommended in adult practice. However, cranial imaging is only rarely justified and it may be hazardous to take a critically ill patient to a radiology department before they have been adequately stabilized and monitored. Occasionally, the CT scan may be helpful in ruling out intracranial hemorrhage in patients where the diagnosis is unclear. Some clinicians may be comforted by a cranial CT scan to exclude the presence of cerebral edema or raised ICP prior to LP. However, clinically significant raised ICP or cerebral odema may not be evident on a CT scan; and the decision to perform a LP should be made on the clinical assessment [94, 95].

22.7 Cardiovascular Shock

Meningococcal septicemia may progress into cardiovascular shock (see Fig. 22.1). Shock results from a combination of hypovolemia caused by capillary leak syndrome, together with myocardial dysfunction, altered vasomotor tone and impaired cellular metabolism [96]. The increased vascular permeability results from endothelial injury causing leakage of water and plasma proteins from the intravascular compartment into the tissues. Plasma proteins are similarly lost into the urine, resulting in a urinary albumin loss equivalent to that found in nephrotic syndrome [97].

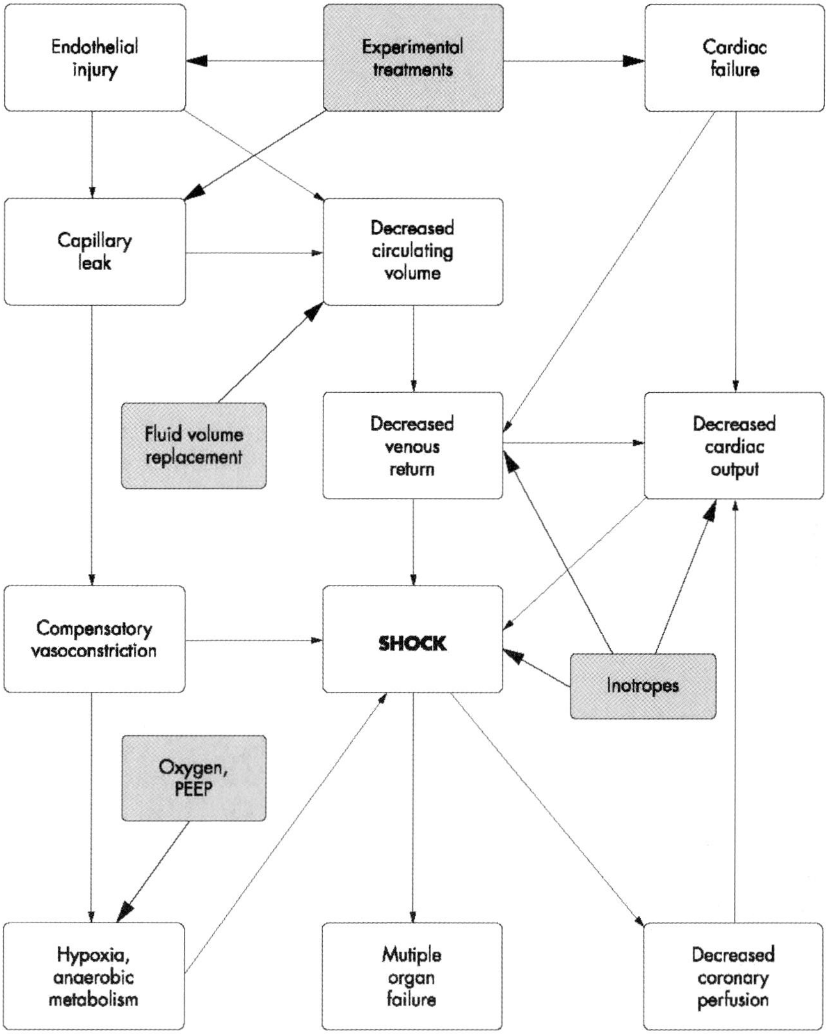

Fig. 22.1 Clinical mechanisms of shock and sites of action of treatment. Reproduced from [92] with permission from the BMJ Publishing Group.

In addition, depressed mental status occurs in patients with raised ICP, who may also have poor peripheral circulation due to altered brainstem function. This may be confusing, even to experienced medical practitioners. However, raised ICP also causes preservation of blood pressure and a normal or relatively slow heart rate for age, which are good signs to distinguish raised ICP from shock.

The clinical features of shock arise because perfusion of vital organs is maintained at the expense of peripheral perfusion and perfusion of nonvital organs.

In early shock, compensatory physiological processes including tachycardia, reduced renal perfusion and decreased skin perfusion maintain circulating volume and consequently cardiac output. Preservation of higher mental function may occur, despite hypotension, which may make observers underestimate the degree of cardiovascular collapse.

Children are able to compensate for the loss of up to 40% of their circulating volume without developing hypotension; and therefore children may have a normal blood pressure until the shock is advanced (compensated shock). Tachypnea reflects the development of tissue hypoxia and metabolic acidosis and, as shock progresses, hypoxia reflects decreased lung perfusion and developing pulmonary edema. Eventually, a decreased level of consciousness indicates loss of cerebral vascular homeostasis and reduced brain perfusion; and hypotension signifies failure of compensatory mechanisms. Although adults, and particularly the elderly, may present with hypotension as an early sign of shock, children who develop decompensated shock have a very high mortality rate [98].

Tachypnea indicates probable onset of pulmonary edema in compensated shock or decreased pulmonary perfusion in decompensated shock. Capillary leak continues during resuscitation; and worsening of tissue edema may occur as hypovolemia is corrected. This accounts for the alveolar edema that increases during resuscitation. Metabolic acidosis may result from poor tissue perfusion and further drive the increased ventilation for respiratory compensation.

The vasoconstriction that occurs as a compensatory mechanism in shock reduces blood flow to the skin, peripheries and some organs, especially the kidneys and gut. As a result, patients with meningococcal septicemia may present with very cool peripheries and prolonged capillary refill time, with sluggish or even absent blood flow to the skin and oliguria. In the most severe cases, ischemia of skin or even a whole limb may occur, particularly if accompanied by thrombosis in areas of vascular stasis. In addition, many patients develop acute renal dysfunction, often leading to acute renal failure.

Although this presentation of "cold shock" is more common in children, some children and adults present with meningococcal shock accompanied by vasodilatation, with warm peripheries and bounding pulses, but with hypotension (so-called "warm shock"). The mechanisms behind these differing responses to endotoxinemia are unknown.

Both procoagulant and anticoagulant pathways of hemostasis are dysregulated in meningococcal septicemia as a consequence of activation of the inflammatory and coagulation cascades and possibly by the loss of anticoagulant plasma proteins into the urine and tissue as a result of capillary permeability changes. Disseminated intravascular coagulation results in thrombocytopenia and both hemorrhage and thrombosis are seen in the skin (as purpura fulminans) [99]. It is likely that the disturbed coagulation seen in meningococcal sepsis arises as a result of the loss of anticoagulant proteins from the plasma (such as proteins C and S) and the failure of anticoagulant mechanisms on the surface of the endothelium. The endothelial receptors required for the activation of protein C (endothelial protein C receptor and thrombomodulin) have been shown to be downregulated on the endothelium of patients with meningococcal septicemia [100]. In addition to this, levels of circulating activated protein C and antithrombin 3 are reduced in patients with severe sepsis. The upregulation of coagulation induced by endotoxin in the plasma is therefore uninhibited. In addition, the normal fibrinolytic mechanisms are suppressed in sepsis, both by the reduced production of endothelial tissue plasminogen activator and by the production of an acute-phase protein (plasminogen activator inhibitor-1) and other fibrinolysis inhibitors. This results in intravascular clot formation, with suppression of the normal mechanisms to degrade intravascular thrombi, and the clinical syndrome of DIC and purpura fulminans.

Myocardial dysfunction arises as a result of a number of different pathological processes that are activated in septic shock [101]. Hypovolemia is probably the major stimulus to tachycardia, but metabolic derangements including hypoxia, acidosis, hypokalemia, hypocalcemia, hypophosphatemia, hypomagnesemia, hypoglycemia and disturbed fatty acid metabolism may also affect myocardial contractility. Bacterial products and inflammatory cytokines also directly suppress myocardial contractility [96, 101–104]. Poorly characterized myocardial depressant factors previously described in the plasma of septic patients were recently clarified in meningococcal plasma and were found to be largely the result of high levels of IL6 in meningococcal plasma [103].

Myocardial contractility improves with volume resuscitation and correction of metabolic derangements in many patients, but patients with persistent poor perfusion and hypotension (despite adequate volume resuscitation) require inotropic support to improve myocardial function. Most patients who survive do regain normal cardiac function during convalescence, despite evidence of myocardial cytotoxic injury in the acute phase of disease [105].

22.8 Initial Assessment and Management

The initial assessment of any individual with potentially critical illness follows the standard algorithms that are widely taught in acute life support training: (a) airway, (b) breathing, (c) circulation, (d) disability. Emergency life support should commence where indicated by this assessment. Unless consciousness is compromised, the airway is usually patent in meningococcal septicemia. Breathing may be compromised by pulmonary edema or oligemia and hypoxia may be present. Most deaths from meningococcal infection result from the consequences of endotoxin-mediated shock. After the standard a,b,c review, careful assessment for signs of shock and attention to management of hypovolemia are paramount.

Management priorities are dictated by the presence of shock or raised intracranial pressure and are discussed in detail below. An algorithm has been developed to assist direction of early management in both children (Fig. 22.2) and adults (Fig. 22.3).

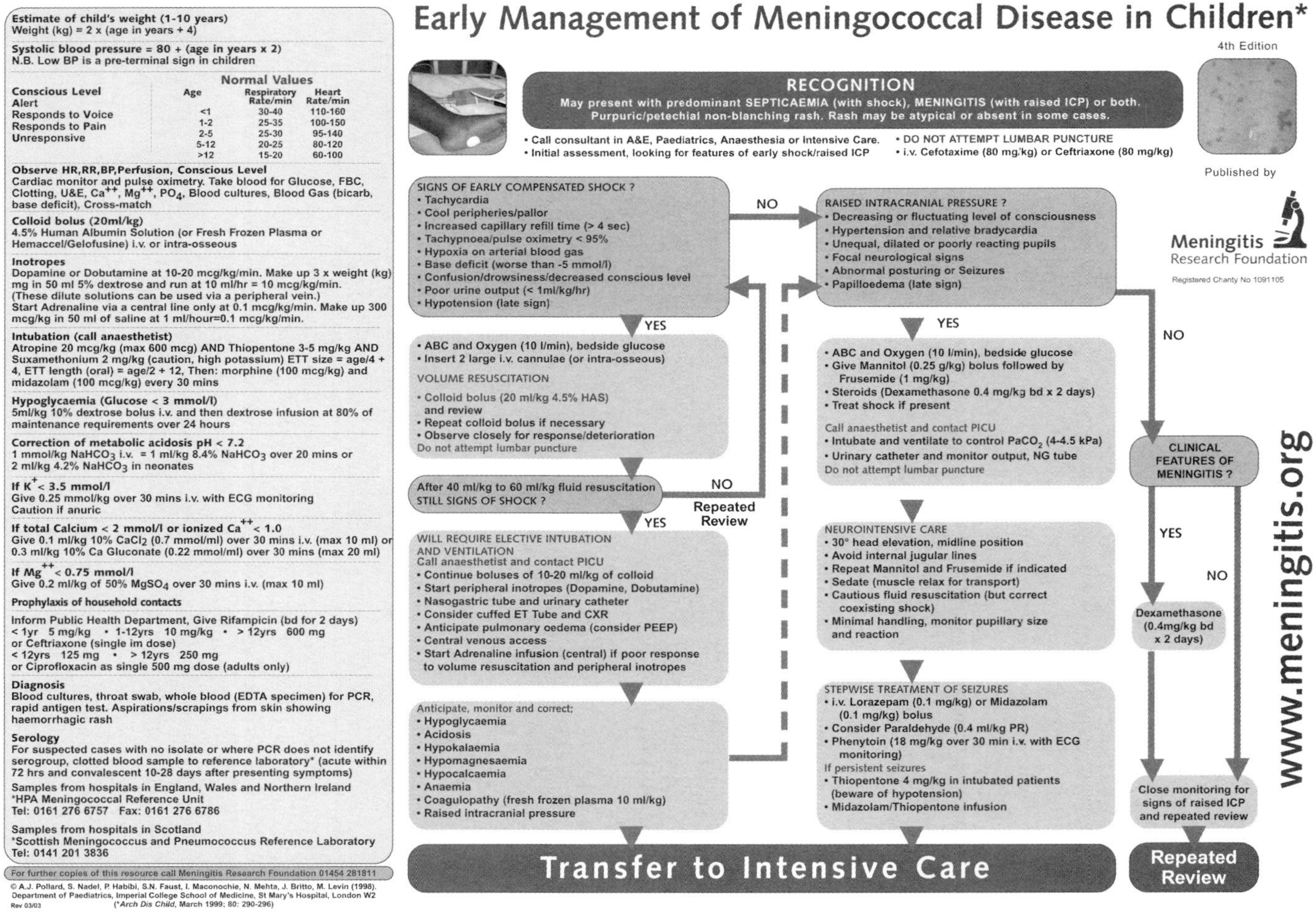

Fig. 22.2 Algorithm for early management of meningococcal disease in children (reproduced with permission of the Meningitis Research Foundation, www.meningitis.org).

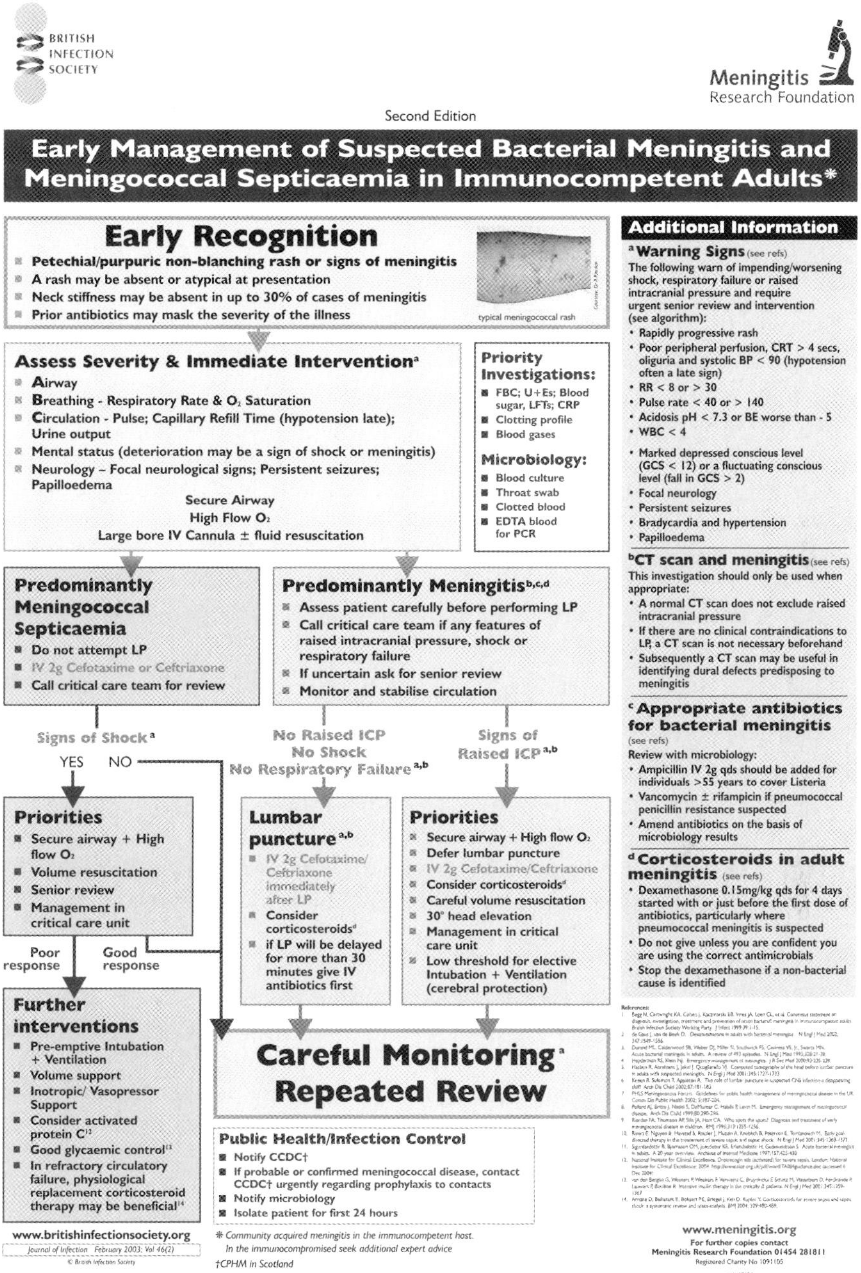

Fig. 22.3 Algorithm for early management of suspected bacterial meningitis and meningococcal septicemia in adults [reproduced with permission of the Meningitis Research Foundation (www.meningitis.org) and the British Infection Society (BIS, www.britishinfectionsociety.org), copyright BIS].

22.8.1 Management of Shock

The goal of circulatory support in shock is the maintenance of adequate tissue perfusion and oxygenation. The priority in achieving this goal is volume resuscitation to restore intravascular volume. Early, aggressive fluid resuscitation is associated with improved survival [106]. In addition, myocardial support with inotropes is frequently necessary in order to maintain end-organ perfusion in more severely ill patients.

Peripheral venous access can be difficult in young children and may be impossible in shock. If attempts at peripheral intravenous cannula placement are unsuccessful after a few minutes, intraosseous access should be secured without delay [107]. Establishment of central venous access, although desirable, can delay resuscitation and should wait until after initial stabilization.

An initial bolus of 20 ml kg^{-1} of colloid should be given over 5 min [108] to children with signs of shock. The expected response to volume replacement is reduction of heart rate and improvement in peripheral perfusion (warming of peripheries, shortening of capillary refill time). In mild cases, where shock is rapidly reversed by this initial fluid bolus, a repeated review is mandatory as the disease may progress and shock may reappear, even after initial stabilization, due to ongoing capillary leak.

When signs of shock persist after an initial 20 ml kg^{-1} colloid, a further 20 ml kg^{-1} should be given over 5–10 min [106, 109]. If signs of shock persist after 40–60 ml kg^{-1} of fluid resuscitation, there is a significant risk of pulmonary edema and elective tracheal intubation; and mechanical ventilation should be initiated, even in the absence of signs of respiratory failure (see below) [109]. This is associated with an improvement in outcome of septic shock [110] by reducing myocardial and respiratory muscle oxygen consumption and improving cardiac output; and it allows the delivery of positive end-expiratory pressure (PEEP) to aid oxygenation and eases placement of intravascular catheters for venous and arterial access.

Continued volume resuscitation is required for persistent signs of shock. As myocardial depression invariably coexists with severe volume depletion, inotropic support should be initiated in patients who have persistent shock after 40 ml kg^{-1} of fluid. It is usually impractical to gain central venous access prior to intubation. Dilute solutions of vasocative agents such as dopamine or dobutamine can be given as an infusion through a peripheral vein until the airway is secured and central venous access is obtained. These drugs must be used cautiously because of the risks associated with extravasation. In refactory meningococcal shock, adrenaline and/or noradrenaline [98], infusion may be required but should only be infused into a central venous catheter unless *in extremis.*

The adequacy of volume replacement therapy should be monitored using heart rate, blood pressure, central venous pressure, urine output, metabolic status and peripheral perfusion as indicators. It can be very difficult to decide whether persistently shocked children require further volume replacement or myocardial support with inotropes. Inotropic support should be initiated concurrently with continued volume resuscitation. There is some evidence to suggest that monitoring of mixed venous or central venous oxygen saturation may indicate cardiac output and help to guide fluid and inotrope requirements [109].

Placement of a urinary catheter is an important part of the emergency management of shocked children, as urine output is a sensitive index of end-organ perfusion.

Some children with severe capillary leak syndrome are only stabilized after replacement of more than twice their circulating volume with colloid solutions and concurrent inotropic support.

Efforts to improve the circulation in refractory shock also include the use of experimental agents or modes of therapy. There is some anecdotal experience with potent vasopressors such as angiotensin II, vasopressin and nitric oxide antagonists. However, experience with these agents is limited and routine use cannot be recommended.

Although there is controversy about the use of human albumin solution (HAS) for volume replacement therapy [111–113], 4.5% human albumin solution has been our major resuscitation fluid used in meningococcal sepsis for several decades. The use of HAS has been associated with a reduction in morbidity and mortality rates in children with severe meningococcal disease [8, 9]. There is some support for the use of HAS as volume expansion in children from a study of malaria-associated shock in children [114]; and, in the absence of evidence that other fluids have an advantage in meningococcal patients with profound capillary leak, it is difficult to justify a change in practice. However, a change to crystalloid use has been made in response to this continuing controversy by some units in the UK. A large randomized controlled study comparing HAS with normal saline in adult patients in intensive care units in Australia and New Zealand [115] has suggested that HAS may be beneficial for the treatment of patients with septic shock. However, no such studies have been performed in children.

In severe capillary leak, it is likely that all resuscitation fluids will readily leak from the circulation into the tissues and the effects of volume resuscitation may be shortlived [116], requiring close monitoring and further volume replacement therapy.

22.8.2
Respiratory Support

High-flow facial oxygen should be delivered routinely during the initial assessment of the patient. If no major problem in airway or breathing is present, priority is given to the assessment and treatment of the circulation. However, early, elective intubation should be considered mandatory in any child who has persistent shock after 40–60 $ml\ kg^{-1}$ of volume resuscitation, since intubation and ventilation protects the airway, reduces the risk of pulmonary edema, facilitates adequate oxygenation and ventilation, and reduces the work of breathing and oxygen consumption [110, 117]. Indications for immediate endotracheal intubation are fluctuating or decreased conscious level (Glasgow coma score <8), signs of raised intracranial pressure, hypoxia and/or respiratory failure, pulmonary edema and hypotension (decompensated shock). Use of positive end-expiratory airways pressure following intubation may reduce hypoxia by limiting pulmonary edema. Nasotracheal intubation should be performed with caution in meningococcal disease, as it may precipitate uncontrollable hemorrhage in the presence of severe coagulopathy.

Rapid sequence intubation using atropine, thiopentone and suxamethonium is preferred [118]. The aim should be to intubate the trachea before decompensated shock or severe hypoxia occurs, as induction of anaesthesia may exacerbate hypotension with worsening of shock as a result of vasodilation and removal of the innate sympathetic drive. Children with decompensated shock may further deteriorate on induction of anesthesia, unless close attention to volume resuscitation and inotropic support is made before, during and after induction. Ketamine is an alternative induction agent in place of thiopentone, as it may cause less cardiovascular compromise. Boluses of colloid and inotropes should be drawn up and available to give if shock worsens during induction.

22.8.3
Biochemical and Hematological Derangements

Children with meningococcal sepsis may have profound derangements in metabolism [50, 119]. These abnormalities in the metabolic environment may contribute to myocardial depression and should be corrected. Anemia and hypoglycemia are common findings and should be detected by repeated blood testing and treated. A 10% glucose infusion should be commenced as maintenance fluid early in resuscitation to prevent hypoglycemia. Hyperglycemia may occur following resuscitation and stabilization. Data from adults on intensive care with sepsis indicates that a reduction in mortality is possible with strict control of blood glucose, using insulin for hyperglycemia, with the greatest benefit being in those with multiorgan failure or a septic focus [120]. Again, there are no data available in children.

Disseminated intravascular coagulopathy is common. There may be bleeding from mucosal surfaces and venepuncture sites. In addition, spontaneous pulmonary, gastric or cerebral hemorrhage may occur, particularly if there is associated thrombocytopenia. Correction of coagulopathy with fresh frozen plasma, platelets and, in severe cases, cryoprecipitate, may prevent life-threatening hemorrhage. In general, correction of thrombocytopenia is not required but, if hemorrhage from venepuncture sites or spontaneous mucous membrane bleeding occurs despite replacement of clotting factors, platelet transfusion may be required.

Recombinant activated protein C has been shown to reduce mortality in adult septic shock [121] and there is a rationale for its use in children with meningococcal disease [99, 100, 122]. A retrospective analysis of its use in adults and children with meningococcal meningitis, septicemia and purpura fulminans has suggested that it is safe to use in these patients, but as yet there are no data to suggest that it may be beneficial in children with severe sepsis [123].

Metabolic acidosis is invariably present in severe shock. Athough the use of bicarbonate replacement is controversial, severe acidosis impairs myocardial contractility and, if pH is <7.2 due to a metabolic acidosis, sodium bicarbonate should be infused (see Fig. 22.2) [98]. Acidosis and oliguria would be expected to cause hyperkalemia but, paradoxically, most patients with meningococcal shock have hypokalemia [124, 125]. In view of the impaired myocardial function and risk of arrhythmia associated with low serum potassium, hypokalemia should be corrected. Hypocalcemia is also common in sepsis [126] and is corrected with the intention of achieving stabilization of myocardial function and improving blood pressure [127–129], though calcium supplementation in sepsis remains controversial [130, 131]. If there is also hypomagnesemia, hypokalemia may be refactory to treatment [132] and potassium homeostasis improves when serum magnesium is maintained at high normal values [133]. Hypomagnesemia may cause cardiac arrhythmias and has been associated with an increased mortality in sepsis [129]. Phosphate is important for tissue oxygen utilization, glycolysis, smooth and striated muscle strength (including diaphragmatic) and left ventricular contractility [134]. Symptoms are unusual until serum phosphate falls below 0.32 mmol l^{-1} [135]. These features of hypoposphatemia are mainly related to ATP depletion. Hypophosphatemia should be corrected if serum phosphate falls below 0.7 mmol l^{-1} as phosphate. Repeated biochemical monitoring to detect electrolyte abnormalities should be undertaken at hourly intervals during resuscitation and derangements corrected, as described in Fig. 22.2.

22.8.4 Impaired Organ Perfusion

The combination of hypovolemia, decreased myocardial contractility, vasoconstriction and thrombosis results in impaired organ perfusion. The kidney may be particularly affected, with the most obvious result being vasomotor nephropathy, causing oliguria or anuria. The severity of the renal impairment relates to the degree of shock and acute tubular necrosis may ensue. Acute renal insufficiency may occur, initially due to renal hypoperfusion. Most children are oligo/anuric until circulation is restored by adequate fluid resuscitation and inotropic support. If these measures are unsuccessful, or there is severe intractable pulmonary edema, massive fluid requirement or severe metabolic derangement, then renal replacement therapy with either hemofiltration or acute peritoneal dialysis may be required. Very rarely, long-term renal replacement therapy may be required. There is some evidence that hemofiltration may be beneficial in patients with septic shock because of a theoretical property of removal of circulating toxins and inflammatory cytokines.

Maintenance of enteral feeding is desirable wherever possible. Attempts should be made to maintain enteral feeding during management of meningococcal shock with intragastric or jejunal feeds, although parenteral nutrition may be necessary in some cases. Intestinal failure results from compromised perfusion of the gastrointestinal tract in combination with bowel wall edema and ascites, with consequent ileus or even intestinal necrosis and perforation in rare cases [136].

The skin may be severely compromised in meningococcal septic shock through inadequate perfusion as a result of endogenous vasoconstriction or the use of therapeutic vasoconstrictors. Areas affected by purpura may also become necrotic and denuded of superficial layers or even full skin thickness injury. Decreased skin perfusion may predispose pressure areas to ischemic damage and tissue edema, or capillary leak, or may cause a limb compartment syndrome. The role of fasciotomy to treat compartment syndrome is not clearly established but has been used in some circumstances [137]. Advice from orthopedic and plastic surgeons may be needed for limb salvage. Fasciotomy and amputation should not be considered until it is felt to be absolutely necessary and only performed following extensive multidisciplinary discussion.

22.8.5 Raised Intracranial Pressure

Although most critically ill children with meningococcal infection have shock as their primary clinical problem, a proportion present with signs of raised intracranial pressure (ICP). Conversely, a majority of patients with meningitis have mildly raised ICP [138], but clinically significant raised intracranial pressure is an uncommon presenting feature of meningococcal disease. Raised intracranial pressure probably arises as a result of central nervous system inflammation and capillary leak, leading to cerebral edema [139]. In addition, rarely in meningococcal meningitis, changes in the dynamics of CSF flow may occur because of increased production or decreased resorption, leading to hydrocephalus.

Signs of raised ICP include a declining level of consciousness, focal neurological signs including unequal, dilated or poorly responsive pupils, hypertension and relative bradycardia. Papilledema is a late finding in acute raised ICP. Patients without significant meningeal inflammation who have profound shock may also present with impaired consciousness as a result of cerebral hypoperfusion. Conversely, patients without shock who have raised intracranial pressure may have clinical features suggesting shock, including peripheral vasoconstriction and poor peripheral perfusion.

Care should be taken not to confuse the poor peripheral circulation seen in shock (see above) with the vasoconstriction often seen with raised ICP, where abnormal neurology may be associated with delayed capillary refill time without evidence of shock. In this circumstance, poor peripheral perfusion associated with absence of a metabolic acidosis in blood gases, together with relative bradycardia, normal or high blood pressure and other neurological signs, it should be assumed that abnormal neurology is due to raised ICP [140].

Sending a child for a CT scan may delay life-saving treatment. Moreover, detection of raised ICP depends more on clinical features and is not reliably shown by CT [86]. In a patient with raised ICP, intravenous infusion of mannitol and elective tracheal intubation is indicated, as suggested in Fig. 22.2.

In the assessment of the child with raised ICP from meningococcal infection, initial assessment may reveal coexistent shock. In this case, the priority of management is to correct the shock before addressing specific measures to control ICP [141, 142]. An adequate blood pressure is necessary in order to maintain brain perfusion, particularly if the intracranial pressure is raised. In this situation, fluid resuscitation may result in improved conscious level. In the presence of raised ICP, the airway should be secured and the child should be intubated and mechanically ventilated in order to control pCO_2 in the normal range [142]. A common error is to undertake intubation but then fail to monitor CO_2 and maintain adequate ventilation. Repeated blood gas analysis and the use of end-tidal CO_2 monitoring is essential following intubation in order to avoid hypercapnia. Failure to do this may cause a rise in CO_2 that would be associated with an increase in cerebral blood flow and a further rise in intracranial pressure.

In the absence of shock, cautious diuretic therapy using mannitol and furosemide may reduce cerebral edema and improve cerebral blood flow. Cautious fluid restriction may be useful, but fluid balance requires careful monitoring and any coexisting shock should be treated aggressively [142].

Sedation is essential following tracheal intubation in order to prevent acute rises in ICP caused by agitation and coughing, but muscle relaxants should generally be avoided, as they may mask seizures. Seizures should be aggressively managed to avoid further increases of intracranial pressure (see Fig. 22.2).

Neurointensive care should be instituted using a 30° head-up position, head midline, minimal suction, deep sedation and strict avoidance of hypercapnia [141]. Ideally, the internal jugular vein should be avoided for central venous line placement, as these catheters themselves (and positioning the patient for their insertion) may reduce venous return from the brain and further raise intracranial pressure. In this situation, the femoral vein is the safest option.

While fluids should be closely managed and may need cautious restriction in the management of raised intracranial pressure to avoid fluid overload, there is evidence that maintenance crystalloid need not be restricted in meningitis [143]. However, close observation should be ensured for the development of inappropriate secretion of antidiuretic hormone (SIADH) or cerebral salt wasting. Hyponatremia may worsen cerebral edema and may precipitate seizures.

22.8.6 Steroids

Steroids given with the first dose of antibiotics reduce the incidence of neurological sequelae in both *Haemophilus influenzae* type b and pneumococcal meningitis in childhood [144]. Data from adult studies indicate that both neurological sequelae and mortality may be reduced by use of steroids in all-cause bacterial meningitis [145] and there is also a trend to improved outcome in meningococcal meningitis. Although data are not specifically available for meningococcal meningitis, the pathophysiological events are likely to be similar to those in other forms of bacterial meningitis. Systemic high-dose dexamethasone should be given in cases of suspected bacterial meningitis with, or shortly before, the first dose of antibiotics in an attempt to reduce the incidence of neuronal damage [146–148]. A dose of 0.15 mg kg^{-1} qds for 4 days has been recommended [148], but 0.4 mg kg^{-1} bd for 2 days is equally effective [147]. High-dose steroid use is not indicated in meningococcal shock in the absence of meningitis [149, 150].

There is some evidence that refractory shock may be more common in children with impaired adrenal gland responsiveness, which may be aided by low-dose replacement hydrocortisone [151, 152].

22.8.7 Antibiotic Therapy

Cefotaxime (80 mg kg^{-1}) or ceftriaxone (80 mg kg^{-1}) is preferred as *initial* therapy in shocked patients with a clinical diagnosis of meningococcal disease. Penicillin resistance is extremely rare amongst clinical isolates of *N. meningitidis* and this antibiotic is the logical choice when the microbiological diagnosis has been made. However, until microbiological information is available, there remains the possibility of both penicillin resistance or alternative bacterial diagnosis that might not be adequately treated by penicillin therapy. Other rare bacterial causes of purpura fulminans include *S. pneumoniae, S. aureus* and Gram-negative bacteria. The duration of antibiotic therapy for meningococcal disease does not need to be prolonged and most centers use a 5–7 day course of intravenous antibiotic therapy for both meningococcal meningitis and septic shock. The efficacy of a daily dose of ceftriaxone for 4 days in the treatment of bacterial meningitis is now well established [153–156] and is probably effective because this drug has a long half-life in blood and CSF concentrations remain above the minimal inhibitory concentration of most organisms for 24–48 h after administration (for a review, see [157]). Indeed, recent studies from an epidemic setting indicated that, in a resource-poor setting, a single dose of ceftriaxone was as effective as standard therapy in sub-Saharan Africa with oily chloramphenicol [157].

22.9 Transfer to Intensive Care or Treatment on the General Ward

The majority of children presenting with meningococcal disease do not require intensive care. However, those with persistent shock after initial volume resuscitation (>40 ml kg^{-1}) or signs of raised intracranial pressure should be managed in a specialist pediatric intensive care unit (PICU).

For those who do not immediately require transfer to an intensive care unit, management on the general ward is undertaken with careful monitoring of vital signs (pulse, blood pressure, respiratory rate, urine output, conscious level) for the first 24–48 h. This may be better facilitated by initial management in a high-dependency unit. The failure of recognition of deterioration by inexperienced medical and nursing staff following hospital admission is associated with increased mortality [7].

The decision to move critically ill children can be difficult. A prolonged period of resuscitation may be necessary in the Emergency Department before a child with profound shock is stable enough to move. Transporting children before they are adequately resuscitated can be hazardous and the child should be fully stabilized and monitored before moving to the PICU. Stabilization includes provision of a secure airway, controlled mechanical ventilation, central venous and arterial catheterization and cardiorespiratory monitoring [92]. Transport-related morbidity and mortality are reduced by the use of a specialist pediatric intensive care team [158].

22.10 Adjunctive Therapy for Sepsis

There have only been two properly conducted randomized controlled studies of adjunctive therapy in meningococcal disease.

The only potentially useful adjunctive therapy studied to date is recombinant bactericidal permeability increasing protein (rBPI), which binds to endotoxin and blocks the inflammatory cascade. There was a suggestion of improved outcome in a randomized multicentre placebo-controlled trial, but unfortunately the study was not sufficiently powered to detect a reduction in mortality [159, 160]. However, the rBPI group had fewer amputations, decreased blood product transfusions and improved functional outcome; and fewer children died who received a full 24-h infusion of rBPI (2% rBPI vs 6% placebo, $P=0.07$) [160].

An antiendotoxin antibody, HA1A, was investigated in a randomized controlled trial as a treatment for children with meningococcal septicemia; but it did not provide any significant reduction in mortality when compared with a placebo [161]. Many other agents have been suggested as possible adjunctive therapies in sepsis, but few have been subjected to rigorous clinical evaluation and only activated protein C (aPC) has been shown to have significant effect on outcome in adults (see Table 22.2) [121, 162, 163].

No randomized controlled trials of aPC have yet been concluded specifically in meningococcal sepsis in children; and it is difficult to make recommendations for its use in this setting [164]. However, uncontrolled case series have indicated the possibility of benefit of this agent in meningococcal disease [121, 123]. In particular, the risk of serious bleeding complications may preclude its use in the some patients with meningococcal septicemia. A recently conducted randomized, placebo-controlled study of the use of activated protein C in children with severe sepsis failed to demonstrate any obvious benefit in children with septic shock [165].

Table 22.2 Phase III trials of drugs in severe sepsis. Reprinted from [162] with permission from Elsevier.

Trial	Reference	Substance studied	Number of patients	Mortality (over 28 days; %)			Adverse events in treatment group
				Patients	Controls	Difference and 95% CI [a]	
Chess	197	HA-1A human monoclonal antibody against endotoxin	1578 [b]	41%	37%	–4.0 (–8.8 to 0.8)	Higher mortality in patients with suspected but not later confirmed Gram-negative sepsis
			621 [c]	33%	32%	–1.0 (–8.6 to 6.2)	
InterSept	198	Anti-tumour necrosis factor α	564	37.3% [d]	39.5%	2.2 (–3.8 to 4.6)	Mild serum-sickness-like reaction and transient hypotension
PAF-AH	199	Platelet-activating factor acetylhydrolase	1425	25%	24%	–1.0 (–25 to 15)	Stopped after interim analysis of 1261 patients
KyberSept	200	Antithrombin III (ATIII)	2314	38.9%	38.7%	–0.2 (–10.9 to 8.9)	Increased risk of bleeding in ATIII group; Increased mortality in patients receiving ATIII and heparin compared with placebo (36.6 *vs* 39.4%)
Prowess	121	Activated protein C (aPC)	1690	24.7%	30.8%	6.1 (1.9 to 10.4)	Serious bleeding, 3.5 vs 2.0% (3.7% for combination of heparin and aPC)
Optimist	201	Tissue-factor-pathway inhibitor (TFPI)	1754	34.2%	33.9%	–0,3 (–11 to 10)	Serious bleeding, 6.5 vs 4.8%

a) Minus sign favours placebo.
b) Shock without confirmed Gram-negative bacteremia.
c) Confirmed gram-negative bacterial sepsis.
d) 57/181 (31.5%) in low-dose group. 87/205 (42%) in high-dose group.

Table 22.3 Treatments for septic shock. RCT = Randomised controlled trial. Reprinted from [163], with permission from Elsevier.

	Target population	Main effects	Evidence
A Controlling the source of infection			
Antibiotics	All patients	Appropriate antibiotics improve survival	Common sense, observational studies
Removal of infected and necrotic tissues	Patients with cellulitis, abscess, purulent wounds, infected devices	Improves survival	Common sense, observational studies
B Management of shock			
Restoration of central venous pressure to 8–12 mmHg, mean arterial pressure 65–90 mmHg and central venous oxygen saturation >70% with fluids, vasopressors, inotropic drugs, red blood cell transfusion and mechanical ventilation	All patients; most effective if goal achieved within 6 h	Prevents organ dysfunction and death	1 RCT ($n=263$)
Fluids			
Crystalloids versus albumin		No difference in any outcome between serum saline and 5% albumin	1 RCT ($n=7000$)
Crystalloids versus synthetic colloids		No evidence for difference in clinical outcomes	27 RCTs ($n=2243$) 1 continuing RCT ($n=3000$)
Vasopressors			
Dopamine, norepinephrine or epinephrine	Persistent hypotension after fluid administration		
Dopamine versus norepinephrine		No evidence for difference in mortality	3 RCTs ($n=62$) 1 continuing RCT
Norepinephrine (dobutamine) versus epinephrine		No evidence for difference in mortality	2 RCTs ($n=52$) 1 continuing RCT ($n=330$)
C. Management of organ dysfunction			
Daily versus alternate-day intermittent renal replacement treatment	Overt acute renal failure	Daily intermittent dialysis better than alternate-day dialysis for time to renal recovery and survival	1 RCT ($n=160$)
Intermittent versus continuous treatment		No evidence for difference in mortality	1 continuing RCT ($n=400$)

Table 22.3 (continued)

	Target population	Main effects	Evidence
Mechanical ventilation with low tidal volume, 6–7 ml kg^{-1} ideal body weight	Acute lung injury or acute respiratory distress syndrome	Ventilation with tidal volume 6–7 ml kg^{-1} better then ventilation with 10–15 ml kg^{-1} more survivors and more ventilator-free days	5 RCTs ($n=1202$)
D. Replacing or enhancing host responses			
Endocrine response			
Low dose corticosteroids	Refractory septic shock and basal cortisol concentrations <150 μg l^{-1} or cortisol response to adrenocorticotrophin <90 μg l^{-1}	Improve hemodynamics; reduce shock duration, organ dysfunction, systemic inflammation and mortality	5 RCTs ($n=465$) 1 continuing RCT ($n=800$)
Low-dose vasopressin	Patients not improving with or not meeting criteria for corticosteroids	Improve hemodynamics, reduce shock duration	4 RCTs ($n=98$) 1 continuing RCT ($n=800$)
Hemostasis response			
Drotrecogin alfa	Undisputable septic shock not improving with or not meeting criteria for corticosteroids and with Apache II >24, and at least one new (<48 h) organ dysfunction (e.g. acute lung injury or acute respiratory distress syndrome or acute renal failure and no risk of bleeding)	Improve hemodynamics, reduce shock duration, organ dysfunction and mortality	1 RCT ($n=1690$)

Other treatments which have been studied in the management of septic shock have mainly enrolled adult patients with sepsis; and the use of these approaches in children is by extrapolation (see Table 22.3) [163].

Low-dose replacement steroid therapy may be appropriate in some patients and is mentioned above. One clinical trial of replacement steroid therapy in adults with adrenal insufficiency found that 53% died in the steroid treated group as compared with 63% in the placebo group ($P=0.04$) [166]. Few of the patients in this trial had meningococcal disease. By contrast, high-dose steroid therapy is not helpful in adults and may even cause harm [150, 167].

One important observation in adult sepsis studies is that treatment with low-dose heparin might be associated with improved outcome (see Table 22.4) [162]. This was not an endpoint in any of these studies but is under further investiga-

Table 22.4 Effects of heparin (%) in three trials of natural anticoagulants in sepsis. Reprinted from [162], with permission from Elsevier.

Trial	Reference	Study drug alone	Heparin alone	Study drug and heparin	Placebo
KyberSept (ATIII)	200	37.8	36.6	39.4	43.6
Prowess (aPC)	121	24.0	28.0	25.0	39.0
Optimist (TFPI)	201	34.0	29.8	34.6	42.7

tion. Specific data from children with meningococcal disease is not available and the risk of bleeding in this population may preclude the routine use of this agent in many patients even if it is later proven to be of benefit. In meningococcal disease, heparin may reduce the severity of distal necrosis [168]. It is also possible that recombinant tissue plasminogen activator may reduce peripheral necrosis and minimize risk of amputation. However, its use in patients with severe meningococcal shock and purpura fulminans was associated with an unacceptably high risk of intracranial hemorrhage; and its use in this scenario cannot be recommended [169].

22.11 Conclusion

The outcome of meningococcal disease has improved in recent years due to improvements in the recognition, resuscitation, stabilization, transfer and ongoing care of individuals with the disease. However, despite these improvements, meningococcal infection remains a major cause of morbidity and mortality throughout the world. The introduction of serogroup C conjugated meningococcal vaccine has been an impressive success, but the challenge remains to develop effective vaccines against all the disease-causing serogroups for use throughout the world for the prevention of this devastating disease.

Acknowledgements

Sections of this text have been adapted and reproduced from [91] with permission from the BMJ Publishing Group. The authors are grateful to Mrs Carole Barr for assistance with preparation of the manuscript, to Ms Linda Glennie of the Meningitis Research Foundation and to Dr Robert Heyderman from the British Infection Society for facilitating permission to include Figs. 22.2, 22.3. The authors are also grateful to colleagues at St Mary's Hospital, London, who helped in development of the approach to early management of meningococcal disease that is described in this manuscript, especially Professor Michael Levin and Dr Parviz Habibi.

References

1 Vieusseaux G. **1805**, Memoire sur le maladie qui a régné a Genêve au printemps de 1805, *J Med Chir Pharm* 2, 163–165.
2 Danielson L, Mann E. **1806**, The history of a singular and very mortal disease, which lately made its appearance in Medfield, *Med Agric Reg* 1, 65.
3 Centers for Disease Control and Prevention **2000**, Serogroup W-135 meningococcal disease among travelers returning from Saudi Arabia to United States, 2000, *Morb Mortal Wkly Rep* 49, 345–346.
4 Lapeyssonnie L. **1963**, La meningite cerebro-spinale en Afrique, *Bull WHO* 28[Suppl.], 3–114.
5 Wang JF, Caugant DA, Li X, Hu X, Poolman JT, Crowe BA, et al. **1992**, Clonal and antigenic analysis of serogroup A Neisseria meningitidis with particular reference to epidemiological features of epidemic meningitis in the People's Republic of China, *Infect Immun* 60, 5267–5282.
6 Decosas J, Koama JB. **2002**, Chronicle of an outbreak foretold: meningococcal meningitis W135 in Burkina Faso, *Lancet Infect Dis* 2, 763–765.
7 Ninis N, Phillips C, Bailey L, Pollock JI, Nadel S, Britto J, et al. **2005**, The role of healthcare delivery in the outcome of meningococcal disease in children: case-control study of fatal and non-fatal cases, *BMJ* 330, 1475.
8 Booy R, Habibi P, Nadel S, de Munter C, Britto J, Morrison A, et al. **2001**, Reduction in case fatality rate from meningococcal disease associated with improved healthcare delivery, *Arch Dis Child* 85, 386–390.
9 Thorburn K, Baines P, Thomson A, Hart CA. **2001**, Mortality in severe meningococcal disease, *Arch Dis Child* 85, 382–385.
10 Bryce J, Boschi-Pinto C, Shibuya K, Black RE. **2005**, WHO estimates of the causes of death in children, *Lancet* 365, 1147–1152.
11 Tikhomirov E, Santamaria M, Esteves K. **1997**, Meningococcal disease: public health burden and control, *World Health Stat Q* 50, 170–177.
12 Mulholland K. **1999**, Strategies for the control of pneumococcal diseases, *Vaccine* 17[Suppl.], S79–S84.
13 Rosenstein NE, Perkins BA, Stephens DS, Lefkowitz L, Cartter ML, Danila R, et al. **1999**, The changing epidemiology of meningococcal disease in the United States, 1992–1996, *J Infect Dis* 180, 1894–1901.
14 Pollard AJ, Scheifele D. **2001**, Meningococcal disease and vaccination in North America, *J Paediatr Child Health* 37, 20–27.
15 Hausdorff WP, Bryant J, Paradiso PR, Siber GR. **2000**, Which pneumococcal serogroups cause the most invasive disease: implications for conjugate vaccine formulation and use, part I, *Clin Infect Dis* 30, 100–121.
16 Offit PA, Peter G. **2003**, The meningococcal vaccine – public policy and individual choices, *N Engl J Med* 349, 2353–2356.
17 Public Health Laboratory Service **1997**, Bacterial meningitis in Europe: surveillance report for 1995, *Commun Dis Rep CDR Wkly* 7, 119, 122.
18 Goldschneider I, Gotschlich EC, Artenstein MS. **1969**, Human immunity to the meningococcus, II. Development of natural immunity, *J Exp Med* 129, 1327–1348.
19 Peltola H, Kataja JM, Mäkelä PH. **1982**, Shift in the age-distribution of meningococcal disease as predictor of an epidemic? *Lancet* 2, 595–597.
20 Whalen CM, Hockin JC, Ryan A, Ashton F. **1995**, The changing epidemiology of invasive meningococcal disease in Canada, 1985 through 1992, Emergence of a virulent clone of *Neisseria meningitidis*, *JAMA* 273, 390–394.
21 Kaczmarski EB. **1997**, Meningococcal disease in England and Wales: 1995, *Commun Dis Rep CDR Rev* 7, R55–R59.
22 Greenwood B. **1987**, The epidemiology of acute bacterial meningitis in tropical Africa, in *Bacterial Meningitis*, 1st edn, Academic Press, London, p. 61–91.
23 De Wals P, Hertoghe L, Borlee-Grimee I, De Maeyer-Cleempoel S, Reginster-Ha-

neuse G, Dachy A, et al. **1981**, Meningococcal disease in Belgium. Secondary attack rate among household, day-care nursery and pre-elementary school contacts, *J Infect* 3[Suppl.], 53–61.

24 Moodley JR, Coetzee N, Hussey G. **1999**, Risk factors for meningococcal disease in Cape Town, *S Afr Med J* 89, 56–59.

25 Baker M, McNicholas A, Garrett N, Jones N, Stewart J, Koberstein V, et al. **2000**, Household crowding a major risk factor for epidemic meningococcal disease in Auckland children, *Pediatr Infect Dis J* 19, 983–990.

26 Berild D, Gedde-Dahl TW, Abrahamsen T. **1980**, Meningococcal disease in the Norwegian armed forces 1967–1979, Some epidemiological aspects, *NIPH Ann* 3, 23–30.

27 Neal KR, Nguyen-Van-Tam J, Monk P, O'Brien SJ, Stuart J, Ramsay M. **1999**, Invasive meningococcal disease among university undergraduates: association with universities providing relatively large amounts of catered hall accommodation, *Epidemiol Infect* 122, 351–357.

28 Yusuf HR, Rochat RW, Baughman WS, Gargiullo PM, Perkins BA, Brantley MD, et al. **1999**, Maternal cigarette smoking and invasive meningococcal disease: a cohort study among young children in metropolitan Atlanta, 1989–1996, *Am J Public Health* 89, 712–717.

29 Fischer M, Hedberg K, Cardosi P, Plikaytis BD, Hoesly FC, Steingart KR, et al. **1997**, Tobacco smoke as a risk factor for meningococcal disease, *Pediatr Infect Dis J* 16, 979–983.

30 Cartwright KA, Jones DM, Smith AJ, Stuart JM, Kaczmarski EB, Palmer SR. **1991**, Influenza A and meningococcal disease, *Lancet* 338, 554–557.

31 Fijen CA, Kuijper EJ, Hannema AJ, Sjöholm AG, van Putten JP. **1989**, Complement deficiencies in patients over ten years old with meningococcal disease due to uncommon serogroups, *Lancet* 2, 585–588.

32 Nielsen HE, Koch C, Magnussen P, Lind I. **1989**, Complement deficiencies in selected groups of patients with meningococcal disease, *Scand J Infect Dis* 21, 389–396.

33 Salit IE. **1981**, Meningococcemia caused by serogroup W135. Association with hypogammaglobulinemia, *Arch Intern Med* 141, 664–665.

34 Locker GJ, Wagner A, Peter A, Staudinger T, Marosi C, Rintelen C, et al. **1995**, Lethal Waterhouse–Friderichsen syndrome in posttraumatic asplenia, *J Trauma* 39, 784–786.

35 Emonts M, Hazelzet JA, de Groot R, Hermans PW. **2003**, Host genetic determinants of Neisseria meningitidis infections, *Lancet Infect Dis* 3, 565–577.

36 Maiden MC, Stuart JM. **2002**, Carriage of serogroup C meningococci 1 year after meningococcal C conjugate polysaccharide vaccination, *Lancet* 359, 1829–1831.

37 Caugant DA, Høiby EA, Magnus P, Scheel O, Hoel T, Bjune G, et al. **1994**, Asymptomatic carriage of Neisseria meningitidis in a randomly sampled population, *J Clin Microbiol* 32, 323–330.

38 Gold R, Goldschneider I, Lepow ML, Draper TF, Randolph M. **1978**, Carriage of Neisseria meningitidis and Neisseria lactamica in infants and children, *J Infect Dis* 137, 112–121.

39 Andersen J, Berthelsen L, Bech Jensen B, Lind I. **1998**, Dynamics of the meningococcal carrier state and characteristics of the carrier strains: a longitudinal study within three cohorts of military recruits, *Epidemiol Infect* 121, 85–94.

40 Ala'Aldeen DA, Neal KR, Ait-Tahar K, Nguyen-Van-Tam JS, English A, Falla TJ, et al. **2000**, Dynamics of meningococcal long-term carriage among university students and their implications for mass vaccination, *J Clin Microbiol* 38, 2311–2316.

41 Marzouk O, Thomson AP, Sills JA, Hart CA, Harris F. **1991**, Features and outcome in meningococcal disease presenting with maculopapular rash, *Arch Dis Child* 66, 485–487.

42 Edwards KM, Jones LM, Stephens DS. **1985**, Clinical features of mild systemic meningococcal disease with characterization of bacterial isolates, *Clin Pediatr* 24, 617–620.

43 Kirsch EA, Barton RP, Kitchen L, Giroir BP. **1996**, Pathophysiology, treatment

and outcome of meningococcemia: a review and recent experience, *Pediatr Infect Dis J* 15, 967–978.
44 Havens PL, Garland JS, Brook MM, Dewitz BA, Stremski ES, Troshynski TJ. **1989**, Trends in mortality in children hospitalized with meningococcal infections, 1957 to 1987, *Pediatr Infect Dis J* 8, 8–11.
45 Lodder MC, Schildkamp RL, Bijlmer HA, Dankert J, Kuik DJ, Scholten RJ. **1996**, Prognostic indicators of the outcome of meningococcal disease: a study of 562 patients, *J Med Microbiol* 45, 16–20.
46 Bigham JM, Hutcheon ME, Patrick DM, Pollard AJ. **2001**, Death from invasive meningococcal disease following close contact with a case of primary meningococcal conjunctivitis – Langley, British Columbia, 1999, *Can Commun Dis Rep* 27, 13–18.
47 Chien SY, Sung TC, Mu SC, Hu CC. **1999**, Endophthalmitis as a complication of meningococcal meningitis: report of one case, *Chung Hua Min Kuo Hsiao Erh Ko I Hsueh Hui Tsa Chih* 40, 116–118.
48 Dillon M, Nourse C, Dowling F, Deasy P, Butler K. **1997**, Primary meningococcal arthritis, *Pediatr Infect Dis J* 16, 331–332.
49 Edwards MS, Baker CJ. **1981**, Complications and sequelae of meningococcal infections in children, *J Pediatr* 99, 540–545.
50 Nadel S, Levin M, Habibi P. **1995**, Treatment of meningococcal disease in childhood, in *Meningococcal Disease*, ed. Cartwright K, John Wiley and Sons, Chichester, p. 207–243.
51 Mandl KD, Stack AM, Fleisher GR. **1997**, Incidence of bacteremia in infants and children with fever and petechiae, *J Pediatr* 131, 398–404.
52 Baker RC, Seguin JH, Leslie N, Gilchrist MJ, Myers MG. **1989**, Fever and petechiae in children, *Pediatrics* 84, 1051–1055.
53 Van Nguyen Q, Nguyen EA, Weiner LB. **1984**, Incidence of invasive bacterial disease in children with fever and petechiae, *Pediatrics* 74, 77–80.
54 Nadel S, Britto J, Booy R, Maconochie I, Habibi P, Levin M. **1998**, Avoidable deficiencies in the delivery of health care to children with meningococcal disease, *J Accid Emerg Med* 15, 298–303.
55 Pollard AJ, DeMunter C, Nadel S, Levin M. **1997**, Abandoning empirical antibiotics for febrile children, *Lancet* 350, 811–812.
56 Stiehm ER, Damrosch DS. **1966**, Factors in the prognosis of meningococcal infection, review of 63 cases with emphasis on recognition and management of the severely ill patient, *J Pediatr* 68, 457–467.
57 Perkins MD, Mirrett S, Reller LB. **1995**, Rapid bacterial antigen detection is not clinically useful, *J Clin Microbiol* 33, 1486–1491.
58 Kaczmarski EB, Ragunathan PL, Marsh J, Gray SJ, Guiver M. **1998**, Creating a national service for the diagnosis of meningococcal disease by polymerase chain reaction, *Commun Dis Public Health* 1, 54–56.
59 Cartwright K, Kroll S. **1997**, Optimising the investigation of meningococcal disease, *BMJ* 315, 757–758.
60 Pollard AJ, Probe G, Trombley C, Castell A, Whitehead S, Bigham JM, et al. **2002**, Evaluation of a diagnostic polymerase chain reaction assay for Neisseria meningitidis in North America and field experience during an outbreak, *Arch Pathol Lab Med* 126, 1209–1215.
61 Carrol ED, Thomson AP, Shears P, Gray SJ, Kaczmarski EB, Hart CA. **2000**, Performance characteristics of the polymerase chain reaction assay to confirm clinical meningococcal disease, *Arch Dis Child* 83, 271–273.
62 Corless CE, Guiver M, Borrow R, Edwards-Jones V, Fox AJ, Kaczmarski EB. **2001**, Simultaneous DETECTION of Neisseria meningitidis, Haemophilus influenzae, and Streptococcus pneumoniae in suspected cases of meningitis and septicemia using real-time PCR, *J Clin Microbiol* 39, 1553–1558.
63 Newcombe J, Cartwright K, Palmer WH, McFadden J. **1996**, PCR of peripheral blood for diagnosis of meningococcal disease, *J Clin Microbiol* 34, 1637–1640.
64 Guiver M, Borrow R, Marsh J, Gray SJ, Kaczmarski EB, Howells D, et al. **2000**, Evaluation of the Applied Biosystems automated Taqman polymerase chain reaction system for the detection of

meningococcal DNA, *FEMS Immunol Med Microbiol* 28, 173–179.

65 Taha MK. **2000**, Simultaneous approach for nonculture PCR-based identification and serogroup prediction of Neisseria meningitidis, *J Clin Microbiol* 38, 855–857.

66 Knight AI, Ni H, Cartwright KA, McFadden JJ. **1992**, Identification and characterization of a novel insertion sequence, IS1106, downstream of the porA gene in B15 Neisseria meningitidis, *Mol Microbiol* 6, 1565–1573.

67 Ni H, Knight AI, Cartwright K, Palmer WH, McFadden J. **1992**, Polymerase chain reaction for diagnosis of meningococcal meningitis, *Lancet* 340, 1432–1434.

68 Borrow R, Guiver M, Sadler F, Kaczmarski EB, Fox AJ. **1998**, False positive diagnosis of meningococcal infection by the IS1106 PCR ELISA, *FEMS Microbiol Lett* 162, 215–218.

69 McLaughlin GL, Howe DK, Biggs DR, Smith AR, Ludwinski P, Fox BC, et al. **1993**, Amplification of rDNA loci to detect and type Neisseria meningitidis and other eubacteria, *Mol Cell Probes* 7, 7–17.

70 Radstrom P, Backman A, Qian N, Kragsbjerg P, Pahlson C, Olcen P. **1994**, Detection of bacterial DNA in cerebrospinal fluid by an assay for simultaneous detection of Neisseria meningitidis, Haemophilus influenzae, and streptococci using a seminested PCR strategy, *J Clin Microbiol* 32, 2738–2744.

71 Kotilainen P, Jalava J, Meurman O, Lehtonen OP, Rintala E, Seppälä OP, et al. **1998**, Diagnosis of meningococcal meningitis by broad-range bacterial PCR with cerebrospinal fluid [in process citation]. *J Clin Microbiol* 36, 2205–2209.

72 Seward RJ, Towner KJ. **2000**, Evaluation of a PCR-immunoassay technique for detection of Neisseria meningitidis in cerebrospinal fluid and peripheral blood, *J Med Microbiol* 49, 451–456.

73 Greisen K, Loeffelholz M, Purohit A, Leong D. **1994**, PCR primers and probes for the 16S rRNA gene of most species of pathogenic bacteria, including bacteria found in cerebrospinal fluid, *J Clin Microbiol* 32, 335–351.

74 Ley BE, Linton CJ, Longhurst S, Jalal H, Millar MR. **1997**, Eubacterial approach to the diagnosis of bacterial infection, *Arch Dis Child* 77, 148–149.

75 Kristiansen BE, Ask E, Jenkins A, Fermer C, Radstrom P, Skold O. **1991**, Rapid diagnosis of meningococcal meningitis by polymerase chain reaction, *Lancet* 337, 1568–1569.

76 Saunders NB, Zollinger WD, Rao VB. **1993**, A rapid and sensitive PCR strategy employed for amplification and sequencing of porA from a single colony-forming unit of Neisseria meningitidis, *Gene* 137, 153–162.

77 Saunders NB, Shoemaker DR, Brandt BL, Zollinger WD. **1997**, Confirmation of suspicious cases of meningococcal meningitis by PCR and enzyme-linked immunosorbent assay, *J Clin Microbiol* 35, 3215–3219.

78 Caugant DA, Høiby EA, Frøholm LO, Brandtzg P. **1996**, Polymerase chain reaction for case ascertainment of meningococcal meningitis: application to the cerebrospinal fluids collected in the course of the Norwegian meningococcal serogroup B protection trial, *Scand J Infect Dis* 28, 149–153.

79 de Filippis I, do Nascimento CR, Clementino MB, Sereno AB, Rebelo C, Souza NN, et al. **2005**, Rapid detection of Neisseria meningitidis in cerebrospinal fluid by one-step polymerase chain reaction of the nspA gene, *Diagn Microbiol Infect Dis* 51, 85–90.

80 Borrow R, Claus H, Chaudhry U, Guiver M, Kaczmarski EB, Frosch M, et al. **1998**, siaD PCR ELISA for confirmation and identification of serogroup Y and W135 meningococcal infections, *FEMS Microbiol Lett* 159, 209–214.

81 Borrow R, Claus H, Guiver M, Smart L, Jones DM, Kaczmarski EB, et al. **1997**, Non-culture diagnosis and serogroup determination of meningococcal B and C infection by a sialyltransferase (siaD) PCR ELISA, *Epidemiol Infect* 118, 111–117.

82 Whiley DM, Crisante ME, Syrmis MW, Mackay IM, Sloots TP. **2003**, Detection of Neisseria Meningitidis in clinical samples by a duplex real-time PCR targeting

the porA and ctrA genes, *Mol Diagn* 7, 141–145.
83 Frosch M, Muller D, Bousset K, Muller A. **1992**, Conserved outer membrane protein of Neisseria meningitidis involved in capsule expression, *Infect Immun* 60, 798–803.
84 Orvelid P, Backman A, Olcen P. **1999**, PCR identification of the group A Neisseria meningitidis gene in cerebrospinal fluid, *Scand J Infect Dis* 31, 481–483.
85 Swartley JS, Liu LJ, Miller YK, Martin LE, Edupuganti S, Stephens DS. **1998**, Characterization of the gene cassette required for biosynthesis of the (alpha16)-linked N-acetyl-D-mannosamine-1-phosphate capsule of serogroup A Neisseria meningitidis, *J Bacteriol* 180, 1533–1539.
86 Rennick G, Shann F, de Campo J. **1993**, Cerebral herniation during bacterial meningitis in children, *BMJ* 306, 953–955.
87 Dezateux CA, Dinwiddie R, Helms P, Matthew DJ. **1986**, Recognition and early management of Reye's syndrome, *Arch Dis Child* 61, 647–651.
88 Berkowitz ID, Berkowitz FE, Newton C, Willoughby R, Ackerman AD. **1996**, Meningitis, infectious encephalopathies and other central nervous sytem infections, in *Textbook of Pediatric Intensive Care*, ed. Rogers MC, Williams and Wilkins, Baltimore, p. 1039–1090.
89 Anon. **1997**, Relative contraindications to lumbar puncture, in *Advanced Paediatric Life Support – The Practical Approach*, ed. Group ALS, BMJ Publishing Group, London, p. 27.
90 Nadel S. **2001**, Lumbar puncture should not be performed in meningococcal disease, *Arch Dis Child* 84, 375.
91 Pollard AJ, Britto J, Nadel S, DeMunter C, Habibi P, Levin M. **1999**, Emergency management of meningococcal disease, *Arch Dis Child* 80, 290–296.
92 Welch SB, Nadel S. **2003**, Treatment of meningococcal infection, *Arch Dis Child* 88, 608–614.
93 Kneen R, Solomon T, Appleton R. **2002**, The role of lumbar puncture in children with suspected central nervous system infection, *BMC Pediatr* 2, 8.
94 Heyderman RS, Robb SA, Kendall BE, Levin M. **1992**, Does computed tomography have a role in the evaluation of complicated acute bacterial meningitis in childhood? *Dev Med Child Neurol* 34, 870–875.
95 Hasbun R, Abrahams J, Jekel J, Quagliarello VJ. **2001**, Computed tomography of the head before lumbar puncture in adults with suspected meningitis, *N Engl J Med* 345, 1727–1733.
96 Mercier JC, Beaufils F, Hartmann JF, Azema D. **1988**, Hemodynamic patterns of meningococcal shock in children, *Crit Care Med* 16, 27–33.
97 Oragui EE, Nadel S, Kyd P, Levin M. **2000**, Increased excretion of urinary glycosaminoglycans in meningococcal septicemia and their relationship to proteinuria, *Crit Care Med* 28, 3002–3008.
98 Tobin JR, Wetzel RC. **1996**, Shock and multiorgan failure, in. *Textbook of Pediatric Intensive Care*, ed. Rogers MC, Williams and Wilkins, Baltimore, p. 555–605.
99 Pathan N, Nadel S, Levin M. **2000**, Pathophysiology and management of meningococcal septicaemia, *J R Coll Physicians Lond* 34, 436–444.
100 Faust SN, Levin M, Harrison OB, Goldin RD, Lockhart MS, Kondaveeti S, et al. **2001**, Dysfunction of endothelial protein C activation in severe meningococcal sepsis, *N Engl J Med* 345, 408–416.
101 Parrillo JE. **1993**, Pathogenetic mechanisms of septic shock, *N Engl J Med* 328, 1471–1477.
102 Pathan N, Sandiford C, Harding SE, Levin M. **2002**, Characterization of a myocardial depressant factor in meningococcal septicemia, *Crit Care Med* 30, 2191–2198.
103 Pathan N, Hemingway CA, Alizadeh AA, Stephens AC, Boldrick JC, Oragui EE, et al. **2004**, Role of interleukin 6 in myocardial dysfunction of meningococcal septic shock, *Lancet* 363, 203–209.
104 Kumar A, Thota V, Dee L, Olson J, Uretz E, Parrillo JE. **1996**, Tumor necrosis factor alpha and interleukin 1beta are responsible for in vitro myocardial cell depression induced by human septic shock serum, *J Exp Med* 183, 949–958.

105 Thiru Y, Pathan N, Bignall S, Habibi P, Levin M. A myocardial cytotoxic process is involved in the cardiac dysfunction of meningococcal septic shock. Crit Care Med 2000;28(8), 2979–2983.

106 Carcillo JA, Davis AL, Zaritsky A. **1991**, Role of early fluid resuscitation in pediatric septic shock, *JAMA* 266, 1242–1245.

107 Hodge D. **1985**, Intraosseous infusions: a review, *Pediatr Emerg Care* 1, 215–218.

108 Dula DJ, Lutz P, Vogel MF, Weaver BN. **1985**, Rapid flow rates for the resuscitation of hypovolemic shock, *Ann Emerg Med* 14, 303–306.

109 Carcillo JA, Fields AI. **2002**, Clinical practice parameters for hemodynamic support of pediatric and neonatal patients in septic shock, *Crit Care Med* 30, 1365–1378.

110 Ledingham IM, McArdle CS. **1978**, Prospective study of the treatment of septic shock, *Lancet* 1, 1194–1197.

111 Cochrane Injuries Group Albumin Reviewers **1998**, Human albumin administration in critically ill patients: systematic review of randomised controlled trials, *Br Med J* 317, 225–240.

112 Nadel S, De Munter C, Britto J, Levin M, Habibi P. 1998, Albumin: saint or sinner, *Arch Dis Child* 79, 384–385.

113 Choi PT, Yip G, Quinonez LG, Cook DJ. **1999**, Crystalloids vs. colloids in fluid resuscitation: a systematic review, *Crit Care Med* 27, 200–210.

114 Maitland K, Pamba A, English M, Peshu N, Marsh K, Newton C, et al. **2005**, Randomized trial of volume expansion with albumin or saline in children with severe malaria, preliminary evidence of albumin benefit, *Clin Infect Dis* 40, 538–545.

115 Finfer S, Bellomo R, Boyce N, French J, Myburgh J, Norton R. **2004**, A comparison of albumin and saline for fluid resuscitation in the intensive care unit, *N Engl J Med* 350, 2247–2256.

116 Ernest D, Belzberg AS, Dodek PM. **1999**, Distribution of normal saline and 5% albumin infusions in septic patients, *Crit Care Med* 1999; 27, 46–50.

117 Hussain SN, Roussos C. **1985**, Distribution of respiratory muscle and organ blood flow during endotoxic shock in dogs, *J Appl Physiol* 59, 1802–1808.

118 Yamamoto LG, Yim GK, Britten AG. **1990**, Rapid sequence anesthesia induction for emergency intubation, *Pediatr Emerg Care* 6, 200–213.

119 Khilnani P. **1992**, Electrolyte abnormalities in critically ill children, *Crit Care Med* 20, 241–250.

120 van den Berghe G, Wouters P, Weekers F, Verwaest C, Bruyninckx F, Schetz M, et al. **2001**, Intensive insulin therapy in the critically ill patients, *N Engl J Med* 345, 1359–1367.

121 Bernard GR, Vincent JL, Laterre PF, LaRosa SP, Dhainaut JF, Lopez-Rodriguez A, et al. **2001**, Efficacy and safety of recombinant human activated protein C for severe sepsis, *N Engl J Med* 344, 699–709.

122 de Kleijn ED, de Groot R, Hack CE, Mulder PG, Engl W, Moritz B, et al. **2003**, Activation of protein C following infusion of protein C concentrate in children with severe meningococcal sepsis and purpura fulminans: a randomized, double-blinded, placebo-controlled, dose-finding study, *Crit Care Med* 31, 1839–1847.

123 Vincent JL, Nadel S, Kutsogiannis DJ, Gibney RT, Yan SB, Wyss VL, et al. **2005**, Drotrecogin alfa (activated) in patients with severe sepsis presenting with purpura fulminans, meningitis, or meningococcal disease: a retrospective analysis of patients enrolled in recent clinical studies, *Crit Care* 9, R331–R343.

124 Mauger DC. **1971**, Hypokalaemia as a consistent feature of fulminant meningococcal septicaemia, *Aust Paediatr J* 7, 84–86.

125 Britto J, Nadel S, Habibi P, Levin M. **1996**, Hypokalaemia in meningococcal disease, *Intensive Care Med* 22, S021.

126 Gauthier B, Trachtman H, Di Carmine F, Urivetsky M, Tobash J, Chasalow F, et al. **1990**, Hypocalcemia and hypercalcitoninemia in critically ill children, *Crit Care Med* 18, 1215–1219.

127 Fuhrman BP. **1989**, Hypocalcemia and critical illness in children, *J Pediatr* 114, 990–991.
128 Chernow B. **1990**, Calcium: does it have a therapeutic role in sepsis? *Crit Care Med* 18, 895–896.
129 Goldhill DR. **1997**, Calcium and magnesium, *Care Crit Ill* 13, 112–115.
130 Zaloga GP, Washburn D, Black KW, Prielipp R. **1993**, Human sepsis increases lymphocyte intracellular calcium, *Crit Care Med* 21, 196–202.
131 Steinhorn DM, Sweeney MF, Layman LK. **1990**, Pharmacodynamic response to ionized calcium during acute sepsis, *Crit Care Med* 18, 851–857.
132 Whang R, Whang DD, Ryan MP. **1992**, Refractory potassium repletion. A consequence of magnesium deficiency, *Arch Intern Med* 152, 40–45.
133 Hamill-Ruth RJ, McGory R. **1996**, Magnesium repletion and its effect on potassium homeostasis in critically ill adults: results of a double-blind, randomized, controlled trial, *Crit Care Med* 24, 38–45.
134 Edwards R, Mitchell M, Twaddle S. **1998**, Hypophosphataemia in the critically ill patient – aetiology and management, *Care Crit Ill* 14, 267–270.
135 Weisinger JR, Bellorin-Font E. **1998**, Magnesium and phosphorus, *Lancet* 352, 391–396.
136 Britto J, Nadel S, Habibi P, Levin M. **1995**, Gastrointestinal perforation complicating meningococcal disease, *Pediatr Infect Dis J* 14, 393–394.
137 Davies MS, Nadel S, Habibi P, Levin M, Hunt DM. **2000**, The orthopaedic management of peripheral ischaemia in meningococcal septicaemia in children, *J Bone Joint Surg Br* 82, 383–386.
138 Odio CM, Faingezicht I, Paris M, Nassar M, Baltodano A, Rogers J, et al. **1991**, The beneficial effects of early dexamethasone administration in infants and children with bacterial meningitis, *N Engl J Med* 324, 1525–1531.
139 Kim KS, Wass CA, Cross AS. **1997**, Blood–brain barrier permeability during the development of experimental bacterial meningitis in the rat, *Exp Neurol* 145, 253–257.
140 Kirkham FJ. **2001**, Non-traumatic coma in children, *Arch Dis Child* 85, 303–312.
141 Poss WB, Brockmeyer DL, Clay B, Dean JM. **1996**, Pathophysiology and management of the intracranial vault, in *Textbook of Pediatric Intensive Care*, ed. Rogers MC, Williams and Wilkins, Baltimore, p. 645–665.
142 Sarnaik AP, Lieh-Lai MW. **1993**, Transporting the neurologically compromised child, *Pediatr Clin N Am* 40, 337–354.
143 Duke T. **1998**, Fluid management of bacterial meningitis in developing countries, *Arch Dis Child* 79, 181–185.
144 McIntyre PB, Berkey CS, King SM, Schaad UB, Kilpi T, Kanra GY, et al. **1997**, Dexamethasone as adjunctive therapy in bacterial meningitis, A meta-analysis of randomized clinical trials since 1988, *JAMA* 278, 925–931.
145 van de Beek D, de Gans J, McIntyre P, Prasad K. **2004**, Steroids in adults with acute bacterial meningitis: a systematic review, *Lancet Infect Dis* 4, 139–143.
146 Schaad UB, Kaplan SL, McCracken GH, Jr. **1995**, Steroid therapy for bacterial meningitis, *Clin Infect Dis* 20, 685–690.
147 Schaad UB, Lips U, Gnehm HE, Blumberg A, Heinzer I, Wedgwood J. **1993**, Dexamethasone therapy for bacterial meningitis in children, Swiss meningitis study group, *Lancet* 342, 457–461.
148 Feigin RD, Pearlman E. **1998**, Bacterial meningitis beyond the neonatal period, in *Textbook of Pediatric Infectious Diseases*, 4th edn, ed. Feigin RD, Cherry JD, WB Saunders, Philadelphia, p. 400–429.
149 Bone RC, Fisher CJ, Jr, Clemmer TP, Slotman GJ, Metz CA, Balk RA. **1987**, A controlled clinical trial of high-dose methylprednisolone in the treatment of severe sepsis and septic shock, *N Engl J Med* 317, 653–658.
150 Lefering R, Neugebauer EA. **1995**, Steroid controversy in sepsis and septic shock: a meta-analysis, *Crit Care Med* 23, 1294–1303.
151 Hatherill M, Tibby SM, Hilliard T, Turner C, Murdoch IA. **1999**, Adrenal

insufficiency in septic shock, *Arch Dis Child* 80, 51–55.
152 van Woensel JB, Biezeveld MH, Alders AM, Eerenberg AJ, Endert E, Hack EC, et al. **2001**, Adrenocorticotropic hormone and cortisol levels in relation to inflammatory response and disease severity in children with meningococcal disease, *J Infect Dis* 184, 1532–1537.
153 Roine I, Ledermann W, Foncea LM, Banfi A, Cohen J, Peltola H. **2000**, Randomized trial of four vs. seven days of ceftriaxone treatment for bacterial meningitis in children with rapid initial recovery, *Pediatr Infect Dis J* 19, 219–222.
154 Scholz H, Hofmann T, Noack R, Edwards DJ, Stoeckel K. **1998**, Prospective comparison of ceftriaxone and cefotaxime for the short-term treatment of bacterial meningitis in children, *Chemotherapy* 44, 142–147.
155 Martin E, Hohl P, Guggi T, Kayser FH, Fernex M. **1990**, Short course single daily ceftriaxone monotherapy for acute bacterial meningitis in children: results of a Swiss multicenter study, Part I: Clinical results, *Infection* 18, 70–77.
156 Kavaliotis J, Manios SG, Kansouzidou A, Danielidis V. **1989**, Treatment of childhood bacterial meningitis with ceftriaxone once daily: open, prospective, randomized, comparative study of short-course versus standard-length therapy, *Chemotherapy* 35, 296–303.
157 Nathan N, Borel T, Djibo A, Evans D, Djibo S, Corty JF, et al. **2005**, Ceftriaxone as effective as long-acting chloramphenicol in short-course treatment of meningococcal meningitis during epidemics: a randomised non-inferiority study, *Lancet* 366, 308–313.
158 Britto J, DeMunter C, Habibi P. **1996**, Specialized pediatric interhospital transfer, in *Intensive Care in Childhood*, ed. Tibbrel D, Van der Voort E, Springer-Verlag, Berlin, p. 146–158.
159 Levin M, Quint PA, Goldstein B, Barton P, Bradley JS, Shemie SD, et al. **2000**, Recombinant bactericidal/permeability-increasing protein (rBPI21) as adjunctive treatment for children with severe meningococcal sepsis: a randomised trial, rBPI21 Meningococcal sepsis study group, *Lancet 2000* 356, 961–967.
160 Giroir BP, Scannon PJ, Levin M. **2001**, Bactericidal/permeability-increasing protein – lessons learned from the phase III, randomized, clinical trial of rBPI21 for adjunctive treatment of children with severe meningococcemia, *Crit Care Med* 29[Suppl], S130–S135.
161 Derkx B, Wittes J, McCloskey R. **1999**, Randomized, placebo-controlled trial of HA-1A, a human monoclonal antibody to endotoxin, in children with meningococcal septic shock, European pediatric meningococcal septic shock trial study group, *Clin Infect Dis* 28, 770–777.
162 Polderman KH, Girbes AR. **2004**, Drug intervention trials in sepsis: divergent results, *Lancet* 363, 1721–1723.
163 Annane D, Bellissant E, Cavaillon JM. **2005**, Septic shock, *Lancet* 365, 63–78.
164 Giroir BP. **2003**, Recombinant human activated protein C for the treatment of severe sepsis: is there a role in pediatrics? *Curr Opin Pediatr* 15, 92–96.
165 U.S. Food and Drug Administration **2005**, Safety alert: xigris [drotrecogin alfa(activated)], http://www.fda.gov/medwatch/safety/2005/Xigris_dearhcp_4-21-05.pdf.
166 Annane D, Sebille V, Charpentier C, Bollaert PE, Francois B, Korach JM, et al. **2002**, Effect of treatment with low doses of hydrocortisone and fludrocortisone on mortality in patients with septic shock, *JAMA* 288, 862–871.
167 Cronin L, Cook DJ, Carlet J, Heyland DK, King D, Lansang MA, et al. **1995**, Corticosteroid treatment for sepsis: a critical appraisal and meta-analysis of the literature, *Crit Care Med* 23, 1430–1439.
168 van Deuren M, Brandtzæg P, van der Meer JW. **2000**, Update on meningococcal disease with emphasis on pathogenesis and clinical management, *Clin Microbiol Rev* 13, 144–166.
169 Zenz W, Zoehrer B, Levin M, Fanconi S, Hatzis TD, Knight G, et al. **2004**, Use of recombinant tissue plasminogen activator in children with meningococcal purpura fulminans: a retro-

spective study, *Crit Care Med* 32, 1777–1780.

170 Smirnova I, Mann N, Dols A, Derkx HH, Hibberd ML, Levin M, et al. **2003**, Assay of locus-specific genetic load implicates rare Toll-like receptor 4 mutations in meningococcal susceptibility, *Proc Natl Acad Sci USA* 100, 6075–6080.

171 Read RC, Pullin J, Gregory S, Borrow R, Kaczmarski EB, di Giovine FS, et al. **2001**, A functional polymorphism of toll-like receptor 4 is not associated with likelihood or severity of meningococcal disease, *J Infect Dis* 184, 640–642.

172 Hubacek JA, Stuber F, Frohlich D, Book M, Wetegrove S, Ritter M, et al. **2001**, Gene variants of the bactericidal/permeability increasing protein and lipopolysaccharide binding protein in sepsis patients: gender-specific genetic predisposition to sepsis, *Crit Care Med* 29, 557–561.

173 Harding D, Baines PB, Brull D, Vassiliou V, Ellis I, Hart A, et al. **2002**, Severity of meningococcal disease in children and the angiotensin-converting enzyme insertion/deletion polymorphism, *Am J Respir Crit Care Med* 165, 1103–1106.

174 Hibberd ML, Sumiya M, Summerfield JA, Booy R, Levin M. **1999**, Association of variants of the gene for mannose-binding lectin with susceptibility to meningococcal disease, Meningococcal research group, *Lancet* 353, 1049–1053.

175 Fijen CA, Kuijper EJ, te Bulte M, Daha MR, Dankert J. **1999**, Assessment of complement deficiency in patients with meningococcal disease in the Netherlands [in process citation], *Clin Infect Dis* 28, 98–105.

176 Biesma DH, Hannema AJ, van Velzen-Blad H, Mulder L, van Zwieten R, Kluijt I, et al. **2001**, A family with complement factor D deficiency, *J Clin Invest* 108, 233–240.

177 van der Pol WL, Huizinga TW, Vidarsson G, van der Linden MW, Jansen MD, Keijsers V, et al. **2001**, Relevance of Fcgamma receptor and interleukin-10 polymorphisms for meningococcal disease, *J Infect Dis* 184, 1548–1555.

178 Domingo P, Muniz-Diaz E, Baraldes MA, Arilla M, Barquet N, Pericas R, et al. **2002**, Associations between Fc gamma receptor IIA polymorphisms and the risk and prognosis of meningococcal disease, *Am J Med* 112, 19–25.

179 Bredius RG, Derkx BH, Fijen CA, de Wit TP, de Haas M, Weening RS, et al. **1994**, Fc gamma receptor IIa (CD32) polymorphism in fulminant meningococcal septic shock in children, *J Infect Dis* 170, 848–853.

180 Platonov AE, Kuijper EJ, Vershinina IV, Shipulin GA, Westerdaal N, Fijen CA, et al. **1998**, Meningococcal disease and polymorphism of FcgammaRIIa (CD32) in late complement component-deficient individuals, *Clin Exp Immunol* 111, 97–101.

181 Fijen CA, Bredius RG, Kuijper EJ. **1993**, Polymorphism of IgG Fc receptors in meningococcal disease, *Ann Intern Med* 119, 636.

182 Fijen CA, Bredius RG, Kuijper EJ, Out TA, De Haas M, De Wit AP, et al. **2000**, The role of Fcgamma receptor polymorphisms and C3 in the immune defence against Neisseria meningitidis in complement-deficient individuals, *Clin Exp Immunol* 120, 338–345.

183 Kondaveeti S, Hibberd ML, Levin M. **1999**, The insertion/deletion polymorphism in the t-PA gene does not significantly affect outcome of meningococcal disease [letter], *Thromb Haemost* 82, 161–162.

184 Hermans PW, Hibberd ML, Booy R, Daramola O, Hazelzet JA, de Groot R, et al. **1999**, 4G/5G promoter polymorphism in the plasminogen-activator-inhibitor-1 gene and outcome of meningococcal disease, Meningococcal research group, *Lancet* 354, 556–560.

185 Westendorp RG, Hottenga JJ, Slagboom PE. **1999**, Variation in plasminogen-activator-inhibitor-1 gene and risk of meningococcal septic shock, *Lancet* 354, 561–563.

186 Haralambous E, Hibberd ML, Hermans PW, Ninis N, Nadel S, Levin M. **2003**, Role of functional plasminogen-activator-inhibitor-1 4G/5G promoter polymorphism in susceptibility, sever-

ity, and outcome of meningococcal disease in Caucasian children, *Crit Care Med* 31, 2788–2793.

187 Kondaveeti S, Hibberd ML, Booy R, Nadel S, Levin M. **1999**, Effect of the Factor V Leiden mutation on the severity of meningococcal disease, *Pediatr Infect Dis J* 18, 893–896.

188 Nadel S, Newport MJ, Booy R, Levin M. **1996**, Variation in the tumor necrosis factor-alpha gene promoter region may be associated with death from meningococcal disease, *J Infect Dis* 174, 878–880.

189 Westendorp RG, Langermans JA, Huizinga TW, Elouali AH, Verweij CL, Boomsma DI, et al. **1997**, Genetic influence on cytokine production and fatal meningococcal disease, *Lancet* 349, 170–173.

190 Read RC, Camp NJ, di Giovine FS, Borrow R, Kaczmarski EB, Chaudhary AG, et al. **2000**, An interleukin-1 genotype is associated with fatal outcome of meningococcal disease, *J Infect Dis* 182, 1557–1560.

191 Stuber F, Petersen M, Bokelmann F, Schade U. **1996**, A genomic polymorphism within the tumor necrosis factor locus influences plasma tumor necrosis factor-alpha concentrations and outcome of patients with severe sepsis, *Crit Care Med* 24, 381–384.

192 Fang XM, Schroder S, Hoeft A, Stuber F. **1999**, Comparison of two polymorphisms of the interleukin-1 gene family: interleukin-1 receptor antagonist polymorphism contributes to susceptibility to severe sepsis, *Crit Care Med* 27, 1330–1334.

193 Balding J, Healy CM, Livingstone WJ, White B, Mynett-Johnson L, Cafferkey M, et al. **2003**, Genomic polymorphic profiles in an Irish population with meningococcaemia: is it possible to predict severity and outcome of disease? *Genes Immun* 4, 533–640.

194 Schluter B, Raufhake C, Erren M, Schotte H, Kipp F, Rust S, et al. **2002**, Effect of the interleukin-6 promoter polymorphism (–174 G/C) on the incidence and outcome of sepsis, *Crit Care Med* 30, 32–37.

195 Carrol ED, Mobbs KJ, Thomson AP, Hart CA. **2002**, Variable number tandem repeat polymorphism of the interleukin-1 receptor antagonist gene in meningococcal disease, *Clin Infect Dis* 35, 495–497.

196 Read RC, Cannings C, Naylor SC, Timms JM, Maheswaran R, Borrow R, et al. Variation within genes encoding interleukin-1 and the interleukin-1 receptor antagonist influence the severity of meningococcal disease. Ann Intern Med 2003;138(7), 534–541.

197 McCloskey RV, Straube RC, Sanders C, Smith SM, Smith CR. **1994**, Treatment of septic shock with human monoclonal antibody HA-1A. A randomized, double-blind, placebo-controlled trial, CHESS trial study group, *Ann Intern Med* 121, 1–5.

198 Cohen J, Carlet J. **1996**, INTERSEPT: an international, multicenter, placebo-controlled trial of monoclonal antibody to human tumor necrosis factor-alpha in patients with sepsis, International sepsis trial study group, *Crit Care Med* 24, 1431–1440.

199 Opal S, Laterre PF, Abraham E, Francois B, Wittebole X, Lowry S, et al. **2004**, Recombinant human platelet-activating factor acetylhydrolase for treatment of severe sepsis: results of a phase III, multicenter, randomized, double-blind, placebo-controlled, clinical trial, *Crit Care Med* 32, 332–341.

200 Warren BL, Eid A, Singer P, Pillay SS, Carl P, Novak I, et al. **2001**, Caring for the critically ill patient. High-dose antithrombin III in severe sepsis: a randomized controlled trial, *JAMA* 286, 1869–1878.

201 Abraham E, Reinhart K, Opal S, Demeyer I, Doig C, Rodriguez AL, et al. **2003**, Efficacy and safety of tifacogin (recombinant tissue factor pathway inhibitor) in severe sepsis: a randomized controlled trial, *JAMA* 290, 238–247.

23
Public Health Management

James Stuart

23.1
Introduction

Dealing with the consequences of meningococcal disease is one of the most challenging situations faced by public health physicians. On diagnosis of a case, especially if the patient is in intensive care or has died, the family and friends are likely to be highly distressed and frightened. There is a need to reassure these contacts of the low risk of further cases, whilst at the same time taking immediate action by giving antibiotic prophylaxis to reduce that risk. Defining a line between those who receive and do not receive prophylaxis is a matter of judgement that may not readily be accepted by those who do not receive antibiotics and who consider themselves at risk. Although immediate action may reduce the risk in those individuals, these urgent public health measures have minimal impact on overall disease incidence as the great majority of cases have no direct connection to any other case [1].

Another issue is that many areas of public health policy, especially relating to antibiotic prophylaxis, lack consistency between and within countries. This can partly be attributed to a lack of evidence to underpin such policies, but recent studies can assist rational decision-making [2, 3].

A major area of recent change in evidence-based policy has been the development and introduction of conjugated vaccines. Conjugated C vaccines have been introduced in the UK, Ireland, Spain and the Netherlands with dramatic effect, not only on disease but also on carriage with consequent herd immunity [4, 5]. Conjugate A vaccines are being developed for application in the African "meningitis belt".

This chapter will focus on the main lines of public health action before and after cases occur. Developments in vaccines and issues around vaccine policy will be addressed in other chapters.

Handbook of Meningococcal Disease. Infection Biology, Vaccination, Clinical Management.
Edited by M. Frosch and M.C.J. Maiden

ISBN: 3-527-31260-9

23.2
Action Before a Case

23.2.1
Public and Professional Awareness

The most important public health action before cases is to raise awareness among the public and also among health professionals. Information should be made available on the main signs and symptoms of meningococcal disease and the importance of seeking early medical attention. As most countries have regular annual fluctuations in seasonal incidence, a good time to do this is at the start of the "high incidence" season each year.

Pressing a glass on the rash is a useful lay method of identifying a non-blanching rash, by inference hemorraghic. Although rashes in meningococcal disease are not necessarily hemorrhagic, especially early in the course of disease [6], this is a simple and practical test that can be applied by parents and may save lives.

Helpful information is available from UK charity websites (e.g. Meningitis Trust, at http://www.meningitis-trust.org.uk, Meningitis Research Foundation, at http://www.meningitis.org).

23.2.2
Promoting Early Treatment to Physicians

Invasive meningooccal disease has a high case fatality. Factors influencing risk of death include age, clinical manifestation, characteristics of organism and case management. In the early 20th century before serum therapy became available, about 70% of cases of invasive disease died. Currently in countries with well funded health care systems, fatality rates usually vary between 5% and 10% [7]. Reduction in case fatality attributed to improved clinical management in paediatric care has been reported from a tertiary care referral center [8].

Since meningococcal disease often progresses very rapidly, it is not surprising that delays in starting antibiotic treatment in hospital have an adverse effect on outcome. However, whether giving antibiotics before admission to hospital improves outcome of meningococcal disease remains theoretical; and studies assessing its effectiveness show inconsistent results [9, 10]. The absence of consensus is reflected in differing policies on preadmission antibiotic treatment. Several European countries advise primary care physicians to give parenteral antibiotics to cases of suspected meningococcal disease before transfer to hospital, others do not.

In a systematic review that included 12 observational studies comparing outcome (death) in those given and not given parenteral antibiotics by injection before admission to hospital, most found higher risk of dying if not treated (Hahne S., unpublished data), but a minority of studies found an opposite effect. There was a lower proportion of patients given antibiotics in studies suggesting an adverse effect. One explanation for a link to adverse outcome is that those severely ill were more likely to receive treatment and more likely to die with or without early treatment than those who were less severely ill. This can be regarded as confounding by indication. Stratification by severity in one study reduced the association with an adverse outcome [10], but such stratification cannot be expected to adjust for all clinical confounders such as speed of progression of illness. Another explanation is that those severely ill were indeed adversely affected by antibiotic treatment. The main concern is that preadmission antibiotic treatment could produce hemodynamic instability from release of endotoxins. This is not supported by research to date [11].

Fear of anaphylactic reactions to benzylpenicillin could prevent general practitioners from treating suspected cases, but genuine anaphylaxis is rare and is estimated to occur only in about 1 in 7000–25 000 cases [12]. Concerns have been raised that preadmission antibiotic treatment may lower the proportion of cases that can subsequently be diagnosed by microbiological tests [13] and delay the start of appropriate in-hospital treatment. Early antibiotic treatment reduces the yield from blood culture but has less effect on the sensitivity of DNA detection tests (see Section 23.3.1).

Further studies in which data on severity of disease, disease evolution and subsequent hospital treatment are collected could allow improved adjustment for confounding. However, since severity of disease and disease evolution are difficult to measure objectively when reviewing information obtained retrospectively from primary care settings, adequate adjustment for these factors may be impossible. Randomized controlled trials investigating the effect of preadmission antibiotic treatment on the outcome of meningococcal disease have not been performed, are probably not feasible and may be unethical.

In the absence of good evidence, it is logical to start treatment with systemic antibiotics as soon as a diagnosis is suspected and, where possible, before admission to hospital. The applicability of this recommendation depends on how patients with meningococcal disease enter the health care system and whether domiciliary visits by general practitioners or emergency services allow the delivery of antibiotics.

23.2.3 Surveillance and Response Systems

Public health departments should ensure that policies are in place so that cases are referred early to hospital, reported promptly, and investigated appropriately. An efficient system is needed for contact tracing, prophylaxis and giving out information. Comprehensive information on cases should be gathered to contribute to local public health management and surveillance. The data set should include epidemiological, laboratory and clinical information (Table 23.1).

Table 23.1 Surveillance dataset.

Subject under surveillance	Data required
Case	Name, address, contact details, date of birth, ethnic group, occupation/workplace, school/college/nursery attended, dates/times of disease onset, hospital admission and reporting, antibiotics given prior to admission, clinical features, whether part of cluster, clinical outcome, vaccination status, name of hospital/ward, name of medical consultant, dates and results of specimens
Contacts	Names, addresses and contact details, antibiotics/vaccine/information given and by whom, primary care physician
Notifier	Name, address and occupation

23.3 After a Case

23.3.1 Laboratory Investigation

Identification and characterization of meningococci causing infection provides important information to assist the public health response. Whilst traditional microbiological techniques remain an important part of investigating suspected cases, molecular methods provide important new tools for diagnosis and further characterisation of strains [14].

Blood samples for culture and polymerase chain reaction (PCR) testing are both recommended where available (Table 23.2). The chance of obtaining laboratory confirmation is increased by taking samples at the earliest available opportunity. Antibiotics before admission reduce yield from blood culture [15] but

Table 23.2 Recommended laboratory tests.

Test	Reason for test
Strongly recommended	Blood for culture. Blood for PCR (EDTA or other unclotted blood specimen). CSF for microscopy, culture, PCR (if condition of patient stable and no sign of raised intracranial pressure). Aspirate from other sterile sites suspected of being infected (e.g. joints) for microscopy, culture, PCR.
Optional	Paired sera (on admission and 2–6 weeks later) for antibody tests. Serum for Latex agglutination. Pharyngeal swab (pernasal if patient unable to cooperate) for culture.

have much less effect on sensitivity of PCR. When meningitis is present, cerebrospinal fluid (CSF) offers the best chance of yielding an organism for culture: meningococcal DNA can be found in the CSF up to 96 h after commencing antibiotics [16]. Lumbar puncture should not be performed until the patient's condition has been stabilized and appropriate assessment has been made to exclude raised intracranial pressure. Latex agglutination on serum, CSF or urine may still have a place, though less sensitive unless enhanced by ultrasound [17].

23.3.2 Prophylaxis: Risk

23.3.2.1 Close Contacts

About 97% of cases are sporadic [1]. Although the risk to contacts is low, the highest absolute and relative risk is to people who live in the same household as a case of meningococcal disease [18]. The risk is highest in the first 7 days after a case and falls rapidly during the following weeks. If prophylaxis is not given, the absolute risk to an individual in the same household 1–30 days after an index case is from about 1:300 to 1:500 [19–21]. Interestingly, these and other studies of risk in contacts have found similar levels of risk that are independent of time, country, incidence or predominant serogroup (Samuelsson S., unpublished data). However, during group A epidemics in Africa, risk to close contacts may be much higher, e.g. 1:50 to 1:140 in one study [22], possibly reflecting the high community risk. Beyond this 4-week period, the risk is probably close to background levels.

23.3.2.2 Contacts in Educational/Work Settings

After a single case of meningococcal disease, the risk of linked cases outside the household is low; and this is presumably related to lower intensity of exposure to virulent strains [23]. This is supported by studies of clusters in educational settings [24, 25]. In England and Wales 1995–2001, after one case in a preschool group, primary and secondary school, the absolute risks to each child/pupil in the same institution of becoming a case within the next 4 weeks were approximately 1:1500, 1:18000 and 1:33000 respectively [25]. Reports of clusters in other settings, e.g. workplace, are rare and the level of risk is considered to be lower than educational settings.

23.3.2.3 Contact in Health Care Settings

Health care workers in contact with cases of meningococcal disease often consider themselves to be at high risk. Although risk of disease in the 10-day period after exposure may be increased relative to the risk among adults in the community, absolute risks are very low. In one study, absolute risk was estimated as 1:125000 [26]. The data from this study and anecdotal reports of cases among health care workers are consistent with a small risk from exposure to nasopharyngeal secretions of cases around the time of admission to hospital.

Clinical laboratory workers are at high risk if exposed to aerosolized cultures. In one UK study, five cases were identified over 15 years: all were working outside a safety cabinet on suspensions of isolates from cases of invasive disease [27].

23.3.2.4 **Contact With a Case**

Terms such as primary, coprimary and secondary are often used to describe cases of meningococal disease. However, the evidence does not support classification of further cases as secondary; and it may reinforce the false impression that the case is an important source of infection. The case is likely to have acquired the invasive strain from a close contact, typically in the same household, who is an asymptomatic carrier [23]. The incubation period is usually 3–5 days [27, 28] and cases do not usually have detectable carriage until admission to hospital or shortly beforehand [29]. As the highest risk of illness in untreated households is observed in the first 48 h after onset of disease in the index case [18], the source of infection in these further cases is most likely to be from the same (or another) close contact and not from the case. Also once disease is diagnosed, antibiotics rapidly suppress carriage, so that the case is only infectious for a short period during acute illness. This short infectious period accounts for the few genuine secondary cases that are documented among health care workers who have been exposed to respiratory secretions of a case around the time of admission to hospital.

It follows that transient contact with the index case before acute illness develops is unlikely to be an important risk factor for disease, so that mere proximity to a subsequently diagnosed case (e.g. during travel in a plane, bus, car) may not increase risk. Although guidance for the United States suggests that passengers seated next to the index case on a plane for more than 8 h are at higher risk, there are no published reports of cases in such contacts [30].

23.3.2.5 **Contact With Saliva**

One question that commonly arises is whether salivary contact through sharing cups or glasses is a risk factor. In one study of 258 college students, swabs were taken from the nasopharynx, tonsils and front of mouth [3]. The site with the highest yield was the nasopharynx (32%), whereas tonsillar carriage was 19%. Only one (0.4%) of the 258 swabs from the front of the mouth was positive. The very low isolation rate from the front of the mouth suggests that low levels of salivary contact are unlikely to transmit meningococci. This is supported by laboratory evidence that saliva inhibits meningococcal growth [31] and by epidemiological evidence of no association between meningococcal acquisition and the sharing of glasses or cigarettes [32]. All the evidence suggests that the main method of transmission of meningococcal infection is through respiratory droplets.

23.3.3 Prophylaxis: Risk Reduction

23.3.3.1 Chemoprophylaxis

Two main approaches to chemoprophylaxis are followed. In one approach, advised in Norway and the Czech Republic, oral penicillin is given to contacts for 1 week. The aim is to reduce the risk of disease directly by early treatment. In the other more widely used approach, short courses or single doses of antibiotics such as rifampicin, ciprofloxacin, and ceftriaxone are given to contacts. This second approach aims to reduce the risk of invasive disease by eradicating carriage in the group of close contacts at highest risk. It may act in two ways: (a) by eradicating carriage from established carriers who pose a risk of infection to others and (b) by eradicating carriage in those who have newly acquired the invasive strain and who may themselves be at risk to reduce risk by eliminating carriage [33].

We do not know the effectiveness of the first approach. The second approach is supported by the findings of a systematic review [2]. Three retrospective observational studies showed a consistent and large reduction in risk of further cases in the household among household members given carriage eradication treatment [20, 21, 34]. Potential confounding factors such as age, sex, passive smoking and lower socioeconomic status may have modified the true effect, but the size and consistency of the risk reduction seen in different countries, different times and with different antibiotic regimens supports benefit from this intervention. The approximate number needed to treat to prevent a case was estimated as about 200 individuals.

A recent retrospective study in European countries compared the impact of prophylaxis to the whole of a nursery school after a single case with that of prophylaxis only to close contacts. The findings suggested possible reduction in risk with wider prophylaxis but the difference was not statistically significant (Boccia D., unpublished data).

23.3.3.2 Vaccination

In cases caused by vaccine preventable strains, vaccination would certainly be expected to reduce the long-term risk of disease in close contacts, but only one randomized controlled trial has evaluated effectiveness of vaccination in household contacts [22]. This Nigerian study showed that vaccination in the absence of chemoprophylaxis was effective in preventing further household cases during a serogroup A epidemic. In other settings where chemoprophylaxis is given, the approximate number of close contacts needed to vaccinate to prevent a case has been estimated as 1000 (Samuelsson S., unpublished data).

23.3.4
Prophylaxis: Costs

The decision process for policy should also include the evaluation of economic cost of prophylaxis [35]. Due to the high concern about meningococcal disease, it is likely that the general public would accept substantial financial costs; but the costs of widespread use of antibiotics are not only financial. Harm may arise from drug side-effects, the development of antibiotic resistance and the eradication of naturally immunizing strains from the nasopharynx. The further one goes outside the case household, the lower the chance of finding a carrier of a pathogenic meningococcal strain and the greater the chance of a treatment doing harm by eradicating the carriage of nonpathogenic organisms that may generate cross-protective immunity. This particularly applies in young children who are more likely to be carrying *N. lactamica* than *N. meningitidis* [36].

23.3.5
Prophylaxis: Policy

23.3.5.1 Chemoprophylaxis

Close Contacts In most countries, chemoprophylaxis is recommended for close contacts. The definition of a close contact is necessarily arbitrary but it seems reasonable to confine prophylaxis to those who live in the same household or have an equivalent level of close prolonged contact. Low-level salivary contact, such as sharing drinks, with a case should not by itself be an indication for chemoprophylaxis.

Previous studies have suggested that some subsequent cases in the household may be caused by reintroduction of the virulent strain to the household by the index patient [37]. About 3% of index patients treated with penicillin and who have not received chemoprophylaxis still carry the virulent strain on discharge from hospital [2]. As carriage is usually suppressed but not eradicated by penicillin treatment, this figure is likely to underestimate the true carriage rate among index cases. So, chemoprophylaxis should also be given to the index patient prior to hospital discharge, unless already treated with an antibiotic which is known to eradicate carriage.

Schools Some counties recommend prophylaxis for all children of a nursery/ kindergarten after a single case. Other do not. After a case in a school, it would be unusual to recommend mass prophylaxis. The benefit of giving antibiotics in these settings is not known, the potential for risk reduction is reduced by delays between diagnosis and administration of prophylaxis and the risk of adverse effects are increased according to the numbers treated. These factors need to be assessed when deciding policy.

Health Care Workers Laboratory studies suggest that surgical masks can protect the wearer against droplet transmission [38, 39]. In the United States, masks are recommended when working within 1 m of patients known or suspected to be infected with microorganisms transmitted by large-particle droplets that can be generated during coughing, sneezing, talking or the performance of clinical procedures [40]. UK guidelines also recommend wearing face masks and eye protection when there is a risk of secretions splashing into face and eyes [41].

Prophylaxis should be restricted to those who are not wearing such protection and whose respiratory tract is exposed to droplets from cases around the time of admission to hospital. After starting treatment with intravenous benzylpenicillin, carriage rates decrease rapidly so that meningococci are undetectable by nasopharyngeal swabbing after 24 h on treatment [42]. Third-generation cephalosporin antibiotics would be expected to have a similar or more rapid effect on suppression of carriage. So, if such exposure occurs more than 24 h of starting antibiotic treatment, prophylaxis would not be indicated.

Laboratory workers should not need prophylaxis after exposure, as long as they are following standard health and safety policies and are only working on meningococcal suspensions within a safety cabinet [27].

Choice of Antibiotic Ciprofloxacin (single oral dose), ceftriaxone (single intramuscular injection) and rifampicin (orally for 2 days) are known to be effective in eradicating carriage [43, 44], whereas penicillin is thought to suppress but not eradicate carriage. Each has advantages and disadvantages (Table 23.3).

23.3.5.2 **Vaccination**

Policy on vaccination of contacts varies by country. Given that chemoprophylaxis is effective in reducing short-term risk, vaccination reduces the relatively lower-medium and long-term risk. National policy should be based on cost-effectiveness relative to other interventions. If vaccination is offered, it is sensible to offer to those individuals who are identified as contacts for the purposes of chemoprophylaxis.

Table 23.3 Advantages and disadvantages of antibiotics used for carriage eradication.

Antibiotic	Advantages and disadvantages
Rifampicin	Effective, well established, can be given at all ages, but caution advised in pregnancy, may reduce effectiveness of other medication (such as anticoagulants, anticonvulsants, oral contrceptives), can stain contact lenses, 2-day course, pediatric formulation not available in some countries, risk of resistance
Ciprofloxacin	Effective, single dose; but not advised in pregnancy, anaphylactic reactions reported. Joint damage in animals, so concern in children
Ceftriaxone	Effective, single dose, can be given all ages, considered safe in pregnancy; but given only by injection and is painful(!)

23.3.6 Information

Giving out information widely after a case is good public health practice. Written information can include an explanation of the action being taken, the risk and the signs and symptoms should a further case occur. Examples of letters and information leaflets to support this information are available [33]. If information is not given out, public reaction can be highly negative. If, for example, parents of a school are not informed of a case and diagnosis in a second case is delayed, legal action may result. If anxiety levels are high, attendance by a public health physician at a community meeting may be helpful.

23.4 Outbreaks

Outbreaks of meningococcal disease often generate high levels of public alarm. Contributing to this alarm are the lack of predictability and the speed at which outbreaks develop that can frustrate the efforts of public health authorities. The speed of public health response is thus important both to implement preventive measures and to reduce public anxiety [45]. The same management principles apply to an outbreak as to a single case.

In educational settings, once a second case has occurred, the risk of a third case may be as high as 30–50% [24, 25]. The risks are highest in the week after the second case. Relative risk of further cases in other settings has not been formally assessed, but outbreaks in definable social groups, civilian communities and military recruits are well described.

Although one trial of mass chemoprophylaxis in a closed community (military barracks) showed a significant effect on disease reduction [46], whether such interventions work in schools or civilian communities is not known [47]. In view of the lack of evidence for benefit and the increased potential for harm, mass chemoprophylaxis is best kept for defined target groups at high risk.

The assessment of benefits and costs of interventions should lead to a decision on public health action. This action is likely to include widespread communication and may also involve targeting a group who are considered to be at high risk of disease and carriage for antibiotic prophylaxis and/or vaccination. If an outbreak is caused by strains of a serogroup for which an effective vaccine exists, vaccination should be considered. Data on school clusters from England and Wales showed that if the serogroup of one case had been identified and another case was diagnosed within 4 weeks in the same school, the second case was likely to be of the same strain as the first case [25]. Thresholds for vaccination may help and have been set in some countries, e.g. $10:10^5$ for 3 weeks during any 12 weeks in the United States [48], $15:10^5$ per week for 2 weeks in the African meningitis belt [49].

External factors such as availability of staff, antibiotics, vaccine and feasibility of action may well influence the decisions made. The importance of considering the geographical and population boundaries of any target group and being able to explain the boundaries to those outside the target group cannot be over-emphasised. Attempts to establish whether or not cases are caused by the same strain by phenotyping and preferably by genotyping can provide important information for the management of ongoing community outbreaks.

During massive epidemics of sub-Saharan Africa, chemoprophylaxis of household contacts is likely to be of limited benefit because of the very high community attack rates. In this situation, efforts should be focused on delivering oily chloramphenicol for treatment and mass vaccination for prevention [50].

23.5 Conclusion

Public health management of meningococcal disease is challenging. Better evidence is now available to help guidance in many areas of intervention, but more research is needed. National guidelines should be developed by an expert group and be clearly evidence-based [33]. Such guidelines are important to underpin policy and to reassure both public and professionals.

References

1 Hastings L, Stuart J, Andrews N, Begg N. **1997**, A retrospective survey of clusters of meningococcal disease in England and Wales, 1993 to 1995: estimated risks of further cases in household and educational settings, *Commun Dis Rep Rev* 7, R195–R200.

2 Purcell B, Samuelsson S, Hahne S, Ehrhard I, Heuberger S, Camaroni I, et al. **2004**, Effectiveness of antibiotics in preventing meningococcal disease after a case: systematic review, *Br Med J* 328, 1339–1342.

3 Orr HJ, Gray SJ, Macdonald M, Stuart JM. **2003**, Saliva and meningococcal transmission, *Emerg Infect Dis* 9, 1314–1315.

4 Maiden MCJ, Stuart JM, UK Meningococcal Carriage Group **2002**, Carriage of serogroup C meningococci 1 year after meningococcal C conjugate polysaccharide vaccination, *Lancet* 359, 1829–1830.

5 Ramsay M.E, Andrews N, Trotter CL, Kaczmarski E, Miller E. **2003**, Herd immunity from meningococcal serogroup C conjugate vaccination in England: database analysis, *Br Med J* 326, 365–366.

6 Riordan FAI, Thomson APJ, Sills JA, Hart CA. **1996**, Who spots the spots? Diagnosis and treatment of early meningococcal disease in children, *Br Med J* 313, 1255–1256.

7 Connolly M, Noah N. **1999**, Is group C meningococcal disease increasing in Europe? A report of surveillance of meningococcal infection in Europe 1993–1996, *Epidemiol Infect* 122, 41–49.

8 Booy R, Habibi P, Nadel S, de Munter C, Britto J, Morrison A et al. **2001**, Reduction in case fatality rate from meningococcal disease associated with improved healthcare delivery, *Arch Dis Child* 85, 386–390.

9 Cartwright KAV, Reilly S, White D, Stuart J. **1992**, Early treatment with parenteral penicillin in meningococcal disease, *Br Med J* 305, 143–147.

10 Norgard B, Sorensen HT, Jensen ES, Faber T, Schonheyder HC, Neilsen GL. **2002**, Pre-hospital parental antibiotic treatment of meningococcal disease and

case fatality: a Danish population, *J Infect* 45, 144–151.
11 Van Deuren M, Brandtzaeg P, Van Der Meer JWM. **2000**, Update on meningococcal disease with emphasis on pathogenesis and clinical management, *Clin Microbiol Rev* 13, 144–166.
12 Idsoe O, Guthe T, Willcox RR, De Weck AL. **1968**, Nature and extent of pencillin side-reactions with particular reference to fatalities from anaphylactic shock, *Bull WHO* 38, 159–188.
13 Sorensen HT, Moller-Petersen J, Krarup HB, Pedersen H, Hansen H, Hamburger H. **1992**, Diagnostic problems with meningococcal diseae in general practice, *J Clin Epidemiol* 45, 1289–1293.
14 Corless CE, Guiver M, Borrow R, Edwards-Jones V, Fox AJ, Kaczmarski EB. **2001**, Simultaneous detection of *Neisseria meningitidis,Haemophilus influenzae* and *Streptococcus pneumoniae* in suspected cases of meningitis and septicemia using real-time PCR, *J Clin Microbiol* 39, 1553–1558.
15 Wylie PAL, Stevens D, Drake W, III, Stuart JM, Cartwright KAV. **1997**, Epidemiology and clinical management of meningococcal disease in west Gloucestershire: retrospective, population based study, *Br Med J* 315, 774–779.
16 Ragunathan PL, Ramsay M, Borrow R, Guiver M, Gray S, Kaczmarski EB. **2000**, Clinical features, laboratory findings and management of meningococcal meningitis in England and Wales: report of a 1997 survey, *J Infect* 40, 74–79.
17 Sobanski MA, Barnes RA, Gray SJ, Carr AD, Kaczmarski EB, O'Rourke A, et al. **2000**, Measurement of serum antigen concentration by ultrasound-enhanced immunoassay and correlation with clinical outcome in meningococcal disease, Eur J Clin Microbiol 19, 260–266.
18 De Wals P, Hertoghe L, Borlee-Grimee I, De Maeyer-Cleempoel S, Reginster-Haneuse G, Dachy A, et al. **1981**, Meningococcal disease in Belgium. Secondary attack rate among household, day-care nursery and pre-elementary school contacts, *J Infect* 3[Suppl. 1], 53–61.
19 Munford RS, De Taunay A, De Morais JS, Fraser DW, Feldman RA. **1974**, Spread of meningococcal infection within households, *Lancet* 1974i, 1275–1278.
20 Scholten R, Bijlmer HA, Dankert J, Valkenburg HA. **1993**, Secondary cases of meningococcal disease in the Netherlands, 1989–1990, A reappraisal of chemoprohylaxis, *Ned Tijdschr Geneeskd* 1993, 1505–1508.
21 Meningococcal Disease Surveillance Group **1976**, Analysis of endemic meningococcal disease by serogroup and evaluation of chemoprophylaxis, *J Infect Dis* 134, 201–204.
22 Greenwood BM, Hassan-King M, Whittle HC. **1978**, Prevention of secondary cases of meningococcal disease in household contacts by vaccination, *Br Med J* 1, 1317–1319.
23 Kristiansen B-E, Tveten Y, Jenkins A. **1998**, Which contacts of patients with meningococcal disease carry the pathogenic strain of *Neisseria meningitidis?* Population-based study, *Br Med J* 317, 621–625.
24 Zangwill KM, Schuchat A, Riedo FX, Pinner RW, Koo DT, Reeves MW, et al. **1997**, School-based clusters of meningococcal disease in the United States. Descriptive epidemiology and a case-control analysis, *J Am Med Assoc* 277, 389–395.
25 Davison KL, Andrews N, White JM, Ramsay ME, Crowcroft NS, Rushdy AA, et al. **2004**, Clusters of meningococcal disease in school and preschool settings in England and Wales: What is the risk? *Arch Dis Child* 89, 256–260.
26 Gilmore A, Stuart J, Andrews N. **2000**, Risk of secondary meningococcal disease in health-care workers, *Lancet* 356, 1654–1655.
27 Boutet R, Stuart JM, Kaczmarski EB, Gray SJ, Jones DM, Andrews N. **2001**, Risk of laboratory-acquired meningococcal disease, *J Hosp Infect* 49, 282–284.
28 Heymann DL. **2004**, *Control of Communicable Disease Manual*, 18th edn, American Public Health Association, Washington, D.C.
29 Edwards EA, Devine LF, Sengbusch CH, Ward HW. **1977**, Immunological investigations of meningococcal disease, *Scand J Infect Dis* 9, 105–110.

30 CDC **2001**, Exposure to patients with meningococcal disease on aircrafts – United States, 1999–2001, *Morbid Mortal Wkly Rep* 50, 485–489.
31 Gordon MH. **1917**, The inhibitory action of saliva on growth of the meningococcus, GB Med Res Comm Spec Rep Ser 3, 106–111.
32 Nelson S J, Charlett A, Orr HJ, Barker RM, Neal KR, Taylor C, et al. **2001**, Risk factors for meningococcal disease in university halls of residence, *Epidemiol Infect* 126, 211–217.
33 Anon. **2002**, Guidelines for public health management of meningococcal disease in the UK, *Commun Dis Public Health* 5, 187–204.
34 Samuelsson S, Hansen ET, Osler M, Jeune B. **2000**, Prevention of secondary cases of meningococcal disease in Denmark, *Epidemiol Infect* 124, 433–440.
35 Round A, Palmer S. **1999**, Should we be doing more to prevent Group C meningococcal infection in school age children? How can we decide? *J Public Health Med* 21, 8–13.
36 Gold R, Goldschneider I, Lepow ML, Draper TF, Randolph M. **1978**, Carriage of *Neisseria meningitidis* and *Neisseria lactamica* in Infants and Children, *J Infect Dis* 137, 112–121.
37 Cooke RPD, Riordan T, Jones DM, Painter MJ. **1989**, Secondary cases of meningococcal infection among close family and household contacts in England and Wales, 1984–1987, *Br Med J* 298, 555–558.
38 Weber A, Willeke K, Marchioni R, Myojo T, McKay R, Donnelly J, et al. **1993**, Aerosol penetration and leakage characteristics of masks used in the health care industry, *Am J Infect Control* 21, 167–173.
39 Chen CC, Willeke K. **1992**, Aerosol penetration through surgical masks, *Am J Infect Control* 20, 177–184.
40 Garner JS, Hospital Infection Control Practices Advisory Committee **1996**, Guideline for isolation precautions in hospitals, *Infect Control Hosp Epidemiol* 17, 53–80.
41 Pratt RJ, Pellowe C, Loveday HP, Robinson N, Smith GW, et al. **2001**, The epic project: developing national evidence-based guidelines for preventing health care associated infections, *J Infect* 47[Suppl.], S1–S82.
42 Abramson JS, Spika JS. **1985**, Persistence of *Neisseria meningitidis* in the upper respiratory tract after intravenous antibiotic therapy for systemic meningococcal disease, *J Infect Dis* 151, 370–371.
43 Broome CV. **1986**, The carrier state: *Neisseria meningitidis*, *J Antimicrob Chemother* 18[Suppl. A] 1986, 25–34.
44 Fraser A, Gafter-Gvili A, Paul M, Leibovici L. **2005**, Antibiotics for preventing meningococcal infections (review), (Cochrane Library), John Wiley & Sons, Chichester.
45 Stuart JM. **2001**, Managing outbreaks, the public health response, in *Meningococcal Disease: Methods and Protocols, (Methods in Molecular Medicine*, vol. 67), ed. Pollard A.J., Maiden MCJ, Humana Press, Totowa, N.J., p. 257–272.
46 Kuhns DM, Nelson CT, Feldman HA, Kuhn LR. **1943**, The prophylactic value of sulfadiazine in the control of meningococcic meningitis, *J Am Med Assoc* 123, 335–339.
47 Shehab S, Keller N, Barkay A, Leitner L, Leventhal A, Block C. **1998**, Failure of mass antibiotic prophylaxis to control a prolonged outbreak of meningococcal disease in an Israeli village, *Eur J Clin Microbiol Infect Dis* 17, 749–753.
48 CDC. **1997**, Control and prevention of meningococcal disease and control and prevention of serogroup c meningococcal disease: evaluation and management of suspected outbreaks, *Morbid Mortal Wkly Rep* 46:1–21.
49 Kaninda AV, Belanger F, Lewis R, Batchassi E, Aplogan A, Yakoua Y, et al. **2000**, Effectiveness of incidence thresholds for detection and control of meningococcal meningitis epidemics in northern Togo, *Int J Epidemiol* 5, 933–940.
50 World Health Organization. **1998**, *Control of Epidemic Meningococcal Disease: WHO Practical Guidelines*, WHO, Geneva.

Subject Index

a

Handbook of Meningococcal Disease. Infection Biology, Vaccination, Clinical Management.
Edited by M. Frosch and M. C. J. Maiden

ISBN: 3-527-31260-9